SALEM HEALTH
CANCER

SALEM HEALTH
CANCER

Volume III
Living will — Self-image and body image

Editor
Jeffrey A. Knight, Ph.D.
Mount Holyoke College

Medical Consultants
Laurie Jackson-Grusby, Ph.D.
Children's Hospital Boston, Harvard Medical School

Wendy White-Ryan, M.D., FAAP
Golisano Children's Hospital at Strong Memorial Hospital

SALEM PRESS, INC.
Pasadena, California   Hackensack, New Jersey

∞ The paper used in these volumes conforms to the American National Standard for Permanence of Paper for Printed Library Materials, Z39.48-1992 (R1997).

Note to Readers

The material presented in *Salem Health: Cancer* is intended for broad informational and educational purposes. Readers who suspect that they or someone whom they know or provide caregiving for suffers from cancer or any other physical or psychological disorder, disease, or condition described in this set should contact a physician without delay; this work should not be used as a substitute for professional medical diagnosis or staging. Readers who are undergoing or about to undergo any treatment or procedure described in this set should refer to their physicians and other health care team members for guidance concerning preparation and possible effects. This set is not to be considered definitive on the covered topics, and readers should remember that the field of health care is characterized by a diversity of medical opinions and constant expansion in knowledge and understanding.

Library of Congress Cataloging-in-Publication Data

Salem health : cancer / Jeffrey A. Knight, Laurie Jackson-Grusby, Wendy White-Ryan.
p. cm.
Includes bibliographical references and index.
ISBN 978-1-58765-505-0 (set : alk. paper) — ISBN 978-1-58765-506-7 (vol. 1 : alk. paper) — ISBN 978-1-58765-507-4 (vol. 2 : alk. paper) — ISBN 978-1-58765-508-1 (vol. 3 : alk. paper) — ISBN 978-1-58765-509-8 (vol. 4 : alk. paper)
1. Cancer. I. Knight, Jeffrey A., 1948- II. Jackson-Grusby, Laurie. III. White-Ryan, Wendy.
RC265.S32 2008
616.99′4—dc22

2008030861

First Printing

PRINTED IN THE UNITED STATES OF AMERICA

▶ Contents

▶ Complete List of Contents

Volume 1

VOLUME 2

Volume 3

VOLUME 4

SALEM HEALTH
CANCER

▶ Living will

Category: Social and personal issues
Also known as: Advanced directives for terminal health care

Definition: A living will is a legal document that indicates the care a person wishes to receive if afflicted by a terminal illness that is irreversible and certain to prove fatal. Patients with certain types of cancers or late-stage cancers may find this document useful for dealing with end-of-life issues.

Who executes a living will? Those establishing living wills are often people in good health who wish to make provision for their end-of-life care should they become gravely ill. However, some gravely ill people (such as a person with late-stage cancer) execute such a document after their health has deteriorated to the point that there is no hope of recovery. The person executing a living will must be of legal age and of sound mind.

Related documents: Besides a living will, it is advisable for those implementing such a document to sign a medical power of attorney (MPOA). This document, signed and notarized, should be held by a trusted friend or relative or by the person's attorney. The MPOA authorizes a designated person or persons to make decisions relating to the an individual's care should that person be unable to make such decisions.

Whoever holds the MPOA should be trustworthy and sufficiently objective to make informed decisions regarding treatment. The person or people holding the MPOA should have a realistic view of what the patient would want if he or she were making the needed medical decisions. It is desirable to have both living wills and MPOAs drawn up by an attorney, although standard forms for executing these documents are available at most hospitals or through the National Hospice and Palliative Care Organization.

Procedures to be specified in a living will: No one can foresee every eventuality in end-of-life situations, but commonly used procedures for extending life should be carefully considered when executing a living will. Sometimes terminally ill patients, especially those suffering from some forms of cancer, experience excruciating pain, so the living will should specify that if medical opinion considers a patient terminal, palliatives available to reduce or control that pain should not be withheld.

Some terminal patients are not conscious, are unaware of their surroundings, or may be brain-dead. When this is the case, ventilators or respirators keep them alive. Even if they are conscious, these instruments may limit their ability to communicate. A living will should specify whether mechanical ventilation should be employed if a patient is unable to make such a decision. The living will might indicate the conditions under which ventilators or respirators should be used and for how long their use should continue.

The hearts of terminally ill patients may stop beating, but often such patients can be revived through cardiopulmonary resuscitation (CPR) or electrical stimulation. The living will can specify that treatments of this sort are not to be employed if the heart stops and that the patient's chart should be clearly marked do not resuscitate (DNR).

Terminally ill patients in comas may be kept alive through the use of some of the measures noted above, but they require nutrients and liquids to sustain their lives. The living will should stipulate whether nutritional and hydration measures should be used if it is clear that they can prolong life. Such treatment can be administered intravenously or through a stomach tube. The living will should indicate the extent to which such measures are to be implemented and, if they are used, for how long their use should continue.

Many patients who suffer renal failure are kept alive through dialysis, a procedure that removes harmful and potentially fatal waste from the blood and controls the body fluids that healthy kidneys control automatically. In addressing the question in a living will, it is important to realize that dialysis may be necessary only temporarily but that some types of kidney failure will require it on a sustained basis. Those with kidney cancer should consider the ramifications for their situation.

The living will should specify how the person signing it wishes to be treated if infections develop that would normally indicate the use of antibiotics. Those making living wills must ask whether they would wish to have an infection controlled through medication, mechanical ventilation, or other means to recover only from the infection but not from the condition that has rendered them terminally ill. A living will can also indicate the postmortem disposition of organs and body parts for transplantation.

Not every eventuality can be foreseen by the person drawing up a living will. It is both desirable and necessary, therefore, to execute a MPOA that leaves medical decisions in the hands of a responsible person.

Legal considerations: If a living will is not on file, medical facilities and their employees risk legal action for malpractice or even manslaughter if a patient dies who might have been kept alive through available treatments. The living will absolves medical facilities and personnel from legal action in cases in which terminally ill patients die because life-prolonging treatments specified in the document have been withheld.

Some physicians have moral reservations about permitting patients to die if they can be kept alive by artificial means. When a living will is on file, patients' desires are clearly stated. Any physician who disagrees with their desires can withdraw from the case.

R. Baird Shuman, Ph.D.

▶ For Further Information

Colen, B. D. *The Essential Guide to a Living Will: How to Protect Your Right to Refuse Medical Treatment*. New York: Prentice Hall, 2001.

Hamas, Edward A. *How to Write Your Own Living Will*. Naperville, Ill.: Sphinx, 2002.

Litin, Scott C., Jr., ed. *Mayo Clinic Family Health Book*. 3d ed. New York: HarperCollins, 2003.

Raymond, Joan. "A Guide for Caregivers." *Newsweek*, June 18, 2007, 62-64.

▶ Other Resources

National Cancer Institute
Advance Directives
http://www.cancer.gov/cancertopics/factsheet/support/advance-directives

National Hospice and Palliative Care Organization
http://www.nhpco.org

See also Advance directives; Cardiopulmonary resuscitation (CPR); Caregivers and caregiving; Case management; Counseling for cancer patients and survivors; Do-not-resuscitate (DNR) order; End-of-life care; Hospice care; Long-distance caregiving; Palliative treatment; Transitional care.

▶ Living with cancer

Category: Social and personal issues

Definition: Living with cancer means being alive and as active as possible to enjoy life after having been diagnosed with and treated for cancer.

Diagnosis: Cancer affects about 10.5 million Americans who are at various stages of living with their cancer. Although cancer mortality statistics are generally improving, people fear the diagnosis of cancer. When people first learn that they have this disease, the response may be disbelief. They may think the worst and feel overwhelmed. Many questions will surface and may not have definite answers. To provide the best care, the health care team will need to make certain tests and stage the cancer to see how far the disease has spread. With this information, patients and their health care providers can make decisions on treatments to cure, to control the disease, or to minimize symptoms. Each person experiences cancer differently; becoming a partner in the treatment plan means making choices in many aspects of life.

Education: C. Everett Koop, former surgeon general of the United States, advised that "the best prescription is knowledge." One effective way for patients to face life with cancer is for them to learn as much as possible about the specific diagnosis. Numerous sources are available to provide further education on cancer in general and in detail. Cancer patients may want to know about statistics, risk factors for their type of cancer, staging terms and what they mean, treatment options, and the likelihood of the patient to survive and recover from the cancer and treatments (prognosis).

The first contact for patient education is the health care provider. These professionals can offer information specific to the patient such as the type of cancer, stage of cancer involvement, and options for therapy. Cancer patients should take the initiative to talk with their health care providers to fully understand their unique situation. With that information, patients can pursue other avenues of education.

There are many sources for learning more about cancer. Information can range from simple explanations to complex scientific documentation. Patients can read articles in popular magazines, buy books on most aspects of cancer care, study health care journals, or look up their cancer on the Internet. Generally, reliable information comes from well-respected and well-established cancer care centers, cancer care organizations, government agencies, or health care organizations.

Another source of education is other cancer patients. Attending local support groups and conversing with others who are at different stages of cancer can support and encourage patients. Online Web sites offer message boards where cancer patients can share their personal experiences. Though these can be useful, it is important to remember that this type of information comes from a particular person's point of view. Cancer patients need to seek further information and clarification from their health care providers or other reliable sources before acting on what another cancer patient says.

Coping with cancer: A cancer diagnosis can be stressful for both patients and their families. Patients respond in different ways to their cancer. Many emotions may surface,

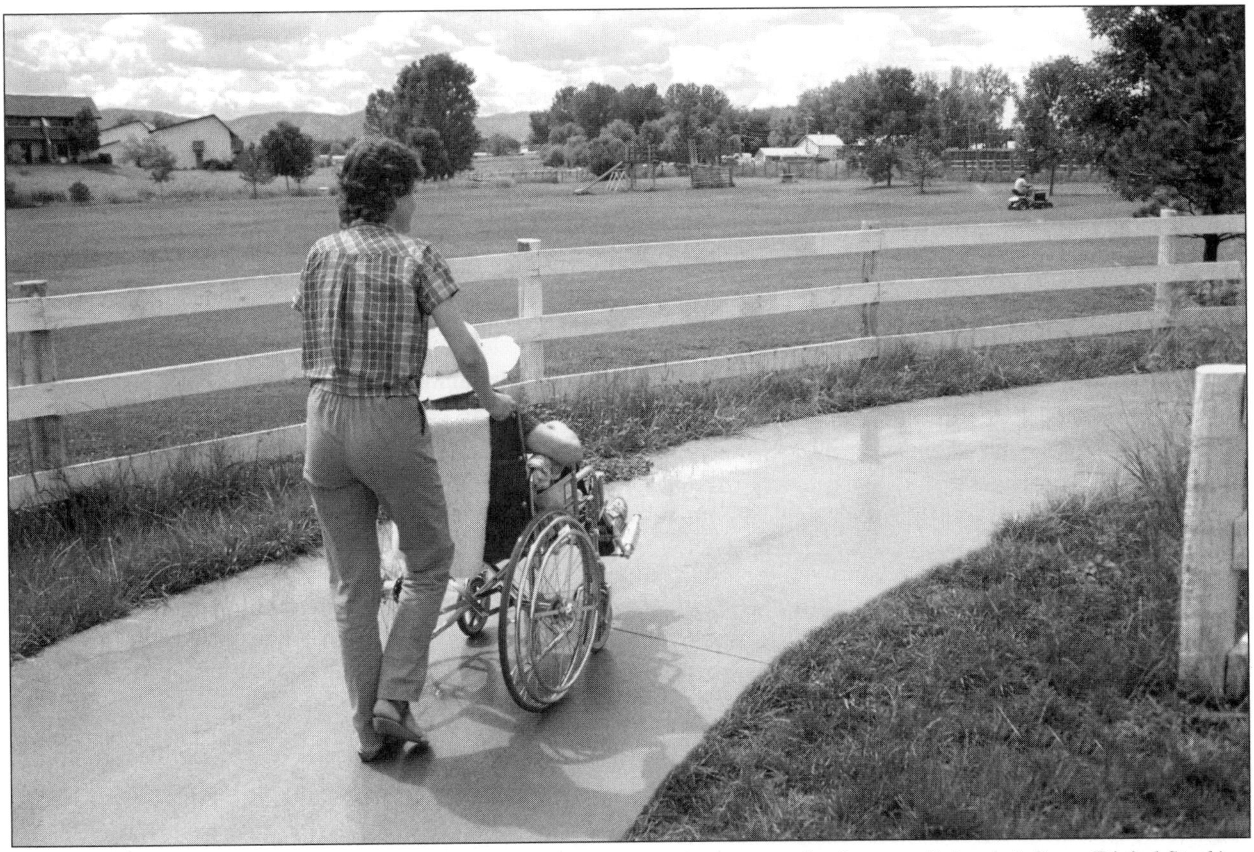

Cancer can be a long-term disease, and patients gradually turn from focusing on the disease to living their lives. (Digital Stock)

such as shock, disbelief, fear, sadness, anxiety, depression, anger, and guilt. Patients may question why they have cancer and what lies ahead. Disbelief may come to those who feel physically well. Fear is a common emotion, but the reasons may range from fear of the treatments and side effects to fear of death and the impact on remaining family members. Fear feeds anxiety, which can interfere with normal daily functioning.

Guilt is another common emotion of cancer patients. Patients may replay their lifestyle choices and wonder if something they did caused the cancer. They may feel guilt over the decisions they made that stole precious time from their life or guilt about their priorities. As some cancers tend to be hereditary, cancer patients may worry about the impact on their children.

Feelings of sadness and hopelessness can block recovery and resumption of meaningful life activities. Depression can come with sleep problems, loss of appetite, feelings of worthlessness, decreased energy, irritability, or lack of interest in activities once enjoyed. Physical symptoms such as headache or digestive problems may occur. Feeling sad is a normal reaction when people learn that they have cancer, but if depression continues and thoughts of suicide surface, patients may require help through counseling and prescribed medications.

Cancer patients experience the feeling of loss—loss of control, autonomy, dreams, choices, or the future. Loss is a normal feeling and allows cancer patients to grieve over actual or perceived interruptions in their lives. Counseling may be useful for both cancer patients and their families.

Taking action: Cancer can be a long-term disease and last for many years. Cancer patients experience an initial adjustment to their diagnosis and treatment. The focus of their first thoughts may be on dying, but as time goes on, these thoughts shift to their normal lives. Taking certain steps can help cancer patients reengage in their usual activities of daily living.

One helpful step is paying attention to personal needs for rest, nutrition, recreation, and relationships. Relaxation activities such as meditation and guided imagery can assist in healing and encourage good mental health. Adequate nutrition is important to keep the immune system at an optimal level.

Participating in activities that patients enjoy, such as going to the movies, listening to music, going to lunch with friends, or pursuing their hobbies, can relieve depression. Creative expression though journaling, writing poetry or stories, reading, or drawing can keep patients' minds off cancer and minimize projecting into the future. Simply going shopping can be a boost to the morale.

Starting or resuming an exercise program can help cancer patients increase strength, improve flexibility, and build endurance. Studies show that exercise can also improve long-term survival. Radiation treatments can result in fatigue, but light or moderate walking can boost energy and stimulate the appetite. Another benefit of exercise is that the release of natural body chemicals, called endorphins, can improve patients' moods and help relieve pain. Various levels of exercise, such as walking, swimming, cleaning the house, gardening, or dancing, can provide pleasure as well as health benefits.

Almost daily the media reports on the value of alternative or complementary therapies. Cancer patients may become interested in these therapies as ways to relax, to reduce side effects of cancer treatment, or to cure their disease. Some of these practices, such as massage, guided imagery, acupuncture, or hypnosis, may be useful when used along with traditional cancer treatments. Vitamins and herbal supplements have gained monumental popularity in the United States. Although some sources claim that herbs and vitamins can cure cancer, these statements are often unfounded. Cancer patients should speak with their health care providers before using alternative therapies.

Sometimes cancer patients are unable to perform activities of daily living without assistance. However, by seeking help they can continue to go to the grocery or to church. Friends and family often welcome the opportunity to provide meals or transportation so that they can show love to the cancer patient. Asking for help is not always comfortable for cancer patients who covet their autonomy. However, taking action to seek help is a healthy behavior.

Sexuality: Having cancer does not alter the human need for sex and intimacy. However, having this disease can temporarily alter people's attitudes and desires. Changes in emotions are normal for cancer patients but can affect their relationship with their partners. Physical side effects from cancer treatments such as nausea, vomiting, and fatigue can decrease interest in sex. Cancer therapies can affect the patients' body image and lessen the confidence in their attractiveness. Women may experience dryness of the vagina, and men may have trouble having or maintaining an erection.

Some people believe that cancer can be passed to another person by intimacy. Partners may be hesitant to engage in sexual intercourse with cancer patients. Also, cancer patients may need to refrain from sex for a period of time because of surgery or a lowered immune system. This can be difficult for both the cancer patient and the partner. Communication is key to resolving misunderstandings. Cancer patients should be open and honest about their concerns with their health care professionals. These professionals can help make referrals for counseling and support when needed.

Family dynamics: Cancer changes all aspects of family life. Priorities change and unresolved emotions may surface. There may be more struggles in the family dynamics. Roles may change as cancer patients must use energy and time to take treatments or care for themselves. A reassignment of roles can be overwhelming, especially for older children or youths who now become caregivers. Patients must be allowed to continue to fill as many parts of their family role as possible and not be treated as an invalid. If the dynamics of family life become dysfunctional, a family counselor can help.

Spiritual support: Cancer is a serious illness that can challenge people's spiritual beliefs. Spiritual distress (unresolved spiritual conflict or doubt) can compromise patients' coping skills. Unlike religion (a set of beliefs, practices, or doctrine), spirituality includes the person's sense of purpose, relationship to others, and beliefs about life's meaning. Some cancer patients may feel they are being punished by a higher power or may lose their faith, while others experience a deepening of their faith during their illness.

Pastors, rabbis, or other faith leaders may be valuable resources during this difficult time. Some home health and hospice care agencies have chaplains on their interdisciplinary teams and offer home support for cancer patients. The best person for cancer patients to talk with is the one who provides compassionate and supportive communication. Spiritual support can create an improved quality of life for cancer patients. Patients may experience decreased stress, anxiety, or pain. Connecting to others results in less isolation. Spirituality can help cancer patients tolerate treatments better and bring peace in a time of chaos.

Life after cancer: Cancer survivors face different challenges. Intensive cancer therapy can leave people with lifelong health concerns. After the treatments or surgery are complete, patients have new questions. Will the cancer come back? Will my life be the same as before I was diagnosed with cancer? Will I need continued observation? Where do I go from here?

There will be follow-up care that includes regular medical checkups, usually with the primary physician. Tests will most likely occur at specific intervals to check for continued remission (when the cancer is reduced or disappears). If any tests indicate concerns, cancer patients are referred to the cancer health care provider for further assessment.

Many survivors say that life has new meaning for them, and they see life in a new light. Priorities have changed. Their bodies have changed. Cancer patients may have made new friends and developed new relationships. Even their diets may have changed. Life and all it has to offer have changed forever.

Marylane Wade Koch, M.S.N., R.N.

▶ For Further Information

Felder, Tamika. "What Cancer Taught Me About Living." *Essence*, July, 2006.

Harpman, Wendy Schlessel. *After Cancer: A Guide to Your New Life*. New York: W. W. Norton, 1994.

Kaelin, Carolyn M., and Francesca Coltrera. "Cancer and Staying Fit." *Newsweek*, March, 2007.

_______. *Living Through Breast Cancer*. New York: McGraw-Hill, 2005.

Krychman, Michael L. *One Hundred Questions and Answers for Women Living with Cancer: A Practical Guide for Survivorship*. Sudbury, Mass.: Jones and Bartlett, 2007.

Ovitz, Joanne K. *Facing the Mirror with Cancer: A Guide to Using Makeup to Make a Difference*. Chicago: Belle Press, 2004.

Stafford, Jacqui. "A Whole New Outlook." *Shape*, October, 2004.

▶ Other Resources

American Psychosocial Oncology Society
http://www.apos-society.org

Cancer Survivor Network
http://www.acscsn.org

Cancer.Net
http://www.cancer.net/portal/site/patient

National Center for Complementary and Alternative Medicine
http://nccam.nih.gov

Still You Fashions
http://www.stillyoufashions.com

The Wellness Community
http://www.thewellnesscommunity.org

See also Advance directives; Anxiety; Caregivers and caregiving; Case management; Cognitive effects of cancer and chemotherapy; Counseling for cancer patients and survivors; Depression; Elderly and cancer; Electrolarynx; Esophageal speech; Family history and risk assessment; Fertility issues; Financial issues; Grief and bereavement; Home health services; Hospice care; Informed consent; Insurance; Integrative oncology; Karnofsky performance status (KPS); Living will; Medical marijuana; Medicare and cancer; Pain management medications; Palliative treatment; Personality and cancer; Poverty and cancer; Prayer and cancer support; Psycho-oncology; Psychosocial aspects of cancer; Relationships; Second opinions; Self-image and body image; Sexuality and cancer; Side effects; Singlehood and cancer; Stress management; Support groups; Survivorship issues; Transitional care; Watchful waiting.

▶ Lobectomy

Category: Procedures
Also known as: Pulmonary lobectomy, lung lobe removal

Definition: Lobectomy is the surgical removal of a lobe of a lung.

Cancers treated: Lung cancer

Why performed: Lobectomy is a surgical procedure used to treat lung cancer when the tumor is limited to one area of the lung. It may also be used to treat bronchiectasis, tuberculosis, lung abscess, localized fungal infections, or blebs associated with emphysema.

Patient preparation: Before surgery, studies are performed to check for abnormalities and establish a baseline for postoperative comparison. These studies include a chest X ray, electrocardiogram (ECG), bleeding time, and blood tests to check kidney function, electrolytes, hemoglobin, oxygen levels, and white blood cell count. Pulmonary function tests are performed to evaluate lung function. A blood sample is also drawn to check the patient's blood type in case a transfusion is needed during surgery. The patient must not eat or drink for at least eight hours before surgery, and an intravenous (IV) catheter is inserted for fluids and medications. An indwelling urinary catheter may also be inserted so that urine output can be monitored closely during and after the procedure.

Steps of the procedure: When the patient arrives in the operating suite, an arterial catheter may be inserted to monitor the patient's blood pressure and oxygenation. Af-

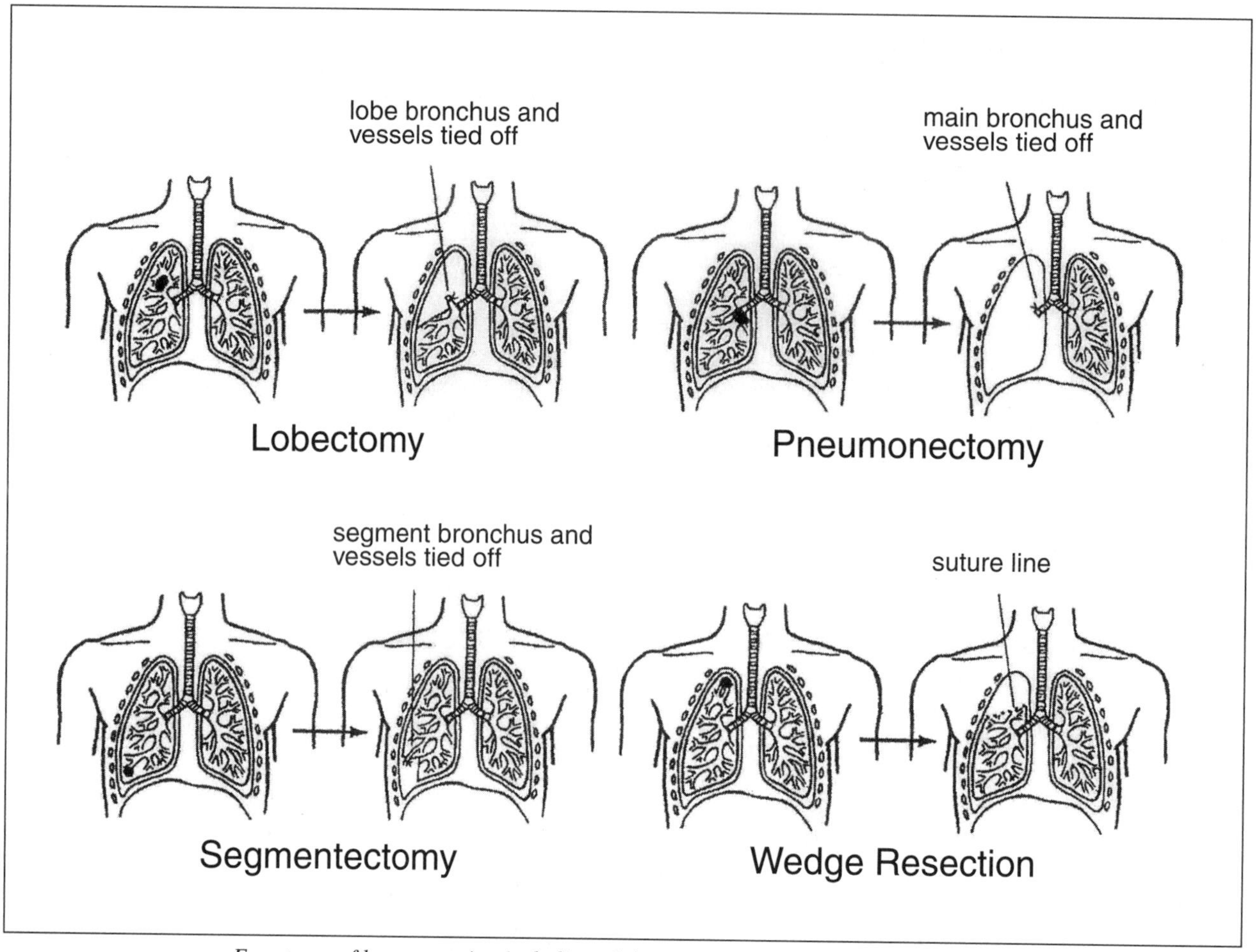

Four types of lung surgeries, including a lobectomy. (Custom Medical Stock Photo)

ter the patient is anesthetized, the surgeon makes an incision into the chest cavity. When the chest cavity is entered, the lung collapses. The surgeon locates and ties off sources of bleeding, spreads the ribs, and exposes the area of the lung for removal. The surgeon removes the affected lung lobe and repairs the vessels and lung passages from where it was removed. The surgeon inserts one or two chest tubes to drain fluid and reexpand the lung. Then, the surgeon closes the chest cavity and applies a sterile dressing.

After the procedure: The patient is typically transferred to the intensive care unit (ICU) and attached to a monitor that displays heart rhythm, blood pressure, and oxygen saturation. These devices help the ICU nurses closely monitor the patient's condition. The patient receives supplemental oxygen and IV fluids. The nurses check the chest tube drainage frequently to monitor for excess bleeding. The patient is encouraged to turn, cough, breathe deeply, and use an incentive spirometer to prevent pneumonia. Sequential compression devices are attached to the patient's legs to help prevent blood clots.

Risks: The risks of lobectomy include surgical site infection, pneumonia, hemorrhage, and respiratory failure.

Results: Pathologic examination of the lung specimen reveals the type of cancer.

Collette Bishop Hendler, R.N., M.S.

See also Bilobectomy; Bronchoalveolar lung cancer; Esophagectomy; Lung cancers; Mesothelioma; Pleural effusion; Pleurodesis; Pneumonectomy; Surgical biopsies; Thoracoscopy; Thoracotomy.

▶ Lobular carcinoma in situ (LCIS)

Category: Diseases, symptoms, and conditions
Also known as: Lobular neoplasia

Related conditions: Lobular carcinoma, atypical lobular hyperplasia, ductal carcinoma in situ (DCIS), ductal carcinoma

Definition: Lobular carcinoma in situ (LCIS) is a type of noninfiltrating breast cancer that originates in the breast lobules. It differs from other breast cancers in its propensity to develop in multiple sites in one or both breasts. Unlike other in situ cancers, LCIS is considered a marker rather than a premalignant lesion for subsequent development of invasive breast cancer. Only 25 to 35 percent of patients with lobular carcinoma in situ develop invasive cancer, compared with patients with other in situ lesions, such as ductal carcinoma in situ (DCIS). Between 25 and 70 percent of those with DCIS will develop invasive breast cancer.

Risk factors: Being a woman is a significant risk factor because men do not possess developed lobular breast tissue. Increasing age (forty and above) also contributes to the risk of LCIS. A family history of breast cancer, especially in first-degree relatives, is another significant risk factor, although not specific to any type of breast cancer. White patients have a twelvefold increased risk of LCIS compared with the general population; however, patients of African American origin have a higher rate of recurrence. Other risk factors include obesity, late (or not) first childbirth (older than thirty years), and a prior history of breast cancer.

Etiology and the disease process: The etiology of LCIS has been linked in some studies to loss of heterozygosity in chromosome 16q, 17p, and17q (*BRCA1* tumor-suppressor gene), which predisposes people to unregulated monoclonal proliferation. An alteration in the E-cadherin adhesion complex has also been noted in LCIS. Lobular carcinoma in situ originates from the terminal duct-lobular apparatus, where it is thought that monoclonal cells from the cellular lining (epithelium) of this apparatus undergo uninhibited proliferation within the lobule. Cells do not possess the atypical findings of other cancer cells, such as increased nucleus-to-cytoplasm ratios, increased cellular division, and loss of cellular cohesion or necrosis. However, the cells are enlarged and possess characteristic mucoid globules that help distinguish LCIS from DCIS. An interesting characteristic of LCIS is that invasion of tissue outside the lobule does not ensue, leaving lobular tissue architecture intact. As a result, LCIS can develop in multiple lobules undetected by clinical breast examinations and mammography. In spite of this, development of invasive cancer from LCIS is slow and may take as long as fifteen to twenty years.

Incidence: The overall incidence of LCIS, as documented by breast biopsies with a suspicious mammogram, is estimated at 2 to 5 percent. LCIS accounts for 9.8 percent of all breast malignancies. The diagnosis of LCIS peaks around the mid-forties. It is also interesting to note that more than 90 percent of women diagnosed with lobular carcinoma in situ are premenopausal, which suggests a plausible role of estrogen in LCIS proliferation.

Symptoms: LCIS is often missed due to the lack of overt signs and symptoms like those associated with other breast lesions, such as incidental discovery of a breast mass on self-examination, changes in the skin or nipples, and the presence of pain or nipple discharge. More often than not, LCIS is an incidental finding in otherwise normal breast biopsies. The presence of "neighborhood calcifications" in normal tissue surrounding the lesion on mammography is unique to LCIS and may aid in diagnosis.

Screening and diagnosis: Screening for all breast cancer follows the American Cancer Society (ACS) recommendations. ACS guidelines recommend that breast examinations be conducted every three years as part of a routine checkup beginning at age twenty (annually beginning at age forty) and that screening mammographies be conducted annually starting at age forty. Diagnosis of LCIS depends on the pathologic findings obtained by needle core biopsy. LCIS may accompany invasive cancer in 5 percent of cases. On microscopic examination, cancer cells may be densely packed and occupy the lobular spaces (acini), terminal ducts, or ductules completely without spread to adjacent structures. The cell nucleus, nucleolus, and cytoplasm are dark-staining and large. Immunohistochemical studies may also reveal E-cadherin-negative cells.

Treatment and therapy: Definitive surgical treatment of LCIS is geared toward removal of the multiple sites presumed to be contained in one breast. This is accomplished by surgical removal of the entire breast (total mastectomy) with optional dissection of axillary lymph nodes. The latter is optional because of the rare (less than 1 percent) occurrence of lymph node spread. Prophylactic removal of the opposite breast in the absence of pathological findings is not recommended in spite of the possibility of development of LCIS. Other treatment options include clinical observation and yearly mammography. Tamoxifen, an estrogen-receptor antagonist may be used in reducing the further development of LCIS in the remaining breast. A bilateral total mastectomy is also an option for patients with a familial inheritance of the *BRCA1* gene as demonstrated by genetic studies.

Prognosis, prevention, and outcomes: Prognosis is generally excellent with complete excision. However, progression to multiple or bilateral LCIS is high, approaching 90 percent and 70 percent, respectively. Simultaneous invasive cancer incidence is 5 percent.

Aldo C. Dumlao, M.D.

▶ For Further Information

Harding, Fred. *Breast Cancer: Cause—Prevention—Cure*. Rev. ed. London: Tekline Publishing, 2007.

Knox, Sally M., and Janet K. Grant. *The Breast Cancer Care Book: A Survival Guide for Patients and Loved Ones*. Grand Rapids, Mich.: Zondervan, 2004.

Simone, John. *The LCIS and DCIS Breast Cancer Fact Book*. Raleigh, N.C.: Three Pyramids Publishing, 2002.

▶ Other Resources

American Cancer Society
http://www.cancer.org

Cancer Backup
Lobular Carcinoma in Situ
http://www.cancerbackup.org.uk/Cancertype/Breast/DCISLCIS/LCIS

National Cancer Institute
Lobular Cancer in Situ
http://www.cancer.gov/cancertopics/pdq/treatment/breast/HealthProfessional/page6

See also Breast cancer in children and adolescents; Breast cancers; Comedo carcinomas; Ductal carcinoma in situ (DCIS); Ductal lavage; Invasive ductal carcinomas; Invasive lobular carcinomas; Mastectomy; Medullary carcinoma of the breast; Microcalcifications; Mucinous carcinomas; Tubular carcinomas.

▶ Long-distance caregiving

Category: Social and personal issues

Definition: Long-distance caregiving is providing for the well-being of another person without being physically present. Caregiving is considered long distance when the caregiver lives an hour's travel or farther from the care receiver. The people who receive care usually live in homes, apartments, and other independent living situations.

Support services: People who provide long-distance caregiving arrange, manage, or hire one or more of several support services:

- Home health care: Physical and respiratory therapy, nursing, home health aides, psychological or psychiatric care, medication assistance, and home medical treatments
- Personal care: Help with activities of daily living, such as dressing, bathing, eating, using the toilet, and grooming
- Homemaker services: Meal preparation, house cleaning, laundry, shopping for food and other items
- Companionship: People who regularly make supportive visits or telephone calls
- Live-in assistance: Help provided by people who cook, clean, and perform other nonmedical services in exchange for housing, meals, and a salary
- Transportation: Rides to and from medical appointments, religious services, and other places

Prevalence: Millions of families and friends live far apart, and millions of people have cancer and other health challenges. Career, education, family situations, and other life demands often separate caregivers from care receivers. Physical distance does not free caregivers from the responsibility of managing the care of others who deal with cancer and other illnesses.

Health care organizations estimate that more than 5 million people in the United States provide long-distance caregiving services for others.

Strategies: Successful long-distance caregivers organize networks of volunteers and professionals, including their care receivers, who are central to the networks. Teamwork and communication are the guiding principles of these networks.

Long-distance caregivers often assign responsibility for components of care. For example, they ask neighbors to do yardwork, or friends to run errands. They stay in contact with these local caregivers to monitor the welfare of the care receiver.

When possible, long-distance caregivers join their care receivers at medical appointments to learn about diagnoses, treatments, and ways to manage needs. They also seek advice about care options from doctors, oncology nurses, and social workers.

Some long-distance caregivers benefit from creating care notebooks on paper or in computers. They use them to write notes, create lists, and organize information, resources, medications, and schedules. They log contact information for doctors, therapists, medical facilities, emergency contacts, friends, neighbors, and clergy.

Resourceful caregivers might use telephone books from care receivers' locations or the Internet to find assistance. They gather information about medical facilities, assisted living facilities, nursing homes, hospice care providers, and other resources.

They also frequently call or send letters and e-mail messages to care receivers to communicate love and support and to monitor needs. They make regular visits to reassure care receivers that they care and to determine whether home care situations work.

Successful long-distance caregivers plan for sudden and unexpected needs. They expect change in care receivers' situations and plan ahead to deal with it. They prepare to make unexpected visits by researching quick and easy ways to travel to their care receivers.

Effective long-distance caregivers make decisions with their care receivers about legal and financial matters. They help organize care receivers' key legal, financial, and insurance documents. They also ensure that living wills, health directives, and medical and legal powers of attorney are in order and communicated to appropriate professionals.

Strengths and limitations: Long-distance caregivers have strengths and limitations. They know that distance creates limitations, and they occasionally feel guilty, stressed, anxious, or overwhelmed by the challenges of their responsibilities. They do not keep their caregiving a secret. They ask for help as a sign of strength and a means to improve care. They stay as flexible as possible and allow themselves to accept others' help. Sometimes they hire a professionally certified care manager to resolve issues before crises arise.

Wise long-distance caregivers are kind, caring, and patient with themselves. They make their own physical, emotional, and spiritual health a priority. They meet their own needs and take respite breaks from caregiving. They accept support from family, friends, and their faith communities. Many of them reach out to caregiver support groups, online bulletin boards, and buddy systems.

They are receptive to care receivers' existing informal support systems—the friends, neighbors, and others on whom care receivers depend. They bring these resources into their care networks and ask the people to contact them when they have new information or learn about problems requiring assistance.

Susan E. Ullmann, M.T. (ASCP), M.A.

▶ For Further Information

American Medical Association. *American Medical Association Guide to Home Caregiving.* New York: John Wiley & Sons, 2001.

Heath, Angela. *Long Distance Caregiving: A Survival Guide for Far Away Caregivers.* Atascadero, Calif.: American Source Books, 1993.

Karp, Freddie, ed. *So Far Away: Twenty Questions for Long-Distance Caregivers.* Bethesda, Md.: National Institute on Aging, National Institutes of Health, U.S. Department of Health and Human Services, 2006.

Rosenblatt, Bob, and Carol Van Steenberg. *Handbook for Long-Distance Caregivers.* San Francisco: Family Caregiver Alliance of the National Center on Caregiving, 2003.

Sparks, Martha E. *Cherish the Days: Inspiration and Insight for Long-Distance Caregivers.* Indianapolis, Ind.: Wesleyan, 2004.

▶ Other Resources

American Cancer Society
http://www.cancer.org

Cancer.Net
http://www.cancer.net/portal/site/patient

National Hospice and Palliative Care Organization
http://www.nhpco.org

See also Advance directives; Aging and cancer; Anxiety; Brief Pain Inventory (BPI); Cancer education; Caregivers and caregiving; Case management; Counseling for cancer patients and survivors; Elderly and cancer; Financial issues; Home health services; Insurance; Living will; Living with cancer; Oncology social worker; Pain management medications; Relationships; Support groups; Transitional care.

▶ Loop electrosurgical excisional procedure (LEEP)

Category: Procedures

Also known as: Large loop excision of the transformation zone (LLETZ), large loop excision of the cervix (LLEC), loop cone biopsy of the cervix

Definition: Loop electrosurgical excisional procedure (LEEP) is a procedure that may be used to excise or cut away abnormal, possibly precancerous cells (cervical intraepithelial neoplasia) on the surface of the cervix as indicated by the results of a Pap test.

Cancers diagnosed or treated: Cervical intraepithelial neoplasia or dysplasia (CIN), abnormal cell changes on the surface of the cervix

Why performed: A LEEP removes abnormal, possibly precancerous cells indicated by results of a Pap test and seen on colposcopy (a noninvasive device used to see inside the cervix) on the surface of the cervix. A LEEP may also be used as a diagnostic procedure when abnormal cells are suspected high in the cervical canal and are not visible using a colposcope.

Patient preparation: While there is no standard preparation needed for a LEEP, the patient should consult with her doctor or provider. A LEEP is not performed while a patient is menstruating.

Steps of the procedure: The patient, unclothed from the waist down, draped with a cloth or paper, lies on an exam table as for a typical pelvic exam with feet raised in stirrups. A speculum is inserted in the vagina to allow the physician to see inside the vagina and cervix to guide the colposcope to the area where the abnormal cells are located. A tube is attached to the speculum to remove any smoke caused by the procedure. Then an electrosurgical dispersive pad is placed on the thigh, which allows the electric current to return safely. The physician will attach a single-use disposable loop electrode to the generator hand piece. A vinegar (acetic acid) or iodine solution will be used to prepare the cervix, allowing the physician to assess the extent of the abnormal cells. If a cervical block or anesthetic will be used to numb the cervix, then a pain medication will be administered beforehand. Once the local anesthetic or block is injected into the cervix, the electroloop is generated and the wire loop will pass through the surface of the cervix. Finally, an electrosurgical generator sends a painless electrical current that cuts away the affected cervical tissue as the loop wire moves through the cervix, causing the abnormal cells to burst. The procedure takes about ten to twenty minutes to complete.

After the procedure: The patient may go home following the procedure. While rare, complications may include mild cramping, mild discomfort or pain, bleeding, heavy vaginal discharge, or strong vaginal odor. The patient should report any significant side effect to her doctor. The patient is typically advised not to engage in sexual intercourse for four weeks following the procedure. Ibuprofen (Motrin, Advil) may be taken for cramping. The patient is advised not to lift heavy objects, douche, or use tampons for four weeks following the procedure and is advised to take showers instead of baths to reduce the risk of infection. The patient's doctor will make a follow-up appointment to perform a colposcopy to check that all abnormal cells have been removed and perform a Pap test to confirm this.

Risks: The LEEP is very safe. The benefits of treating potentially precancerous cells with the procedure outweigh its minimal risks. Those risks may include heavy bleeding, bleeding with clots, severe abdominal cramping, fever, foul-smelling discharge, incomplete removal of abnormal tissue, cervical stenosis (narrowing of the cervix), infection, and possibly cutting or accidental burning of normal tissue if the patient moves during the procedure.

Results: Typically, the patient returns to normal activity within one to three days after the LEEP. The doctor will disclose the results of the histologic specimen obtained from the LEEP regarding whether invasive cancer may have developed deep in cervical tissue. A follow-up appointment is made to perform a colposcopy to confirm that all abnormal cells have been removed, a Pap test is repeated to confirm their removal, and the patient is advised to return on a regular basis for Pap tests to track the possible recurrence of abnormal cervical cells.

Susan H. Peterman, M.P.H.

See also Afterloading radiation therapy; Antiviral therapies; Benign tumors; Biological therapy; Birth control pills and cancer; Carcinomas; Carcinomatosis; Cervical cancer; Colposcopy; Conization; Diethylstilbestrol (DES); Endometrial cancer; Exenteration; Fertility drugs and cancer; Gynecologic cancers; Human papillomavirus (HPV); Hysterectomy; Hystero-oophorectomy; Infectious cancers; Pap test; Pelvic examination; Pregnancy and cancer; Vaccines, preventive; Vaginal cancer; Virus-related cancers.

▶ Lumbar puncture

Category: Procedures
Also known as: Spinal tap

Definition: Lumbar puncture is the insertion of a needle between two vertebrae in the lower back (lumbar region) into the spinal canal in order to obtain a sample of cerebrospinal fluid (CSF) for analysis.

Cancers diagnosed or treated: Cancers of the central nervous system (brain and spinal cord), such as meningeal carcinomatosis

Why performed: Although usually used for diagnosing disease, sometimes the procedure is used to provide a mechanism for the introduction of medications to treat dis-

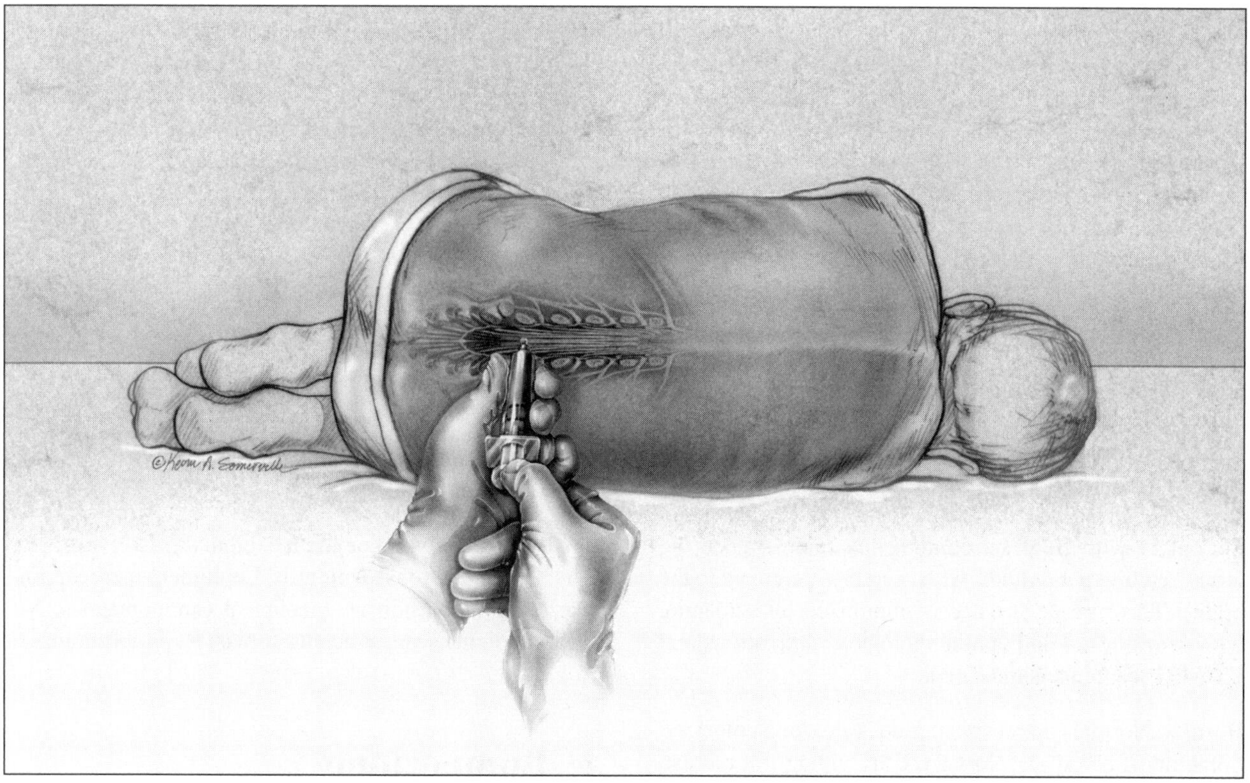

A lumbar puncture. (©Kevin A. Somerville/Phototake—All rights reserved)

ease, to introduce agents for further study of possible disease, or as actual treatment for some disease. Lumbar puncture results are used to help diagnose diseases such as meningitis, subarachnoid hemorrhage, Guillain-Barré syndrome, and multiple sclerosis. In addition, dyes for myelograms or anesthetics for pain relief may be introduced using lumbar puncture.

Patient preparation: A computed tomography (CT) scan or magnetic resonance imaging (MRI) scan is sometimes completed prior to lumbar puncture, but these scans are not always indicated. Certain blood tests are taken to compare the results from the blood to the results from the cerebrospinal fluid collected during the lumbar puncture, including serum chemistry panels (glucose) and complete blood counts (white blood cell count). Ideally, medications such as aspirin, ibuprofen, or other antiplatelet agents should be discontinued forty-eight to seventy-two hours before an elective lumbar puncture.

Steps of the procedure: The patient is placed on his or her side with knees drawn up toward the chest and back flexed toward the legs. Sterile procedure is completed, including sterile gloves, alcohol swabbing, iodine preparation, and isolation of the puncture area with sterile towels or paper drapes. The health care professional performing the procedure palpates (feels) the spine to locate the best position to insert the needle in the patient's lower back. In adults, the spinal cord extends down to the first lumbar vertebra (five lumbar vertebrae are present, with the highest on the back labeled as number 1), so the health care professional locates an area below vertebra11, usually between the third and fourth lumbar vertebrae or the fourth and fifth lumbar vertebrae. Infants require a 14-15 insertion area since the spinal cord terminates at a lower level in infants than in adults. A local anesthetic with a tiny needle is used to numb the insertion site for the larger lumbar puncture needle.

After the procedure: The patient should lie flat on the back for about two hours following the procedure. Rising too fast after a lumbar puncture can increase the risk of the most frequent complication of an lumbar puncture, a positional headache.

Risks: A headache that changes with position is the most frequent complication, occurring in about 25 percent of cases. These headaches usually resolve with rest and hydration. Uncommon complications include damage to nerves in the head and facial region that typically resolve within four months. Rare complications include tumors and cysts that form in the area of the needle insertion site.

People with leukemia may have an increased risk of hematoma (clot) formation at or near the insertion site of the lumbar puncture needle. Lenworth N. Johnson and Michael A. Meyer have reported in *Neuro-ophthalmology* (2005) that leukemia patients who have a traumatic lumbar puncture can suffer contamination of the CSF with cancer cells, and the median survival time of these patients can be reduced in this situation.

The gravest complication of a lumbar puncture is herniation of the brain stem, where the lower portion of the brain is suddenly pulled down by the pressure release of opening the spinal canal to remove fluid. This can happen if a brain tumor or growth has increased pressure in the spinal canal, since the fluid in the spinal canal is physically in contact with fluid surrounding the brain (hence the term "cerebrospinal fluid," with "cerebro" referring to the brain). This rare occurrence is minimized by screening with neurological and ophthalmologic examinations and CT/MRI scanning as indicated.

Results: Normal cerebrospinal fluid is clear and colorless. Sometimes, blood discolors the CSF, giving it a reddish color. If blood is present, then it can indicate a very serious condition known as subarachnoid hemorrhage. Usually, if blood is present in the CSF, then the blood comes from what is known as a "traumatic tap," resulting from the inadvertent puncture of small blood vessels with the lumbar puncture needle. A traumatic tap is not usually a serious problem, but the blood source requires identification. Four or five small tubes of CSF are collected from a typical lumbar puncture. Blood from a traumatic tap diminishes from the first tube collected to the last tube collected. Other tests can be completed to help determine the source of blood found in a lumbar puncture.

Laboratory tests routinely completed on CSF include protein, glucose, and white and red blood cell counts. Cultures and studies for bacteria, fungi, and viruses may be completed. Cells found in the CSF may be microscopically examined to determine if cancers of the brain or spinal cord are present. The pressure of the fluid as it initially drains out of the spinal canal, called the opening pressure, is measured, as is the closing pressure at the end of the procedure. Elevated pressures can indicate tumors or masses in the cranial cavity.

Richard P. Capriccioso, M.D.

▶ For Further Information

Fischbach, Frances Talaska, and Marshall Barnett Dunning III. *A Manual of Laboratory and Diagnostic Tests*. 7th ed. Philadelphia: Lippincott Williams & Wilkins, 2004.

Johnson, Lenworth N., and Michael A. Meyer. "Lumbar Puncture." In *Neuro-ophthalmology: The Practical Guide*, edited by Leonard A. Levin and Anthony C. Arnold. New York: Thieme Medical, 2005.

Pagana, Kathleen Deska, and Timothy J. Pagana. *Mosby's Manual of Diagnostic and Laboratory Tests*. 3d ed. St. Louis: Mosby Elsevier, 2006.

▶ Other Resources

WebMD

Lumbar Puncture
http://www.webmd.com/brain/Lumbar-Puncture?page=1

See also Acute lymphocytic leukemia (ALL); Blood cancers; Carcinomatous meningitis; Leptomeningeal carcinomas; Medulloblastomas; Meningeal carcinomatosis; Nuclear medicine scan; Pineoblastomas; Retinoblastomas.

▶ Lumpectomy

Category: Procedures
Also known as: Breast-conserving surgery, partial mastectomy

Definition: A lumpectomy is breast-conserving surgery and is the most common form of breast surgery performed for cancer. It is usually done as an inpatient procedure, or as "day surgery," under general or local anesthesia, when a lump or mass is found in only one section of the breast by physical examination, mammogram, ultrasound, or magnetic resonance imaging (MRI) of the breast. During a lumpectomy, the lump and some of the surrounding normal-appearing breast tissue are removed and the margins between the lumpectomy and the rest of the breast are examined for any residual tumor.

Cancers diagnosed or treated: Breast cancer

Why performed: A lumpectomy is performed to remove cancer as a breast-conserving method; it is also sometimes called partial mastectomy, as opposed to complete removal of the breast, known as mastectomy. Patients may not be candidates for lumpectomy and radiation if they have more than one cancer in the same breast, have a connective tissue disease such as lupus or vasculitis, are pregnant, or have already had radiation to the same breast.

Sentinel node biopsy may also be performed on the same day of the operation in order to examine the lymph nodes in the armpit or axilla of the breast affected for the presence of cancer that may have spread from the primary lump or site in the breast to the lymph nodes.

Patient preparation: Lumpectomy is usually preceded by a breast biopsy performed by a radiologist or breast surgeon that confirms the presence of breast cancer and in most cases tells the surgeon the type of breast cancer present. This latter information allows the surgeon to decide on the need for the surgery and the type of operation necessary.

Patient instructions are NPO (from the Latin *nulla per os*, or "nothing by mouth") after midnight on the day before the surgery. If sentinel node biopsy is performed in conjunction with lumpectomy, then the patient will need to be injected with radionuclide the day before the breast surgery. The injection is usually done around the nipple or areola by a nuclear medicine physician or radiologist. In the operating room the next day, the surgeon then uses a probe that is sensitive to small doses of gamma radiation emitted by the radiotracer to identify and remove the main draining node or nodes in the axilla, thereby eliminating the need to sample all the nodes in the axilla and thus reducing the risk of lymphedema, a swelling of the affected arm that can occur after full axillary node dissection.

Steps of the procedure: If the lump cannot be felt, then a procedure to mark the location of the mass will be performed, usually in the radiology suite the morning of the surgery. A thin wire or needle is inserted using mammography or ultrasound to guide the radiologist, depending on if the lesion was visible on prior mammogram or ultrasound. This is called a breast needle (or wire) localization. The surgery itself lasts about an hour. After general anesthesia is given, the surgeon will make a curved incision in the breast, usually in the form of a smile or frown which follows the contour of the breast in order to minimize scarring. After the lump and the surrounding breast tissue are removed with a scalpel, a drain may be left in place to collect excess fluid or blood, and the surgeon will then close the wound with stitches and apply a sterile dressing over the wound.

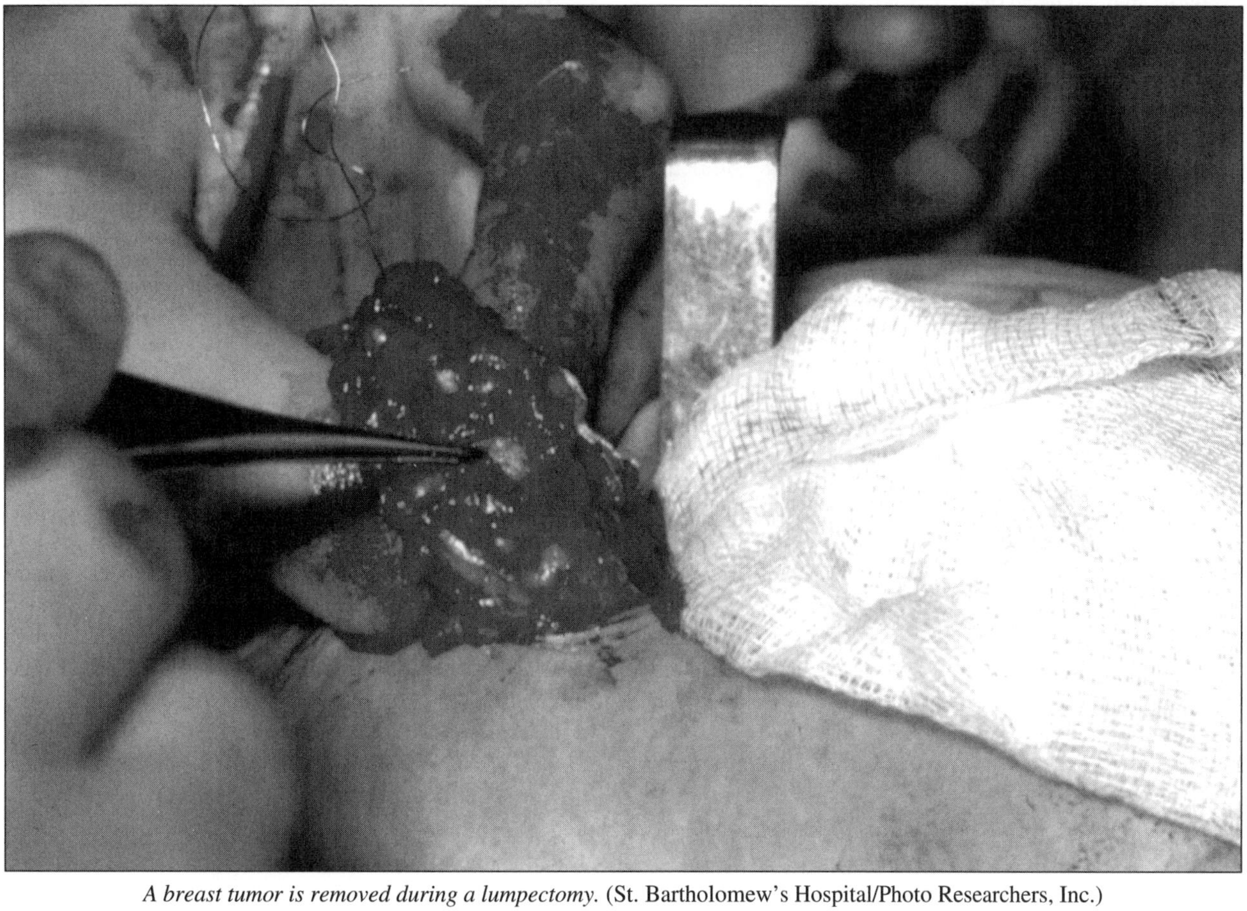

A breast tumor is removed during a lumpectomy. (St. Bartholomew's Hospital/Photo Researchers, Inc.)

After the procedure: The patient will awake in the recovery room and may be required to stay overnight, depending on many factors, including the procedure itself, the general health of the patient, and how easily the patient recovers from anesthesia.

Risks: The risks of general anesthesia are the same regardless of the procedure; patients who have any questions about anesthesia or any part of the operation should discuss these issues with their referring physician or health care provider. There may be some loss of sensation in the affected breast, and the breasts may not match in size and shape after the surgery, which may or may not be acceptable to the patient.

Results: Once the pathology results are back, the doctor will review the pathology report and discuss the next steps, including the need for additional therapy.

Lumpectomy is usually, but not always, followed by radiation therapy to eliminate any possibility of microcancers (cancer that are too small to identify by physical examination or radiologic means). If the margins are not clean of cancer, then a second operation, called a reexcision, may be necessary.

Debra B. Kessler, M.D., Ph.D.

▶ For Further Information

Benedet, Rosalind. *Understanding Lumpectomy: A Treatment Guide for Breast Cancer*. Omaha, Nebr.: Addicus Books, 2003.

Dewar, J. A., R. Arriagada, S. Benhamous, et al. "Local Relapse and Contralateral Tumor Rates in Patients with Breast Cancer Treated with Conservative Surgery and Radiotherapy." *Cancer* 76 (1995): 2260-2265.

Giulano, A., D. M. Kirgan, J. M. Guenther, et al. "Lymphatic Mapping and Sentinel Lymphadenectomy for Breast Cancer." *Annals of Surgery* 220 (1994): 439-442.

Reiber, A., K. Schramm, G. Helms, et al. "Breast-Conserving Surgery and Autogeneous Tissue Reconstruction in Patients with Breast Cancer: Efficacy of MRI of the Breast in the Detection of Recurrent Disease." *European Journal of Radiology* 13 (2003): 780-787.

See also Accelerated partial breast irradiation (APBI); Biopsy; Breast cancers; Breast self-examination (BSE); Breast ultrasound; Clinical breast exam (CBE); Lumps; Mammography; Mastectomy; Needle biopsies; Needle localization; Sentinel lymph node (SLN) biopsy and mapping; Stereotactic needle biopsy; Surgical biopsies; Surgical oncology; Wire localization.

▶ Lumps

Category: Diseases, symptoms, and conditions
Also known as: Masses

Related conditions: Cysts, fibromas

Definition: Lumps are abnormal masses or swellings on the skin or in the body.

Risk factors: There are many conditions that may cause lumps, such as a cyst, fibroma, injury, or cancer.

Etiology and the disease process: The likely causes of lumps include benign breast diseases, a lipoma (collection of fatty tissue), exostoses (new bone formation), cancer, an injury, an enlarged organ, or a swollen lymph node. Lymph nodes often swell in response to various infections or diseases, including the common cold, infections, viruses, mononucleosis, tonsillitis, lymphoma, Hodgkin disease, and leukemia. A variety of tissues in the body respond to hormonal changes, and as a result, certain lumps are transient. As an example, breast lumps may appear at all ages. Male or female infants may develop breast lumps temporarily in response to receiving estrogen from the mother's milk. Breast-feeding women are prone to benign breast lumps from mastitis (inflammation of the mammary gland). Other underlying conditions for breast lumps include fibrocystic breasts, fibroadenoma, cyst, abscess, fat necrosis, gynecomastia (male breasts), duct papilloma (epithelial tumor growth), sclerosing adenosis (excess growth of breast tissues), and ductal ectasia (dilatation of the subareolar ducts). Fibrocystic breasts and fibroadenomas often occur in women during the reproductive years and are considered a normal variation of breast tissue. Cysts are fluid-filled sacs that can become tender.

Incidence: Lumps commonly occur and often spontaneously resolve.

Symptoms: The signs and symptoma of lumps are swelling or pain, often in the breast, under the skin, and in the groin.

Screening and diagnosis: Lumps are detected by touch, visually, or by the perception of pain. Medical examination can reveal their cause and whether they are benign or malignant. Most common potentially cancer-related lumps develop in the breasts. Although typically lumps in the breast are benign breast cysts, they may be indicators of breast cancer. As a result, lumps found in the breast should be immediately examined to detect potential cases of breast cancer.

Treatment and therapy: The nature and causes of lumps determine how they are treated. Cysts can easily be drained by a physician, but if they do not disappear, surgery may be needed. Generally, if the fluid removed from the cyst is relatively clear and the lump disappears, no further treatment is necessary. However, if the fluid is bloody, the cyst must be inspected for the possible presence of cancer cells.

Prognosis, prevention, and outcomes: Lumps tend to be benign. However, if a malignancy is detected, the survival rate with early diagnosis tends to be higher than after delayed detection.

Anita Nagypál, Ph.D.

See also Accelerated partial breast irradiation (APBI); Biopsy; Breast cancer in children and adolescents; Breast cancer in men; Breast cancers; Breast self-examination (BSE); Breast ultrasound; Clinical breast exam (CBE); Fibrocystic breast changes; Fibrosarcomas, soft-tissue; Head and neck cancers; Lumpectomy; Mammography; Surgical biopsies; Symptoms and cancer.

▶ Lung cancers

Category: Diseases, symptoms, and conditions
Also known as: Carcinomas of the lung, small-cell lung cancer (SCLC), oat cell carcinoma, non-small-cell lung cancer (NSCLC)

Related conditions: Mesothelioma

Definition: Lung cancer is an uncontrolled cell growth in lung tissues, which may lead to metastasis and infiltration of other tissues beyond the lungs.

Risk factors: Long-term exposure to tobacco smoke is the main risk factor (90 percent of the cases) for the development of lung cancer. The lifetime risk of developing lung cancer among male smokers is 17.2 percent, and among female smokers the risk is 11.6 percent. This lifetime risk is significantly lower among nonsmokers, accounting for 1.3 percent of cases of lung cancers in men and for 1.4 percent of cases in women. The occurrence of lung cancer in nonsmokers (less than 10 percent of the cases) may be due to genetic factors, secondhand smoke, air pollution, and exposure to occupational respiratory carcinogens such radon gas, chromium, asbestos, and inorganic arsenic. There are more than four thousand chemicals in tobacco smoke, making the identification of the contributing factors to lung carcinogenesis challenging.

Genetic predisposition might also contribute to the risk of lung cancer development. First-degree relatives of patients with lung cancer have an increased risk of lung cancer compared with those of controls. However, familial aggregation of lung cancer might in part be caused by shared exposure to tobacco smoke. A major autosomal susceptibility locus for inherited lung cancer was found at chromosome 6q23-25, which contains numerous potential genes of interest, including *SASH1*, *LATS1*, *IGF2R*, *PARK2*, and *TCF21*. Genetic aberrations associated with lung cancer often encompass multiple genetic aberrations, including deoxyribonucleic acid (DNA) sequence alterations, copy number changes, allele loss, and abnormal promoter methylations.

Etiology and the disease process: The lung is a common place for metastasis of tumors that originate from tissues other than the lung. The site of origin identifies these nonprimary lung cancers. For example, a breast cancer metastasis to the lung is still called breast cancer. These metastatic lung cancers usually have a distinctive round appearance on chest X ray. Primary lung cancers typically metastasize to the adrenal glands, liver, brain, and bone.

The majority of lung cancers arise from epithelial cells. The two main types of lung carcinomas are histologically defined as SCLC and NSCLC. At diagnosis, it is essential to distinguish which type of lung cancer is present because their treatment varies. SCLC is usually treated with chemotherapy, while NSCLC is often treated with surgery.

There are three main subtypes of NSCLC: squamous cell lung carcinoma, adenocarcinoma, and large-cell lung carcinoma. Squamous cell lung carcinoma, which accounts for 31 percent of lung cancers, usually originates near a central bronchus and often grows more slowly than other cancer types. Adenocarcinoma is associated with smoking, accounts for about 29 percent of lung tumors, and usually arises in peripheral lung tissue. Despite its link to smoking, adenocarcinoma is the most common form of cancer among patients who have never smoked. Variants of adenocarcinoma are adenocarcinoma (not otherwise specified), bronchoalveolar carcinoma, pdenosquamous carcinoma, papillary adenocarcinoma, mucoepidermoid carcinoma, adenoid cystic carcinoma, and other specified adenocarcinomas. Bronchoalveolar carcinoma is more common in women who have never smoked. Large-cell lung carcinoma often develops around the surface of the lung, and it is an aggressive, fast-growing type of NSCLC that tends to metastasize early. This type of malignancy accounts for about 11 percent of lung cancers.

SCLCs are strongly associated with smoking, but they are less common than NSCLCs. SCLCs usually originate in the larger breathing tubes and develop rapidly. Although SCLCs respond well to chemotherapy initially, they often are metastatic at diagnosis and have a worse prognosis than NSCLCs.

Incidence: Lung cancer is the most common cause of cancer-related death in men and the second most common in women worldwide. Lung cancer is responsible for 1.3 million deaths worldwide annually. The incidence of the disease increases with age up to about age seventy. Worldwide, approximately twice as many men as women develop lung cancer. This ratio decreases in areas in which the prevalence of cigarette smoking among women is high. The highest numbers of new lung cancers are found in the United States and Europe. In 2005, the estimated number of new cases in the seven major commercial markets was 393,000, and by 2015 new cases of lung cancer are estimated to reach approximately 561,000. About 80 percent of lung cancers are NSCLC, and 17 percent are SCLC. Over 50 percent of NSCLC patients are diagnosed with an advanced stage of the disease.

Symptoms: Lung cancer symptoms may include dyspnea (shortness of breath), hemoptysis (coughing up blood), chronic coughing or change in regular coughing pattern, wheezing, pain in the chest or abdomen, cachexia (weight loss), fatigue, loss of appetite, dysphonia (hoarse voice), clubbing of the fingernails (uncommon), and dysphagia (difficulty swallowing). At the time of diagnosis, the most common symptom of lung cancer (occurring in more than half of patients) is coughing. Other common symptoms at the time of diagnosis are weight loss and intermittent aching chest pain, which occurs in up to 50 percent of patients. Approximately 60 percent of lung cancer patients develop dyspnea, and up to 35 percent of patients have hemoptysis.

Symptoms and signs of development depend on the organ involved in the spread of disease. With a tumor in the mainstem bronchi, the initial symptom is most often wheezing that may be accompanied by a cough. If the cancer spreads to the left pharyngeal nerve, resulting in left vocal cord paralysis, and hoarseness of the voice occurs, this indicates an unresectable tumor. In addition to laryngeal nerve involvement, the left phrenic nerve is also commonly affected, which could result in paralysis of the left hemidiaphragm. Right paratracheal adenopathy or central

Incidence of Lung Cancer per 100,000 People, by Gender

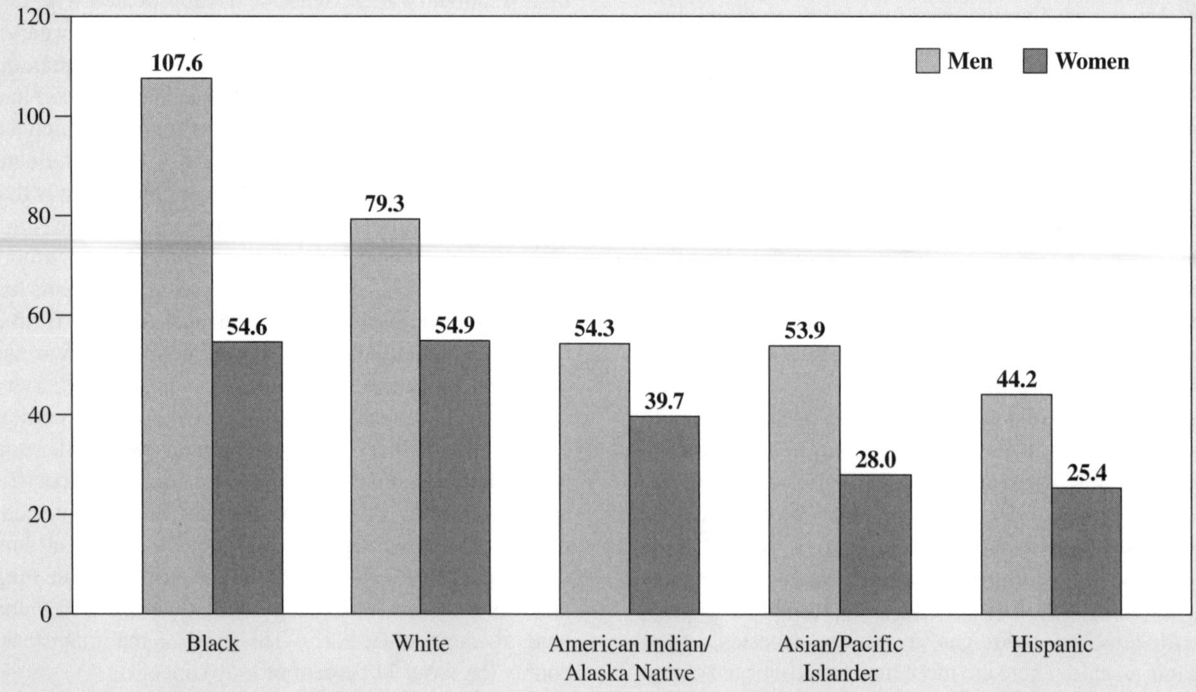

Source: Data from National Cancer Institute, Surveillance Epidemiology and End Results, Cancer Stat Fact Sheets, 2008
Note: Based on cases diagnosed in 2000-2004

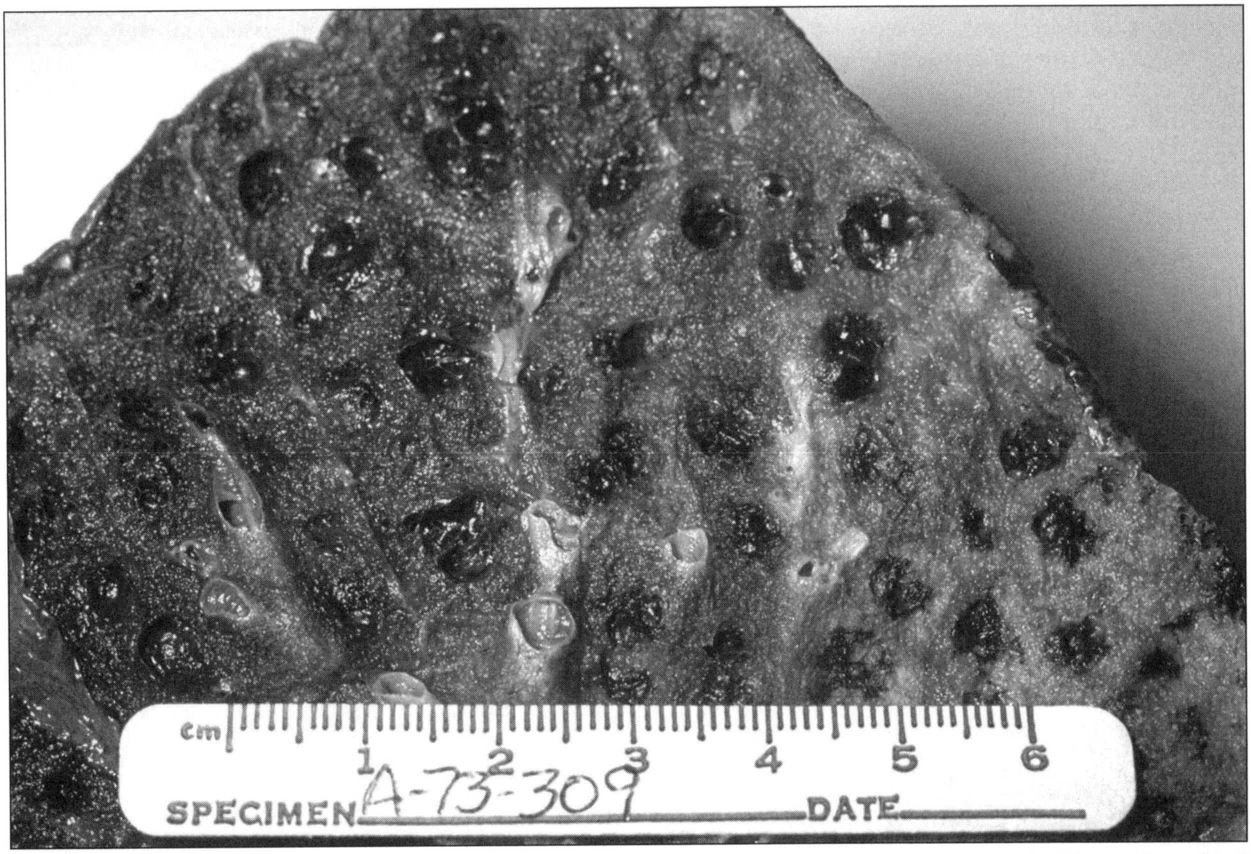

Centrilobular emphysema in a lung, characteristic of smoking, a major risk factor for lung cancer. (Centers for Disease Control and Prevention)

enlargement of a tumor in the right upper lobe of the lung often obstructs the superior vena cava. Such a tumor position often causes the patient to have facial or upper extremity swelling, venous swelling in the neck or chest, a cough, and dyspnea. A tumor localized in the apex of the lung usually causes shoulder and upper chest pain. Tumors located in the top of the lung may also cause damage to the brachial plexus and result in Horner syndrome (injury to the sympathetic nerves). Approximately 8 to 15 percent of lung cancer patients have pleural involvement and experience pleuritic chest pain or dyspnea.

Screening and diagnosis: Lung tumors are typically detected by chest radiography done during a general checkup or in response to reported symptoms. When a neoplasm is confirmed, staging of disease is required to develop the appropriate treatment plan and prognosis. Computed tomography (CT) scans and whole-body positron emission tomography (PET) scans are noninvasive staging methods. If clinical symptoms indicate the disease may have spread, other parts of the body may also be scanned.

Invasive staging modalities are used for confirmation of the diagnosis. Pathological diagnosis of neoplastic growth is obtained by sputum (mucus) cytology of tissues extracted from the tumor. Specimen sampling is crucial for diagnostic accuracy of cytology. Typically, transthoracic needle aspiration or endoscopic ultrasound with fine needle aspiration is used for sensitive diagnosis confirmation. For centrally located tumors, flexible bronchoscopy is one of the most common techniques, and it is often accompanied by bronchial washings. Transbronchial needle aspiration with fluoroscopic or CT scan guidance is used for submucosal or peribronchial tumors. In case of peripheral lung lesions, transthoracic lung biopsy offers high sensitivity sampling, and mediastinoscopy is the preferred method to evaluate a tumor in the mediastinal lymph node. Pulmonary function tests are also used.

Lung cancer staging is an assessment of the disease's progression from its original source. Precise staging of lung cancers is essential to develop prognosis and treatment. The most widely used staging system for NSCLC is the International Staging System (ISS), which uses TNM (tumor/lymph node/metastasis) categories that describe four stages of disease. SCLC is classified as limited-stage if it is confined to one half of the chest; otherwise it is extensive-stage.

Treatment and therapy: Treatment depends on the histological type of cancer, the stage, and the patient's performance status (how well the patient is able to perform daily living activities). Treatments include surgery, chemotherapy, and radiotherapy.

Commonly used systemic agents are bevacizumab (Avastin), carboplatin, cisplatin, docetaxel (Taxotere), erlotinib (Tarceva), etoposide, gemcitabine (Gemzar), ifosfamide (Mitoxana), irinotecan (Camptosar), mitomycin (Mutamycin), paclitaxel (Taxol), pemetrexed (Alimta), vinblastine (Velban), and vinorelbine (Navelbine).

The gold-standard therapy for advanced or metastatic disease is platinum-based chemotherapy, a cytotyic theropy that prolongs survival, controls symptoms, and improves quality of life compared with best supportive care (treatment to prevent, control, or relieve side effects or complications and to improve the patient's quality of life). However, patients with poor performance status do not benefit from cytotoxic chemotherapy. Bevacizumab (a monoclonol antibody) plus chemotherapy or chemotherapy alone is beneficial in patients with low performance status, as indicated by the Eastern Cooperative Oncology Group (ECOG) score of 0 to 1. In cases of advanced NSCLC, concurrent chemotherapy with radiation (chemoradiation) is better than sequential chemoradiation, and it is superior to radiation alone. Carboplatin or cisplatin is effective in combination with docetaxel, etoposide, gemcitabine, irinotecan, paclitaxel, vinblastine, and vinorelbine. Erlotinib is often used for nonsmoker patients with active epidermal growth factor receptor mutations or gene amplification. Single agents, such as docetaxel, pemetrexed, tyrosine kinase inhibitor, or erlotinib, are offered for second-line patients. Docetaxel is superior to best supportive care as second-line therapy in terms of quality of life. In addition, erlotinib is also superior to best supportive care in terms of survival as second- and third-line therapy.

Prognosis, prevention, and outcomes: The primary way to prevent lung cancer is to eliminate tobacco smoking. Approximately 42 percent of lung cancer patients survive for at least one year. Worldwide, the five-year survival rate is 14 percent with treatment. In particular, the five-year survival is 16 percent in the United States and 10 percent in Europe. Five-year survival decreases when advanced disease or NSCLC is present at diagnosis. For both men and women, age-standardized lung cancer mortality rates are highest in the United States compared with Japan and many European countries, including France, Germany, Italy, Spain, and the United Kingdom.

Anita Nagypál, Ph.D.

▶ For Further Information

American Cancer Society. *Quick Facts Lung Cancer: What You Need to Know—Now*. Atlanta: Author, 2007.

Desai, Sujal R., ed. *Lung Cancer*. New York: Cambridge University Press, 2007.

Eckardt, John R., and Julia E. Kimmis. *Understanding Lung Cancer: A Guide for Patients and Their Families*. Manhasset, N.Y.: CMP Healthcare Media, 2005.

Gilligan, David, and Robert Rintoul. *Your Guide to Lung Cancer*. London: Hodder Arnold, 2007.

Hunt, Ian, Martin Muers, and Tom Treasure, eds. *ABC of Lung Cancer*. Malden, Mass.: Blackwell, 2008.

Mountain, C. F. "Revisions in the International System for Staging Lung Cancer." *Chest* 111 (1997): 1710-1717.

Roth, Jack A., James D. Cox, and Waun Ki Hong, eds. *Lung Cancer*. 3d ed. Malden, Mass.: Blackwell, 2008.

▶ Other Resources

American Cancer Society
http://www.cancer.org

American Lung Association
Facts About Lung Cancer
Http://www.lungusa.org/site/pp.asp?c=dvLUK9O0E&b=35427

Lung Cancer Online Foundation
http://www.lungcanceronline.org/

LungCancer.org
http://www.lungcancer.org

National Cancer Institute
Lung Cancer
http://www.cancer.gov/cancertopics/types/lung

See also Air pollution; Bilobectomy; Bronchoalveolar lung cancer; Bronchography; Bronchoscopy; Coughing; Hemoptysis; Klinefelter syndrome and cancer; Lambert-Eaton myasthenic syndrome (LEMS); Lobectomy; Mesothelioma; Pleural biopsy; Pleural effusion; Pleurodesis; Pneumonectomy; Pneumonia; Smoking cessation; Soots; Thoracentesis; Thoracoscopy; Thoracotomy; Tobacco-related cancers.

Lutein

Category: Lifestyle and prevention
Also known as: Xanthophyll, non-provitamin A carotenoid

Definition: Lutein is a yellow pigment and micronutrient found in some vegetables, fruits, and eggs, and also in the human retina. It is best known as a carotenoid, a plant phytochemical thought to have antioxidant properties that protect against cell-damaging molecules known as free radicals.

Cancers treated or prevented: Prostate, breast, colon, lung, and ovarian cancers

Delivery routes: Oral via food or dietary supplements. The most significant food sources for lutein are broccoli, brussels sprouts, collards, kale, peas, pumpkin, spinach, turnip, mustard and dandelion greens, summer and winter squash, and sweet yellow corn. Egg yolks contain a more quickly absorbed form of lutein. Lutein absorption is increased from the intestine when combined with a dietary fat source, such as oil or margarine.

How this substance works: Lutein is chemically similar to the micronutrient zeaxanthin, and they often work together to provide protective benefits. Lutein, also known as a non-provitamin A carotenoid, cannot convert into vitamin A when needed by the body. Most studies find that lutein protects the eyes from disease, such as age-related macular degeneration and cataracts. Some studies find lutein effective against cancer because it decreases the growth of blood vessels to cancerous tumors, increases cancer cell destruction, and improves cell deoxyribonucleic acid (DNA) repair. Overall study results are mixed, however, with one study showing lutein reduced prostate cancer by 25 percent (and as much as 32 percent when combined with the carotenoid lycopene) and another showing an increase in stomach cancer. In general, most studies find that lutein provides some protection against breast, colon, lung, ovarian, and prostate cancers. The dosage and safety of lutein dietary supplements are still unknown. Doses of lutein up to 20 milligrams per day have been determined to be safe. Consuming lutein from food sources is advised, however, because of its interaction with other compounds found within these foods.

Side effects: Caution is advised for individuals with allergies or sensitivities to eggs or lutein-containing vegetables. In general, no toxicities or drug interactions have been reported with lutein from food sources. Caution, especially in pregnant or lactating women, should be used with lutein supplements because the risks are still unknown.

Alice C. Richer, R.D., M.B.A., L.D.

See also Amenorrhea; Antiandrogens; Antioxidants; Carotenoids; Complementary and alternative therapies; Craniopharyngiomas; Dietary supplements; Free radicals; Fruits; Lycopene; Nutrition and cancer prevention; Pituitary tumors.

Lycopene

Category: Lifestyle and prevention
Also known as: Non-provitamin A carotonoid

Definition: Lycopene is the red pigment in some fruits and vegetables that gives them their colorful appearance. It is best known as a carotenoid, a plant-produced phytochemical well known for its antioxidant properties.

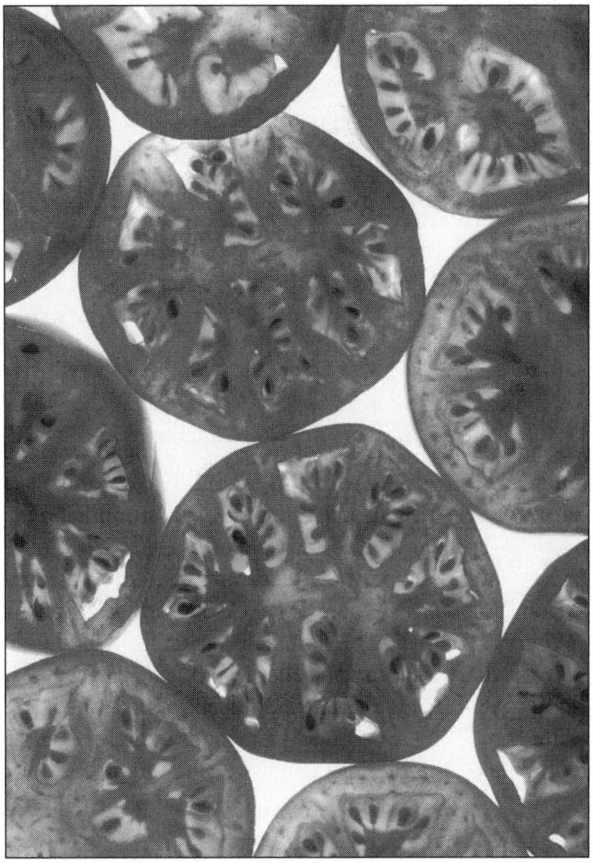

Tomatoes are a major source of lycopene. (U.S. Department of Agriculture)

Cancers treated or prevented: Prostate, lung, and stomach cancers

Delivery routes: Oral via food or dietary supplements. The most common food sources for lycopene are tomatoes and tomato products. Other significant food sources are apricots, guava, watermelon, papaya, and pink grapefruit. Processed tomatoes and tomato products provide more available lycopene than raw forms. The absorption of lycopene is increased when combined with a dietary fat source, such as the oil used in preparing pizza or tomato sauce.

How this substance works: Lycopene is believed to act as an antioxidant, blocking the destructive action of cell-damaging molecules known as free radicals. Also known as a non-provitamin A carotenoid, it cannot convert into vitamin A in the body, like some other carotenoids, when needed. Lycopene is fat-soluble; thus it is stored in the body and broken down in the intestine for use. Because of this, including dietary fat with a lycopene source increases its absorption. Lycopene is believed to play a role in preventing many diseases, such as cancer, heart disease, and macular degeneration, and it may slow the progression of some cancers. Some studies show the strongest protective evidence against lung, stomach, and prostate cancers. Other nutrients and compounds in fruits and vegetables are thought to combine with lycopene, however, and this synergy may actually be responsible for the protective benefits seen in these studies. The dosage and safety of dietary lycopene supplements are still unknown. Many studies have found positive benefits from consuming lycopene from fruit and vegetable sources, rather than dietary supplements, with no known safety issues.

Side effects: Caution is advised for individuals with allergies or sensitivities to tomatoes and tomato products or to fruits, vegetables, and dietary supplements that include lycopene. The high level of acid in tomatoes may irritate stomach disorders. While there is some belief that lycopene could decrease the side effects of radiation and chemotherapy, it may also decrease their effectiveness. As a rule, lycopene dietary supplements should be avoided during cancer treatment. Lycopene from food sources, however, has not been found to interfere with treatment. Some drugs may also decrease lycopene absorption.

Alice C. Richer, R.D., M.B.A., L.D.

See also Antioxidants; Carotenoids; Chemoprevention; Complementary and alternative therapies; Dietary supplements; Free radicals; Fruits; Lutein; Nutrition and cancer prevention.

▶ Lymphadenectomy

Category: Procedures
Also known as: Lymph node dissection

Definition: Lymphadenectomy is the surgical removal of lymph nodes. It is used to diagnose and treat almost all types of cancers because lymph nodes are found throughout the body and are one of the first places to which cancer spreads. Lymphadenectomy is an especially common procedure in diagnosing and treating breast cancer because of the number of lymph nodes located near the breast.

Cancers diagnosed and treated: Most, especially breast cancer

Why performed: The lymphatic system is part of the immune system, which helps keep the body free of disease. Lymph is a clear, yellowish fluid that oozes out of blood vessels and is carried in channels throughout the body. Eventually it is funneled back into a vein and reenters the blood circulatory system. Interspersed along the lymph channels are about six hundred enlarged areas called lymph nodes.

Lymph nodes filter bacteria, viruses, and cancer cells out of the lymph. These undesirable cells are then destroyed by white blood cells (lymphocytes) stored in the lymph nodes. There are many lymph nodes in the head and neck, another large cluster near the breast and under the armpit, and another group in the groin. When bacteria, viruses, or cancer cells overwhelm lymph nodes, the nodes swell and can be felt on the surface of the body. For example, when the lymph nodes behind the ears and along the throat are enlarged, people often say they have "swollen glands," although lymph nodes are not true glands.

Lymph nodes can be surgically removed either as a diagnostic tool or as a therapeutic procedure to treat cancer. In a lymph node biopsy, several samples of lymph node tissue are removed and examined under the microscope to see if they contain cancer cells. Based on the results of the biopsy, full removal of some nodes (a lymphadenectomy) may be performed.

One newer approach to lymphadenectomy aimed at preventing unnecessary surgery involves identifying sentinel nodes and removing them first. Sentinel nodes are the first nodes to which lymph travels after it leaves the area where cancer is present. They provide an early warning that the cancer has begun to spread. The location of sentinel nodes is determined before surgery by lymphangiography and other imaging tests. Lymphangiography involves slowly injecting a fluorescent dye into the lymphatic system and tracing its progress using X rays.

If no cancer is found in the sentinel nodes, then the cancer probably has not spread to the lymphatic system and no additional nodes need to be removed. If cancer has spread to the sentinel nodes and beyond, then lymphadenectomy becomes a treatment for cancer and lymph nodes suspected of containing malignant cells are surgically removed.

Patient preparation: Before a lymphadenectomy, various tests such as a lymphangiogram (dye injected into the lymphatic system) and other imaging scans are done to locate the cancer, determine where it is likely to have spread, and indicate to the surgeon which lymph nodes should be removed.

The patient is prepared for major surgery. In addition to tests to locate the cancer, the patient is given standard preoperative blood and liver function tests, meets with an anesthesiologist, and is required to fast for about eight hours before surgery.

Steps of the procedure: Lymphadenectomy is usually performed under general anesthesia in a hospital. An incision is made in the appropriate area, and lymph nodes and surrounding tissue are removed. Often the sentinel lymph nodes or a sampling of other lymph nodes are removed and examined under a microscope while the patient is still on the operating table. The condition of these nodes then dictates how much other tissue the surgeon will remove. Temporary drains are inserted under the skin to remove excess lymph that accumulates, and the incision is closed.

After the procedure: This procedure normally requires a hospital stay. The length of stay and the recovery period depend on the number of nodes removed and the general health of the patient. The patient may feel temporary numbness or a tingling or burning sensation in the region where the lymph nodes were removed. Radiation therapy or chemotherapy may be given after lymphadenectomy to help kill any cancer cells that remain in the body.

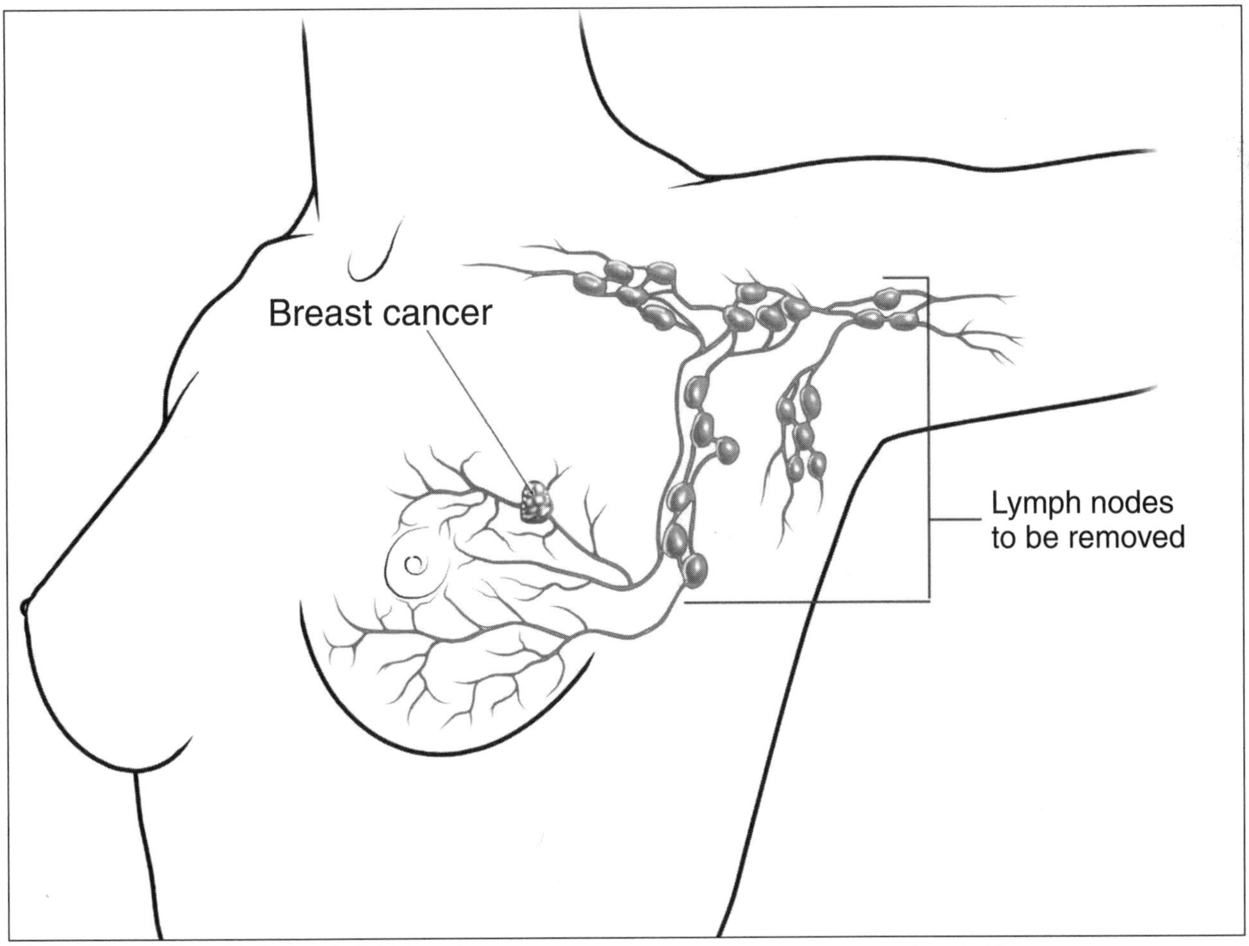

Removal of axillary lymph nodes during lymphectomy. (©Visuals Unlimited/Corbis)

Risks: All surgery carries the risk of bleeding, infection, and allergic reaction to anesthesia. Nevertheless, the greatest risk related to lymphadenectomy is the development of lymphedema after the operation. Lymphedema occurs when the lymphatic system is overwhelmed by large amounts of lymph. The lymph seeps into the surrounding tissue and causes swelling. About 15 percent of individuals have mild lymphedema, with 1 to 2 percent reporting severe swelling. Postoperative radiation therapy increases the risk of developing lymphedema.

Results: For diagnostic lymphadenectomy, if no malignant cells are found in the removed lymph nodes, then it is unlikely that cancer has spread beyond the primary tumor. If lymph nodes are enlarged and malignant cells are found, then there is a high chance that the cancer may metastasize. Therapeutic lymphadenectomy may slow cancer but does not, by itself, cure it. The success of this treatment depends on the stage of the cancer and how many lymph nodes are involved.

Martiscia Davidson, A.M.

▶ For Further Information

Khatri, Vijay P., ed. *Lymphadenectomy in Surgical Oncology*. Philadelphia: Saunders, 2007.

Leong, Stanley P. L. *Selective Sentinel Lymphadenectomy for Human Solid Cancer*. New York: Springer, 2007.

Sato, K., R. Shigenaga, S. Udea, et al. "Sentinel Lymph Node Biopsy for Breast Cancer." *Journal of Surgical Oncology* 96, no. 4 (September 15, 2007): 322-329.

▶ Other Resources

BreastCancer.org
Lymph Node Removal
http://www.breastcancer.org/treatment/surgery/lymph_node_removal/index.jsp

WebMD Cancer Health Center
Lymph Node Biopsy
http://www.webmd.com/cancer/lymph-node-biopsy

See also Axillary dissection; Biopsy; Breast cancers; Lumpectomy; Lymphangiography; Lymphangiosarcomas; Lymphedema; Lymphocytosis; Lymphomas; Metastasis; Sentinel lymph node (SLN) biopsy and mapping; Surgical oncology.

▶ Lymphangiography

Category: Procedures

Definition: Lymphangiography is the injection of a dye or radioactive material into the lymphatic system so that the location and condition of lymph nodes and lymph vessels can be determined using X rays.

Cancers diagnosed: Most often used to determine the location of sentinel lymph nodes in breast cancer or to determine the condition of lymph nodes prior to biopsy or removal; sometimes used to diagnose lymphomas

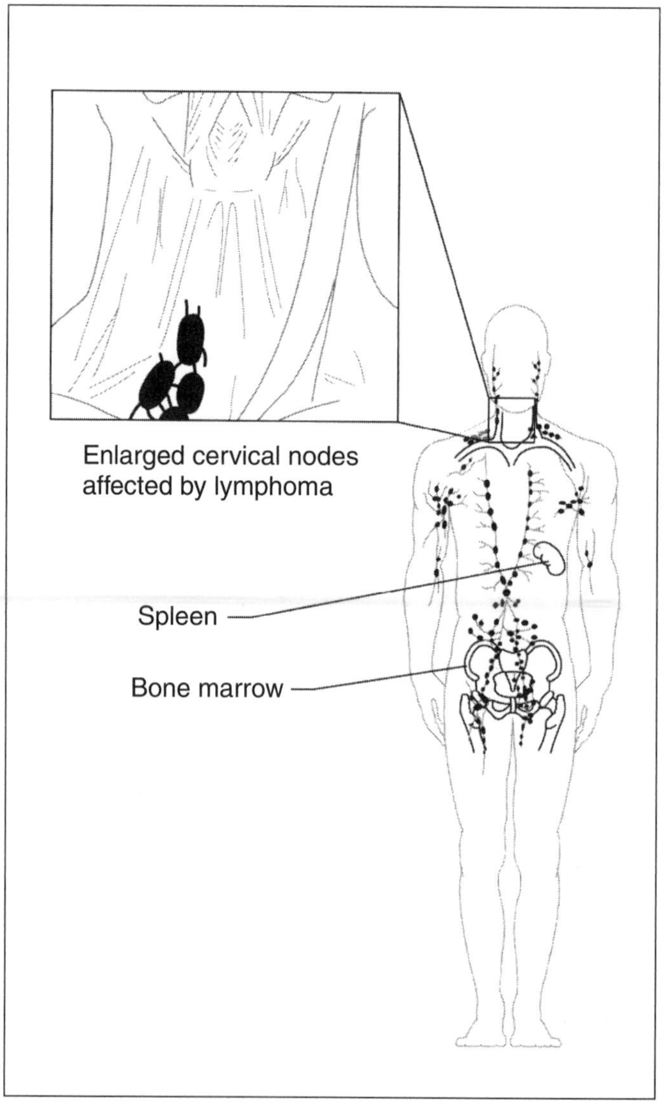

Major nodes of the lymphatic system; enlarged nodes can be caused by lymphomas and other cancers.

Why performed: The lymphatic system is part of the immune system. It consists of a network of channels that carries lymph, a clear, yellowish fluid, and about six hundred nodes, or enlarged spaces. The lymph nodes trap bacteria, viruses, and cancer cells so that they can be destroyed by white blood cells stored in the nodes. Lymph nodes are one of the first places to which cancer spreads, so knowing if there are cancer cells in the nodes is important in staging and treating all cancers.

Lymphangiography helps the surgeon determine where to biopsy or which lymph nodes to remove. The sentinel nodes are the first nodes through which lymph flows after it passes the primary tumor. In some women with breast cancer, the sentinel node is located using lymphangiography and then removed. If no cancer is found, then no additional nodes need to be removed, thus reducing the amount of surgery that the patient needs.

Patient preparation: Minimal preparations are needed for lymphangiography. The patient may be asked not to drink for several hours before the test, since the lymphangiography takes up to seven hours and requires that the patient remain still.

Steps of the procedure: A dye is infused into the hand or foot. The dye enters the lymph system and highlights the lymph channels and nodes. The dye may cause a mild burning feeling. It enters the body very slowly, and the patient must remain still during this time.

After the procedure: The site where the dye was infused is cleaned and closed. The patient's urine may be bluish for several days. Dye can remain in the body for up to two years.

Risks: Allergic reaction to the dye and infection at the infusion site are the main risks.

Results: From this test, the physician can tell if the lymph nodes are swollen or clogged, a condition that may indicate cancer. The surgeon can also determine which nodes are sentinel nodes.

Martiscia Davidson, A.M.

See also Biopsy; Breast cancers; Cystography; Embolization; Imaging tests; Lymphadenectomy; Lymphangiosarcomas; Lymphedema; Lymphocytosis; Lymphomas; Metastasis; Sentinel lymph node (SLN) biopsy and mapping; Testicular cancer; X-ray tests.

▶ Lymphangiosarcomas

Category: Diseases, symptoms, and conditions
Also known as: Lymphatic vessel tumors, angiosarcomas, lymphangioendotheliomas, Stewart-Treve syndrome, hemangiosarcomas

Related conditions: Primary or secondary lymphedemas, classical radical mastectomy

Definition: A lymphangiosarcoma is a rare malignant tumor that begins in the cells of the lymph vessels, usually in the upper extremities of individuals who have lymphedema.

Risk factors: Risks factors for lymphangiosarcomas are a history of primary or secondary lymphedema, having had a classical radical mastectomy, or having radiation or chronic infections in a lymphodemous limb.

Etiology and the disease process: Lymphangiosarcoma begins in the cells of the lymphatic vessels. This tumor is seen in the upper arms approximately five to fifteen years after a classical radical mastectomy, specifically in individuals who have long-standing lymphedema. Although the breast cancer may have been cured with the radical mastectomy, a secondary cancer diagnosis of lymphangiosarcoma has a poor prognosis. The radical mastectomy procedure is now outmoded and has been replaced with a more conservative surgical procedure. Lymphangiosarcomas can also arise in individuals with long-standing idiopathic lymphedema of several years. The signs of lymphangiosarcoma are a purple or bruised area on an extremity (usually the upper arm) that becomes a sore that does not heal with necrosis (breakdown) of the skin and underlying tissue. There are often satellite spots from the original site. The tumor metastasizes quickly.

Incidence: Lymphangiosarcoma is rare; the occurrence in patients who had a radical mastectomy for breast cancer is less than 1 percent.

Symptoms: Symptoms of lymphangiosarcoma are purple or bruised areas on the skin of the arms or legs.

Screening and diagnosis: The appearance of purplish, bruised-looking areas on the extremities of an individual with long-standing lymphedema is an indication for further evaluation. A biopsy is taken from the site; diagnosis is made by histologic examination and rules out metastatic disease from a primary tumor or another sarcoma (such as Kaposi sarcoma).

Treatment and therapy: There is not an effective treatment or therapy for lymphangiosarcoma. The lymphangiosarcoma site is removed surgically, and amputation of the affected limb may be necessary. Chemotherapy may also be given after surgical treatment.

Prognosis, prevention, and outcomes: The rate of recurrence is high, and the long-term survival rate is poor, in large part because of the rapid spread of the tumor to the chest wall, the liver, and to bone.

Vicki Miskovsky, B.S., R.D.

See also Angiosarcomas; Breast cancers; Fibrosarcomas, soft-tissue; Lymphadenectomy; Lymphedema; Mastectomy.

▶ Lymphedema

Category: Diseases, symptoms, and conditions
Also known as: Lymphatic obstruction

Related conditions: Cancer, malformations of the lymph system

Definition: Lymphedema is a blockage in the lymphatic system that results in swelling, or edema. The lymph system is a network of channels that move lymph, a clear fluid, around cells and through nodes that filter harmful substances such as bacteria.

Risk factors: Surgery and radiation are most often associated with lymphedema. If the patient receives radiation to the underarm or has lymph nodes removed during surgery or as part of a sentinel lymph node biopsy, the lymph channel may be damaged. Lymph node removal for biopsy related to cancer spread is common and may also be done in the chest, groin, pelvic, and neck areas. Tumor growth may also cause lymphedema by compression.

Etiology and the disease process: There are two kinds of lymphedema, primary and secondary. Primary lymphedema is a rare condition inherited at birth, and secondary lymphedema is caused by blockages from infection, surgery, radiation therapy scar tissue, pressure on lymph nodes from a growing tumor, or removal of lymph nodes during surgery. Primary lymphedema is due to a malformation in the lymph system present at birth. Secondary lymphedema is a mechanical interruption in the normal flow of lymph.

When an interruption in the lymph system occurs, the ability to transport fluid is impaired, leading to swelling as the fluid collects in the tissues below the area of blockage. For example, if lymph nodes under the arm or in the groin are removed, the arm or leg may swell. The fluid that collects is interstitial fluid, which causes inflammation. As the fluid collects, the swelling progresses, and the patients note an increase in the size of their arms, legs, or abdomen depending on the site of the blockage. Because the disease is progressive, the swelling continues and may lead to fatigue, the inability to fit clothing over the affected area, and the inability to carry on the activities of daily living. As the disease progresses, the skin in the affected area may become thickened and begin to resemble an orange peel, known as peau d'orange. The skin may break down easily, leading to oozing of fluid through the skin and ultimately infection.

Incidence: Incidence rates for secondary lymphedema vary significantly by site. Some 10 to 40 percent of breast cancer patients with lymph node removal under the arm develop lymphedema. In women with major gynecologic surgery for ovarian and other cancers, the incidence rate ranges from 15 to 44 percent. A limited number of studies of head and neck cancer patients report that up to 5 percent experience lymphedema.

Symptoms: Swelling is the most common and obvious symptom of lymphedema. The patient may also report a feeling of heaviness in the affected body part. Pain and weakness in the limb may be obvious to the patient. Sensations may decrease, including an inability to feel heat or cold. As the disease progresses, the skin becomes hard and loses its elasticity, and the limb may become two to three times its normal size. Lymphedema in the abdominal area may result in bowel and bladder problems. If untreated, fluid oozing from the skin may be noticed, and the skin may seem to disintegrate, leading to open sores.

Screening and diagnosis: Patients at risk for lymphedema should be screened at each doctor's visit and educated to the signs and symptoms of lympedema. Diagnosis of lymphedema is generally made after patients complain of symptoms, such as swelling and fullness. Physical examination, a medical history including medicines taken, and changes since the previous examination are important in diagnosis. There are no specific tests for diagnosing lymphedema. There is no staging of lymphedema, but measurement and recording of the circumference of the affected area are important to monitor progression of the disease.

Treatment and therapy: Treatment of lymphedema is primarily mechanical: elevation of the affected area, manual lymphatic drainage using gentle massage to move fluid toward the center of the body (decongestive therapy), wearing of custom-fitted compression garments on the affected limb, and practicing good skin care and injury protection. Antibiotics may be necessary to prevent or treat infections, but other drugs are not generally effective. Patients are often encouraged to watch their weight, exercise appropriately, and eat protein-rich foods. Bowel and bladder complications such as constipation and urine retention may require treatment. Surgery for lymphedema is not recommended. Because the disease is progressive and treatment is based on symptoms, management and control are the therapies of choice. Patient education is critical to treatment and must be an important part of the therapy for lymphedema.

Prognosis, prevention, and outcomes: There are no clinical studies that support actions to prevent lymphedema. There is no cure for lymphedema so the prognosis depends on the patient's compliance with treatment measures. The use of sentinel lymph node biopsy rather than aggressive lymph node removal may be contributing to a decreasing incidence of the disease. The key to an optimal outcome is early recognition and treatment of the symptoms and compliance with ongoing treatment.

Patricia Stanfill Edens, R.N., Ph.D., FACHE

▶ For Further Information

Fu, M. R. "Breast Cancer Survivors' Intentions of Managing Lymphedema." *Cancer Nursing* 28, no. 6 (2005): 446-457.

Golshan, M., and B. Smith. "Prevention and Management of Arm Lymphedema in the Patient with Breast Cancer." *Journal of Supportive Oncology* 4, no. 8 (2006): 381-386.

▶ Other Resources

American Cancer Society
http://www.cancer.org

National Cancer Institute
Lymphedema
http://www.nci.nih.gov/cancertopics/pdq/supportivecare/lymphedema/patient

National Lymphedema Network
http://www.lymphnet.org

See also Axillary dissection; Edema; Endotheliomas; Lumpectomy; Lymphadenectomy; Lymphangiosarcomas; Mastectomy; Radiation therapies; Side effects.

▶ Lymphocytosis

Category: Diseases, symptoms, and conditions
Also known as: Raised lymphocyte count

Related conditions: Lymph symptoms, absolute lymphocytosis, hematological malignancy, lymphoma, leukemia, lymphoproliferative disorders

Definition: Lymphocytosis is an abnormal excess of lymphocytes in the blood. Lymphocytes are a type of white blood cell that help fight infections. A healthy adult has an absolute lymphocyte count (ALC) of 1,300 to 4,000 per microliter of blood. ALC over 4,000 indicates lymphocytosis; however, this number may be higher in children up to six years of age, as their ALC is significantly higher than in adults.

Risk factors: There are more than thirty medical condition that may underlie lymphocytosis. The most common causes include viral and bacterial infections, such as mononucleosis (glandular fever), influenza, pertussis (whooping cough), or tuberculosis. Malignant blood diseases, such as chronic lymphocytic leukemia, follicular lymphoma, hairy cell leukemia, and leukopenia, may also cause lymphocytosis.

Etiology and the disease process: Lymphocytosis indicates an underlying problem, but it is not a disease in itself. The lymph nodes are the most commonly affected organs. Transient stress lymphocytosis may also occur after trauma or extensive psychological or physical stress, and it typically resolves within two days of diagnosis. Transient stress lymphocytosis may be in part mediated by modulation of catecholamine and steroid hormones and cell adhesion molecules.

Incidence: Lymphocytosis is common and occurs in most people throughout life, usually in association with viral infections.

Symptoms: Symptoms of lymphocytosis may include sore throat, fever, and fatigue. However, lymphocytosis typically causes no symptoms and is often discovered incidentally via a routine blood test.

Screening and diagnosis: A complete blood count will identify lymphocytosis. Further investigation is done by assessing the major lymphocyte subsets, such as T cells, B cells, and natural killer cells. The subgroups of T cells are CD4 T cells (helper cells) and CD8 T cells (cytotoxic cells). In a healthy person, approximately 75 percent of lymphocytes are T cells, with a 2:1 ratio of CD4 to CD8, and about equal proportions of the remainder cells are B cells and natural killer cells. A marked increase in lymphocytes may indicate a serious condition, such as the presence of chronic lymphocytic leukemia. Many types of blood cancer are often identified after diagnosing lymphocytosis.

Treatment and therapy: For the best therapy, it is necessary to address the underlying issue that caused lymphocytosis. If a malignant blood disease is detected, cancer treatment may be needed.

Prognosis, prevention, and outcomes: Depending on the cause of lymphocytosis, it may spontaneously resolve or may need medical interaction to relieve its symtoms.

Anita Nagypál, Ph.D.

See also Acute lymphocytic leukemia (ALL); Ataxia tel angiectasia (AT); Biological therapy; Blood cancers; Childhood cancers; Chronic lymphocytic leukemia (CLL); Complete blood count (CBC); Cutaneous T-cell lymphoma (CTCL); Edema; Hairy cell leukemia; Hodgkin disease; Immune response to cancer; Leukemias; Leukopenia; Non-Hodgkin lymphoma; Richter syndrome; Sézary syndrome; Thymomas; Thymus cancer.

▶ Lymphomas

Category: Diseases, symptoms, and conditions
Also known as: Hodgkin disease, non-Hodgkin lymphoma, Burkitt lymphoma

Related conditions: Cancer of the lymph nodes, cancer of the spleen, leukemia, acquired immunodeficiency syndrome (AIDS)

Definition: Lymphatic cancer is a blood cancer that involves the lymphocytes (white blood cells). Cancerous cells grow and multiply, mostly in the lymph nodes and spleen, where they cause swelling and a suppression of the body's natural immune system. Lymphoma occurs in two forms, Hodgkin disease and non-Hodgkin lymphoma. The presence of abnormal cells known as Reed-Sternberg cells after the scientists who discovered them indicates Hodgkin disease and differentiates this lymphoma from all other types, including Burkitt lymphoma, which are designated non-Hodgkin lymphoma.

Risk factors: As the causes of both Hodgkin disease and non-Hodgkin lymphoma are unknown, the risk factors cannot be definitively determined. However, in non-Hodgkin lymphoma, it is thought that the suppression of the immune system, particularly in high-risk patients such as those who have undergone organic transplantation and are on antirejection medications, is a significant risk factor. A spike in the incidence of non-Hodgkin lymphoma has been detected among people who have had the human immunodeficiency virus (HIV) for four or more years, largely because their immune systems have been compromised.

A link has been detected between the development of lymphoma and exposure to flour in some agricultural jobs. Also, in more advanced cases of the disease, a link has been found to exposure to X rays and to certain forms of chemotherapy.

Heredity appears to have little effect in the development of lymphomas, although physicians who diagnose the disease do record genetic details in their diagnoses.

Etiology and the disease process: The causes of lymphoma are not fully understood. The fact that lymphoma is not a single disease with clear-cut boundaries has made it difficult to understand and assess. Some lymphomas are relatively easy to treat and have good survival rates, whereas other forms of the disease grow very rapidly and aggressively so that successful treatment is more problematic. In the United States, lymphoma has been found most often among the well educated and those in more affluent socioeconomic situations.

The lymphatic system contains two types of cells, the B cells and the T cells. The former manufacture antibodies designed to fight infections. The T cells, on the other hand, regulate the immune system. More than 90 percent of lymphomas in the United States originate in the B cells. Lymphatic cancer cells can be present in the stomach and the intestines, the bones, the skin, the sinuses, and in the lymph nodes.

More than thirty types of non-Hodgkin lymphomas have been identified microscopically, each unique in its morphology. As a result, treatment is most effective if it is directed toward a specific variety of the disease.

Incidence: In 2007, 71,380 were estimated to be diagnosed with lymphoma, and 19,730 were estimated to die of it. The age-adjusted incidence rate was 22 per 100,000 people per year. Both Hodgkin disease and non-Hodgkin lymphoma are found more often in men than in women. Non-Hodgkin lymphoma affects more people in their twenties and in the fifty-five to seventy age group. One variety of non-Hodgkin lymphoma, Burkitt lymphoma, is found largely in the Tropics and in Africa. It is thought to be related in some way to the Epstein-Barr virus. Non-

Hodgkin lymphoma is the fifth most frequently occurring cancer in the United States. It is also the third fastest-growing cancer worldwide, with the highest incidence of the disease found in North America, western Europe, and Australia.

Symptoms: The most frequent symptom is a swelling in the lymph nodes in the neck, under the arms, or in the groin, usually referred to as swollen glands. In some cases, particularly in young children, the thymus gland in the upper chest may also be swollen.

The swelling is clearly visible in most cases and usually is not painful. It is sometimes accompanied by other symptoms—loss of appetite, fever, weight loss, and night sweats—that are frequently mistaken for influenza. These symptoms may disappear after a short time, only to reappear.

People suffering from lymphoma often have an overall feeling of illness characterized by lethargy, headaches, and ulceration of the skin accompanied by itching. If the disease has spread to the abdominal area, it may be accompanied by pain and bleeding as well as by swelling. In such cases, the patient may vomit blood or have blackened stools indicating internal bleeding.

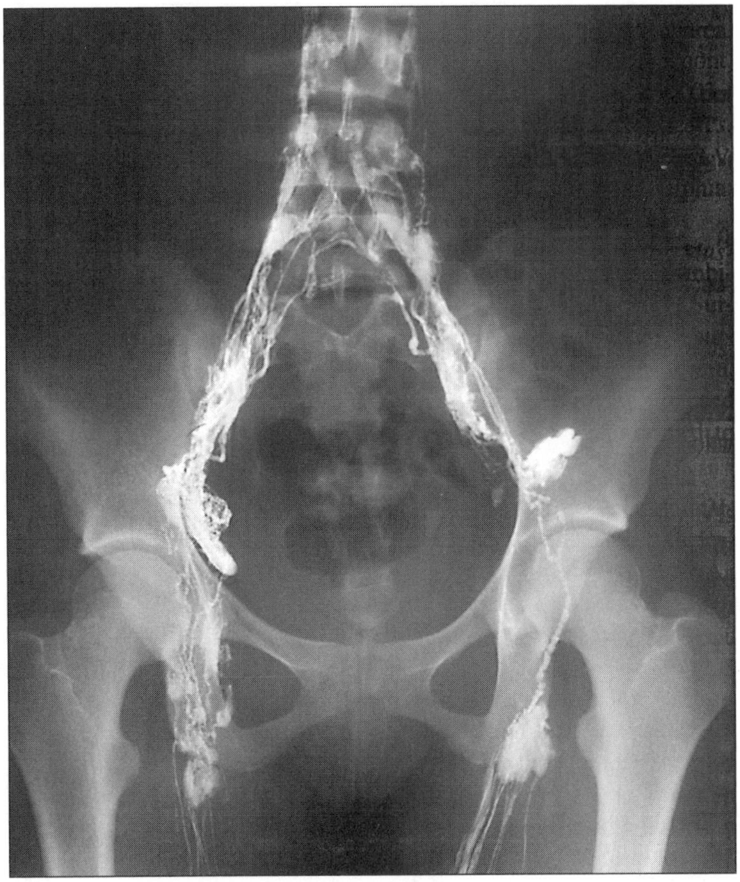

A lymphangiogram reveals lymphoma in a child's pelvic lymph glands. (Zephyr/Photo Researchers, Inc.)

Because non-Hodgkin lymphoma usually grows slowly, it may be asymptomatic or may produce only minor symptoms that can easily be ignored in the early stages of the disease. Therefore, this type of lymphoma is frequently diagnosed at Stage III or IV rather than in the earliest stages when the cure rate is greatest. Hodgkin disease, on the other hand, grows and spreads rapidly. Its early symptoms may cause its victims to seek medical intervention in the earlier stages of the disease.

Screening and diagnosis: The usual method for diagnosing lymphoma involves the removal and microscopic examination of tissue from the lymph nodes for biopsy. If cancer cells are found, further diagnosis may be indicated and usually will involve X rays of the chest or lymph glands, removal of bone marrow to be biopsied, ultrasound, and scanning by computed tomography (CT), magnetic resonance imaging (MRI), or positron emission tomography (PET).

The Ann Arbor staging system is used for Hodgkin disease and non-Hodgkin lymphoma:

- Stage I: Cancer cells have been found in only one section of the lymph nodes or in just one confined area outside the lymph nodes.
- Stage II: Cancer has been detected in two or more lymph nodes on the same side of the diaphragm.
- Stage III: Cancer cells have been found on both sides of the diaphragm and may have spread to surrounding areas, notably the spleen, the lungs, the liver, or the bone marrow.
- Stage IV: Cancer cells are found in more than one spot within the lymphatic system or in organs located at a significant distance from the lymphatic area.

Treatment and therapy: A biopsy not only determines whether cancer cells are present but also can more specifically identify the kinds of cancer cells that are present. It is important to customize treatment for each individual patient to the greatest degree possible; therefore, identification of the precise kinds of cancerous cells is vital.

For patients with Stage I and Stage II lymphomas, the first avenue of treatment is radiation therapy. If there are

Age at Death for Lymphoma, 2001-2005

Age Group	*Deaths (%)*
Under 20	0.6
20-34	2.4
35-44	3.4
45-54	7.6
55-64	13.9
65-75	22.9
76-84	32.8
85 and older	16.5

Source: Data from National Cancer Institute, Surveillance Epidemiology and End Results, Cancer Stat Fact Sheets, 2008

Note: The median age at death from 2001 to 2005 was seventy-four, with an age-adjusted death rate of 7.8 per 100,000 men and women per year.

signs that the malignancy has spread, radiation may be supplemented by chemotherapy. If the disease has advanced considerably or is likely to, the treatment of choice may be a bone marrow transplant.

When a bone marrow transplant—considered a treatment of last resort—is used, it is also combined with continued radiation therapy and chemotherapy. The patient undergoing such treatment usually has a badly compromised immune system so that the postoperative treatment involves isolation under sterile conditions for an extended period to prevent infection from some of the opportunistic diseases that are found in hospitals.

An alternative treatment is the mini bone marrow transplant. This method involves the use of low-level, minimally toxic chemotherapy or radiation therapy to kill some of the patient's bone marrow, leaving some cancer cells. Cancer-free bone marrow from a donor is then introduced into the patient's bone marrow. In time, this cancer-free bone marrow produces cancer-free cells that attack and destroy the remaining cancerous cells. Stem cell research also appears to have considerable promise in the treatment of lymphoma.

Prognosis, prevention, and outcomes: There is no clear-cut way to prevent lymphoma, although avoiding some occupational and environmental hazards may decrease the likelihood that it will develop. Links have been made between increases in the spread of the disease and such environmental hazards as hydrocarbons and noxious fumes. Avoiding polluted air and water is certainly essential.

Also, diet has profound effects in combating many forms of cancer, including lymphoma. A diet low in fats, limited in animal protein, and containing few refined carbohydrates will strength the immune system and lead to a sense of overall well-being. People should routinely eat at least five servings of fruits and vegetables every day.

The outlook for those suffering from lymphoma depends largely on the stage at which the cancer was detected. Many Stage I patients are cured of the disease. The five-year survival rate among Stage I and Stage II patients approaches 80 percent. Among Stage IV patients, the two-year survival rate is about 50 percent. Each year the statistics are more encouraging as new medications and techniques are developed and employed in treating the disease.

Certainly the key to survival is early diagnosis. Any symptoms should receive the attention of a qualified physician. Particularly dangerous are phantom symptoms, those that disappear after a short time but then return. The interval between their first appearance and their return is crucial because this is the period in which the disease is most susceptible to treatment designed to eliminate it.

R. Baird Shuman, Ph.D.

▶ For Further Information

Adler, Elizabeth M. *Living with Lymphoma: A Patient's Guide*. Baltimore: Johns Hopkins University Press, 2005.

Freedman, Jeri. *Lymphoma: Current and Emerging Trends in Detection and Treatment*. New York: Rosen, 2006.

Holman, Peter, Jodi Garrett, and William Jansen. *One Hundred Questions and Answers About Lymphoma*. Sudbury, Mass.: Jones and Bartlett, 2004.

Litin, Scott C., Jr., ed. *Mayo Clinic Family Health Book*. 3d ed. New York: HarperCollins, 2003.

National Institutes of Health. *What You Need to Know About Hodgkin's Disease*. Bethesda, Md.: National Institutes of Health, 1999.

_______. *What You Need to Know About Non-Hodgkin's Lymphoma*. Bethesda, Md.: National Institutes of Health, 1999.

Park, Alice. "The Cancer Test: Exposing a Growing Tumor's Secrets May Be as Simple as Drawing Blood." *Time*, June 25, 2007, 53.

Teetley, Peter, and Philip Bashe. *Cancer Survival Guide*. Rev. ed. New York: Broadway Books, 2005.

▶ Other Resources

American Cancer Society
http://www.cancer.org

The Leukemia and Lymphoma Society
http://www.leukemia-lymphoma.org

Lymphoma Information Network
http://www.lymphomainfo.net/lymphoma/whatis.html

Lymphoma Research Organization
http://www.lymphoma.org

MedlinePlus
Lymphoma
http://www.nlm.nih.gov/medlineplus/lymphoma.html

See also Burkitt lymphoma; Castleman disease; Cutaneous T-cell lymphoma (CTCL); Epstein-Barr virus; Hemolytic anemia; Hepatitis C virus (HCV); HIV/AIDS-related cancers; Hodgkin disease; Human T-cell leukemia virus (HTLV); Immune response to cancer; Immunocytochemistry and immunohistochemistry; Immunotherapy; Klinefelter syndrome and cancer; Lambert-Eaton myasthenic syndrome (LEMS); Leukapharesis; Lymphangiography; Lymphocytosis; Malignant fibrous histiocytoma (MFH); Mantle cell lymphoma (MCL); Mucosa-associated lymphoid tissue (MALT) lymphomas; Mycosis fungoides; Myeloma; Nijmegen breakage syndrome; Non-Hodgkin lymphoma; Organ transplantation and cancer; Primary central nervous system lymphomas; Richter syndrome; Sézary syndrome; Simian virus 40; Sjögren syndrome; Thymomas; Thymus cancer; Virus-related cancers; Waldenström macroglobulinemia (WM); Young adult cancers.

▶ M. D. Anderson Cancer Center

Category: Organizations

Definition: M. D. Anderson Cancer Center is an academic and patient care facility that is in the Texas Medical Center in Houston and part of the University of Texas system of academic institutions. The center's mission statement is "to eliminate cancer in Texas, the nation, and the world through outstanding programs that integrate patient care, research and prevention, and through education for undergraduate and graduate students, trainees, professionals, employees and the public." M. D. Anderson Cancer Center is one of thirty-nine comprehensive cancer centers in the United States as designated by the National Cancer Institute, National Institutes of Health. It is also one of twenty-one member institutions that make up the National Comprehensive Cancer Network, a nonprofit consortium of patient care facilities dedicated to improving the quality of cancer care.

History: Munroe Dunaway Anderson, a wealthy banker and cotton merchant, created a sizable charitable foundation several years before his death that would eventually fund the cancer hospital bearing his name along with other institutions within the Texas Medical Center. In 1941, the Texas state legislature appropriated $500,000 for the creation of a center for cancer research and treatment within the University of Texas system. Originally funded as the Texas State Cancer Hospital and the Division of Cancer Research, the institution was renamed the following year after the trustees of the M. D. Anderson Foundation proposed matching the state's grant to launch the center on the condition that the institute would be located in Houston. Biomedical research at the new institution commenced in 1943, and patient care services began the following year. By the mid-2000's, M. D. Anderson employed more than

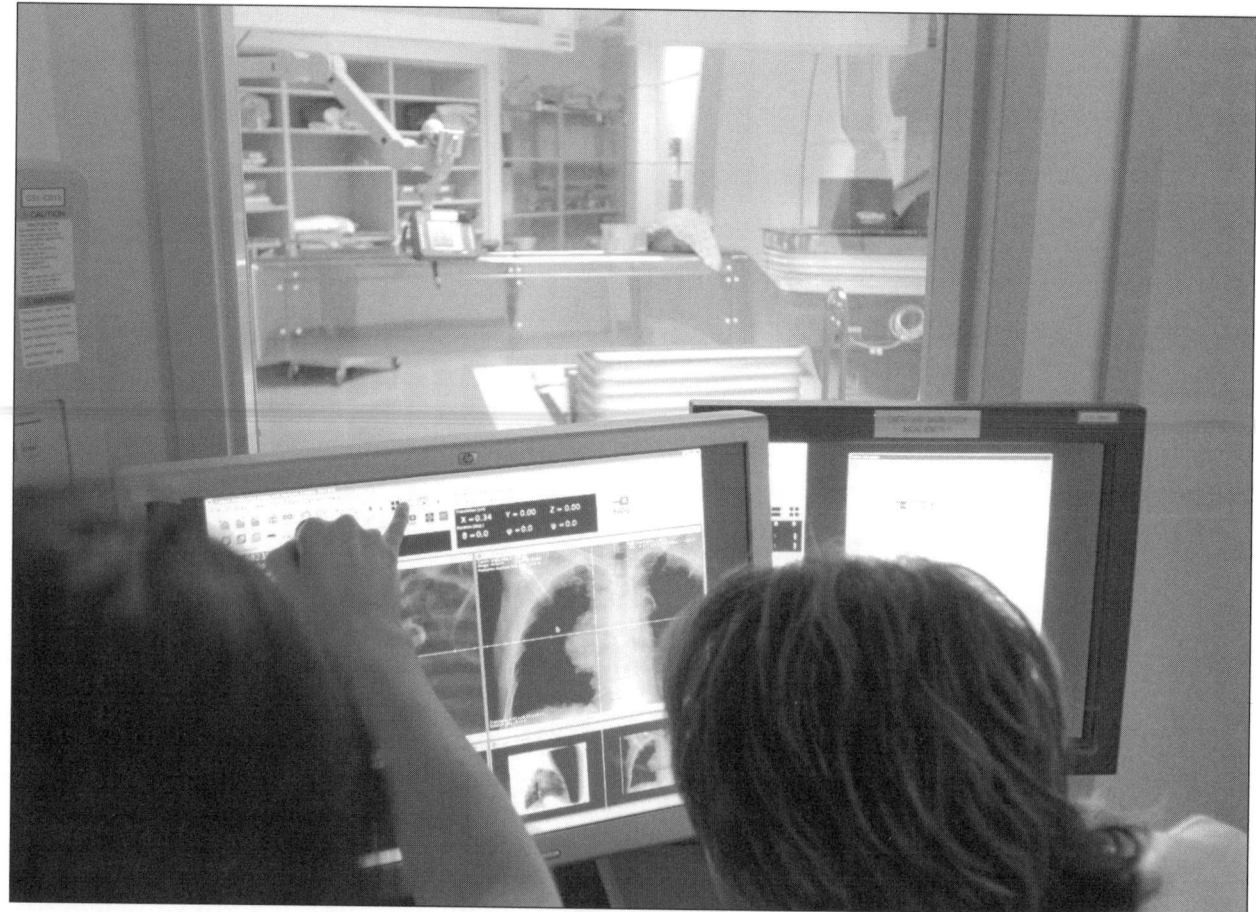

At the M. D. Anderson Proton Therapy Center, a radiation therapist and oncologist use X rays to determine the position of a patient's tumor in the left lung before using a proton beam to attack the tumor. (AP/Wide World Photos)

15,000 faculty and staff, and its annual operating budget exceeded $2 billion.

Patient care: M. D. Anderson Cancer Center's patient care resources include 512 inpatient beds, an emergency center, and numerous outpatient clinics organized primarily by specialty. M. D. Anderson provides patient care to more than 74,000 people each year, with about one-third of patients coming from outside the state of Texas. In addition to its services for patients with known cancers, the facility also operates a cancer prevention clinic that offers diagnostic evaluation, risk assessment, genetic testing, and counseling in risk reduction and preventive medicine. Most patient care activities are conducted on the main campus within the Texas Medical Center, although M. D. Anderson also coordinates care in several satellite clinics in the Houston metropolitan area.

M. D. Anderson patients have access to several types of support services to accompany their treatment, including patient education classes, a resource library, psychosocial and pastoral care services, and complementary therapies such as nutritional counseling and massage. For patients who have completed treatment, M. D. Anderson operates a rehabilitation program and a medical clinic for long-term follow-up. A number of nonhealth-related patient services are provided for patient comfort and convenience, such as an onsite hotel, a travel agency, and activities for patients and family members.

Research: In 2005, M. D. Anderson Cancer Center spent approximately $342 million on medical research. The center has been consistently among the top recipients of research grants from the National Cancer Institute. Of note, the institution houses ten National Cancer Institute Specialized Programs of Research Excellence focusing on leukemia, melanoma, and cancers of the bladder, breast, endometrium, head and neck, lung, ovary, pancreas, and prostate.

Research at the center is organized within several divisions that in turn are subdivided into more focal research areas. For example, the Division of Basic Research houses scientific programs in areas such as cancer genetics, biomedical engineering, and immunology. Other divisions are organized according to clinical specialty, such as medicine, surgery, imaging, and prevention science. Research efforts are closely integrated with patient care services. Accordingly, M. D. Anderson houses the largest clinical trial program of any cancer center in the United States. In 2005, more than 12,000 of the center's patients participated in basic, clinical, and population-based research studies.

Education: Through supervised rotations, residencies, and fellowships, M. D. Anderson offers clinical training to medical students, physicians, nurses, pharmacists, and other health professionals. More recently, the center began offering undergraduate degrees and certificates in several allied health professions through its own School of Health Sciences. Baccalaureate degrees and certificates are granted in clinical laboratory science, cytogenetic technology, cytotechnology, diagnostic imaging, histotechnology, medical dosimetry, molecular genetic technology, and radiation therapy.

M. D. Anderson offers formal research training aimed primarily at graduate and postdoctoral students. The center contributes to graduate-level research training programs in health sciences as a partner within the multiinstitutional University of Texas Graduate School of Biomedical Sciences. The graduate school awards master's and doctoral degrees in a variety of disciplines, including basic sciences such as cell biology and genetics as well as applied sciences such as medical physics and pathology.

Andrea Bradford, M.A.

▶ For Further Information

Elliott, Frederick C. *The Birth of the Texas Medical Center: A Personal Account*. College Station: Texas A&M University Press, 2004.

M. D. Anderson Hospital and Tumor Institute. *The First Twenty Years of the University of Texas, M. D. Anderson Hospital and Tumor Institute*. Houston: Author, 1964.

Slaga, Thomas J. "Fifty Years of the University of Texas M. D. Anderson Cancer Center and the Study of Carcinogenesis." *Molecular Carcinogenesis* 4, no. 6 (1991): 417-418.

▶ Other Resources

M. D. Anderson Cancer Center
http://www.mdanderson.org

National Cancer Institute
Cancer Centers Program
http://cancercenters.cancer.gov/index.html

National Comprehensive Cancer Network
M. D. Anderson Cancer Center
http://www.nccn.org/members/profiles/mda.asp

Texas Medical Center
http://www.texmedctr.tmc.edu/root/en

See also American Association for Cancer Research (AACR); American Cancer Society (ACS); American Institute for Cancer Research (AICR); Dana-Farber Cancer Institute; Duke Comprehensive Cancer Center; Fox Chase Cancer Center; Fred Hutchinson Cancer Research Center; Jonsson Comprehensive Cancer Center (JCCC); Mayo Clinic Cancer Center; Memorial Sloan-Kettering Cancer Center; National Cancer Institute (NCI); National Science Foundation (NSF); Prevent Cancer Foundation; Robert H. Lurie Cancer Center.

▶ Macrobiotic diet

Category: Lifestyle and prevention

Definition: Macrobiotics is a lifestyle and philosophy that includes an approach to nutrition based on whole grains, beans, vegetables, and the Chinese principle of yin and yang. A macrobiotic diet usually consists of organic and locally grown foods, seasonal vegetables, complex carbohydrates, and fewer fats, sugars, and chemically processed foods than in a typical Western diet. The philosophy also promotes physical activity, avoidance of pesticides and other chemicals, and stress reduction.

History: The word "macrobiotic" comes from the Greek words for "great life" and was first used by Hippocrates, the father of medicine. In the eighteeth century, German physician Christoph Hufeland to used this term describe a program for good health. The modern macrobiotic diet was developed in the twentieth century by George Ohsawa and has evolved under Michio Kushi. It was further popularized in the 1980's when a number of books were published—including books by several medical professionals—who credited the diet for their recovery from cancer and other illnesses.

The diet: On a typical day, the standard macrobiotic diet includes complex carbohydrates from brown rice, millet, barley, whole wheat, oats, and other whole grains (40 to 60 percent of calories), vegetables (20 to 30 percent of calories), beans and bean products (such as tofu), sea vegetables, pickles, vegetable oil, and seasonings. Fruit, fish or seafood, and sweets are eaten occasionally (once a week), and red meat, eggs, poultry, and dairy are consumed on a limited basis (once a month or less). The diet is modifiable based on a person's age, sex, activity level, personal needs, and environment.

Benefits: Few studies have been done on the macrobiotic diet for cancer prevention, and most of the research to date has been inconclusive. The diet may affect hormone metabolism; for example, women consuming a macrobiotic diet have much higher levels of phytoestrogens (plant hormones) in their urine than women consuming an omnivorous diet. This may result in a lower risk for hormonally influenced cancers (such as breast cancer). In addition, the macrobiotic diet is consistent with general cancer prevention guidelines of reducing fat intake, animal products, and processed foods while increasing intake of whole grains, vegetables, and fruits.

Risks: In the late 1980's, there were reports that children and adolescents eating a macrobiotic diet showed below-average growth and some nutrient deficiencies (vitamins B_{12} and D). Most nutritionists recommend that people on macrobiotic and vegan diets make sure to get enough vitamins B_{12} and D from fortified foods or supplements.

Lisa M. Lines, M.P.H.

See also Antioxidants; Carotenoids; Complementary and alternative therapies; Dietary supplements; Green tea; Herbs as antioxidants; Integrative oncology; Sun's soup.

▶ Magnetic resonance imaging (MRI)

Category: Procedures

Definition: Magnetic resonance imaging (MRI) is a noninvasive and pain-free diagnostic imaging test performed using powerful magnets and radio waves rather than ionizing radiation. The magnets cause the protons in the hydrogen ions found in the body's water to arrange themselves in a certain way in relation to the magnetic field. Once the protons are aligned, the radio waves are bounced off the tissues. This is the "resonance" part of the test. The signals that return to the scanner are analyzed by computer. An MRI takes slicelike images of the body, but it is able to acquire these images in several planes, so that it provides three-dimensional images. MRI can provide high image resolution and significant detail. Consequently, it provides more information than computed tomography (CT).

Most MRI machines consist of a large cylinder, called a bore, with a thick casing around it. The magnets surround the patient when he or she is being scanned. Open MRI units have been developed, but they are not available everywhere. In open MRI machines, the magnets do not surround the patient, as there are gaps in the magnets. This change does affect the quality of the images created to some degree, but it also permits the scanning of very obese patients and those with claustrophobia (fear of closed spaces).

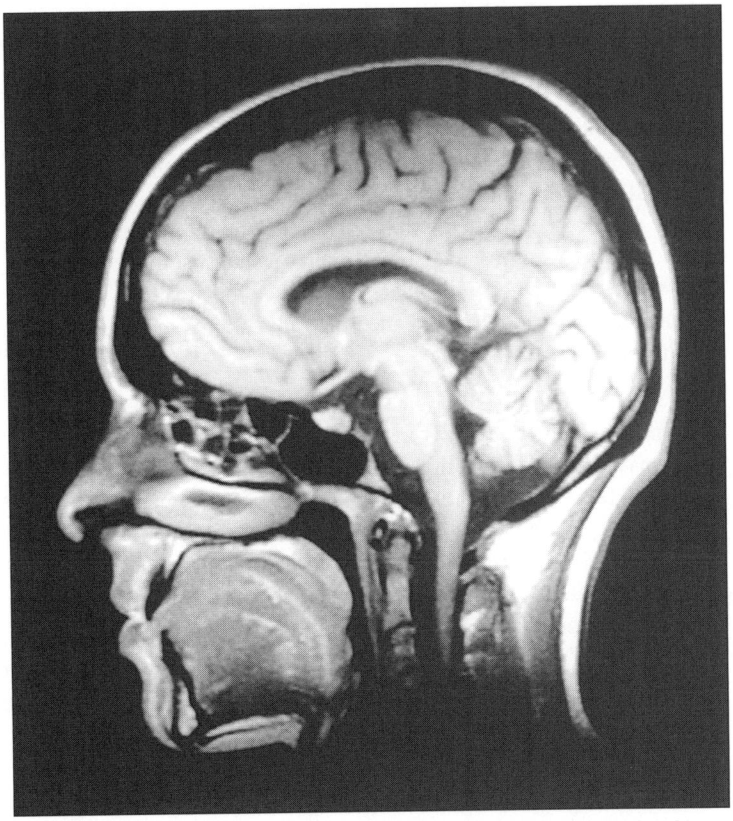
An MRI allows doctors to see soft tissues in the brain. (Digital Stock)

In order to receive a clear image, several types of magnets are used in an MRI machine: resistive magnets, permanent magnets, superconducting magnets, and gradient magnets. Resistive and superconducting magnets consist of coils of wire around a cylinder. They become magnetic only when electrical current is passed through them. Superconducting magnets are bathed in liquid helium, which is extremely cold at a temperature of –452.4 degrees Fahrenheit. This greatly decreases the resistance of the wire coil. As a result, superconducting magnets require a great deal less electrical current to magnetize. A permanent magnet is always a magnet and requires no electrical current to flow through it. The gradient magnets are very low-strength magnets and are used to localize the magnetic field to the portion of the body being examined.

There are several drawbacks to MRI. A large percentage of patients are excluded from MRI testing because the test cannot be performed if the patient has any metal in or on the body or if he or she is on any machinery for monitoring or life support. Patients with pacemakers, cochlear implants, clips in the brain, artificial heart valves, older vascular stents, intrauterine devices, metal plates or screws, surgical staples, implanted drug infusion ports, and recently replaced artificial joints should not have MRIs. Patients who are on a ventilator, a cardiac monitor, or an infusion pump or in traction should not have an MRI.

Another drawback is that the patient must lie perfectly still during the exam in order for the imaging to be clear. An MRI can be difficult for a patient with claustrophobia because the scan is performed with the part to be examined in the center of the tube. Another drawback is that extremely obese patients cannot be scanned by the closed scanner if they are too large for the bore. In addition, MRIs usually are not performed on pregnant patients because there has not been enough research done to ensure the safety of the fetus.

Cancers diagnosed: An MRI can diagnose most kinds of cancer. It can be used to assess the blood vessels, lungs, liver, heart, stomach, large and small intestines, biliary tract, kidneys, brain and nerves, spleen, pancreas, male testes and prostate, female uterus and ovaries, and the pelvic, knee, and hip bones. To identify structures in the abdomen, it is helpful to use oral contrast, such as liquid barium, and/or intravenous dyes, such as gadolinium. MRI is particularly effective at evaluating tumors in the central nervous system, spine, joints, extremities, breasts, and liver.

Why performed: An MRI is performed to evaluate abnormalities in body tissue. These abnormalities include tumors, congenital abnormalities, vascular abnormalities, tissue inflammation, infection, bleeding, and edema.

Patient preparation: Before an MRI, a patient must remove all metal from the body, such as jewelry, watches, belt buckles, hearing aids, removable dental work, and hairpins. The clothing must have no metal on it, such as zippers or metal decorations. The patient is also asked to empty the pockets prior to the MRI. Since the MRI uses a strong magnet, any metal objects could become projectiles once the MRI is turned on, potentially causing injury to the patient. The patient may be asked to wear hospital pajamas if there is metal on the clothing. The patient is asked to remove any makeup before the MRI because the iron in some makeup can be affected by the MRI. Also, medication patches should be removed prior to an MRI because the procedure can cause a burn on the site of the patch.

The patient is often given earplugs because the MRI

scanner makes loud noises. It is essential that the patient lie still while in the scanner, so he or she may be given a sedative prior to the test. This is more likely if the patient has claustrophobia or is confused. Positioning devices are used to keep the body part to be scanned in a stationery position. If the patient is to receive contrast dye, then an intravenous line will be inserted into the arm. The patient may be given a liquid contrast to drink before the test. For some parts of the body, small coils are positioned by the area to be scanned. These devices enhance the radio waves and thus improve the MRI images.

Steps of the procedure: For an MRI, the patient lies on a table in the center of the MRI machine. Foam blocks and straps may be used to position the patient. If intravenous contrast is to be used, then it will be injected at this time.

Once the patient is positioned, the table slides into the bore of the MRI. The MRI scanner is turned on and the scan is performed. The scan usually includes several runs and can take from fifteen to forty-five minutes depending on what part of the body is being scanned and the reason for the scan. There is a microphone in the room with the MRI machine so that the patient can communicate with the technician. The patient may be given prism glasses to wear so that he or she can see the MRI technician.

After the procedure: After the procedure, there is no special follow-up care required unless the patient has received a sedative prior to the MRI. In this case, the patient will need to be driven home.

Risks: There are few risks associated with an MRI, unless the person has metal on or in the body or there are metal objects in the room where the test is performed. There is a small risk that a patient might be allergic to the radioactive dye, if it is used.

Results: The MRI yields multidimensional computer images of the tissue being examined. A radiologist who reviews these images is able to differentiate between cancer, edema, infection, bleeding, and inflammation. The patency of blood vessels can also be exhibited. MRI is particularly effective for examining the central nervous system.

Christine M. Carroll, R.N., B.S.N., M.B.A.

▶ For Further Information

Westbrook, Catherine. *MRI in Practice*. 3d ed. Malden, Mass.: Blackwell, 2005.

Huettel, Scott, et al. *Functional Magnetic Resonance Imaging*. Sunderland, Mass.: Sinauer Associates, 2004.

Pagana, Kathleen Deska, and Timothy J. Pagana. *Mosby's Manual of Diagnostic and Laboratory Tests*. 3d ed. St. Louis: Mosby Elsevier, 2006.

▶ Other Resources

How Stuff Works
How MRI Works
http://health.howstuffworks.com/mri.htm

Neurosciences on the Internet
Use of Functional Magnetic Resonance Imaging to Investigate Brain Function
http://www.neuroguide.com/gregg.html

Radiology Info
MRI of the Body
Http://www.radiologyinfo.org/en/info.cfm?pg=bodymr&bhcp=1

WebMD
Magnetic Resonance Imaging (MRI)
http://www.webmd.com/a-to-z-guides/magnetic-resonance-imaging-mri

See also Angiography; Bone scan; Brain scan; Bronchography; Computed tomography (CT)-guided biopsy; Computed tomography (CT) scan; Cystography; Ductogram; Endoscopic retrograde cholangiopancreatography (ERCP); Gallium scan; Hysterography; Imaging tests; Lymphangiography; Mammography; Nuclear medicine scan; Percutaneous transhepatic cholangiography (PTHC); Positron emission tomography (PET); Radionuclide scan; Thermal imaging; Thyroid nuclear medicine scan; Urography; X-ray tests.

▶ Malignant fibrous histiocytoma (MFH)

Category: Diseases, symptoms, and conditions
Also known as: MFH, sarcoma, histiocytoma

Related conditions: Lymphoma, multiple myeloma, hematologic diseases

Definition: Malignant fibrous histiocytoma (MFH) is the most common primary malignant soft-tissue tumor of adulthood. It can also be present in bone. It is usually seen in late adulthood with a peak at age fifty. These are aggressive tumors with a tendency to recur and metastasize.

Risk factors: Malignant fibrous histiocytoma is the most common radiation-induced sarcoma; MFH of bone is more frequent in whites, with a male-to-female ratio of 1.5:1.

Etiology and the disease process: Malignant fibrous histiocytomal cells is thought to derive from primitive mesenchymal cells, with four cell types predominating: storiform/pleomorphic, myxoid, giant cell, and inflammatory.

Incidence: Malignant fibrous histiocytoma accounts for 20 to 30 percent of all soft-tissue sarcomas. It is the most common malignant sarcoma of older adults.

Symptoms: Soft-tissue malignant fibrous histiocytoma usually presents as a painless soft-tissue mass with progressive enlargement over months. Any deep-seated, painless, invasive intramuscular mass in a patient over the age of fifty is most likely MFH. Patients with retroperitoneal MFH have symptoms of fatigue, weight loss, abdominal pressure, fever, and malaise. Osseous MFH usually presents with pain over several months with or without swelling and can be associated with pathologic fracture.

Screening and diagnosis: Soft-tissue malignant fibrous histiocytoma is best diagnosed with magnetic resonance imaging (MRI) with gadolinium contrast. This tumor usually appears as a well-defined hypervascular heterogeneous soft-tissue mass with areas of hemorrhage and necrosis. Osseous MFH usually presents as an aggressive Stage IIb lesion associated with pathologic fracture in approximately 20 percent of cases. Staging depends on pathology, compartmentalization, and presence or absence of metastases:

- Stage Ia: Low grade, intracompartmental
- Stage Ib: Low grade, extracompartmental
- Stage IIa: High grade, intracompartmental
- Stage IIb: High grade, extracompartmental
- Stage III: Presence of metastases

Treatment and therapy: Treatment for Stage I tumors involves surgical resection with wide margins, whereas treatment for Stage II involves surgical resection with adjuvant radiation or chemotherapy.

Prognosis, prevention, and outcomes: Prognosis depends on tumor size, depth, location, histologic subtype, and presence of metastases. Local recurrence is seen in approximately 20 to 31 percent of cases. The five-year survival rate is 80 percent if the tumor is under 5 centimeters (cm) but drops to approximately 40 percent if the tumor is greater than 10 cm at diagnosis (however, for retroperitoneal tumors, the five-year survival is 15 to 20 percent). Metastases can occur to the lung, lymph nodes, bone, and the liver.

Debra B. Kessler, M.D., Ph.D.

See also Amputation; Fibrosarcomas, soft-tissue; Limb salvage; Liposarcomas; Mesenchymomas, malignant.

▶ Malignant rhabdoid tumor of the kidney

Category: Diseases, symptoms, and conditions
Also known as: Rhabdoid tumor of the kidney, MRT

Related conditions: Wilms' tumor

Definition: Malignant rhabdoid tumor of the kidney is an extremely aggressive and lethal cancer that occurs only in infants and young children.

Risk factors: Malignant rhabdoid tumor of the kidney is caused by a mutation or deletion of the *INI1* gene. However, there are no known risk factors associated with its development.

Etiology and the disease process: Malignant rhabdoid tumor of the kidney is made up of an overgrowth of rhabdoid (rod-shaped) cells. These cells may appear like epithelial (skin), neural (nerve), muscle, or mesenchymal (rare soft-tissue tumor) cells. A single rhabdoid tumor may include all these types of cells or only one or two. The cells tend to infiltrate the kidney tissue and to metastasize early. A common site of metastasis is the brain.

Incidence: Malignant rhabdoid tumor of the kidney is a rare tumor. According to the National Wilms' Tumor Study (NWTS) group data, only 1.6 percent of cases of childhood renal tumors are malignant rhabdoid tumors. Malignant rhabdoid tumors are equally common in both sexes, and the median age at which it occurs is eleven months.

Symptoms: The most common symptoms observed are fever, hematuria (blood in the urine), fussiness, and hypertension. Other symptoms are those of brain metastasis, such as seizures and loss of previously achieved motor skills.

Screening and diagnosis: There is no routine screening for malignant rhabdoid tumor of the kidney. The most definitive testing includes abdominal ultrasound and abdominal computed tomography (CT) scan. Then the tumor is biopsied.

The staging for malignant rhabdoid tumor of the kidney was devised by the NWTS group and then modified by the Children's Oncology Group (COG). The stages are as follows:

- Stage I: The tumor has not spread beyond the one kidney.
- Stage II: The tumor is localized to the area around the kidney, and there is no evidence of tumor spread.
- Stage III: The tumor has spread into the abdomen.

- Stage IV: There are metastases outside the abdominal or pelvic cavities.
- Stage V: There are bilateral tumors.

Treatment and therapy: The primary treatment is surgical removal of the kidney. It is usually removed through direct incision, to avoid any spillage of cancer cells. At this time, lymph nodes are sampled and the adrenal gland may be removed. Bilateral tumors are not removed. Chemotherapy is performed on all patients with malignant rhabdoid tumor of the kidney.

Prognosis, prevention, and outcomes: The prognosis for malignant rhabdoid tumor of the kidney is poor, with an average survival time of less than one year. There is no way to prevent it.

Christine M. Carroll, R.N., B.S.N., M.B.A.

See also Childhood cancers; Wilms' tumor.

▶ Malignant tumors

Category: Diseases, symptoms, and conditions
Also known as: Cancerous tumors

Related conditions: Most cancers

Definition: Malignant tumors are those that invade surrounding tissue. Commonly known as cancer, cells of malignant tumors are abnormal in morphology, tend to be larger than normal, and have odd shapes and large and irregular nuclei. By entering into the bloodstream or the lymphatic system, these cells spread to surrounding tissue, where they damage the tissues and organs. A sarcoma is a cancer of the connective tissue, and carcinomas are of epithelial origin. Malignant tumors are named using the Latin or Greek root of the organ of origin as a prefix and "sarcoma" or "carcinoma" as the suffix. For example, a malignant tumor of the liver is called hepatocarcinoma; a malignant tumor of the fat cells is called liposarcoma.

Risk factors: The most common risk factors for development of malignant tumors include tobacco use; exposure to ultraviolet (UV) radiation, ionizing radiation, certain chemicals, and viruses; and family history.

Etiology and the disease process: A mutated cell that continues to divide is a hallmark of cancer. The deoxyribonucleic acid (DNA) repair mechanisms are damaged, and the immune system is compromised such that the tumor cells rapidly multiply undeterred. Additionally, the tumor has an extensive vasculature that provides nutrients and oxygen for its growth.

Symptoms: Unusual bleeding or discharge, a change in the shape or coloration of a wart or mole, a sore throat that does not heal, unexplained weight loss, persistent cough, and anemia are some warning signs. Many symptoms are caused by the fatigue, pain, and stress imposed on the body by malignant tumors.

Screening and diagnosis: X rays, ultrasound, magnetic resonance imaging (MRI), and computed tomography (CT) scans are used to detect changes in tissues or organs, and blood tests are used to monitor abnormal cell counts. Presence of tumor markers such as prostate specific antigen (PSA), carcinoembryonic antigen (CEA), and human chorionic gonadotropin hormone in the blood are used to screen high-risk individuals.

Treatment and therapy: Malignant tumors can be removed before they metastasize (spread), but frequently they grow back. Besides a person's age, general health, and response to treatment, the outcome depends on the type and location of the cancer, the stage of the disease (the extent to which the cancer has spread), or its grade (how abnormal the cancer cells look and how quickly the cancer is likely to grow and spread). Treatment includes surgery, radiation therapy, chemotherapy, hormone therapy, or biological therapy. However, most often a combination of therapies is required for complete eradication of the malignancy. Choice of a healthy, active, tobacco-free lifestyle with a minimum exposure to harmful UV rays can go a long way in preventing cancer.

Banalata Sen, Ph.D.

See also Cancer biology; Carcinomatosis; Invasive cancer; Metastasis; Tumor markers.

▶ Mammography

Category: Procedures
Also known as: Breast X ray

Definition: Mammography is a radiographic procedure used to examine internal breast tissue for possible abnormalities. Three types of mammograms are performed: screening mammogram, diagnostic mammogram, and digital mammogram.

In a screening mammogram, X-ray images of the breast are recorded on X-ray film (conventional method) or electronically (digital method). The recommendation for screening mammograms is once every two years for those women who are forty to forty-nine years old and once every year for women fifty years old and above. Patients with

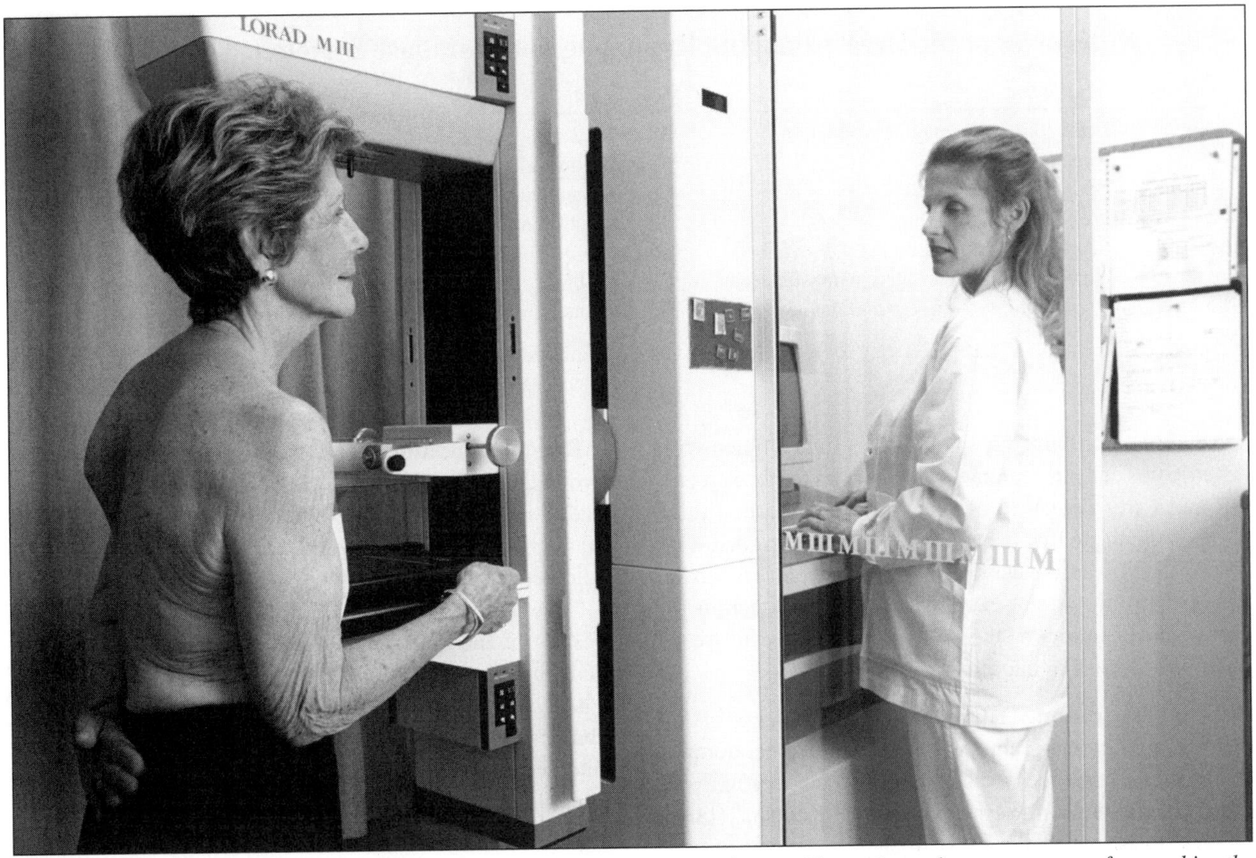

Women are advised to have mammograms once every two years between ages forty and forty-nine and once every year after reaching the age of fifty. (PhotoDisc)

a family history of breast cancer, however, should have the first mammogram before forty years of age and should continue to have them yearly. Also, regardless of age, patients who have been diagnosed as having breast cancer should have a mammogram yearly.

In a diagnostic mammogram, a series of X-ray images of the breast from various angles are recorded on X-ray film (conventional method) or electronically (digital method). Diagnostic mammograms are used to diagnose lumps that a woman feels during self-examination or a health care provider detects during a clinical breast examination if other unexpected symptoms—such as change in breast shape or size, or occurrence of nipple discharge, breast pain, or thickening of breast skin—are present. During a diagnostic mammogram, more X rays are taken than during a screening mammogram in order to get views from many angles. A diagnostic mammogram may be required if the patient has breast implants in order to be able to view breast tissue that can be hidden by the implant.

In a digital mammogram, X-ray images of the breast are recorded electronically and are stored on a computer. The images can then be manipulated via computer software for further evaluation. The average dose of radiation used is lower than that for film mammography. In terms of cancer detection, no differences between digital imaging and traditional film imaging have been found for the general population. Digital mammography is considered preferable, however, for those women who are under the age of fifty, have dense breasts, or are premenopausal or perimenopausal.

In addition, the National Cancer Institute (NCI) is supporting research to develop new procedures for detecting breast tumors. Technologies currently being investigated are magnetic resonance imaging (MRI) and positron emission tomography (PET). Other methods being investigated are those to detect genetic markers for breast cancer, which involve analysis of blood, urine, or fluid aspirated from the nipple.

Cancers diagnosed: Breast cancer

Why performed: In the United States, the most frequently occurring cancer for women is breast cancer. By

Categories of the Breast Imaging Reporting and Database System (BI-RADS)

Category	*Assessment*	*Follow-up*
0	Need additional imaging evaluation	Additional imaging needed before a category can be assigned
1	Negative	Continue annual screening mammography (for women over age 40)
2	Benign (noncancerous)	Continue annual screening mammography (for women over age 40)
3	Probably benign	Receive a 6-month follow-up mammogram
4	Suspicious abnormality	May require biopsy
5	Highly suggestive of malignancy (cancer)	Requires biopsy
6	Known biopsy—proven malignancy (cancer)	Biopsy confirms presence of cancer before treatment begins

age eighty, approximately one of every nine women will develop this cancer. Mammography allows for the screening and early detection of breast-tissue abnormalities. Statistics indicate that use of mammography can result in detection of breast cancer one to two years before it can be detected by breast self-examination. Early detection of breast cancer improves the chances for successful treatment of this form of cancer.

Patient preparation: The patient should shower or bathe prior to the mammogram and should not use deodorant, body lotions, sunscreens, creams, powders, or perfume on the chest or underarms, as they may cause "artifacts" (false images) to appear on the X-ray image.

Steps of the procedure: Patients who have breast implants should mention that fact when making the mammogram appointment. Both the technologist who performs the mammogram and the radiologist who interprets the mammogram must have experience in working with implants.

Prior to undergoing mammography, the patient will be asked if she has undergone any type of breast surgery, as this may affect the way in which the X-ray films are interpreted. She will then be asked to remove all clothing and jewelry from the waist up. The patient will be given a short gown and asked to put it on so that it opens in the front.

The procedure begins with the radiologic technologist placing one of the breasts on a platform and lowering a plastic plate onto the breast until it is flattened as much as possible. This allows for the successful X-ray visualization of as much breast tissue as possible. The technologist then positions the X-ray machine, stands behind a protective barrier, and takes the image. A front-view X ray (from the upper surface down) and a side-view X ray of the breast will be taken. Next, the technologist repeats this procedure with the other breast. While the patient may feel uncomfortable when the breast is being flattened, this discomfort is short in duration.

After the procedure: The patient will be asked to wait while the X-ray films are developed and then viewed by a radiologist to make sure that none of the images need to be retaken. Once this has been confirmed, the patient will be allowed to redress and use deodorant.

The patient should ask how long it will take to get the results of the mammography and whether those results will be sent to the patient as well as to the doctor. She may also want to ask where the "films" will be stored, so that they can be retrieved if the patient moves out of the area and needs to have future mammograms performed at another location. This is important because the new radiologist may use those earlier images as a reference to determine if there have been any changes in breast tissue over time.

Risks: Mammography uses low-dose radiation and is considered to be very safe. Patients who are pregnant or think they may be pregnant, however, should not have a mammogram. A pregnant woman should not be exposed to X rays because of the possible risk to the fetus.

The safety and reliability of mammograms are mandated by a federal law called the Mammography Quality Standards Act (MQSA). This law requires that all mammography facilities in the United States meet stringent quality standards, including those for the medical physicist, who tests the mammography equipment; the technologist, who takes the mammogram; and the radiologist, who interprets the mammogram. The facilities must also maintain certification by the Food and Drug Administration (FDA) and undergo an annual inspection.

Results: A normal result means that the X-ray films revealed no obvious signs of breast cancer. In certain instances, however, breast cancer may still be present. This false negative result is more common for those women with breast tissue that is more dense, as is typical for younger women. The more dense the breast tissue, the more difficult it is to visualize abnormal spots on the X-ray image.

An abnormal result means that something has been identified that needs to be looked at more closely. The abnormality may be an unusual-looking area of breast tissue or a type of cyst or lump. Even the presence of a lump, however, does not necessarily indicate cancer. A lump can be either benign (noncancerous) or malignant (cancerous). Therefore, additional testing—such as a diagnostic mammogram, ultrasound, or biopsy—may be required to determine if the abnormality is the result of breast cancer. The most common type of biopsy is known as a needle biopsy. This procedure consists of inserting a small-gauge needle into the area in question and removing a small tissue sample. That sample is then sent to a laboratory for determination if any cancerous cells are present. An abnormality that is interpreted as breast cancer when none is present is called a false positive result. Like the false negative result, it is more common for younger women. It is also more common for those women who have a family history of breast cancer, have had a previous breast biopsy, or are taking estrogen.

The American College of Radiology (ACR) has established a system for uniform reporting of mammogram results called the Breast Imaging Reporting and Database System (BI-RADS) that consists of seven categories. Radiologists and physicians use it to help determine appropriate patient care.

Cynthia L. De Vine, B.A.

▶ For Further Information

Lanyi, M. *Mammography: Diagnosis and Pathological Analysis*. New York: Springer, 2003.

Pisano, E. D., C. Gatsonis, E. Hendrick, et al. "Diagnostic Performance of Digital Versus Film Mammography for Breast-Cancer Screening." *New England Journal of Medicine* 353 (October 27, 2005): 1773-1783.

Qasee, A., et al. "Screening Mammography for Women Forty to Forty-nine Years of Age: A Clinical Practice Guideline from the American College of Physicians." *Annals of Internal Medicine* 146, no. 7 (April 3, 2007): 511-515.

▶ Other Resources

American Cancer Society
http://www.cancer.org

American College of Radiology
http://www.acr.org/index.asp

National Breast and Cervical Cancer Early Detection Program
http://www.cdc.gov/cancer/nbccedp/index.htm

National Cancer Institute
Cancer Information Service
http://cis.nci.nih.gov

National Women's Health Information Center
http://www.womenshealth.gov

Susan G. Komen Breast Cancer Foundation
http://www.komen.org

See also Accelerated partial breast irradiation (APBI); Breast cancer in children and adolescents; Breast cancer in men; Breast cancer in pregnant women; Breast cancers; Breast implants; Breast ultrasound; Calcifications of the breast; Childbirth and cancer; Clinical breast exam (CBE); Comedo carcinomas; Duct ectasia; Ductal carcinoma in situ (DCIS); Ductal lavage; Ductogram; Estrogen-receptor-sensitive breast cancer; Fibroadenomas; Fibrocystic breast changes; Hormone replacement therapy (HRT); Invasive ductal carcinomas; Invasive lobular carcinomas; Lobular carcinoma in situ (LCIS); Lumpectomy; Medullary carcinoma of the breast; Microcalcifications; Needle biopsies; Needle localization; Nipple discharge; Peutz-Jeghers syndrome (PJS); Phyllodes tumors; Tubular carcinomas; Wire localization.

▶ Managed care

Category: Social and personal issues
Also known as: Health maintenance organizations (HMOs), preferred provider organizations (PPOs)

Definition: Managed care is a process used by health insurance plans to pay for and coordinate the delivery of health care services to people covered under the managed care plan.

Prevalence of managed care: Managed care is the most predominant form of health insurance in the United States. The majority of private health insurance plans are managed care plans. The Kaiser Family Foundation and the Health Research and Educational Trust survey estimated that 97 percent of employees enrolled in an employer's group health insurance were covered under a managed care plan in 2006. The prevalence of managed care in public health insurance plans has grown rapidly since 1990. Approximately 60 percent of people enrolled in Medicaid receive services through managed care, representing a 900 percent increase from 1991. The Medicare program, which has traditionally provided public health insurance through an indemnity plan, has seen increasing enrollments in its managed care Medicare Advantage plans.

Principles of managed care: Health insurance was once primarily organized as an indemnity or fee-for-service system. Persons covered under an indemnity health insurance plan can visit any physician or medical facility they choose and submit a claim to the insurer for reimbursement of a certain percentage of the medical expenses. In response to escalating health care costs, managed care systems were developed and promoted as a way to pay for medical services and control the quality, accessibility, utilization, and cost of those services. As a result, persons covered under a managed care plan have limitations on which health care providers they can use and must follow the plan's procedures in accessing the health care providers to receive coverage.

Managed care has many different forms, but there are a few fundamental principles and processes shared by all managed care plans. Managed care plans control the access of persons covered under the plan (covered persons) to medical services. Medical services are covered only if they are provided by certain health care providers that are either on the staff of the managed care plan or under contract with the plan. Covered persons are assigned to or can choose from a list of primary care physicians, who are usually family doctors, internists, pediatricians, or obstetricians/gynecologists. The primary care physician's role in coordinating care is to eliminate inappropriate and unnecessary services; he or she provides preventive and routine care to covered persons and acts as a gatekeeper to arrange for and authorize care from other health care providers. The patient must therefore obtain a referral from the primary care physician before seeking nonemergency medical care from a specialist, hospital, or outpatient facility.

Managed care plans also use "utilization reviews" to determine the medical necessity or appropriateness of services. Reviews can take place before, during, or after services have been rendered. Because these reviews determine whether or not the plan will cover the medical expenses, patients are encouraged to seek "preauthorization" for services requiring review. For example, a cancer patient who has been advised to undergo an operation to biopsy or remove a tumor may need to arrange for preauthorization of the surgery in order to determine the amount of coverage the plan will provide, if any.

Clearly, therefore, managed care plans can influence the quality of care delivered to covered persons. The plans impose standards for selection of health care providers that are associated with the plan. The plans also have formal programs of quality assurance and provide incentives for plan doctors to use best practice protocols or treatment guidelines, which are based on standards of care set by medical experts. Through case or disease management programs, plans identify covered persons with chronic health care needs and coordinate with the primary care physician to establish a cost-effective treatment plan and monitor patient outcome.

At the same time, to manage costs, plans may restrict certain treatments or limit inpatient admissions and lengths of stay, favoring outpatient care when possible. Health care providers associated with managed care plans are reimbursed at negotiated rates. Some plans pay a fixed amount, called a "capitation payment," for each health care provider providing services to covered persons, regardless of the number or type of services rendered. Other plans negotiate with providers and reimburse them for actual expenses based on a discounted rate. Clearly, then, the incentives built into such plans can be financial as well as oriented toward a good health outcome for the patient.

Types of plans: Three primary types of managed care plans exist: health maintenance organization (HMO) plans, point-of-service (POS) plans, and preferred provider organization (PPO) plans.

HMOs are the oldest and strictest form of managed care. Enrollment in HMO plans peaked in 1996 and began to decline thereafter, but HMOs are still a prevalent form of managed care. HMOs pay for services delivered by health care providers who are employees of the HMO or health care providers who are under contract with an HMO as so-called network providers. The covered person is usually responsible only for a fixed copayment. Care is delivered through a primary care physician, and care from other providers must be authorized by the primary care physician in order for it to be covered. Typically, the other providers must also be associated with the HMO.

A POS plan is usually offered by an HMO and may be referred to as an "open-ended" HMO plan. Under a POS plan, the covered person can receive services from a health care provider who is not an employee or network member of the HMO. These services are available at higher cost to the covered person through a deductible and coinsurance and frequently do not require a referral from a primary care physician.

A PPO plan is a form of managed care offered by insurers other than HMOs and is currently the most popular form of managed care plan. The insurer contracts with a network of area health care providers who agree to accept set fees for services given to covered persons. The plan offers financial incentives for covered persons to receive care from in-network providers, such as low copayments. Covered persons can receive care from health care providers, including primary care physicians, who are not members of the PPO network, but only at a higher cost through deductibles and coinsurance. Covered persons may also be responsible for paying the difference between what the insurer paid the out-of-network health care provider and what the provider charged. Covered persons can often make self-referrals and do not need to get a referral from a primary care physician.

Consumer protections: Because managed care plans make coverage decisions that can ultimately restrict access to care, many states have passed consumer protection laws governing managed care practices. These laws apply only to managed care plans that are state-regulated. Many states allow a covered person with a chronic illness to pick a specialist as a primary care physician, since going through a primary care physician for referrals is time-consuming. Other states allow primary care physicians to give standing referrals to persons with chronic illnesses, such as cancer, who need special medical care over a long period of time.

Managed care plans can deny coverage of a service based on their assessment that coverage is not provided for under the contract, the proper procedures in obtaining the services were not followed, or the services were not appropriate or medically necessary. Managed care plans must follow state and federal rules for internally reviewing covered persons' complaints and appeals concerning denial of coverage. Most states have enacted procedures for external or independent reviews, especially when denial of coverage was based on a determination by the insurer that services rendered were not appropriate or medically necessary. Several states require persons employed by insurance companies who make decisions on medical necessity of care to have medical credentials or have a current in-state medical license. Many states have established an ombudsman office to act on behalf of covered persons during disputes with insurers over denial of coverage.

States have prohibited managed care plans from compromising physicians' medical opinions. Most states prohibit gag clauses in health care provider contracts that would keep doctors from informing patients of their treatment options. Federal law bans the use of gag clauses in Medicaid and Medicare plans. States have also banned the practice of rewarding doctors for performing less costly procedures or prescribing less costly drugs.

Finally, many states produce a report card on the performance of managed care plans. The report cards detail how well a managed care plan handles complaints, covers and delivers care, and gives access to specialized care. Some reports also include measurers of health care providers associated with managed care plans.

Amanda McQuade, Ph.D.

▶ For Further Information

Buckley, John F., and Nicole D. Prysby. *2005 State by State Guide to Managed Care Law*. New York: Aspen, 2005.

Kongstvedt, Peter R. *Managed Care: What It Is and How It Works*. 2d ed. New York: Aspen, 2004.

Marcinko, David E., and Hope R. Hetico, eds. *Dictionary of Health Insurance and Managed Care*. New York: Springer, 2006.

▶ Other Resources

Agency for Healthcare Research and Quality
http://www.ahrq.gov

Centers for Medicare and Medicaid Services
U.S. Department of Health and Human Services
http://www.cms.hhs.gov

Kaiser Family Foundation
http://www.kff.org

Kaiser State Health Facts
http://www.statehealthfacts.org

MedlinePlus
http://www.nlm.nih.gov/medlineplus/managedcare.html

Patient Advocate Foundation
http://www.patientadvocate.org

See also Financial issues; Health maintenance organizations (HMOs); Insurance; Medicare and cancer; Preferred provider organizations (PPOs); Second opinions; Social Security Disability Insurance (SSDI).

▶ Mantle cell lymphoma (MCL)

Category: Diseases, symptoms, and conditions
Also known as: Non-Hodgkin lymphoma, B-cell lymphoma

Related conditions: Hodgkin lymphoma

Definition: Mantle cell lymphoma (MCL), or B-cell lymphoma, is a rare form of non-Hodgkin lymphoma (NHL), with 6 to 8 percent of cases of NHL accounting for MCL. MCL primarily affects the B lymphocytes of the lymphatic system. The lymphatic system is made up of lymph nodes that are linked by lymph vessels responsible for delivering fluid throughout the body, as well as collecting waste from tissues, purifying it, and then returning it to the blood.

MCL has two distinct groups: indolent or low-grade lymphoma and aggressive or high-grade lymphoma.

Risk factors: There are no risk factors for MCL.

Etiology and the disease process: Causes for MCL have not been identified; however, it is known that Caucasian males are more susceptible to MCL and that it is most prevalent in adult populations. It has been determined that patients with MCL have an overexpression of cyclin D1, which is a protein that encourages cellular growth. This cyclin D1 overexpression has been traced to a translocation between chromosomes 11 and 14.

Incidence: MCL is found typically in adults in their sixties, affecting males more often than females at a ratio of 3:1. Cases of MCL have been steadily increasing since the 1970's. As the initial symptoms of MCL often go undetected, upon diagnosis the majority of patients already have Stage IV disease.

Symptoms: MCL is often detected because of swelling in the lymph nodes of the neck, groin, or armpit that is painless yet noticeable either visibly or to the touch. Accompanying symptoms often include fatigue, decreased appetite, fever, night sweating, weight loss, itchiness, and breathlessness.

Screening and diagnosis: MCL is diagnosed following surgical removal of a portion of the swollen lymph node. The tissue collected is then sampled to review its cells under a microscope to make the diagnosis. Additional supportive tests may include blood tests, bone scans, marrow biopsies, and X rays to provide information on the extent of the spread of the lymphoma and its type. The information gained from these tests will assist the doctor in determining the appropriate treatment plan for the cancer.

The Ann Arbor staging for non-Hodgkin lymphoma, which is the definitive disease process guide for lymphomas, defines four stages of the disease. Stage I is lymphoma limited to a primary lymph node, organ, or tissue site in one body area. Stage II includes two or more lymph nodes or regions of lymph nodes either on the upper or lower half of the body. Stage III includes two or more lymph nodes or regions of lymph nodes on both the upper and lower parts of the body, and Stage IV includes lymphoma that has spread from the lymph nodes to one or more organs in the body. Each stage also includes a subclassification of either A or B, to identify either the absence of symptoms (A) or the presence of symptoms (B). Additionally, lymphoma that has spread beyond the lymph nodes to the organs can be classified with an E for extranodal.

Relative Survival Rates for Mantle Cell Lymphoma, 1988-2001

Years	*Survival Rate (%)*
1	83.9
2	72.6
3	65.2
5	51.1
8	37.4
10	34.3

Source: Data from L. A. G. Ries et al., eds., *Cancer Survival Among Adults: U.S. SEER Program, 1988-2001—Patient and Tumor Characteristics*, NIH Pub. No. 07-6215 (Bethesda, Md.: National Cancer Institute, 2007)

Treatment and therapy: Treatment for MCL is dependent upon the patient's stage of disease. Patients with indolent MCL who are asymptomatic often manage their disease with a "watch and wait" approach without medication until symptoms appear. As most patients with MCL are diagnosed, however, already at Stage IV, aggressive therapy is often prescribed. Aggressive therapy can consist of chemotherapy alone; however, this is often not enough to treat the cancer. Aggressive therapy typically includes a combination of chemotherapy and radiation. Allogenic stem cell transplantation has also been used to introduce stem cells that are not cancerous into the body to assist the body in its fight against the cancer. Allogenic stem cell transplantation, however, causes side effects which are often deemed intolerable by the patient, is difficult to perform, and is rarely used as a treatment option. Additional therapy, such as treatment with a monoclonal antibody, can also be used in combination with chemotherapy, to target and kill select cancer cells.

The patient may also be given medications to counteract the side effects caused by the first-line therapies, such as steroids to combat nausea, or interferons to allow the body to increase its immune response.

Prognosis, prevention, and outcomes: Prognosis for MCL can be determined by its classification as either indolent or aggressive, and indolent MCL typically has a better prognosis than aggressive MCL. As the majority of cases of MCL are diagnosed as Stage IV, MCL has only a moderate prognosis. Patients diagnosed with MCL most often have an average survival of three to four years. Even in patients with a good or fair prognosis, curing MCL is uncommon.

Anna Perez, M.Sc.

▶ For Further Information

Clarke, C. A., and S. L. Glaser. "Changing Incidence of Non-Hodgkin Lymphomas in the United States." *Cancer* 94 (2002): 2015-2023.

Norton, A. J., J. Matthews, V. Pappa, et al. "Mantle Cell Lymphoma: Natural History Defined in a Serially Biopsied Population over a 20-Year Period." *Annals of Oncology* 6 (1995): 249-256.

▶ Other Resources

American Cancer Society
http://www.cancer.org

Leukemia and Lymphoma Society
http://www.leukemia-lymphoma.org

National Cancer Institute
www.cancer.gov/search/geneticsservices

See also Angiogenesis inhibitors; Burkitt lymphoma; Non-Hodgkin lymphoma; Proteasome inhibitors; Richter syndrome; Virus-related cancers.

▶ Mastectomy

Category: Procedures

Definition: A mastectomy is the surgical removal of a breast.

Cancers diagnosed or treated: Breast cancer

Why performed: A mastectomy is performed to remove a breast that has been affected by cancer. It is very important to remove all the cancerous tissue so that the cancer cannot spread to other parts of the body. Many women who have been diagnosed with breast cancer are given the option to choose between mastectomy and breast-conserving surgery (lumpectomy) plus radiotherapy. For these women, many factors may need to be weighed before making a decision. Mastectomy is usually recommended for certain types of patients, including women who have previously had radiotherapy to the affected breast, women with two or more areas of cancer in the same breast, women with connective tissue diseases (such as scleroderma) that make them inappropriate candidates for radiotherapy, and male breast cancer patients. Although breast cancer in men (accounting for less than 1 percent of cancer cases in men), is relatively rare its treatment, including mastectomy, is the same as it is in women.

Women believed to be at moderate or high risk of developing breast cancer may choose to have one or both breasts removed prophylactically to prevent, rather than to treat, breast cancer. It is believed that preventive mastectomy reduces the chance of developing breast cancer by about 90 percent in such women.

Patient preparation: The patient will probably meet with the surgeon a few days before the surgery. The surgeon will want to know about any medications the patient is taking that could interfere with surgery. A routine blood workup, urinalysis, and an electrocardiogram (ECG) may be performed a few days before the surgery. Patients will normally be instructed not to eat or drink for at least eight hours before surgery.

If the patient is to have a sentinel lymph node biopsy during the procedure, then a small amount of a radioactive substance and a blue dye will be injected into the area several hours before surgery.

Steps of the procedure: There are four types of mastectomy. A simple mastectomy involves removal of all of the breast tissue. A simple mastectomy with node sampling involves removal of the breast tissue and some of the lymph nodes from under the arm. A modified radical mastectomy involves removal of all breast tissue plus all lymph nodes from under the arm. A radical mastectomy involves removal of all breast tissue and all lymph nodes from under the arm, plus the muscles from the chest wall. This procedure was the most commonly performed type of mastectomy in the past, but it is rarely performed today. Studies have shown that the modified radical mastectomy is equally effective, and therefore it has become the most common type of procedure for removing the entire breast.

The procedure is performed under general anesthesia. A diagonal or horizontal cut is made across the breast, and the breast tissue is removed. Small nerves are cut between the breast tissue and the skin area. Some of the lymph nodes from under the arm on the side of the cancer are usually removed during the procedure, so that the surgeon can check them for cancer cells. The exact number of lymph nodes under the arm will vary from person to person, but there are approximately twenty. A few lymph nodes may be removed to check for cancer cells, a procedure known as axillary gland sampling. Sometimes all of the lymph nodes under the arm are removed, a procedure known as axillary clearance.

Sometimes a procedure known as sentinel lymph node biopsy is used. In this procedure, a small amount of radioactive liquid and a blue dye are injected into the area before the operation. This allows the surgeon to identify the draining lymph nodes for the area, the ones most likely to contain cancer cells if the cancer has started to spread. These sentinel lymph nodes are usually one to three in number. They will contain radioactivity that can be detected with a handheld Geiger counter and will appear blue in color. These lymph nodes are removed and tested to see whether they contain cancer cells. If a sentinel lymph node contains cancerous cells, then more lymph nodes will need to be removed. If it is obvious that a sentinel lymph node contains cancer, then the surgeon can proceed to the remove additional lymph nodes at the time of the mastectomy. If cancer is detected in a sentinel lymph node after the mastectomy through microscopic study by a pathologist, then additional lymph nodes will need to be removed in another procedure. If the sentinel nodes are cancer-free, then it is very unlikely that the cancer has spread to other lymph nodes. In this case, the patient can avoid the potential side effects of full lymph node surgery.

A plastic or rubber drainage tube will most likely be inserted to drain fluid from the wound area before the incision is closed up with stitches. A pressure dressing is placed over the wound area to minimize oozing after the surgery.

After the procedure: The patient will experience short-term pain and swelling and will have a scar. Possible complications include wound infection. The patient will most likely have one or more drainage tubes coming from the wound area to drain blood and tissue fluid to prevent them from collecting and causing swelling or infection. These tubes will be removed several days after the surgery. Occasionally, fluid collects around the wound after the tubes have been removed and needs to be drained.

The extent of the surgery will determine the length of hospital stay, but it will probably be from one to several days. After going home, the patient will need considerable rest. Lifting or carrying of heavy objects should be avoided, and the patient should not drive for a few weeks. Gentle

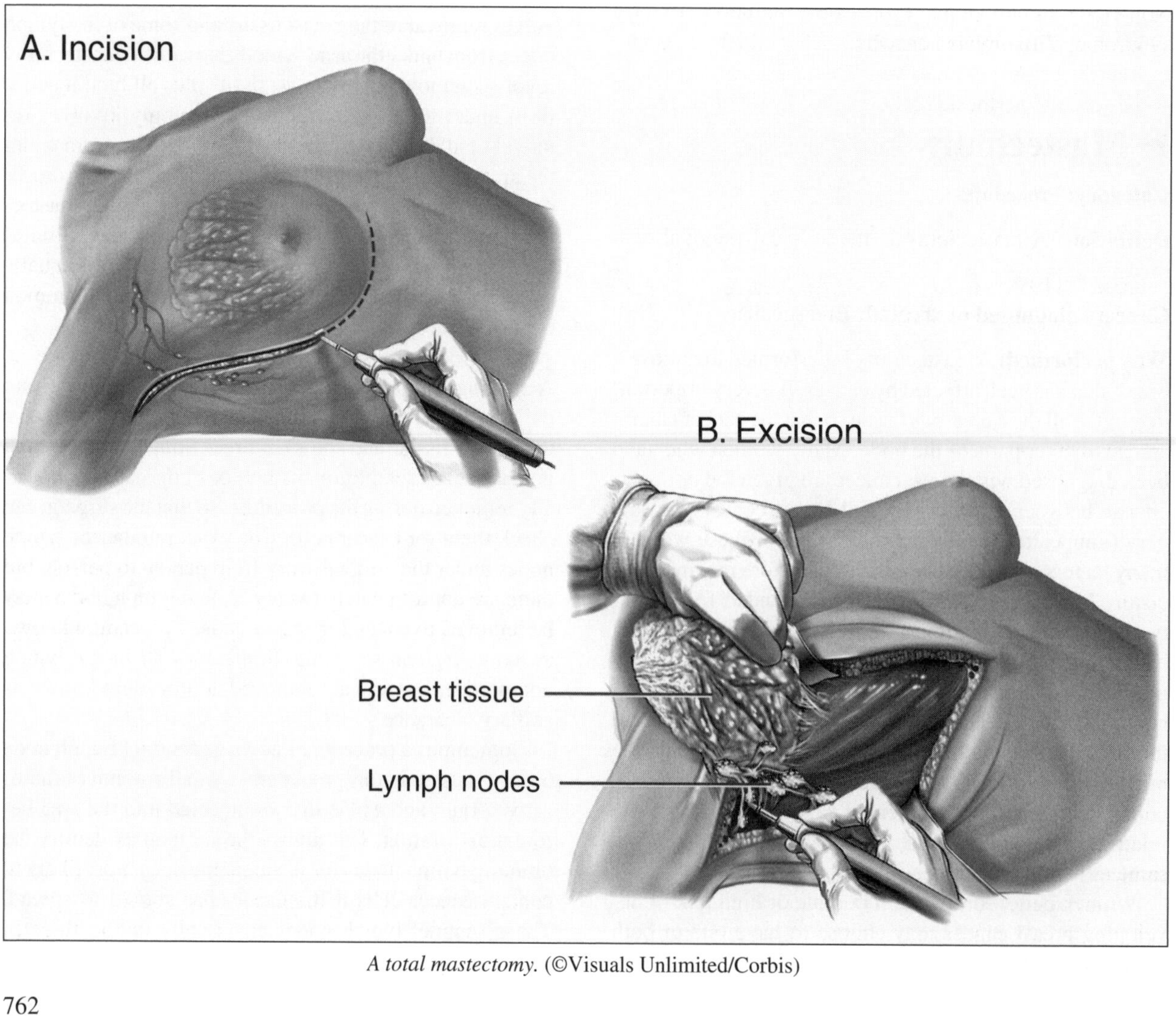

A total mastectomy. (©Visuals Unlimited/Corbis)

exercises may be recommended to relieve pain and stiffness and to encourage circulation to the area.

Many patients experience a pulling sensation near or under the arm after a mastectomy. Patients may experience phantom breast sensations such as unpleasant itching, "pins and needles," pressure, or throbbing after a mastectomy. One study showed that more than one-third of the patients experienced such sensations and that the incidence was similar whether or not the patient had had breast reconstruction. These sensations are believed to be caused by the cutting of small nerves during the procedure and are analogous to phantom pains that can occur after limb amputations.

Undergoing a mastectomy can be an emotional time for a patient. Patients may find it helpful to talk to others who have been through the operation, both before and after the surgery. If a breast reconstruction procedure is not done at the time of the mastectomy, then the patient can use a prosthesis inside her bra to provide the shape of a breast.

Risks: A mastectomy is normally a safe and effective operation. There are extremely rare risks associated with the use of general anesthesia. In rare cases, hematoma, an accumulation of blood in the wound area, or seroma, an accumulation of clear fluid in the wound area, may occur. Both of these conditions can be treated.

Removing lymph nodes can sometimes lead to fluid buildup and swelling in the affected arm, which can cause pain and tenderness in the arm and hand. This condition, called lymphedema, usually starts months or years after the surgery and develops slowly over time. It is more likely to occur if all of the lymph nodes and vessels are removed. Lymphedema cannot be cured, but the symptoms can be reduced by early recognition of the condition and careful management. Other possible side effects of the removal of lymph nodes are limitation of arm and shoulder movement and numbness of the upper arm.

Results: If breast cancer is detected early, then mastectomy results in a ten-year survival rate of more than 90 percent.

Jill Ferguson, Ph.D.

▶ For Further Information

Dickson, R. B., and M. E. Lippman. "Cancer of the Breast." In *Cancer: Principles and Practice of Oncology*, edited by Vincent DeVita, Jr., et al. 6th ed. Philadelphia: Lippincott Williams & Wilkins, 2001.

Singletary, S. E. "Techniques in Surgery: Therapeutic and Prophylactic Mastectomy." In *Diseases of the Breast*, edited by J. R. Harris et al. 3d ed. Philadelphia: Lippincott Williams & Wilkins, 2004.

Vazquez, B., D. Rousseau, and T. C. Hurd. "Surgical Management of Breast Cancer." *Seminars in Oncology* 34 (2007): 234-240.

▶ Other Resources

American Cancer Society
Surgery for Breast Cancer
http://www.cancer.org/docroot/CRI/content/CRI_2_4_4X_Surgery_5.asp?sitearea=

Cancer Backup
Breast Cancer Information Centre
http://www.cancerbackup.org.uk/Cancertype/Breast

Imaginis: The Breast Cancer Resource
Mastectomy
http://www.imaginis.com/breasthealth/mastectomy.asp

National Cancer Institute
Preventive Mastectomy: Questions and Answers
http://www.cancer.gov/cancertopics/factsheet/Therapy/preventive-mastectomy

See also Breast cancers; Breast implants; Breast reconstruction; Lumpectomy; Lymphedema; Mammography; Sentinel lymph node (SLN) biopsy and mapping.

▶ Mastocytomas

Category: Diseases, symptoms, and conditions
Also known as: Mast cell tumors

Related conditions: Mastocytosis

Definition: Mastocytomas are lesions found in mastocytosis, a disease characterized by an abnormal increase in tissue mast cells. Mastocytomas do not lead to the hematogenous spread of mast cells; there is no known association with mastocytomas and a predilection to develop mast cell leukemia.

Risk factors: Mastocytomas typically develop only in people with mastocytosis.

Etiology and the disease process: Mast cells are ubiquitous throughout the body and are found in almost all body tissues. They release proinflammatory mediators such as histamine on activation. Mastocytosis may be limited to the skin, in which case it is referred to as cutaneous mastocytosis, or may involve systemic organ systems, in which case it is referred to as systemic mastocytosis. Mastocytomas—along with urticaria pigmentosa, diffuse cutaneous mastocytosis, and telangiectasia macularis eruptive perstans—make up the spectrum of cutaneous disease. Accumulations of mast cells in the skin result in these conditions.

Mastocytomas can appear as solitary or multiple lesions and typically affect only children before the age of six months. Mastocytomas more commonly appear as solitary lesions, and if a second lesion or multiple lesions develop, they typically do not occur more than two months after the first lesion. They are rare in adults because they usually resolve early in life. Although mastocytomas most commonly are localized to the skin, other organs, such as the gastrointestinal system, may be affected. They are nodular, usually range in size from three to four centimeters, and frequently occur on an extremity.

Incidence: The incidence of mastocytomas is unknown.

Symptoms: Lesions may be asymptomatic or may intermittently become itchy, red, and swollen if the lesions are stroked. More commonly, lesions are symptomatic.

Screening and diagnosis: The lesions typically demonstrate Darier's sign. Darier's sign occurs when a lesion is stroked and the lesion and the surrounding area become itchy, red, and swollen. On histological examination, mastocytomas show marked tumorlike aggregates of mast cells throughout the dermis.

Treatment and therapy: Mastocytomas that cause mechanical problems or systemic problems can be treated locally with PUVA therapy (psoralen combined with long-wave ultraviolet light). Potent topical steroids under occlusive dressings are also utilized. Surgical excision is also an option but should be considered only as a last option, as the natural course of the lesions is to resolve.

Prognosis, prevention, and outcomes: Mastocytomas usually appear in infancy, and the occurrence of the lesions resolves by adolescence.

Sarah Kasprowicz, M.D.

See also Benign tumors; Veterinary oncology.

▶ Matrix metalloproteinase inhibitors

Category: Chemotherapy and other drugs

Definition: Matrix metalloproteinase inhibitors suppress the enzymatic activity of extracellular matrix metalloproteinases secreted by cancer cells.

Cancers treated: Several matrix metalloproteinase inhibitors are currently in clinical trials. Their efficacies in treating cancers are unknown at this time.

Delivery routes: Oral, intraperitoneal, intrapleural

How these drugs work: Matrix metalloproteinases are a family of enzymes normally secreted by connective tissue cells and inflammatory cells (phagocytes). They are called *metallo*proteinases because they contain a zinc atom at their catalytic (active) site. These enzymes play a role in several normal physiologic processes, including embryo implantation and normal angiogenesis associated with tissue growth and wound healing.

Malignant tumors undergo invasive growth and metastasis. The viscous connective tissue matrix, composed of collagens, laminins, fibronectins, elastins, and proteoglycans, forms the scaffolding for cellular organization in tissues and provides a barrier to cancer cell migration. Cancer cells, however, can also secrete matrix metalloproteinases, which allows metastasis to proceed by breaking down the connective tissue extracellular matrix. Matrix metalloproteinases are also important contributors to abnormal angiogenesis, the process by which cancer cells stimulate the production of new blood capillaries that deliver nutrients to the tumor cells and are essential for their continued growth.

Researchers identified compounds in tissues that inhibited the activity of the matrix metalloproteinases and have developed new inhibitors by chemical synthesis. The inverse relation between matrix metalloproteinase activity and clinical outcome in cancer has led to the development and testing of these inhibitors in pancreatic, colon, and liver tumor model systems. Since 1993, matrix metalloproteinase inhibitors have undergone rapid clinical development for efficacy in treating colon, ovarian, pancreatic, prostate, gastric, skin, and both non-small-cell and small-cell lung cancers. The most promising inhibitors are those that can be administered orally, making them suitable for chronic administration, which appears to be necessary for optimal effect.

Targeting matrix metalloproteinases in cancer is complicated by the fact that they are absolutely necessary for normal physiological processes; thus researchers must find a delicate balance between disease treatment and the progression of these processes. Unfortunately, clinical trials conducted on synthetic broad-spectrum inhibitors (those targeting several matrix metalloproteinases) have yielded disappointing results in cancer pathology. Nevertheless, researchers are making intensive efforts to find new classes of matrix metalloproteinase inhibitors that have high (rather than broad) selectivity against specific metalloproteinases.

Side effects: Reported side effects from matrix metalloproteinase inhibitors include abdominal pain, fever, elevated liver enzymes, musculoskeletal pain and stiffness, mild thrombocytopenia, skin rash, and cutaneous phototoxicity.

Bernard Jacobson, Ph.D.

See also Angiogenesis; Cancer biology; Carcinomatosis; Malignant tumors; Metastasis.

▶ Mayo Clinic Cancer Center

Category: Organizations

Definition: The Mayo Clinic is the first and largest integrated group practice in the world. Based in Rochester, Minnesota, it contains hospital facilities, research laboratories, and a medical school. Together with its satellite hospitals and practices in Jacksonville, Florida, and Scottsdale, Arizona, the clinic treats more than half a million patients annually and operates by the philosophy that the needs of the patient come first. Mayo Clinic is consistently ranked as one of the best hospitals in the United States by authorities throughout the world. It began as a small outpatient operation but now is a comprehensive health care institution for southern Minnesota and its neighboring states, providing a full range of inpatient and outpatient services. Its research department is also world-renowned, publishing more than 2,800 publications a year in biomedical journals. The Mayo Clinic College of Medicine offers programs in graduate education and clinical medicine.

Statistics: Mayo Clinic is Minnesota's second-largest not-for-profit organization. In 2004 it acquired $5.6 billion. In 2007, it employed more than 3,300 physicians, scientists, and researchers, and 46,000 allied health staff. Between its founding in 1915 and 2007, the oldest of Mayo Clinic's five graduate medical schools trained more than 17,000 students. Mayo medical school trained more than 1,000 physicians between 1972 and 2007.

History: Mayo Clinic began as a small practice founded by William Worrall Mayo and his two sons, William James Mayo and Charles Horace Mayo. W. W. Mayo, originally from the United Kingdom, immigrated to the United States in 1846. He began practicing medicine as the examining surgeon for the Union Army in southern Minnesota. His sons, William and Horace, returned to Rochester to join their father's practice after graduating from medical school. In 1883, a devastating tornado struck, leaving many casualties and Rochester in ruins. The trio and a nun, Mother Alfred Moes from the Sisters of St. Francis, recognized the need for a large facility to treat the ill and injured and built the twenty-seven-bed Saint Mary Hospital in 1889. This hospital remains in operation in the twenty-first century with 1,157 beds. Two years later, Henry Stanley Plummer joined the practice. Ideologies and systems of group practice that Plummer developed and incorporated then are still widely used. The most notable examples include the centralized, individual, dossier-style medical record and the interconnecting telephone communication system. In 1905, Louis B. Wilson joined the clinic to implement and run the experimental laboratories. He is considered the father of research in Rochester and is known for his contribution of the fresh-frozen tissue method for pathological diagnosis. In 1914 Wilson was appointed as the first director of the Mayo Foundation for Medical Education and Research.

W. W. Mayo's philosophy, "No one is big enough to be independent of others," greatly influenced his sons. From the outset of their professional careers, the Mayo brothers encouraged collaboration and learning among the medical practitioners. In 1906 six visiting surgeons established the Surgeons Club and formalized the open-door policy. The brothers' practice has not always been called the Mayo Clinic. The brothers originally included their names in the title and the name Mayo Clinic was coined by their medical colleagues who visited the Mayo brothers and preferred to refer to the duo practice as the Mayo Brothers' Clinic or the Mayos' Clinic. In 1939 the brothers passed away two months apart. Charlie Mayo passed away from lobar pneumonia, and William Mayo died in his sleep because of complications of his stomach cancer.

Even after the passing of the founders, Mayo Clinic continued to contribute greatly to society. During World War II, the clinic offered its aero-medical research services to the military for one dollar per year. During this time, the antiblackout suit was developed for military pilots. The suit technology is still in use. In 1950, Edward Kendall and Philip Hensch became corecipients of the Nobel Prize in Physiology or Medicine for their work in isolating hormones of the adrenal cortex.

Oncological services: Every year, thousands of patients flock to Mayo Clinic oncology departments, which treat more than two hundred different kinds of cancer. The medical oncology department administers chemotherapy and immunotherapy, and the radiation oncology department administers radiation therapy. These departments work in sync with the Mayo Clinic Comprehensive Cancer Center, which conducts cancer research, clinical trials, clinical treatments, and education. Innovative and advanced cancer care is available at Mayo Clinic. Patients also have access to novel drug, immunologic, and gene therapies through ongoing clinical trials. The oncology department services include bone marrow transplantation, electronic portal imaging device (EPID) target localization, familial cancer genetics screening and counseling, stereotactic radiosurgery, high-dose-rate (HDR) brachytherapy, hyperthermia, intensity-modulated radiation therapy (IMRT), intraoperative radiation therapy, intravascular brachytherapy, low-dose-rate brachytherapy, permanent prostate brachytherapy, radiofrequency ablation of tumors, and small field conformal radiation therapy.

Institutional features: The Mayo Clinic employs a comprehensive patient financial counseling system. First, patients are provided an estimate of costs and informed of financial support that could be provided by their insurance companies. Although fees tend to be higher than those in standard practice, the costs are well managed by the clinic's financial counseling system. Mayo Clinic also operates by group practice principles, which tend to reduce future health costs.

Rena C. Tabata, M.Sc.

▶ For Further Information

Braasch, W. F. *Early Days in the Mayo Clinic*. Springfield, Ill.: Thomas, 1969.

Sheperd, J. T. *Inside the Mayo Clinic: A Memoir*. Afton, Minn.: Afton Historical Society Press, 2003.

Wilder, L. *The Mayo Clinic*. New York: Harcourt, Brace, 1942.

▶ Other Resources

Mayo Clinic Cancer Center
http://cancercenter.mayo.edu/

National Cancer Institute
Cancer Centers Program: Mayo Clinic Cancer Center
http://cancercenters.cancer.gov/cancer_centers/mccc.html

See also American Association for Cancer Research (AACR); American Cancer Society (ACS); American Institute for Cancer Research (AICR); Dana-Farber Cancer Institute; Duke Comprehensive Cancer Center; Fox Chase Cancer Center; Fred Hutchinson Cancer Research Center; Jonsson Comprehensive Cancer Center (JCCC); M. D. Anderson Cancer Center; Memorial Sloan-Kettering Cancer Center; National Cancer Institute (NCI); National Science Foundation (NSF); Prevent Cancer Foundation; Robert H. Lurie Cancer Center.

▶ Mediastinal tumors

Category: Diseases, symptoms, and conditions
Also known as: Mediastinal neoplasias

Related conditions: Pericardial cysts, ectopic thyroid, bronchiogenic cysts

Definition: Mediastinal tumors are benign or malignant growths in the mediastinum, which is the central chest cavity that separates the lungs and contains the heart, aorta, esophagus, thymus, and trachea.

Risk factors: Risk factors include neurofibromatosis (von Recklinghausen disease), Li-Fraumeni syndrome, and a family history of Hodgkin disease.

Etiology and the disease process: The mediastinum is divided into the front, middle, and posterior mediastinum. The anterior mediastinum lies between the heart and the sternum. The middle mediastinum extends from the surface of the heart to the trachea (windpipe), and the posterior mediastinum begins behind the trachea and ends at the front of the vertebral column (backbone). Each mediastinal compartment is subject to specific types of tumors.

Anterior mediastinal tumors include tumors of the thymus (thymomas), lymphomas, teratomas, and thyroid tumors. Thymomas usually occur in adults, but 15 percent of them occur in children. Lymphomas account for 10 to 20 percent of anterior mediastinal tumors. Hodgkin disease causes most adult cases of mediastinal lymphomas.

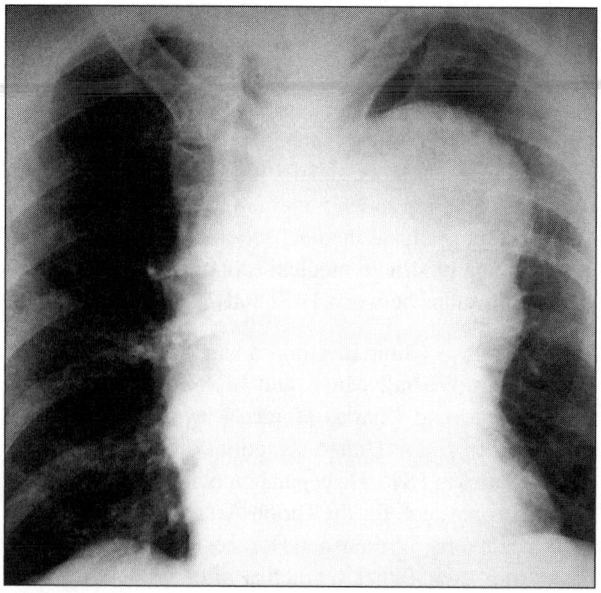

Mediastinal tumors. (LifeART© 2008 Wolters Kluwer Health, Inc.-Lippincott Williams &Wilkins. All rights reserved.)

Teratomas (germ-cell tumors) account for 10 to 15 percent of mediastinal tumors. Thyroid tumors grow from goiters and primarily occur in women.

Tumors of the middle mediastinum include lymphomas (most common), mesenchymal tumors, and carcinomas. Mesenchymal tumors account for 6 percent of primary mediastinal tumors and are also called soft-tissue tumors that originate in connective tissue within the chest (about half are malignant).

Neurogenic tumors (derived from nerve cells) are the most common tumors of the posterior mediastinum and include malignant schwannomas and neuroblastomas. Some 19 to 39 percent of mediastinal tumors are neurogenic and are usually benign in adults but malignant in children. Endocrine and mesenchymal tumors are also found in the posterior mediastinum.

Though typically diagnosed in people between the ages of thirty and fifty, mediastinal tumors can occur at any age and in any tissue that passes through the chest.

Incidence: Thymomas occur at a rate of 3 cases per million people per year. Lymphoblastic lymphomas in children occur at a rate of 6 cases per million. There are about 6 cases of mediastinal germ-cell tumors per million in children per year. Some 125 children per year in the United States are diagnosed with mediastinal neuroblastomas.

Symptoms: Half of mediastinal tumors produce no symptoms, but masses in the chest can compress other tissues and prevent proper functioning. The most common symptoms are cough, shortness of breath, and chest pain. Accompanying symptoms include trouble swallowing (dysphagia), chest pain, fever, chills, night sweats, coughing up blood (hemoptysis), hoarseness, unintentional weight loss, wheezing, tender or swollen lymph nodes (lymphadenopathy), and stridor (high-pitched, noisy respiration).

Between 35 and 50 percent of people with thymomas experience myasthenia gravis-like symptoms that include weakness of eye muscles, drooping of one or both eyelids (ptosis), and fatigue. Certain mediastinal tumors can produce neurotransmitters (catecholamines) that significantly raise blood pressure (hypertension). Other types of neurosarcomas can make insulinlike substances that can cause low blood sugar concentrations (hypoglycemia).

Blood work may show abnormally high levels of serum calcium (hypercalcemia) and abnormally low levels of antibodies (hypogammaglobulinemia), circulating blood cells (cytopenia), and normal red blood cells (pernicious anemia).

Screening and staging: Many different types of imaging tests can detect mediastinal tumors. Chest X rays are essential to determine the location of mediastinal tumors. Computed tomography (CT) and magnetic resonance imaging (MRI) scans are common imaging methods for detecting mediastinal masses. CT scans are also used to direct needle biopsies of potentially tumorous masses. Positron emission tomography (PET) scans are used to determine the spread of the tumor to other parts of the body. If the tumor is located in a difficult-to-reach spot, then laparoscopic surgery called mediastinoscopy is used to biopsy the mass.

Most mediastinal tumors are solid tumors, which are graded by TNM (tumor/lymph node/metastasis) staging. T refers to the primary tumor and grades it from 0 to 4. N specifies the spread of the cancer to nearby lymph nodes (ranked 0 to 3). M represents metastasis or spread of the tumor beyond the lymph nodes to other parts of the body (0 or 1).

Treatment and therapy: Thymomas are primarily treated with surgery, followed by radiation or chemotherapy. For lymphomas, chemotherapy followed by radiation is the treatment of choice. For neurogenic tumors, surgery is the treatment of choice. It is possible to surgically resection some mesenchymal tumors and radiation can help in some cases, but some fibrosarcomas are not treatable with surgery or chemotherapy. Malignant schwannomas are very aggressive tumors that require multiagent chemotherapy.

Prognosis, prevention, and outcomes: The outcome is highly dependent on the type of tumor. If untreated, the prognosis is very poor. If properly treated, the prognosis for thymomas, lymphomas, thyroid tumors, teratomas, and some neurogenic tumors is generally quite good. Mesenchymal tumors tend to have a poor prognosis.

Michael A. Buratovich, Ph.D.

▶ For Further Information

Duwe, Beau V., Daniel H. Sterman, and Ali I. Musani. "Tumors of the Mediastinum." *Chest* 128 (2005): 2893-2909.

Huang, Tsai-Wang, et al. "Middle Mediastinal Thymoma." *Respirology* 12, no. 6 (2007): 934-936.

Quint, Leslie E. "Imaging of Anterior Mediastinal Masses." *Cancer Imaging* 7 (2007): S56-S62.

Strollo, Diane C., Melissa L. Rosado de Christenson, and James R. Jett. "Primary Mediastinal Tumors: Part 1, Tumors of the Anterior Mediastinum." *Chest* 112 (1997): 511-522.

_______. "Primary Mediastinal Tumors: Part 2, Tumors of the Middle and Posterior Mediastinum." *Chest* 112 (1997): 1344-1357.

▶ **Other Resources**

American Cancer Society
http://www.cancer.org

National Cancer Institute
http://www.cancer.gov

See also Klinefelter syndrome and cancer; Lung cancers; Mediastinoscopy; Stent therapy; Superior vena cava syndrome; Surgical biopsies; Thoracoscopy.

▶ Mediastinoscopy

Category: Procedures
Also known as: Thoracoscopic mediastinal biopsy

Definition: Mediastinoscopy is an endoscopic procedure used to examine the mediastinum (space between and in front of the lungs). Compared to open-chest surgery, which requires one 6-inch to 8-inch incision, mediastinoscopy uses several small, 1-inch incisions to access the mediastinum, thereby minimizing trauma, decreasing postoperative pain, and promoting a shorter hospital stay and a quicker recovery.

Cancers diagnosed or treated: Sarcoidosis, lung cancer, lymphoma, Hodgkin disease, myasthenia gravis, mesothelioma, mediastinal or neurogenic tumors, thymomas

Why performed: Mediastinoscopy is performed with a biopsy to evaluate abnormal mediastinal tissue, lymph nodes, inflammation, or infection. It can be used as a staging procedure to evaluate non-small-cell lung cancer.

Mediastinoscopy is also used to remove malignant lymph nodes and mediastinal tumors. Benign and malignant mediastinal tumors that are not removed can interfere with the normal function of the organs in the mediastinum, including the aorta, vena cava, heart, and pericardium.

Patient preparation: Tests may include a chest X ray, computed tomography (CT) scan, and magnetic resonance imaging (MRI). One week before the procedure, patients must stop taking anticoagulants, as directed by the physician. In general, patients must not eat or drink for eight to ten hours before the procedure.

Steps of the procedure: A sedative may be given before the patient receives general anesthesia. A mediastinoscope (small videoscope) is inserted under the sternum through a small incision at the base of the neck. The mediastinoscope is manipulated, and images of the abnormal area are displayed on a computer screen to guide the surgeon during the procedure. CT may also be used during the procedure. Other surgical instruments are inserted through two or three small chest incisions, and a tissue sample is removed.

After the procedure: The hospital recovery is about one to two days, and some patients may be able to go home the day of the procedure. Before going home, the patient receives a follow-up schedule and aftercare instructions. The patient can generally return to normal activities within three to four weeks after discharge.

Risks: The risks of mediastinoscopy include bleeding, infection, allergic reaction to the anesthetic, blood vessel damage, a tear in the esophagus, laryngeal nerve injury that can cause permanent vocal hoarseness, or collapse of a lung (pneumothorax). The overall complication rate is reportedly low, at under 2.5 percent, with major complications under 0.5 percent and mortality under 0.5 percent.

Results: The biopsy tissue is examined for malignancy, inflammation, or infection. The type and extent of disease will help determine the patient's treatment.

Angela M. Costello, B.S.

See also Bronchoalveolar lung cancer; Endoscopy; Lung cancers; Mediastinal tumors; Mesothelioma; Pneumonectomy; Surgical biopsies; Thoracoscopy.

▶ Medical marijuana

Category: Social and personal issues

Definition: Medical marijuana involves use of the plant *Cannabis sativa*, and its chemical derivatives, for treating medical complaints and conditions.

In the United States, at the federal level, marijuana for medicinal purposes currently comes in the form of dronabinol (Marinol) and nabilone (Cesamet). Marinol comes in capsule form and is a synthetic version of delta-9-tetrahydrocannabinol (THC), the active ingredient in *Cannabis sativa*. Cesamet is a derivative of THC that also comes in pill form. Individuals also use marijuana in dried form, such as by eating it, smoking it, or using it in a vaporizing device, to attempt to achieve certain medicinal effects.

Access to medical marijuana: Federal law in the United States supports the use of Marinol and Cesamet but does not support the use of other forms of marijuana for medicinal purposes. There are some conflicts, however, between state and federal law in the United States. By 2008, twelve states had passed legislation legalizing medical marijuana in one way or another. In some cases, there were state-level rules governing possession of dried forms of the drug and/or plants in varying quantities for patients and care providers; in others, circumstances varied county by county. Many required users of medical marijuana to obtain the drug in certain ways and/or maintain registration for medical purposes. Rules varied from country to country as well. Holland, for instance, permitted use of marijuana by the public for any purpose in establishments called coffee shops. Even in Holland, however, there were strict guidelines on where it could be used, the amount permitted to be given to each user or to be present in each shop, and other matters, such as the impact of the coffee shop on the surrounding community.

Medicinal effects and uses: Marinol and Cesamet address appetite problems, as well as nausea and its associated vomiting. In terms of nausea, they are used typically in individuals undergoing chemotherapy for cancer, and particularly in individuals who have not responded to other forms of treatment for those conditions. In terms of appetite, they are used typically in clients with acquired immunodeficiency syndrome (AIDS) to combat a loss of appetite and its associated weight loss. Other, diverse conditions have been reported as potentially benefiting from medical marijuana, including Alzheimer's disease, anorexia, cancer, chronic or debilitating pain, cramping, Crohn disease, glaucoma, human immunodeficiency virus (HIV), multiple sclerosis, seizures, muscle spasms, and wasting syndrome (cachexia). This list does not include all conditions that varying state laws recognize as eligible for marijuana use. Many of the states that have legalized medical marijuana have, as part of the law, clauses that either allow the list of treatment-eligible conditions to be amended or are open-ended and subject to physician approval. Scientific reports continue to generate speculation about conditions that may receive benefit from treatment, such as depression. Use of marijuana for all of these conditions, however, remains the subject of great debate and is illegal in most states.

Controversies of medical marijuana: Despite the fact that synthetic THC and THC derivatives serve medical purposes, and despite the fact that twelve states allowed the use of marijuana for medicinal purposes as of 2008, medical marijuana is a controversial topic. Opponents of medical marijuana are quick to point out that Marinol and Cesamet exist as pharmaceuticals regulated by the Food and Drug Administration (FDA) and are adequate to cover the conditions most often treated with marijuana. Proponents of medical marijuana counter that those drugs do not work well for everyone and that they are only to be used for certain conditions. In the light of pain and suffering caused by other conditions, they argue, why not allow medical marijuana use? Again, opponents answer that other viable treatments exist that are better to try as treatment options, that the evidence for marijuana's efficacy in treating these other conditions is weak, and that there are strong social, physical, mental, and behavioral cons to the use of marijuana and its alternative forms.

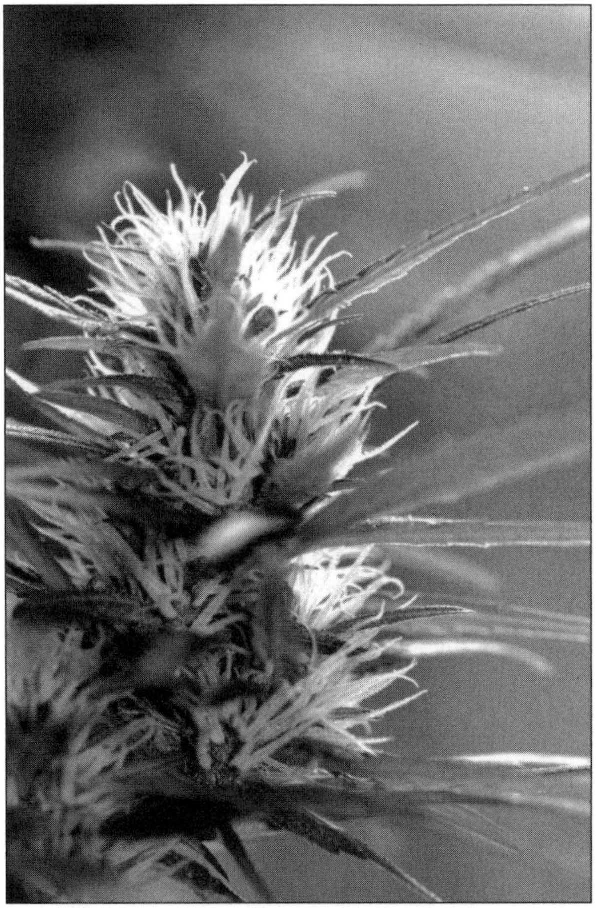

Cannabis sativa *in flower.* (©Gary Boisvert/Dreamstime.com)

Typical cons cited are posed in terms of short-term and long-term risks. In the short term, these may include memory and learning difficulties, panic, anxiety, coordination problems, and impaired problem solving. In the long term, these may include problems related to addiction, such as abuse or dependence, motivational problems, daily cough, phlegm problems, respiratory problems, impact on the immune system, and possibly cancer. Proponents argue that the pros outweigh the cons and that, despite evidence that some may consider weak, this method of treatment for such debilitating conditions deserves further study.

The debate continues, however, from state to state and country to country. Future studies focusing on the risk impacts of marijuana use are to be expected. Expanding the use of Marinol to other conditions may be on the horizon. The fight to allow studies examining the utility of marijuana for treating health conditions faces continued struggles in the United States and elsewhere.

Nancy A. Piotrowski, Ph.D.

▶ For Further Information

Earleywine, Mitch. *Understanding Marijuana: A New Look at the Scientific Evidence*. New York: Oxford University Press, 2002.

Gerber, Rudolph Joseph. *Legalizing Marijuana: Drug Policy Reform and Prohibition Politics*. Westport, Conn.: Praeger, 2004.

Rosenthal, Ed, and Steve Kubby. *Why Marijuana Should Be Legal*. New York: Thunder's Mouth Press, 2003.

Russo, Ethan B., and Franjo Frotenhermen, eds. *Handbook of Cannabis Therapeutics: From Bench to Bedside*. Binghamton, N.Y.: Haworth Press, 2006.

Russo, Ethan B., Melanie Dreher, and Mary Lynn Mathre, eds. *Women and Cannabis: Medicine, Science, and Sociology*. Binghamton, N.Y.: Haworth Press, 2002.

Selvanathan, Saroja, and Eliyathamby A. Selvanathan. *The Demand for Alcohol, Tobacco, and Marijuana: International Evidence*. Burlington, Vt.: Ashgate, 2005.

See also Antinausea medications; Appetite loss; Delta-9-tetrahydrocannabinol.

▶ Medical oncology

Category: Medical specialties
Also known as: Chemotherapy, immunotherapy, biological therapy

Definition: Medical oncology is the medical specialty for the treatment of cancerous diseases with chemotherapy, hormonal therapy, biological therapy, and other drugs. Medical oncology complements other cancer treatment modalities, including surgery, radiation therapy, rehabilitation, and palliative care. Medical oncologists are physicians who specialize in the assessment and management of patients with cancer and are trained to administer chemotherapy and other cancer medications. Medical oncology practices can be found in university medical centers, community hospitals, specialized cancer hospitals, and comprehensive cancer centers.

Subspecialties: Gynecological oncology, medical oncology/hematology, pediatric oncology/hematology, radiation oncology

Cancers treated: Various, especially blood-related cancers such as acute leukemia as well as gastric, breast, bladder, testicular, colorectal, lung, prostate, and ovarian cancers

Training and certification: Medical oncologists first obtain a four-year medical degree from an accredited program and board certification from the American Board of Internal Medicine, then complete a one-year internship in a clinical setting, followed by three years of postgraduate residency training in the use of medical and chemotherapeutic treatments of adult cancerous conditions. Oncology fellows who specialize in combined hematology and oncology receive an additional year of training.

Medical oncology fellows are eligible to take a Certification Exam in Medical Oncology, offered by the American Board of Internal Medicine, after completing a minimum of three years of successful training. They become certified as diplomates of the American Board of Internal Medicine after passing this exam. Once certified, medical oncologists may further their training by participating in one or more years of clinical or laboratory research.

Medical oncologists are trained in the basic science and clinical expression of cancer in adults. They are involved in patient care, teaching, and research. They study the etiology of cancer as well as its evaluation, diagnosis, and management in ambulatory and hospitalized patients. Medical oncologists acquire experience in treating a wide variety of neoplastic diseases and in managing the entire spectrum of medical complications of cancer and its treatments. Specific areas of study include chemotherapy, surgery, radiation therapy, and biological therapy. Medical oncologists may specialize in certain types of cancer or certain therapies such as immunotherapy, but they have the expertise to treat all forms of cancer with a variety of drug therapies.

Oncology clinical practice guidelines, quality care standards, and quality assurance measures in the United States have been established primarily by the American Society of Clinical Oncology (ASCO), a nonprofit organization representing more than 25,000 cancer professionals worldwide. It offers scientific and educational programs and a wide range of initiatives to promote the exchange of cancer information. ASCO publishes clinical practice guidelines and the National Initiative on Cancer Care Quality, which includes quality-of-care indicators. It also supports the Quality Oncology Practice Initiative, an oncologist-led, practice-based quality improvement program to promote excellence in cancer care.

Services and procedures performed: A medical oncologist is often the main health care provider for adults diagnosed with cancer. The medical oncologist plans and coordinates the diagnosis and treatment of new or recurrent malignancies. Oncologists coordinate the patient's diagnostic tests, develop a treatment plan, determine the appropriate systemic or adjunctive drug regimen to treat the patient's condition, and supervise the dosage, schedule, and administration of cancer drugs to treat localized or metastatic malignancies. Medical oncologists also develop cancer treatment protocols, participate in clinical trials and research, and ensure that quality standards for chemotherapy delivery are followed.

Medical oncologists are part of a multidisciplinary team of cancer health care providers whose goals are to provide early detection; accurately diagnose the condition; offer prompt, appropriate treatment to improve quality of life and survival; provide psychological guidance through complex treatment phases; reduce long-term effects of chemotherapy and radiation therapy; and provide long-term follow-up. Medical oncologists are trained in chemotherapy drug indications and toxicities so that they can safely administer these therapies while minimizing side effects and appropriately managing complications.

Related specialties and subspecialties: Medical oncologists work with a multidisciplinary team that includes the primary care physician and other specialists, such as clinical oncologists; oncologist surgeons including urologic surgeons, orthopedic surgeons and neurosurgeons; diagnostic radiologists; radiation oncologists; infectious disease specialists; pathologists; oncology nurses; physical therapists; and oncology social workers and other allied health care professionals, such as educational specialists, registered dietitians, and pharmacologists.

Communication between the medical oncologist and the patient's primary care physician is essential to ensure the continuum of care. Medical oncologists consult with radiation oncologists and oncologist surgeons so that chemotherapy can be combined with radiation and surgery to ensure the best outcome for the patient.

Oncologist surgeons use surgical techniques such as laparoscopy and thoracoscopy to diagnose and treat cancers. They first obtain a four-year medical degree from an accredited program and board certification from the American Board of Surgery, then complete five years of residency training in an accredited general surgery program and at least two years of fellowship training in oncological surgery.

Diagnostic radiologists obtain and interpret medical images to determine what disease the patieint has. They obtain a four-year medical degree from an accredited program and board certification from the American Board of Radiology or the American Osteopathic Board of Radiology, then must pass a licensing examination and complete at least four years of residency training in an accredited radiology program.

Radiation oncologists, also known as clinical oncologists, treat cancers using radiation. In the United States, most radiation oncologists complete residency training in radiation oncology in a program approved by the American Council of Graduate Medical Education or the American Board of Radiology.

Infectious disease specialists are physicians who concentrate on the diagnosis and treatment of infectious diseases. Their training consits of a four-year medical degree from an accredited program, board certification from the American Board of Pediatrics, three or more years of residency training, and two to three years of additional training in infectious diseases.

Pathologists are physicians who specialize in the pathology of hematologic malignancies and solid tumors. They use immunochemistry and molecular techniques to assess malignancies. Their training consists of a four-year medical degree from an accredited program, board certification from the American Board of Internal Medicine, three or more years of residency training, and one to two years of additional training in pathology.

The Oncology Nurses Society facilitates the professional development of oncology nurses. Oncology nurses educate patients and family, provide medical care, and administer medications. Oncology clinical nurse specialists are registered nurses with a master's degree in oncology nursing. They understand treatment protocols and how to manage treatment complications and prepare and administer medications, including chemotherapy. Oncology nurse practitioners are registered nurses with a master's or doctoral degree.

Angela M. Costello, B.S.

▶ For Further Information

Abeloff, M. D., et al. *Clinical Oncology*. 3d ed. Edinburgh, Scotland: Churchill Livingstone, 2004.

Cavalli, F., et al., eds. *Textbook of Medical Oncology*. 3d ed. New York: Informa Healthcare, 2004.

Kantarjian, H. M., et al. *The M. D. Anderson Manual of Medical Oncology*. New York: McGraw-Hill, 2006.

▶ **Organizations and Professional Societies**

American Board of Internal Medicine
http://www.abim.org

American Society of Clinical Oncology
http://www.asco.org
1900 Duke Street, Suite 200
Alexandria, VA 22314

National Comprehensive Cancer Network
http://www.nccn.org
275 Commerce Drive, Suite 200
Fort Washington, PA 19034

Oncology Nurses Society
http://www.ons.org
125 Enterprise Drive
Pittsburgh, PA 15275

▶ **Other Resources**

CancerCare
http://www.cancercare.org

Cancer.Net
http://www.cancer.net/portal/site/patient

Chemocare.com
http://www.chemocare.com

National Cancer Institute
Chemotherapy and You: Support for People with Cancer
http://www.cancer.gov/cancertopics/chemotherapy-and-you

See also Dermatology oncology; Endocrinology oncology; Gastrointestinal oncology; Gynecologic oncology; Hematologic oncology; Molecular oncology; Neurologic oncology; Occupational therapy; Oncology; Oncology clinical nurse specialist; Oncology social worker; Pediatric oncology and hematology; Pharmacy oncology; Psycho-oncology; Radiation oncology; Surgical oncology; Urologic oncology; Veterinary oncology; Viral oncology.

▶ Medicare and cancer

Category: Social and personal issues

Definition: Medicare is the health insurance program of the United States government for people aged sixty-five or older and for younger citizens who have specific disabilities or end-stage renal disease (ESRD), a condition in which the person has permanent kidney failure and requires dialysis or transplant.

History: The Medicare program has affected the lives of millions of Americans since President Lyndon B. Johnson signed into law the Medicare bill of 1965. The roots of this universal health care coverage for seniors and the disabled reach back to 1935, when the federal government introduced the first government health insurance bill. In 1945 President Harry S. Truman became the first president to endorse government health insurance for the elderly and would become the first person to enroll twenty-one years later, receiving the first issued Medicare card.

In 1972 benefits for disabled and end-stage renal disease (ESDR) patients were added. The Supplemental Security Income (SSI) program came next, and then benefits for hospice were added temporarily in 1982 and confirmed permanent in 1986. With the threat of budgetary problems, the diagnosis-related group (DRG) prospective payment system began in 1983. Until that time, Medicare reimbursed for most covered medical charges that were of a "reasonable cost." Several other changes evolved over time, including provisions for Medicare health maintenance organizations (HMOs) and the voluntary Part D outpatient prescription drug program, available to beneficiaries in 2006.

Medicare is funded by the Social Security Administration. To receive benefits, participants must have paid into the plan through their employers. The Medicare budget is about 10 percent of the entire budget of the Unites States government. In the mid-2000's, about 40 million Americans were receiving health insurance under the Medicare program.

Medicare basics: The Medicare program is divided into several parts. Part A is hospital insurance and covers inpatient stays with some follow-up costs after hospitalization. Also covered is care in a skilled nursing facility. Part B is medical insurance and pays for physicians, nurse practitioners, and outpatient services. Part C offers several plans as options, and Part D covers outpatient prescription drugs. Anyone who has worked and paid into the social security plan has the Part A benefit, but Parts B and D are optional, provided for a monthly fee. For some benefits, the Medicare patient must meet annual deductibles before full plan coverage takes place.

Medicare is less comprehensive than many private insurance plans available to younger Americans. Many seniors opt to pay for secondary insurance coverage to pay the difference or gap in Medicare coverage for provision of needed services. Unfortunately, the high costs of many therapies and drugs have left many seniors and disabled persons without adequate insurance coverage and without access to new modalities of treatment.

Coverage for cancer prevention and screening: In 2005, the Centers for Medicare and Medicaid Services (CMS) launched two national decisions for improving the care of cancer patients. Insurance coverage was expanded to include diagnostic tests and chemotherapy treatments for Medicare beneficiaries. One part of the preventive program is coverage for a "Welcome to Medicare" physical examination. This one-time benefit is designed to reduce the risk of serious health problems in the future.

Other services are now covered as preventive health. For example, research shows that breast cancer risk increases with age. To screen for breast cancer, annual mammograms with digital technology are covered for all women the age of forty or older on Medicare. Any Medicare recipient between the ages of thirty-five and thirty-nine receives one baseline mammogram. The participant pays 20 percent of the Medicare-approved amount with no Part B deductible.

Cervical cancer screening is provided through a Pap smear and pelvic examination (with breast examination) every twenty-four months. If the participant has an established high risk for cervical or vaginal cancer, arrangements can be made for these tests each year. The Pap test itself is covered, but the participant pays 20 percent of the Medicare-approved cost with no Part B deductible.

Discovery of precancerous polyps (growths in the colon) and removal can decrease the incidence of colon cancer. Medicare participants the age of fifty or older and at average risk for colorectal cancer are allowed fecal occult blood tests every year, flexible sigmoidoscopy once every four years, colonoscopy once every ten years (but not within four years of a sigmoidoscopy), and barium enema once every four years (instead of a colonoscopy or sigmoidoscopy). If the age fifty or older Medicare recipient is at high risk for cancer, the colonoscopy is provided every two years and barium enema once every two years (instead of the colonoscopy or sigmoidoscopy). The fecal test is free but for other tests, the Medicare recipient pays 20 percent of the Medicare-approved amount after meeting the annual Part B deductible. The flexible sigmoidoscopy or colonoscopy costs 25 percent of Medicare-covered charges if done on an outpatient basis.

The last cancer-screening procedure included in Medicare is the prostate cancer test for men over the age of fifty. Coverage includes a digital exam and prostate-specific antigen (PSA) test every year or more often if needed for diagnostic purposes. The digital exam requires a 20 percent copay with no coinsurance or Part B deductible for the PSA.

Coverage in clinical trials: Medicare offers members more choices to participate in clinical trials for the diagnosis and treatment of cancer. In a clinical trial, research is conducted with participants to improve new ways of providing quality and effective cancer care. Participants have access to promising new therapies as researchers find better and more effective ways to treat cancer. Many positives can come from participation, including being the first to benefit from a new treatment, gaining access to new treatments not available to the general public, having access to high-quality physician specialists, and helping future patients. The less attractive part of clinical trials is that new drugs may have unknown side effects, the new treatment may be less effective than the traditional one, and being in a clinical trial may require more doctor visits.

Although clinical trials are not for everyone, Medicare recipients now have choices with assurance of insurance coverage. To be covered, clinical trials must be funded by the National Cancer Institute (NCI) or NCI-sponsored groups.

Medicare Modernization Act: The Medicare Modernization Act of 2006 provided prescription drug coverage for Medicare recipients as Medicare Part D coverage. Drugs listed on the approved formulary are covered in this voluntary plan. Key drugs needed by cancer patients such as oral chemotherapy, immunotherapy, and hormonal therapy are covered. Other useful medications on this plan are drugs for the side effects of cancer treatments such as nausea and low blood counts.

The plan is administered by diverse companies with variation in coverage, deductibles, and out-of-pocket expenses. Medicare patients have options but need to research which plan is best for them. It is recommended that Medicare participants keep a complete updated list of their prescription drugs and ask if a less expensive brand is available that is as effective. Local Social Security Offices have information to help participants compare plans to meet specific needs.

Even with Medicare drug insurance, medications used by the cancer patient can be expensive. Sometimes state pharmaceutical assistance programs provide additional assistance to complement Medicare coverage. Sometimes the cancer patient can qualify for a low-income subsidy through Social Security. The oncology social worker can assist the participant to identify ways to get help for drug coverage and other services.

Robert W. Koch, D.N.S., R.N.

▶ For Further Information

Field, Marilyn J., Robert L. Lawrence, and Lee Zwanziger, eds. *Extending Medicare Coverage for Preventive and*

Other Services. Washington, D.C.: National Academy Press, 2000.

Muller, Charlotte, et al. *Costs and Effectiveness of Cervical Screening in Elderly Women*. Washington, D.C.: Office of Technology Assessment, 1990.

U.S. Congress. Office of Technology Assessment. *Breast Cancer Screening for Medicare Beneficiaries*. Washington, D.C.: Author, 1987.

_______. *Cost and Effectiveness of Prostate Screening in Elderly Men*. Washington, D.C.: Author, 1995.

▶ Other Resources

AARP

Centers for Medicare and Medicaid Services
http://www.cms.hhs.gov

Medicare
http://www.medicare.gov

AARP.org
Medicare Prescription Drug Coverage
http://www.aarp.org/research/medicare/drugs/

Medicare Rights Center
http://www.medicarerights.org

Social Security Online
http://www.ssa.gov

State Health Insurance Assistance Programs
http://www.shiptalk.org

See also Advance directives; Aging and cancer; Elderly and cancer; Financial issues; Health maintenance organizations (HMOs); Insurance; Managed care; Preferred provider organizations (PPOs); Second opinions; Social Security Disability Insurance (SSDI).

▶ Medullary carcinoma of the breast

Category: Diseases, symptoms, and conditions
Also known as: Infiltrating breast cancer

Definition: Medullary carcinoma is a rare but invasive breast cancer distinguished microscopically by a well-defined boundary, presence of cells from the immune system at its edges, and large, misshapen cancer cells.

Related conditions: Familial breast cancer

Risk factors: Medullary breast carcinoma is more frequent in women with a genetic predisposition. Mutations in tumor-suppressor genes, whether genetic or unknown in origin, can prevent their normal function of suppressing abnormal growth. This mutation occurs at the *BRCA1* and *BRCA2* genes. In some studies, medullary carcinomas account for up to 19 percent of all cancers in women with a *BRCA1* mutation. In women with a family history of reproductive-system cancers, smoking increases breast cancer risk significantly.

Estrogen can stimulate breast cancers. Changes in deoxyribonucleic acid (DNA), which carries the instructions for all cells, can cause normal cells to become cancerous, and such changes are more likely to occur with age.

Etiology and the disease process: Estrogen exposure tends to encourage breast cancer, and hormones can boost breast cancer growth. Gene mutations can inhibit the body's defenses.

Incidence: These infrequent cancers make up 2 to 7 percent of breast cancer cases.

Symptoms: Most cancers start without symptoms, detectable if at all by only mammography or ultrasound. As the cancer develops, a lump or thickening may begin. An unusual lump in the breast or armpit area, one that feels firm or unlike other breast tissue, or a lump that seems "fixed" and immobile, needs to be investigated.

Screening and diagnosis: Medullary carcinomas are distinguishable by histology (microscopic examination). Monthly self-examination and regular mammography increase early detection. Staging for medullary carcinomas is as follows:

- Stage I: Cancerous cells have invaded nearby tissue.
- Stage II: Cancerous cells are in lymph nodes in the armpit.
- Stage III: Cancerous cells have invaded lymph nodes, breastbone, and other tissues above the waist.

Treatment and therapy: Treatment is the same as for invasive ductal carcinoma: usually a combination of local therapy (affecting only the cancer site, such as surgery and radiation) and systemic therapy using drugs (chemotherapy, hormone therapy, and immunotherapy), either by mouth or intravenously, to kill cancer cells that might have spread elsewhere but are not yet detectable.

Prognosis, prevention, and outcomes: When caught early, medullary breast cancers are curable and prognosis is good, with 70 percent of patients surviving for ten years. Good, balanced nutrition with avoidance of dietary fat and a healthy lifestyle that avoids smoking and includes exercise are among the best strategies for decreasing the chance of developing cancer.

Jackie Dial, Ph.D.

See also *BRCA1* and *BRCA2* genes; Breast cancer in men; Breast cancer in pregnant women; Breast cancers; Carcinomatosis; Invasive ductal carcinomas; Invasive lobular carcinomas.

▶ Medulloblastomas

Category: Diseases, symptoms, and conditions

Related conditions: Supratentorial primitive neuroectodermal tumors, neurofibromatosis (von Recklinghausen disease), Gorlin syndrome

Definition: Medulloblastomas are malignant (cancerous) or benign (noncancerous) tumors that form in the cerebellum of the brain. The cerebellum controls balance and movement, posture, and speech. These tumors occur more often in children but may rarely appear in adults.

Risk factors: There is no known cause of medulloblastomas, but, scientists are uncovering changes in genes and chromosomes that may influence the development of these tumors. A small percentage of tumors may tend to occur in families, particularly in families with neurofibromatosis (von Recklinghausen disease), an inherited disease that causes benign tumors to occur on peripheral nerves in the body. A few individuals with Gorlin syndrome, an inherited disease related to basal cell carcinoma and other conditions, also develop medulloblastoma.

Etiology and the disease process: Medulloblastoma is a relatively rare disease, with no known cause other than a familial tendency. The tumor is considered fast growing. Because of the location of the tumor, walking and talking disruptions are common as the disease progresses.

Incidence: The tumor occurs more often in boys than girls, and generally before the age of eight, with a peak incidence between five and ten years of age. In the United States, the incidence of medulloblastoma is 1.5 to 2 cases per 100,000 population (children). Approximately 1,000 cases are diagnosed annually, with 1 in 5 brain tumors in children diagnosed as medulloblastoma.

Symptoms: The classic, initial symptoms of medulloblastoma are morning headaches, nausea, vomiting, and other flulike symptoms. Because the symptoms mimic flu, the tumor may go undiagnosed until symptoms progress to balance problems. Older children may be more easily diagnosed than infants, as infants may initially exhibit an increase in head size and irritability, both common in infants as they grow and develop. Vomiting may make the person feel better, as the intracranial pressure is temporarily relieved. Symptoms increase as the tumor grows.

Screening and diagnosis: There is no screening test for medulloblastoma. Diagnosis begins with a history of symptoms and neurological examination. Radiology studies include magnetic resonance imaging (MRI), including the use of a contrast dye, to identify the presence of a brain tumor, and a positron emission tomography (PET) scan, used to determine if the tumor is active and growing. Other procedures, such as a lumbar puncture to take cerebrospinal fluid (CSF), a bone marrow aspiration and biopsy, and a bone scan, may be done to look for signs of cancer. A confirmed diagnosis is made during surgery, and pathologic examination of the tumor specimen removed determines if the tumor is benign or malignant.

Two risk groups are used in childhood medulloblastoma to determine treatment management, rather than the adult staging process. The average risk group and the poor risk group are differentiated based on the tumor remaining after surgery, spread of cancer cells within the brain and spinal cord, or distant spread of tumor cells to other parts of the body. Adults are staged based on the remaining tumor and whether the tumor has spread using the TNM (tumor/lymph node/metastasis) staging system.

Treatment and therapy: Treatment of medulloblastoma is with surgery, radiation therapy, chemotherapy, and, if necessary, mechanical diversion of cerebrospinal fluid with a shunt to carry blocked fluid out of the brain. Surgery is used to remove as much of the tumor as possible. Imaging studies may show that the tumor is inoperable. A bi-

Relative Survival Rates for Medulloblastoma, 1988-2001

Years	*Survival Rate (%)*
1	89.2
2	84.6
3	78.4
5	66.4
8	56.8
10	52.5

Source: Data from L. A. G. Ries et al., eds., *Cancer Survival Among Adults: U.S. SEER Program, 1988-2001—Patient and Tumor Characteristics*, NIH Pub. No. 07-6215 (Bethesda, Md.: National Cancer Institute, 2007)

opsy will still be done to determine the type of tumor and whether it is malignant. If the tumor has grown into the brain stem, removal may not be an option, as the side effects of removal are life-threatening. Steroids are used to decrease swelling in the brain. A shunt, or tube to drain CSF away from the brain, usually to the abdomen, may be placed during surgery. Radiation therapy to the brain and the spinal cord is then used to kill any cells remaining. Radiation may be done with stereotactic radiosurgery, intensity-modulated radiation therapy, or external beam radiation. Chemotherapy may be used in infants to postpone the use of radiation, as cranial radiation side effects may be severe. Chemotherapy may be given either intravenously (into a vein) or intrathecally (into the cerebrospinal fluid) by use of an Ommaya reservoir. In adults, chemotherapy effectiveness is less clear.

Prognosis, prevention, and outcomes: The prognosis for medulloblastoma varies with the patient's age at diagnosis, the size of the tumor, the amount remaining after surgery, and the level of tumor cell spread to other sites in the brain, spinal cord, or elsewhere in the body (metastasis). Approximately 70 percent of adults are alive at five years after diagnosis, and up to 80 percent of children with average-risk classification can be expected to reach five years. With poor risk classification, up to 65 percent of children may survive to five years. The outcome for infants is poor, with a 30 to 50 percent survival. There is no prevention for medulloblastoma. Quality of life may be negatively affected by the side effects of therapy, including learning disabilities, hearing loss from drug therapy, obesity, thyroid deficiency, and other problems depending on treatment and site. Recurrence is always a risk as tumors may be difficult to remove completely.

Patricia Stanfill Edens, R.N., Ph.D., FACHE

▶ For Further Information

Hargrave, D. R., and S. Zacharoulis. "Pediatric CNS Tumors: Current Treatment and Future Directions." *Expert Review of Neurotherapeutics* 7, no. 8 (August, 2007): 1029-1042.

Parker, W., E. Filion, D. Roberge, and C. R. Freeman. "Intensity-Modulated Radiotherapy for Craniospinal Irradiation: Target Volume Considerations, Dose Constraints, and Competing Risks." *International Journal of Radiation Oncology, Biology, Physics* 69, no. 1 (September 1, 2007): 251-257.

▶ Other Resources

American Brain Tumor Association
http://www.abta.org

American Cancer Society
http://www.cancer.org

National Cancer Institute
Childhood Medulloblastoma Treatment
http://www.cancer.gov/cancertopics/pdq/treatment/childmedulloblastoma/patient/

See also Brain and central nervous system cancers; Craniotomy; Neuroectodermal tumors; Turcot syndrome.

▶ Melanomas

Category: Diseases, symptoms, and conditions
Also known as: Skin cancer

Related conditions: Basal cell cancer, squamous cell cancer

Definition: Melanomas are malignant tumors of the skin that occur in the melanocytes, the cells that produce melanin (skin pigment).

Risk factors: Melanomas occur most commonly in fair-skinned people, particularly natural blonds and redheads, especially those with a history of sun exposure or multiple serious sunburns. A history of serious sunburns in childhood is a particular risk. Risk for the disease is strongly related to having a family history; which is characteristic of about 1 in 10 of patients with melanoma. Additional risk factors include large or multiple moles and past personal history of melanoma or of less serious skin cancers, known as basal cell or squamous cell cancers. People with diseases that suppress the immune system are at added risk for melanoma. Occupational exposure to coal tar, pitch, creosote, arsenic compounds, or radium increase a person's risk for the disease. Celtic descent, male gender, and older age are also risk factors.

Etiology and the disease process: Repeat exposure to harmful ultraviolet rays from the sun or artificial sources such as sunlamps or tanning booths appears to be the most significant factor contributing to the development of melanoma. This is borne out by the fact that the incidence of melanoma increases in the lower latitudes of the world where the sun is strongest. Additionally, in parts of the world where the ozone layer is thin, the incidence is higher. In Queensland, Australia, for example, where there is a hole in the ozone, between 1979 to 1987, the rate of melanoma doubled to 55.8 per 100,000 men and rose to 42.9 per 100,000 women.

Melanomas can occur on parts of the body not usually

exposed to the sun, including the soles of the feet and the genitals. Melanoma starts with an abnormal skin growth, which is generally quite small. When discovered at this early stage, melanomas can be easily removed and the cancer cured. If the growth is not removed, it thickens and invades surrounding tissue and nearby lymph nodes. The cancer can then spread through the lymph nodes to sites distant from the original growth, including vital organs, soft tissues, and other lymph nodes.

Incidence: In the 1970's, the incidence rate of melanoma rose dramatically to about 6 percent a year. Incidence continues to rise but at a slower rate; from 1981 to 2001 the rate of growth was about 3 percent a year.

The American Cancer Society estimated that 59,940 men and women in the United States would be newly diagnosed with melanoma in 2007. Melanoma affects adults of all ages as well as teenagers. Based on statistics for the years 2001 to 2003, the probability of a man in the United States developing melanoma is 1 in 49. For a woman in the United States, the probability is 1 in 73. Rates for whites are ten times higher than for African Americans. However, one type of melanoma, which develops on the palms of the hands, soles of the feet, and nail beds, occurs more frequently in African Americans and Asians.

Symptoms: Melanoma generally first appears as a new mole or a change in the shape, size, or color of an existing mole. The American Cancer Society describes the warning signals in terms of a mnemonic: ABCD. "A" for asymmetry, meaning that the mole is not uniformly round; "B" for border, in that the edges of the mole are irregular; "C" for color, referring to the varied colors (generally in tones of tan, brown, and black) throughout the mole; and "D" for diameter, meaning that the mole is larger than 6 millimeters (mm).

Screening and diagnosis: People with serious risk factors or symptoms should have regular full body exams by a dermatologist to identify any skin abnormalities, and baseline photographs should be taken so that any changes can be tracked. Suspect moles or skin abnormalities should be removed and analyzed for cancer cells.

Incidence of Melanoma per 100,000 People, by Gender

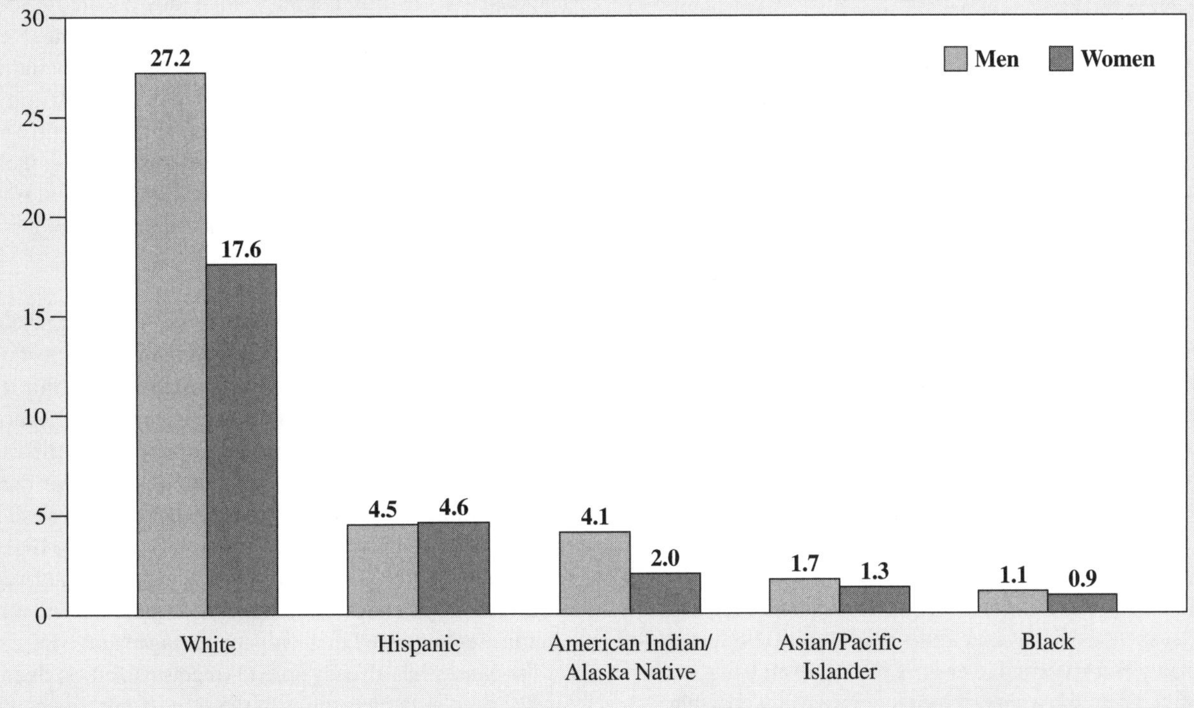

Source: Data from National Cancer Institute, Surveillance Epidemiology and End Results, Cancer Stat Fact Sheets, 2008
Note: Based on cases diagnosed in 2000-2004

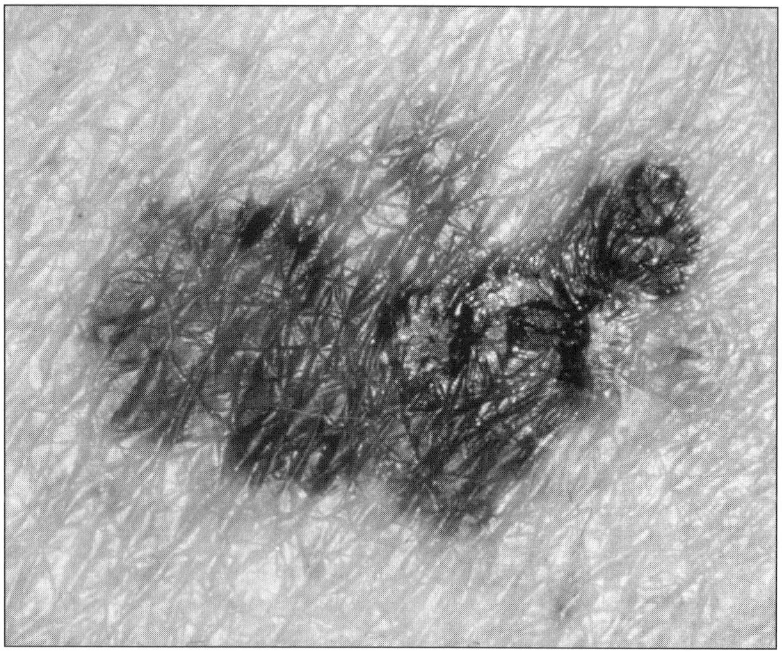

Melanoma. (National Cancer Institute)

The stages of melanoma are defined as follows:

- Localized, Stage 0: These melanomas involve only the top layer of skin, the epidermis.
- Localized, Stages I and II: These melanomas involve the underlying layer of skin, the dermis, and are rated according to the depth they penetrate the skin (known as the Breslow depth) and their degree of ulceration (how much the epidermis is eroded and exposes the dermis below). Ulceration is determined by a pathologist, using a microscope.
- Regional, Stage III: These melanomas include those in which the cancer has spread to nearby lymph nodes.
- Advanced, Stage IV: These melanomas include those where cancer has spread beyond the region of the skin growth to distant sites in the body, including internal organs and distant lymph nodes.

Treatment and therapy: Significant advances have been made in the early detection of melanoma. All suspect moles or skin growths should be removed and tested for cancerous cells. Removal of localized growths (Stages 0-II) can be done one of three ways: surgically, cutting out the suspect tissue; by electrodessication and curettage, using an electric current to destroy the tissue and then scraping the area with a special tool to remove any possible remaining cancer cells; or by cryosurgery, which freezes the tissue. About 83 percent of melanomas are diagnosed in these early stages while the cancer is still confined to the primary skin growth. Surgery successfully removes the cancer for the majority of patients with early-stage melanoma. In some cases, radiation therapy may be directed at the area following surgery to kill any cancer cells that may remain. Patients with Stages 0 to II melanoma have an excellent prognosis.

If the growth is extensive, the surgeon will remove lymph nodes to determine if the cancer has spread. After their removal, Stage III and IV melanomas may be treated with radiation or immunotherapy (agents that attempt to harness the human body's own disease-fighting properties to kill cancer cells) or chemotherapy (toxic agents targeted to kill cancer cells). Two therapeutic agents approved by the U.S. Food and Drug Administration (FDA) for the treatment of Stage III and IV melanoma are dacarbazine (DTIC, chemotherapy) and interleukin-2 (IL-2, immunotherapy). Some patients with Stage III and IV disease experience a full recovery with chemotherapy; however, positive responses to the drug therapy, when they occur, are most often partial and brief. Much research is being done to explore other possible treatments for melanoma, including combinations of different chemotherapies and new immunotherapies. Some of these agents are not specifically approved by the FDA to treat melanoma. Patients with melanoma may be eligible to become subjects in clinical trials in which these experimental agents or combinations of agents are tested.

Prognosis, prevention, and outcomes: The thickness of a patient's tumor is the best single indicator of the prognosis. After having melanomas of less than 0.76 mm removed, about 96 to 99 percent of patients are cured. About 1 in 10 patients with melanoma is diagnosed after the cancer has already spread to nearby lymph nodes. For these patients in the regional stage (Stage III), the prognosis is not as good, but survival rates for patients with Stage III disease range widely, depending on how many lymph nodes are affected by the cancer. About 3 of 10 patients with melanoma are diagnosed in an advanced stage (Stage IV), after the cancer has already spread (metastasized) to distant sites. Those with metastases to the skin or soft tissue or to distant lymph nodes appear to fare better than those with lung or other vital organ metastases.

Recommended measures to prevent melanoma include

avoiding excessive direct sunshine, especially during the hours when the sun is high in the sky (from about 10 A.M. to 2 P.M.); using sunscreen and protective clothing to prevent sunburn; and not using sunlamps; tanning booths, or other artificial sources of ultraviolet light. People should become familiar with the moles and spots on their bodies and report any changes that could indicate melanoma to their doctors.

Charlotte Crowder, M.P.H., ELS

▶ For Further Information

Kaufman, Howard. *The Melanoma Book: A Complete Guide to Prevention and Treatment*. New York: Gotham Books, 2005.

Poole, Catherine M., and I. V. DuPont Guerry. *Melanoma: Prevention, Detection, and Treatment*. 2d ed. New Haven, Conn.: Yale University Press, 2005.

Schofield, Jill R., and William A. Robinson. *What You Really Need to Know About Moles and Melanoma*. Baltimore: Johns Hopkins University Press, 2000.

▶ Other Resources

Melanoma Center
http://www.melanomacenter.org

Melanoma Research Foundation
http://www.melanoma.org/

National Cancer Institute
Melanoma
http://www.cancer.gov/cancertopics/types/melanoma

Skin Cancer Foundation
Melanoma
http://www.skincancer.org/melanoma/index.php

See also Breslow's staging; Dermatology oncology; Dysplastic nevus syndrome; Merkel cell carcinomas (MCC); Moles; Premalignancies; Risks for cancer; Skin cancers; Squamous cell carcinomas; Sunlamps.

▶ Melphalan

Category: Carcinogens and suspected carcinogens
RoC status: Known human carcinogen since 1980
Also known as: Alkeran

Related cancers: Acute leukemia

Definition: Melphalan is a highly toxic anticancer drug that belongs to a family of drugs known as alkylating agents. It is a derivative of nitrogen mustard.

Exposure routes: Orally or by intravenous injection as part of medical treatment. Skin contact or dust inhalation is possible during the manufacturing process and in handling of the drug during preparation and administration.

Where found: Used in the treatment of various cancers including multiple myeloma and ovarian and breast cancer

At risk: People who have been previously treated with melphalan alone or in association with other chemotherapy drugs; health professionals (nurses, pharmacists, physicians) who handle the drug during preparation, administration, and cleanup; workers involved in the manufacturing process. The general population is not considered to be at risk.

Etiology and symptoms of associated cancers: Melphalan is used to treat cancer but can itself cause a secondary cancer as a long-term side effect. It is a cytotoxic drug that affects the growth of cancer cells by interfering with the deoxyribonucleic acid (DNA) within the cells. It is the damage to cellular DNA that can lead to a secondary cancer months or years after treatment with melphalan. Studies of melphalan (and other alkalating agents) indicate that the risk of secondary leukemia increases with the cumulative dose and chronicity of treatment. In one study, the ten-year cumulative risk of developing acute leukemia or myeloproliferative syndrome after melphalan therapy was 19.5 percent for cumulative doses ranging from 730 to 9,652 milligrams (mg). In this same study, as well as in an additional study, the ten-year cumulative risk of developing acute leukemia or myeloproliferative syndrome after melphalan therapy was less than 2 percent for cumulative doses under 600 mg. However, there is no known cumulative dose below which there is no risk of developing a secondary malignancy. The symptoms of secondary acute leukemia include recurrent infections, bone and joint pain, swollen lymph nodes, and shortness of breath.

History: The nitrogen mustards were developed as a derivative of sulfur mustard gas, which was first used as a weapon of war in 1917. Observation of military personnel exposed to sulfur mustard showed that it lowered the white blood cell count. Drugs derived from nitrogen mustard, such as melphalan, were introduced into the clinical setting in 1946.

Melanie Hawkins, B.S.N., R.N., O.C.N.

See also Hyperthermic perfusion; Multiple myeloma.

▶ Memorial Sloan-Kettering Cancer Center

Category: Organizations

Also known as: New York Cancer Hospital, Memorial Hospital for the Treatment of Cancer and Allied Diseases, MSKCC

Definition: The Memorial Sloan-Kettering Cancer Center, developed from the initial U.S. cancer hospital, provides comprehensive oncology treatment and research. Its four campuses are located in Manhattan; Basking Ridge, New Jersey; Long Island; and Westchester.

History: The Memorial Sloan-Kettering Cancer Center originated as the New York Cancer Hospital in Manhattan. In 1880, physician J. Marion Sims demanded the establishment of a local cancer hospital after Women's Hospital administrators prevented him from admitting cancer patients. Philanthropists funded a medical facility specifically for cancer, which started treating patients in 1887. Twelve years later, that facility was renamed General Memorial Hospital for the Treatment of Cancer and Allied Diseases.

In 1936 John D. Rockefeller gave land for construction of a new Memorial Hospital. Alfred P. Sloan, Jr., and Charles Franklin Kettering financed the Sloan-Kettering Institute (SKI) to conduct medical research next to that hospital. In 1980, SKI and Memorial Hospital joined to form the Memorial Sloan-Kettering Cancer Center, which offered pioneering U.S. oncology facilities and services and diagnostic centers specifically for breast and prostate cancers. Donors financed additional construction, such as the Rockefeller Research Laboratories.

Services and procedures performed: Diverse cancer specialties practiced at the Memorial Sloan-Kettering Cancer Center and innovative procedures and technology developed by its experts benefit patients. Its radiologists evaluate malignant tumors with computed tomography (CT) scanning or magnetic resonance imaging (MRI) to determine their three-dimensional shape so that intensity-modulated radiation therapy (IMRT) can hit tumors directly without damaging other organs. Memorial Sloan-Kettering Cancer Center personnel devised ways to deliver chemotherapy and radiation simultaneously. The center's High-Throughput Screening (HTS) Core Facility enables physicians to identify chemicals most effective to fight specific cancers. Its surgical centers incorporate robotic processes.

The Memorial Sloan-Kettering Cancer Center operates affiliated outpatient clinics in New York and New Jersey. The center's staff developed the Symptom Tracking and Reporting (STAR) Web site for patients outside the office to alert physicians regarding symptoms and side effects.

The Memorial Sloan-Kettering Cancer Center offers the Clinical Genetics Service, which evaluates people's hereditary risks for specific cancers. The center's counselors provide individual discussion and support groups. Survivor services for adult and children encourage patients' continued contact during remission to monitor their cancer-free status.

Education: In addition to providing cancer education services for patients and the community, the Memorial Sloan-Kettering Cancer Center promotes advanced oncology educational opportunities for scientists, physicians, and other medical professionals. Postdoctoral fellows conduct research in its laboratories. Clinical fellowships enable physicians to interact with patients in various departments within the center. The center created the Louis V. Gerstner, Jr., Sloan-Kettering Graduate School of Biomedical Services in 2004 for students to earn doctorates specializing in biological aspects of cancer. This program educates scientists to envision how their research might aid patients.

Other Memorial Sloan-Kettering Cancer Center educational resources include such publications as the Sloan-Kettering Institute cancer series, conference proceedings, annual reports, and books written by center's medical professionals. The center's site posts Web casts of Cancer-Smart lectures from the center.

Outreach: Memorial Sloan-Kettering Cancer Center medical professionals have provided free screening for breast and cervical cancers at the Breast Examination Center of Harlem since 1979. The center and North General Hospital in Harlem offer cancer screening and treatment at the Ralph Lauren Center for Cancer Care and Prevention. A Memorial Sloan-Kettering Cancer Center mobile van has also made mammograms available.

Research: Memorial Sloan-Kettering Cancer Center research and clinical trials contribute to more effective cancer therapies and drugs that oncology professionals have adopted worldwide. Center scientists tested implanting radioactive seeds in cancers. Researchers have investigated using magnetic resonance spectroscopy with MRI for more effective tumor evaluation chemically and physically. The center's personnel devised nomograms in which breast cancer patients' responses to health questionnaires revealed how malignancies might spread.

The center's Human Oncology and Pathogenesis Program (HOPP) applies molecular investigation results to strengthen cancer prevention, diagnosis, and treatment. Its scientists analyze how pharmaceuticals affect detrimental proteins in genes they detect in breast cancer and other malignant cells. The center's experts contribute to improving the Information Hyperlinked over Proteins database, which maintains information regarding how genes and proteins interact. Specialized units such as the Brain Tumor Center enhance Memorial Sloan-Kettering Cancer Center's research efforts. In 2001 the Memorial Sloan-Kettering Cancer Center began presenting the biennial Paul A. Marks Prize for Cancer Research.

Elizabeth D. Schafer, Ph.D.

▶ For Further Information

Bevilacqua, José Luiz B., et al. "Doctor, What Are My Chances of Having a Positive Sentinel Node? A Validated Nomogram for Risk Estimation." *Journal of Clinical Oncology* 25, no. 24 (August 20, 2007): 3670-3679.

Horner, Peter. "O.R. in the O.R.: Saving Lives as Well as Money, Memorial Sloan-Kettering Center Earns the Edelman with Breakthrough Modeling and Computational Techniques for Treating Prostate Cancer." *OR/MS Today* 34, no. 3 (June, 2007): 18-22.

Kovner, Abba. *Sloan-Kettering: Poems*. Translated from the Hebrew by Eddie Levenston. New York: Schocken Books, 2002.

Lang, Joan. "Making Comfort Healthy: Cancer Center's New Chef Finds Ways to Satisfy Patients' Need for Comfort." *Food Service Director* 20, no. 8 (August, 2007): 40.

Pérez-Peña, Richard. "A $100 Million Gift to Sloan-Kettering." *New York Times*, May 10, 2006, p. B3.

Straus, Joan Sutton. *A Legacy of Caring: The Society of Memorial Sloan-Kettering Cancer Center*. New York: The Society of Memorial Sloan-Kettering Cancer Center, 1996.

Winawer, Sidney J., Moshe Shike, Philip Bashe, and Genell Subak-Sharpe. *Cancer Free: The Comprehensive Cancer Prevention Program*. New York: Fireside/Simon & Schuster, 1996.

▶ Other Resources

Information Hyperlinked over Proteins
http://www.ihop-net.org

Memorial Sloan-Kettering Cancer Center
http://www.mskcc.org

National Comprehensive Cancer Network
Memorial Sloan-Kettering Cancer Center
http://www.nccn.org/members/profiles/memorial.asp

See also American Association for Cancer Research (AACR); American Cancer Society (ACS); American Institute for Cancer Research (AICR); Dana-Farber Cancer Institute; Duke Comprehensive Cancer Center; Fox Chase Cancer Center; Fred Hutchinson Cancer Research Center; Jonsson Comprehensive Cancer Center (JCCC); M. D. Anderson Cancer Center; Mayo Clinic Cancer Center; National Cancer Institute (NCI); National Science Foundation (NSF); Prevent Cancer Foundation; Robert H. Lurie Cancer Center.

▶ Meningeal carcinomatosis

Category: Diseases, symptoms, and conditions
Also known as: Carcinomatous meningitis, leptomeningeal carcinomatosis

Related conditions: Almost any type of cancer can be associated with this condition, but it is generally seen with breast, melanoma, and lung cancers.

Definition: Carcinomatous meningitis is the spread of tumor cells from a primary central nervous system (CNS) source, such as a brain tumor, or from a distant source, such as a lung or breast tumor, via the blood to the subarachnoid space, where it spreads via the fluid covering the brain, called the cerebral spinal fluid (CSF) fluid, to involve the coverings of the brain, known as the leptomeninges.

Risk factors: In adults, primary brain tumors such as oligodendroglioma or secondary tumors, also called metastases, from lung, breast, melanoma, lymphoma, ovarian, or gastric cancer can spread to the brain surfaces.

Etiology and the disease process: Unlike other forms of meningitis, where the invading organism is a bacterium, fungus, or virus, the invaders in carcinomatous meningitis are cancer cells. In adults, meningeal carcinomatosis is usually the result of the metastasis of a primary brain tumor or a secondary cancer in a person who has lymphoma, melanoma, or lung, breast, or gastric tumors.

Incidence: The incidence of meningeal carcinomatosis is increasing because cancer patients are surviving longer. It is seen in about 3 to 5 percent of patients who have cancer.

Symptoms: Patients usually complain of nonspecific symptoms of headache, back pain, or weakness in an extremity.

Screening and diagnosis: Meningeal carcinomatosis can be diagnosed by magnetic resonance imaging (MRI) or myelography together with computed tomography (CT). A spinal tap (also called a lumbar puncture), whereby a needle is inserted into the cerebral spinal fluid within the subarachnoid space and the fluid is sampled, is the usual form of diagnosis, although cerebral spinal fluid cytology is negative in 10 percent of cases.

Treatment and therapy: Meningeal carcinomatosis is difficult to cure and the aim of treatment is usually to ameliorate symptoms, usually by chemotherapy injected into the spinal fluid via lumbar puncture (intrathecal methotrexate) or by radiotherapy to the brain.

Prognosis, prevention, and outcomes: Some patients respond to treatment; however, the prognosis is generally poor with death occurring within one month if the disease is untreated.

Debra B. Kessler, M.D., Ph.D.

See also Carcinomatous meningitis; Leptomeningeal carcinomas; Lumbar puncture.

▶ Meningiomas

Category: Diseases, symptoms, and conditions
Also known as: Meningeal tumors

Related conditions: Intracranial and spinal tumors, extra-axial brain tumors, neurofibromatosis

Definition: Meningiomas are tumors of the meninges, the thin layers of tissue that surround the brain and spinal cord. This type of neoplasm most likely originates from cells of the arachnoid matter, the middle element of the three meningeal coverings, and occur mainly at the base of the brain and around the cerebral convexities. Meningiomas are visibly demarcated from the brain tissue and thus are classified as extra-axial tumors. They can extend from the surface of the dura matter, the outer meningeal layer, and erode the cranial bones, causing exostosis, or growth of the bone. In general, these are solitary lesions, and more than 80 percent of them are benign. However, multiple lesions are common in patients with neurofibromatosis type 2 (NF2), a genetic disorder that affects the nervous system. Several different histological types have been described, with the meningothelial, fibrous, and transitional forms as the most frequently found.

Risk factors: Although the risk factors for meningiomas are largely unknown, evidence suggests an association of risk with a family or personal history of neurofibromatosis type 2, exposure to ionizing radiation (during full-mouth dental radiographs), and use of sex hormones (oral contraceptives or hormone replacement therapy). Other risks factors that have been explored without conclusive results are head trauma, cell phone use, breast cancer, and allergic diseases.

Etiology and the disease process: The precise origin of the majority of the meningiomas is uncertain. However, several forms of this disease are clearly associated with the loss of a tumor-suppressor gene on chromosome 22, known as merlin and encoded by the *NF2* gene. Merlin belongs to the 4.1 family of proteins, a group of molecules with roles in maintaining cell structure. Genetic defects in merlin account for many sporadic meningioma cases. In addition to merlin, other members of the 4.1 protein family with tumor-suppression activity have been involved in meningioma initiation (for example, 4.1B and 4.1R). However, meningioma progression seems to involve genetic changes in chromosomes other than chromosome 22.

The presence of a high density of progesterone receptors in the vast majority of meningiomas suggests a functional role of progesterone-signaling pathways in the pathogenesis and might explain the twofold and tenfold higher incidence respectively of cranial and spinal meningiomas in women. Other proteins that might participate in the disease process of meningioma include telomerase, transforming growth factor-beta, and somatostatin.

Incidence: Meningiomas are the most common nonglial and most common extra-axial tumors of the brain, with an annual age-adjusted incidence rate of 5 per 100,000 individuals. The relatively frequent autopsy finding of small asymptomatic undiagnosed meningiomas suggests that the actual incidence rate is significantly higher. They are more common in women, and the highest incidence is observed in the sixth and seventh decades of life. Childhood cases of meningioma are rare.

Symptoms: Symptoms of meningiomas depend on the location and size of the lesion and result from increased intracranial pressure and edema of the brain structures adjacent to the tumor. The most common symptoms are headache, unilateral sensory disturbances (for example, hearing or visual loss), vertigo, imbalance, focal seizures, spastic weakness, numbness of the limbs, and painless proptosis or "bulging" eyes, among others.

Screening and diagnosis: No screening tests are available. The tendency of meningiomas to calcify and their abundant blood supply allow their diagnosis by contrast-enhanced computed tomography (CT), magnetic resonance imaging (MRI), and arteriography. On both CT and MRI scans, meningiomas appear as homogeneous, smoothly outlined masses, with attachments to the dura matter. Their extra-axial location differentiates them from common intra-axial tumors of the central nervous system, and their unique image density characteristics differentiate them from Schwannoma, another extra-axial tumor.

The World Health Organization (WHO) classifies meningiomas into three grades based on their histological features and the likelihood of recurrence.

- Grade I: Benign meningiomas, with low risk of recurrence and aggressive growth
- Grade II: Atypical meningiomas, with greater risk of recurrence and aggressive growth
- Grade III: Anaplastic or malignant meningiomas, with the greatest risk of recurrence and aggressive growth

Some 80 percent of all meningiomas are of WHO Grade I on diagnosis.

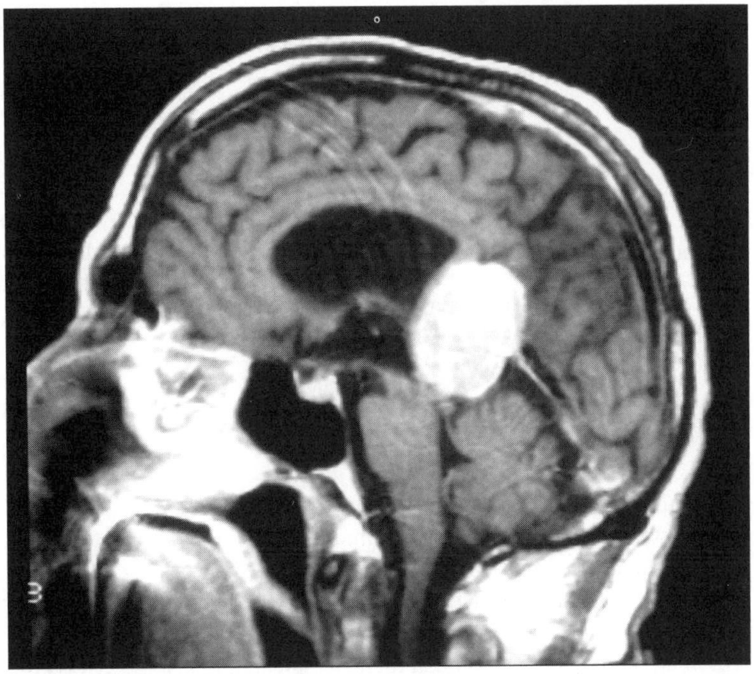

An MRI image of a meningioma in the brain's pineal region. (Living Art Enterprises, LLC/Photo Researchers, Inc.)

Treatment and therapy: The primary treatment is complete surgical excision of the tumor. Focused radiation by Gamma Knife or proton beam is used when the lesion is located around vital structures or when it is a high-grade or recurrent tumor. Although effective chemotherapy has not yet been developed, studies on the use of hormonal antagonists and other molecules are ongoing.

Prognosis, prevention, and outcomes: Complete removal of the tumor is achieved in more than 70 percent of the cases, and in most patients, hearing and other functions of the nervous system are preserved. Recurrence depends on the grade of the tumor, ranging from 5 percent for WHO Grade I tumors up to 80 percent for WHO Grade III after five years of treatment. Prevention of meningiomas is difficult since the etiology is poorly understood.

Reyniel Cruz-Aguado, Ph.D.

▶ For Further Information

Claus, E. B., et al. "Epidemiology of Intracranial Meningioma." *Neurosurgery* 57 (2005): 1088-1095.

Lusis, E., and D. H. Gutmann. "Meningioma: An Update." *Current Opinion in Neurology* 17 (2004): 687-692.

Riemenschneider, M. J., A. Perry, and G. Reifenberger. "Histological Classification and Molecular Genetics of Meningiomas." *Lancet Neurology* 5 (2006): 1045-1054.

▶ Other Resources

Brain Tumor Foundation
http://www.braintumorfoundation.org/about.asp

MayoClinic.com
Meningioma
http://www.mayoclinic.com/health/meningioma/DS00901

See also Acoustic neuromas; Brain and central nervous system cancers; Carcinomatous meningitis; Cell phones; Endotheliomas; Leptomeningeal carcinomas; Meningeal carcinomatosis; Neurofibromatosis type 1 (NF1); Pheochromocytomas; Spinal axis tumors.

▶ Merkel cell carcinomas (MCC)

Category: Diseases, symptoms, and conditions
Also known as: Neuroendocrine carcinoma of the skin

Related conditions: Ectodermal dysplasia

Definition: Merkel cell carcinomas (MCC) are fast-growing cancers in Merkel cells, which are found in the deepest part of the outermost skin layer and are believed to be associ-

Relative Survival Rates for Merkel Cell Carcinoma, 1988-2001

Years	*Survival Rate (%)*
1	87.4
3	68.6
5	62.8
10	57.5

Source: Data from L. A. G. Ries et al., eds., *Cancer Survival Among Adults: U.S. SEER Program, 1988-2001—Patient and Tumor Characteristics*, NIH Pub. No. 07-6215 (Bethesda, Md.: National Cancer Institute, 2007)

ated with the sense of touch. The structure of Merkel cells is characteristic of cells that assist in impulse transmission between an initial stimulus and the nerve impulse that carries messages to the brain. This cancer appears on the face, head, or neck as a firm, painless, shiny bump that can be red, pink, or blue, and it has been found to spread quickly to other parts of the body. Considered rare, MCC has become the second most common cause of non-melanoma skin cancer deaths, with most deaths from the disease occurring within the first three years after diagnosis.

Risk factors: Risk factors include being over the age of sixty-five and having a history of repeated or prolonged sun exposure. People with weakened immune systems, such as those with human immunodeficiency virus (HIV) infection, patients with organ transplants, and those on medications that suppress the immune system, are also at increased risk of developing MCC.

Etiology and the disease process: Although the exact cause of MCC is not known, it is believed that ultraviolet radiation from the sun and other sources plays a significant role in its development. One theory proposes that stem cells in the skin become cancerous and take on the characteristics of Merkel cells. Genetic abnormalities have been found in the cancer cells, leading to speculation that MCC is genetically linked. MCC grows rapidly, typically beginning on the face (especially around the eye), neck, and head. Metastasis to nearby lymph nodes, other areas of skin, liver, bone, and lungs is common and occurs early in the disease. When MCC spreads to other areas of the skin, the lesions grow rapidly and are flesh-colored to red-purple, firm, and deeper in the skin than the primary lesion.

Incidence: Statistics from the National Cancer Institute indicate that about 1,200 new cases of MCC are diagnosed each year in the United States. Although the number of cases is increasing, it still accounts for less than 1 percent of all skin cancers. The average age at diagnosis is sixty-nine. MCC is substantially more common among white people and affects women more often than men.

Symptoms: The primary skin lesions in MCC usually produce no symptoms. They usually occur as solitary, dome-shaped nodules that are smaller than 2 centimeters (cm) in diameter, but can be larger than 15 cm. The skin surface is typically shiny and the color of the lesions is red, pink, or blue. Although they can develop on any skin surface, they are found on the head or neck in about 50 percent of cases. In 40 percent of the cases, they are found on the arms and legs.

Because metastasis is common with MCC, other symptoms that may be reported include swollen lymph glands and fatigue. New growths, with a different appearance than the primary site, may also be reported.

Screening and diagnosis: Screening for MCC should be performed as part of an annual physical. In addition, people at high risk for MCC should perform routine self-examination. When a nodule is found, a biopsy should be performed to determine its cell type and whether it is benign tissue, MCC or, possibly, another form of cancer. If it is found to be MCC, further testing should follow as soon as possible because of how rapidly it spreads. Additional testing should include sentinel lymph node biopsy, a complete blood count, liver function tests, and a chest X ray. Computed tomography (CT) and positron emission scanning (PET) should also be performed to determine the extent of the cancer's spread.

MCC is divided into three stages depending on the severity of disease.

- Stage I: The disease is localized to the skin at the primary site.
- Stage IA: The primary lesion is less than or equal to 2 cm.
- Stage IB: The primary lesion is greater than 2 cm.
- Stage II: The cancer involves nearby lymph nodes.
- Stage III: The cancer is found beyond the nearby lymph nodes.

The stage at diagnosis is important in determining the possibility of tumor metastasis, the patient's treatment options, and prognosis.

Treatment and therapy: Treatment of MCC is based on the stage of the disease at diagnosis. Most commonly, surgery is performed to remove the primary lesion, along with some normal skin around the lesion's edges. Lymph nodes are also removed to test for cancer cells and spread of the disease. Radiation therapy is usually given to the site of the primary lesion and the lymph nodes. When the cancer has spread beyond the lymph nodes, treatment is mainly palliative to relieve pain. The use of chemotherapy, typically with etoposide and carboplatin, is controversial. Some studies have demonstrated positive results but recommend that it be reserved for metastatic MCC, whereas others have found that, especially with this disease, there was a trend toward decreased survival rates.

Prognosis, prevention, and outcomes: Overall, the two-year survival rate for MCC is 50 to 70 percent. Most recurrences and most deaths from this disease occur within the first three years. The only prevention for MCC is to reduce exposure to ultraviolet light, including the sun.

Dorothy P. Terry, R.N.

▶ For Further Information

Allen, P. J., et al. "Merkel Cell Carcinoma: Prognosis and Treatment of Patients from a Single Institution." *Journal of Clinical Oncology* 23, no. 10 (April 1, 2005): 2300-2309.

Brady, Mary S. "Current Management of Patients with Merkel Cell Carcinoma." *Dermatologic Surgery* 30, no. 2 (February, 2004): 321-325.

Hodgson, N. C. "Merkel Cell Carcinoma: Changing Incidence Trends." *Journal of Surgical Oncology* 89, no. 1 (January, 2005): 1-4.

▶ Other Resources

American Cancer Society
Treating Merkel Cell Carcinoma
http://www.cancer.org/docroot/CRI/content/CRI_2_4_4X_Treatment_of_Merkel_Cell_Carcinoma_51.asp

MayoClinic.com
Merkel Cell Carcinoma
http://www.mayoclinic.com/health/merkel-cell-carcinoma/DS00802

National Cancer Institute
Merkel Cell Carcinoma Treatment
http://www.cancer.gov/cancertopics/pdq/treatment/merkelcell/patient

See also Skin cancers.

▶ Mesenchymomas, malignant

Category: Diseases, symptoms, and conditions
Also known as: Mixed-cell sarcomas

Related conditions: Soft-tissue sarcomas

Definition: Malignant mesenchymomas are a type of soft-tissue sarcoma composed of two or more unrelated malignant forms. These rare tumors contain at least two non-epithelial mesenchymal tissues that are neoplastic, with differing histologies, that are not normally associated together in the same tumor.

Risk factors: There are no readily identifiable risk factors particular to malignant memenchymoma, although several risk factors associated with soft-tissue sarcomas in general have been identified. These include exposure to chlorophenols in wood preservatives and phenoxyacetic acid in herbicides, exposure to ionizing radiation, and very rare genetic predispositions in some families. Sporadic cases of malignant mesenchymoma in patients previously treated with radiation for breast cancer have been reported.

Etiology and the disease process: Etiology is not at all well understood, and connections with diet, smoking, alcohol, or preexisting conditions have not been established.

Incidence: Only about 1 percent of newly diagnosed cancers are soft-tissue sarcomas, and malignant mesenchymomas represent only a small fraction of these. These tumors can develop at any age. Reports from the literature indicate ages of onset from one and a half years to eighty-four, with a median age of forty-six years and a slight preponderance of men.

Symptoms: These tumors can arise in any of the connective tissues of the body, although they are most frequently encountered in the arms, legs, hands, feet, and retroperitoneum. Unusual locations such as the neck, fibula, and uterus have also been reported. They are usually first detected as a painless swelling of the soft tissue. Retroperitoneal tumors may become quite massive before detection and may be diagnosed only after the functions of adjacent organs such as the liver or kidneys have been compromised.

Screening and diagnosis: No screening tests exist, although a few mesenchymomas are known to produce excessive amounts of insulin-like growth factor 2 precursor. Diagnosis is always based on direct histological examination of tumor tissue because other sarcomas of single somatic origin can develop in the same locations.

Treatment and therapy: Surgical removal of the tumor, whenever possible, is the treatment of choice. This can be followed by radiation therapy or chemotherapy (with doxorubicin), although the benefits of these postsurgical treatments are questionable.

Prognosis, prevention, and outcomes: Malignant mesenchymomas are usually described as high-grade sarcomas with a poor prognosis, although small tumors 5 centimeters or less in diameter have a much better prognosis. None of these tumors are encapsulated, so recurrence following excision is relatively common.

Jeffrey A. Knight, Ph.D.

See also Fibrosarcomas, soft-tissue.

▶ Mesothelioma

Category: Diseases, symptoms, and conditions
Also known as: Malignant mesothelioma (MM), pleural mesothelioma, peritoneal mesothelioma, pericardial mesothelioma

Related conditions: Lung cancer, pericardial effusion

Definition: Mesothelioma is a rare cancer of the mesothelium, the collective name for the membranes that surround the body's internal organs. Particular mesothelia—the pleura (which covers the lungs), the peritoneum (which lines the abdominal cavity), and the pericardium (the sac that surrounds the heart)—lend their names to forms of mesothelioma. Pleural mesothelioma and peritoneal mesothelioma are the most common forms. At the cellular level, mesothelioma takes three main forms: epithelioid (50 to 70 percent of cases), in which the cancer cell is typically uniform and cube shaped, with a visible nucleus; sarcomatoid (7 to 20 percent), in which the cells are more irregular and oval shaped, with less visible nuclei; and biphasic (20 to 35 percent), a mixture of the two.

Risk factors: About 80 percent of cases strike those exposed to asbestos, a name that refers to six silicate minerals: the serpentine mineral chrysotile and the amphibole minerals actinolite, amosite, anthophyllite, crocidolite, and tremolite. These minerals were heavily used in many industries and products from the late nineteenth century to the 1980's. Today, although more strictly regulated, they remain components of materials for roofing, thermal and electrical insulation, cement pipe and sheets, flooring, gaskets, friction materials, coatings, plastics, textiles, paper, and other products. Those who work with these materials—in asbestos mining and milling, shipyards, building demolition, heating and insulation, brake repair, and asbestos abatement—as well as family members exposed to their clothing, are at risk.

Etiology and the disease process: Asbestos fibers generally do their damage when inhaled, although ingestion also poses risks. The microscopic fibers pierce the pleural lining and harm its mesothelial cells, resulting in the formation of malignant plaques. These fibers may be transported by the lymphatic system to the abdomen, or the infected person may cough, produce fiber-infested sputum, and reingest it into the abdomen, leading to the peritoneal form of mesothelioma. The worst asbestos fibers seem to be the long, thin fibers of the amphibole minerals. The serpentine mineral chrysotile possesses a feathery fiber that may do less damage, although it is more easily suspended in the air and possibly more subject to inhalation.

Researchers do not completely understand the mechanisms whereby the fibers transform normal cells into cancerous ones, but it is believed that the fibers' mechanical action on mesothelial cells, followed by inflammation as macrophages gather during the immune response, sets the stage. Asbestos has also been shown to mediate the entry of foreign deoxyribonucleic (DNA) into cells, resulting in mutations that lead to the activation of oncogenes, the deletion of tumor-suppressor genes, increased production of free radicals, inactivation of natural cell death (hence uncontrolled cell growth), and other errors. This process may be followed by interactions between the fibers and chromosomes that result in abnormalities, particularly of chromosome 22.

Incidence: Although mesothelioma is a rare form of cancer, its incidence increased in the last two decades of the twentieth century, ranging from 7 to 40 per 1 million in Western, industrialized nations, with several thousand cases diagnosed each year in the United States. (Lung cancer from smoking, by way of comparison, typically strikes 1,000 in 1 million.) Perhaps because of the occupational risk factors, mesothelioma strikes men more often than women, and because it takes years to develop, it is diagnosed most often in those aged sixty and older. Cases in younger persons or with shorter onsets have, however, been reported, and the difficulties of diagnosis (mesothelioma is often misdiagnosed as adenocarcinoma) may mask a higher incidence. Pleural mesothelioma accounts for about 75 percent of all cases, peritoneal mesothelioma about 20 percent, and pericardial mesothelioma about 5 percent.

Symptoms: Pleural mesothelioma is marked by fatigue, anemia, shortness of breath, wheezing, hoarseness, cough, sputum containing blood, and chest pain resulting from the accumulation of fluid in the pleural space. Peritoneal mesothelioma is accompanied by weight loss, cachexia (wasting), abdominal swelling, and pain due to ascites (fluid buildup in the abdominal cavity); bowel obstruction, abnormal blood clotting, anemia, and fever may also appear. In advanced cases of mesothelioma, symptoms may include blood clots in the veins and consequent thrombophlebitis, severe bleeding in many body organs resulting from disseminated intravascular coagulation, jaundice, low blood sugar level, pleural effusion, blood clots in the arteries of the lungs (pulmonary emboli), and severe ascites. Other types of pain, problems in swallowing, and swelling of the neck or face may accompany metastatic tumors.

Screening and diagnosis: Because the symptoms of mesothelioma are common to many conditions and because the disease takes so long to cause severe symptoms, it often remains undetected until well advanced. Unfortunately, no screening tests exist, although researchers are investigating blood levels of osteopontin, a protein associated with mesothelioma, as one means of early detection.

For those whose symptoms have prompted a visit to the doctor, a history of exposure to asbestos, along with a physical examination, lung-function tests, and an X ray, are the first diagnostic steps. If the X ray reveals pleural thickening, computed tomography (CT) or magnetic resonance imaging (MRI) scans usually follow. If these scans show an abnormal amount of fluid or a tumor, aspiration will follow, via pleural tap or chest drain, paracentesis or ascitic drain, or pericardiocentesis, depending on the area affected. Cytology performed on the fluid will reveal or rule out cancer; the absence of abnormal cells would suggest another disease, such as tuberculosis or congestive heart failure.

Even these tests, however, are not sufficient to confirm anything more than the presence of cancerous cells. To diagnose mesothelioma, a biopsy must be performed: thoroscopy if the area is located in the chest, laparoscopy if in the abdomen. These procedures involve small incisions that allow both examination of the cavity and retrieval of tissue samples. Bronchoscopy, in which the physician examines the lung's airways by means of a bronchoscope, and mediastinoscopy, a method of examining the lymph nodes, are also used. Open surgery may be required if the samples retrieved are insufficient to confirm the diagnosis.

If pathology confirms the suspicion of mesothelioma, the disease will require staging. The precise TNM (tumor/lymph node/metastasis) system is usually employed:

- Stage I: Mesothelioma is confined to the right or left pleura, perhaps in addition involving the lung, pericardium, and diaphragm.
- Stage II: Mesothelioma extends to the chest wall and esophagus, both sides of the pleura, and perhaps the heart.
- Stage III: Mesothelioma extends through the diaphragm into the abdominal cavity.
- Stage IV: Mesothelioma has spread through the bloodstream to distant organs.

For pleural mesothelioma, the Butchart system is most commonly used:

- Stage I: Malignant melanoma is confined to the right or left pleura, perhaps in addition involving the lung, pericardium, and diaphragm.
- Stage II: Malignant melanoma extends to the chest wall and esophagus, both sides of the pleura, and perhaps the heart.
- Stage III: Malignant melanoma extends through the diaphragm into the abdominal cavity.
- Stage IV: Malignant melanoma has spread through the bloodstream to distant organs.

Treatment and therapy: Treatment options for advanced mesothelioma include surgery, most often pleurectomy and decortication (removal of the chest lining) and less often extrapleural pneumonectomy (removal of the lung, interior chest lining, hemidiaphragm, and pericardium). These are followed by radiation and chemotherapy. Chemotherapy for pleural mesothelioma includes a combination of pemetrexed, cisplatin, and folic acid to mitigate pemetrexed's side effects. A technique known as "heated intraoperative intraperitoneal chemotherapy," using a heated chemotherapy agent to perfuse affected abdominal and

Relative Survival Rates for Mesothelioma by Area Affected, 1988-2001

	Survival Rate (%)	
Years	*Pleura and Lung*	*Peritoneum and Retroperitoneum*
1	38.2	41.8
3	10.5	25.9
5	6.4	18.4
10	4.3	9.5

Source: Data from L. A. G. Ries et al., eds., *Cancer Survival Among Adults: U.S. SEER Program, 1988-2001—Patient and Tumor Characteristics*, NIH Pub. No. 07-6215 (Bethesda, Md.: National Cancer Institute, 2007)

pelvic areas immediately after surgery, has been developed for peritoneal mesothelioma. Investigations into immunotherapies have seen little success, although interferon alpha has shown some promise.

Prognosis, prevention, and outcomes: Because diagnosis generally occurs late and the disease is aggressive, survival rates are low, tending to average between six and nine months following diagnosis, depending on the type of mesothelioma. In the United States, the death rate from mesothelioma increased from 2,000 to 3,000 per year between 1980 and the late 1990's.

Radiation and chemotherapy are offered as palliative treatments in advanced cases. A thin tube or needle may be installed in the affected region (via paracentesis for the abdomen and thoracentesis for the chest cavity) to relieve fluid buildup and consequent pain.

A diagnosis of mesothelioma is not necessarily a death sentence, however: Paleontologist Stephen Jay Gould, who was diagnosed with peritoneal mesothelioma, lived two decades after his diagnosis and succumbed to a different disease. Fortunately, mesothelioma remains a rare and highly preventable disease if asbestos exposure is identified and eliminated.

Christina J. Moose, M.A.

▶ For Further Information

Galateau-Sallé, Françoise, ed. *Pathology of Malignant Mesothelioma*. London: Springer, 2006.

Pass, Harvey I. *One Hundred Questions and Answers About Mesothelioma*. Sudbury, Mass.: Jones and Bartlett, 2004.

Pass, Harvey I., Nicholas J. Vogelzang, and Michele Carbone, eds. *Malignant Mesothelioma: Advances in Pathogenesis, Diagnosis, and Translational Therapies*. New York: Springer, 2005.

Treasure, T., et al. "Radical Surgery for Mesothelioma: The Epidemic Still to Peak and We Need More Research to Manage It." *British Medical Journal* 328 (2004): 237-238.

▶ Other Resources

Mesothelioma Applied Research Foundation
http://www.marf.org

Mesothelioma Center
http://www.mesotheliomacenter.org

See also Acrylamides; Air pollution; Asbestos; Continuous hyperthermic peritoneal perfusion (CHPP); Erionite; Lung cancers; Mediastinoscopy; Paracentesis; Pericardiocentesis; Pleural biopsy; Pleurodesis; Pneumonectomy; Sarcomas, soft-tissue; Simian virus 40; Surgical biopsies; Thoracoscopy.

▶ Metastasis

Category: Diseases, symptoms, and conditions
Also known as: Metastatic disease, metastatic cancer

Related conditions: Bone cancer, lung cancer, nodal involvement

Definition: Metastasis is the movement or spreading of cancer cells from their original site to other areas of the body. The capacity to metastasize is a characteristic of all malignant tumors. Cancer cells have the ability to enter the bloodstream and flow to any part of the body, making a new home for themselves. Different cancers have different patterns of spreading. When cancer comes back in a patient at a site distant from the original location although the patient appeared to be free of cancer, this is called metastatic recurrence.

Risk factors: Whether cancer cells will metastasize to other parts of the body depends on many factors, including the type of cancer, the stage of the cancer, and the original location of the cancer. Tumors are usually classified as either benign or malignant. Malignant tumors can spread by invasion and metastasis, while benign tumors just grow locally. Often the term "cancer" is used only in reference to malignant tumors, not benign ones.

Etiology and the disease process: Metastasis can occur through the circulatory system, the lymphatic system, or both routes. Common sites for metastasis are the adrenals, the liver, the brain, and the bones. Different cancer types have different metastatic tendencies; that is, the origin of the cancer can often predict the location of metastatic tumor formation. For example, colon cancer will often metastasize to the liver, while prostate cancer tends to metastasize to the bones. Similarly, in women, stomach cancer will often metastasize to the ovaries. It is believed that the migrating cancer cells attempt to find new organs that resemble the local environment of the primary (original) tumor, where they can engraft and thrive. Breast cancer cells, in a high-calcium environment due to the proximity of calcium-containing breast milk, will often metastasize to the bone marrow (also a site of high calcium content).

Cancer will often spread to neighboring lymph nodes; however, this may be referred to as "nodal involvement" or "regional disease" rather than as metastasis. Cancers that are highly metastatic (and therefore particularly dangerous) have been found to secrete proteins that degrade the extracellular matrix that connects cells and separates the organs. Such cells may have greater ability to leave the primary tumor location, migrate into the blood vessels, and then leave the circulation at a remote site. Once cancer cells engraft at a new location, they must induce the growth and infiltration of new microscopic blood vessels to grow in size. Some treatment approaches have attempted to target and interfere with the ability of metastatic tumors to induce new blood vessel growth.

Incidence: Metastatic disease is common in many late-stage cancers. Cancers that frequently are the source of metastasis are melanomas and cancers of the lung, breast, colon, kidney, prostate, and pancreas. Therefore, the incidence of metastatic cancer is similar to the incidence of these common cancers after they progress to a metastatic stage.

Symptoms: The exact symptoms experienced by patients with metastatic cancer depend on the type of disease. For instance, lung metastasis can cause coughing or shortness of breath. Brain metastasis can cause symptoms of confusion, seizures, or even coma. Liver metastasis can reveal itself as abdominal pain or jaundice. Bone metastasis is associated with pain in the bones.

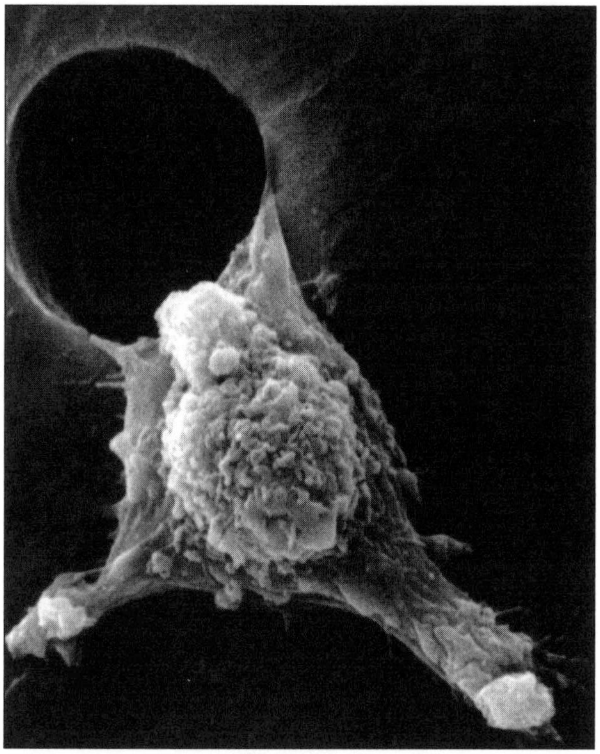

A protein called autocrine motility factor (AMF) causes cancer cells to grow pseudopodia, which enable them to move to other parts of the body. (Science Source/Photo Researchers, Inc.)

Screening and diagnosis: Early metastatic disease may have no signs at all. The more advanced a cancer, the easier it usually is to detect. Each diagnosis of metastasis must be evaluated individually and with care. The extent of each cancer must be determined and all the potential sites of metastasis studied. Metastatic tumors are quite common in the late stages of cancer. Cells collected from a secondary metastatic tumor, when examined under a microscope, can often be identified as cells of the type found in the primary cancer. Therefore, an appropriate treatment regimen may be one that is known to be effective in treating the primary tumor type. The terminology used to describe a metastatic tumor refers to the primary tumor type. For example, breast cancer cells that metastasize to the bone are referred to as "metastatic breast cancer" instead of "bone cancer."

Treatment and therapy: Treatment of metastatic cancer varies widely, depending on the type of cancer and where it has metastasized. Common treatment options include surgery, radiation, and chemotherapy. Biological therapy, radiosurgery, hormone therapy, and laser-immunotherapy can also be treatment options for specific types of metastatic cancer. Treatment must address the symptoms of the metastatic disease along with the primary cancer. Other factors that must be considered in selecting the most appropriate treatment include the size of the metastatic tumor and the patient's age and well-being.

Prognosis, prevention, and outcomes: When a patient is diagnosed with cancer, it is important to determine whether the disease is local or has spread to other locations. The tendency of cancer to spread to secondary organs is what makes the disease potentially life-threatening.

Michael R. King, Ph.D.

▶ For Further Information

Icon Health. *Metastasis: A Medical Dictionary, Bibliography, and Annotated Research Guide to Internet References*. San Diego, Calif.: Author, 2004.

Liotta, L. A., and I. R. Hart, eds. *Tumor Invasion and Metastasis*. Boston: Kluwer, 1982.

Weiss, Leonard. *Principles of Metastasis*. San Diego, Calif.: Academic Press, 1985.

▶ Other Resources

American Cancer Society

What Is Bone Metastasis?

http://www.cancer.org/docroot/CRI/content/CRI_2_4_1X_What_Is_bone_metastasis_66.asp?sitearea=

Children's Hospital Boston
How Cancer Grows and Spreads
http://www.childrenshospital.org/research/Site2029/Documents/CHB_cancer_map.pdf

MetaCancer Foundation
http://www.metacancer.org

See also Cancer biology; Carcinomatosis; Invasive cancer; Malignant tumors; Tumor markers.

▶ Metastatic squamous neck cancer with occult primary

Category: Diseases, symptoms, and conditions
Also known as: Metastatic squamous cell carcinoma of the neck from an unknown primary

Related conditions: Head and neck cancers

Definition: Metastastic squamous neck cancer with occult primary is a cancer in which squamous cells (cells from tissues that line the outside of many body organs) metastisize to lymph nodes in the neck or around the collarbone, and the location of the primary tumor is unknown.

Risk factors: The risk factors for metastatic cancer are the same as those for cancer in general. They include tobacco use, unhealthful diet, alcohol abuse, and genetic factors. In addition, the human papillomavirus as a risk factor has been extensively studied in head and neck cancers.

Etiology and the disease process: In the course of the disease, the cancer cells—cells that divide too quickly and without any order—travel from the organ in which they develop (the primary site), through the blood or lymphatic vessels to the lymph nodes in the neck or around the collarbone.

Incidence: Metastastic squamous neck cancer with occult primary is a rare disease that afflicts less than 200,000 individuals in the United States.

Symptoms: Symptoms may include a lump in the neck or throat, pain in the neck or throat, and metastasis.

Screening and diagnosis: Screening tests to diagnose metastatic squamous neck cancer and the primary tumor include physical exams, biopsies, and different imaging procedures. A diagnosis of the disease is made if the primary tumor is not found during testing. Staging is the process used to determine how far the tumor has spread to other body organs, such as the liver or lungs. There is no standard staging process for metastatic squamous neck cancer with occult primary. The tumors are described as untreated or recurrent.

Treatment and therapy: The treatment of the disease depends on how many lymph nodes are affected, on whether the primary tumor has been detected, and on the patient's age and overall health. Surgery is a common treatment, during which the physician cuts out the cancerous lymph nodes and some of the healthy ones around them. Radiation therapy, to kill the cancer cells and to shrink the tumors, may be given alone or before surgery. Chemotherapy is currently administered only in clinical trials, before or at the same time as radiation therapy. Another treatment option is participation in clinical trials of new treatments.

Prognosis, prevention, and outcomes: Prognosis and outcome depend on many factors, for example, the extent of metastasis in the lymph nodes or the response of the cancer to treatment. Avoiding preventable risk factors, such as smoking, may help reduce the disease risk.

Silke Haidekker, Ph.D.

See also Carcinoma of unknown primary origin (CUP); Epidermoid cancers of mucous membranes; Head and neck cancers.

▶ Microcalcifications

Category: Diseases, symptoms, and conditions
Also known as: Calcifications

Related conditions: Ductal cancer in situ (DCIS)

Definition: Microcalcifications are tiny deposits of calcium phosphate or calcium oxylate found in soft tissues of the body such as the breast. On a mammogram, microcalcifications are seen as fine white flecks with a diameter of less than 1 millimeter. Based on their physical characteristics and location, microcalcifications may be classified as skin, vascular, eggshell, popcornlike, rodlike, punctate (round or oval), milk of calcium, or suture. Although they are very common and most often benign, microcalcifications may be a sign of precancerous changes in the breast.

Risk factors: The incidence of microcalcifications increases with age. However, they are found in women and men of all ages and races.

Etiology and the disease process: Microcalcifications are not associated with dietary calcium. It is thought that they are secreted by the breast cells or are mineralized residue from either normal breast metabolism or abnormal, rapid cell division. They may be related to previous trauma, surgery, infection, or radiation, or they may be an indication of ductal cancer in situ, a noninvasive Stage 0 cancer found in milk ducts of the breast.

Incidence: Microcalcifications and larger macrocalcifications are seen in approximately two-thirds of all mammograms.

Symptoms: The deposits are generally too small to be felt during clinical examinations and do not cause pain.

Screening and diagnosis: Screening mammograms are the standard tool for detecting microcalcifications. Diagnostic mammography, computer-assisted detection software, ultrasound, and comparisons with previous mammograms are used by radiologists to analyze the structure, size, number, shape, and distribution of microcalcifications. The findings are then assigned an assessment category (from 0 to 5), which determines what, if any, follow-up is recommended.

Treatment and therapy: Mammograms classified as categories 1 and 2 are considered negative and require no extraordinary follow-up. Category 3 microcalcifications have a high probability of being benign, but repeat mammograms are typically scheduled to watch for changes in size, number, or shape of deposits. A stereotactic or surgical biopsy of suspicious microcalcifications may be recommended with a category 4 assessment, whereas a category 5 designation indicates a likely malignancy that requires biopsy and surgery or other treatment. Category 0 is used when additional testing is needed before a diagnosis can be made.

Prognosis, prevention, and outcomes: Most microcalcifications are benign. Of those biopsied, more than 80 percent are noncancerous. However, any microcalcifications (especially if they occur in both breasts) are thought to put women at greater risk for breast cancer.

Judy Majewski, M.S.

See also Breast cancer in children and adolescents; Breast cancer in men; Breast cancers; Breast ultrasound; Calcifications of the breast; Cold nodule; Comedo carcinomas; Ductal carcinoma in situ (DCIS); Ductogram; Fibroadenomas; Hormone replacement therapy (HRT); Invasive ductal carcinomas; Mammography; Mastectomy; Medullary carcinoma of the breast; Tubular carcinomas; Wire localization.

▶ Microwave hyperthermia therapy

Category: Procedures
Also known as: Heat therapy

Definition: Microwave hyperthermia therapy is a procedure in which microwaves are used to heat an area in which cancer is present. It is considered an experimental therapy and is not widely available, and it is usually used in combination with radiation therapy or chemotherapy.

Cancers treated: A wide variety of cancers, including prostate, breast, bladder, lung, and liver cancers

Why performed: Microwave hyperthermia therapy aims either to kill tumor cells or to make them more susceptible to other cancer treatments.

Patient preparation: Patient preparation for microwave hyperthermia therapy depends on the area in which the therapy will be done and whether the therapy will be localized or regional. Patients should discuss carefully with their cancer care team the possible outcomes of the therapy and what the realistic outcome expectations are.

Steps of the procedure: In localized hyperthermia, a rod containing coils that produce microwaves is introduced to the tumor. The rod is then turned on and the microwaves heat up the tumor cells. The tumor cells may be heated to such an extent that they die, or they may be heated only to an extent that makes them more susceptible to chemotherapy drugs. It is very difficult to heat only the tumor cells, and normal cells surrounding the tumor may also be affected.

In regional microwave hyperthermia therapy, a device that produces microwaves is aimed at a region, such as an arm or leg. The machine is then started and produces microwaves that heat the entire region. In this case the cells are heated enough to make chemotherapy drugs more effective but not enough to kill the cells.

After the procedure: If the microwave hyperthermia is administered in conjunction with chemotherapy or radiation, then the patient will experience the effects that he or she usually experiences after such therapy. The patient may experience temporary feelings of pain or discomfort from the procedure.

Risks: Microwave hyperthermia therapy is considered an experimental procedure. The risks will depend on the specific procedure being performed but may include pain, infection, swelling, blood clots, and nerve or muscle damage.

Results: The goal of microwave hyperthermia therapy is usually to improve the effectiveness of chemotherapy drugs or radiation therapy. In these cases, the results of the treatment may be hard to define because many other things can also affect the effectiveness of such treatments. The results will also vary depending on the area in which the tumor is located, the extent of the cancer, and whether the procedure was done on a localized or regional area.

Helen Davidson, B.A.

See also Bladder cancer; Breast cancers; Chemotherapy; Hyperthermia therapy; Liver cancers; Lung cancers; Prostate cancer; Radiation therapies; Radiofrequency ablation.

▶ Mineral oils

Category: Carcinogens and suspected carcinogens
RoC status: Known human carcinogen since 1980
Also known as: Petroleum distillate, untreated and mildly refined oils

Related cancers: Skin cancers, particularly squamous skin cell cancers of the scrotum, as well as stomach, bladder, pancreatic, large intestine, rectal, mouth, throat, and lung cancers

Definition: Mineral oils include lubricant-based oils and other products derived from them. They are insoluble in water and are composed of complex mixtures of aliphatic hydrocarbons, naphthenics, and aromatics. Among those that are considered to be most carcinogenic are the polycyclic aromatic hydrocarbons (PAH), particularly benzopyrene, as well as nitrosamines, chlorinated paraffins, long-chain aliphatics, sulfur, N-phenyl-2-naphthylamine, and formaldehyde.

Exposure routes: Mineral oils can be absorbed directly through dermal contact, via inhalation, and by ingestion of substances containing or contaminated with untreated or mildly treated mineral oils.

Where found: Minerals are found at industry work sites and in the environment because about two billion liters of used (and potentially contaminated) lubricating oils are released every year. At least 750 million of these are used as road oil or in asphalt.

At risk: These commonly in contact with mildly treated or untreated mineral oils include workers in the metal, glass, newspaper printing, and automobile and airplane manufacture, and cotton and jute spinning industries.

Etiology and symptoms of associated cancers: Mineral oils generally cause skin cancers by dermal contact, resulting in red, swollen, and possibly painful marks or tumors on or beneath the skin. Stomach and pancreatic cancers often cause abdominal pain. Bladder, large intestine, and rectal cancers, often caused by ingestion of harmful levels of mineral oils, effect excretion of waste, making urination or excretion painful. Cancers of the mouth, throat, and lung are generally caused by inhalation or ingestion of toxic substances in mineral oils. First symptoms are flulike or coldlike irritation of breathing passages, which progressively increases to the point at which breathing and speaking are affected, eventually severely.

History: Mineral oils are used as a base in the manufacture of many types of refined lubricant oils. These refined oil products are then used in construction work, metalwork, manufacturing diesel oils, and mining. Nearly half of the lubricating oils are used in automobile manufacturing and operation. These include engine oils, transmission oils, lubricating oils for gears, bearing oils, and transmission fluids. Highly refined and purified white mineral oils are used for certain medicinal, food, and pharmacological purposes.

Most of the studies on mineral oils as carcinogens have involved relationships between cancers and metalworkers in the West Midlands district of the United Kingdom. Case studies revealed an excess incidence of skin cancers in these metalworkers as well as higher levels of gastrointestinal and bladder cancers. Similarly, studies of cancer incidence in printing occupations have shown increased incidence of and mortality related to a variety of respiratory cancers, including buccal cavity, pharyngeal, and lung cancers.

Results from a number of animal studies show similar relationships. For example, mice treated with repeated application of mineral oils directly to the skin had dramatically increased incidence of skin cancer. Similar applications of mineral oils to rabbits and rhesus monkeys produced tumors typically associated with the skin.

Despite these concerns, mineral oils are still widely used in the United States and elsewhere across the globe and are for sale everywhere. Roughly 85 percent of the manufactured mineral oil products are used for lubricants, another 12 to 14 percent are used as aromatic oils, and the remaining are produced for greases. Finally, refined mineral oils are still an important component of many industries in which lubricants are necessary.

Dwight G. Smith, Ph.D.

See also Carcinogens, known; Lung cancers; Occupational exposures and cancer; Pancreatic cancers; Rectal cancer; Skin cancers; Squamous cell carcinomas; Stomach cancers; Throat cancer.

▶ Mistletoe

Category: Complementary and alternative therapies
Also known as: *Viscum album Lorantaceae*, all heal

Definition: European and American varieties of mistletoe are semiparasitic, woody evergreen plants with white berries that grow on deciduous trees. Mistletoe has a long history of use in Europe and Asia as a medicinal cure-all, and the species *Viscum album Lorantaceae* in particular has been studied for the treatment of multiple types of cancer.

Cancers treated or prevented: Breast, pancreatic, and other cancers

Delivery routes: Intrauscular, subcutaneous, or intravenous (IV) injection of water-based or water-and-alcohol-based extracts

How this substance works: American and European mistletoe plants both contain toxins that provide pharmacologic effects on multiple organ systems. The *Viscum album* species is the primary one used medicinally and provides activity via four viscotoxins, three distinct lectins (M11-3), and the specific lectin viscumin. These toxins are found in the main standardized product Iscador, available in Europe and Asia but not in the United States. The cytotoxic viscotoxins and lectins provide the plant's potential direct anticancer activity by inhibiting protein synthesis in cancer cells and by inducing programmed cancer cell death, respectively.

Immunomodulation is another possible mechanism of cancer treatment and of chemotherapy side effect control. Mistletoe extract may increase white blood cell counts, protect deoxyribonucleic acid (DNA) in white blood cells exposed to damaging chemotherapy, and stimulate cellular secretions of cytokines, including tumor necrosis factor (TNF)-alpha, interleukin (IL)-1, and IL-6, from white blood cells. Increased natural killer cell activity has also been noted in breast cancer patients administered a single intravenous dose of standardized mistletoe preparation.

Varying effects have been observed with different extracts, doses, and types of cancer. Clinical trials have been conducted in Europe, but evidence supporting mistletoe's immune-boosting effect does not yet support the concept that enhanced immunity will help the body fight cancer cells.

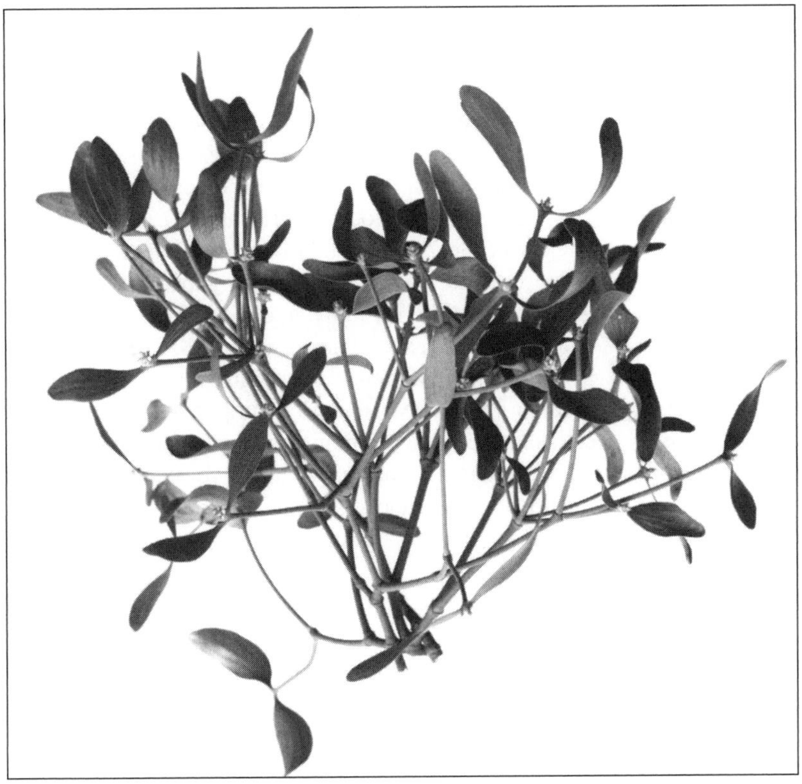

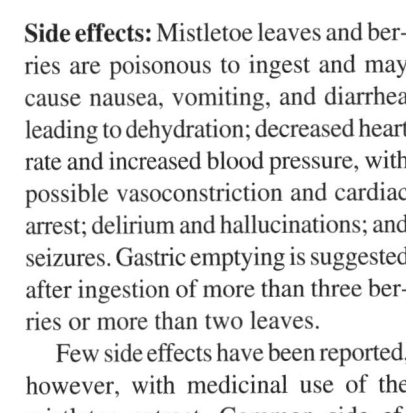

Mistletoe. (©Witold Krasowski/Dreamstime.com)

Side effects: Mistletoe leaves and berries are poisonous to ingest and may cause nausea, vomiting, and diarrhea leading to dehydration; decreased heart rate and increased blood pressure, with possible vasoconstriction and cardiac arrest; delirium and hallucinations; and seizures. Gastric emptying is suggested after ingestion of more than three berries or more than two leaves.

Few side effects have been reported, however, with medicinal use of the mistletoe extract. Common side effects observed with extract administration include injection site reactions, headache, fever and chills, and some cases of anaphylactic shock or allergic reaction. Mistletoe is a uterine stimulant and should be avoided during pregnancy and lactation.

Nicole M. Van Hoey, Pharm.D.

See also Breast cancers; Complementary and alternative therapies; Pancreatic cancers.

▶ Mitochondrial DNA mutations

Category: Cancer biology
Also known as: Mitochondrial heteroplasmy (different mitochondrial mutations are present), homoplasmy (only a single type of mitochondrial DNA, or deoxyribonucleic acid, sequence is present)

Related conditions: Warburg effect

Definition: Mitochondria are organelles in eukaryotic cells that produce energy (adenosine triphosphate, or ATP) by oxidative phosphorylation. Mitochondria are made from the proteins encoded by both nuclear genes and genes from the mitochondrion's own genome. The mitochondrial genome is sixteen kilobase pairs and encodes thirty-seven genes, which function in the mitochondrion. The majority of proteins in the mitochondrion are products of nuclear-encoded genes. There are multiple copies of the mitochondrial genome in each mitochondrion and multiple mitochondria in each cell. Mitochondrial DNA mutates at a high rate, and mitochondrial dysfunction is a factor in the development of cancers. Many defects in mitochondrial function are found in tumors.

The mutation process: Mitochondrial DNA (mtDNA) mutates at a rate about ten times greater than that of nuclear DNA. Likely reasons for this high mutation rate are an error-prone DNA polymerase, inefficient DNA repair enzymes, and exposure to mutagens such as oxygen radicals that are present in the mitochondrion.

Cancer cells have metabolic imbalances and a decrease in mitochondrial apoptosis (programmed, or planned, cell death). In cancer, the rapid growth of tumors is possible because of the shift in the mitochondria to glycolysis rather than the normal respiration (oxidative phosphorylation) to make ATP. Changes are observed in cancer cells, including the production of more of the rate-limiting enzymes of glycolysis and the accumulation of mutations in mitochondrial DNA. Often these mutations are in genes involved in mitochondrial respiration and ATP generation. In addition, sometimes people have mitochondrial mutations (germ-line mutations) that predispose that person to develop cancer. It is thought that most mtDNA mutations are acquired during or after the start of the cancer.

Mitochondrial DNA mutations are divided into two classes. The first class is severe mutations that inhibit oxidative phosphorylation and cause an increase in reactive oxygen species. Such mutations will promote tumor growth. The second class is milder mutations, which will allow tumors to adapt to new microenvironments as a tumor progresses and metastasizes.

Cancer cells are resistant to apoptosis because the induction of mitochondrial outer membrane permeabilization (MOMP) is inhibited. MOMP is a process that mediates apoptosis. In hematological cancers, when this process is inhibited, a neoplasm will occur. Some genes that code for proteins that function in the mitochondrion are located on nuclear chromosomes.

Associated cancers: Changes in mtDNA sequences have been found in many different types of cancers, including lung, breast, pancreatic, gastric, colorectal, thyroid, cervical, and prostate cancers. Mutations in the nuclear DNA-encoded mitochondrial genes for fumarate hydratase and succinate dehydrogenase are associated with uterine leiomyomas and paragangliomas. Studies have shown that the presence of certain mitochondrial DNA sequences (single nucleotide polymorphisms) is associated with an increase (or for other sequences, a decrease) in the risk of developing breast cancer. Germ-line mutations in mitochondrial DNA at nucleotides 10398 and 16189 are linked to breast and endometrial cancer. If the mitochondrial electron transport chain reactions are not functioning well, reactive oxygen species are made that cause oxidative stress and increase the risk of developing breast cancer. Other germ-line mtDNA mutations are associated with an increased risk of prostate cancer. Note that mutations in mtDNA show maternal inheritance because sperm mitochondria are generally eliminated from the embryo, so that mtDNA comes from the mother via the egg.

Mutations and monitoring: Somatic mutations in the displacement loop (D-loop, where the mtDNA starts replication) occur frequently in colorectal cancers. There are hot spots in the D-loop where mtDNA mutations frequently occur. A colorectal tumor with a mutation in the D-loop is associated with a poor prognosis and resistance to fluorouracil-based adjuvant chemotherapy in Stage III colon cancers. Thus changes in mtDNA sequences are involved in the initiation and progression of cancers. Examining the mtDNA mutations in populations of cancer cells may be useful to monitor tumor progression. Analysis of these mutations may be useful for the diagnosis and treatment of the cancer. Targets for drug treatment might include glycolysis and inducing apoptosis in mitochondria.

Susan J. Karcher, Ph.D.

▶ For Further Information

Alirol, E., and J. C. Martinou. "Mitochondria and Cancer: Is There a Morphological Connection?" *Oncogene* 25 (2006): 4706-4716.

Bai, R. K., et al. "Mitochondrial Genetic Background

Modifies Breast Cancer Risk." *Cancer Research* 67, no. 10 (2007): 4687-4694.

Brandon, M., P. Baldi, and D. C. Wallace. "Mitochondrial Mutations in Cancer." *Oncogene* 25, no. 34 (2005): 4647-4662.

Chatterjee, A., E. Mambo, and D. Sidransky. "Mitochondrial DNA Mutations in Human Cancer." *Oncogene* 25, no. 34 (2006): 4663-4674.

Garber, K. "Energy Boost: The Warburg Effect Returns in a New Theory of Cancer." *Journal of the National Cancer Institute* 96, no. 24 (2004): 1805-1806.

_______. "Energy Deregulation: Licensing Tumors to Grow." *Science* 312 (2006): 1158-1159.

Kroemer, G. "Mitochondria in Cancer." *Oncogene* 25 (2006): 4630-4632.

Maitral, Anirban, et al. "The Human MitoChip: A High-Throughput Sequencing Microarray for Mitochondrial Mutation Detection." *Genome Research* 14 (2004): 812-819.

Ohta, S. "Contribution of Somatic Mutations in the Mitochondrial Genome to the Development of Cancer and Tolerance Against Anticancer Drugs." *Oncogene* 25 (2006): 4768-4776.

Ruiz-Pesini, Eduardo, et al. "An Enhanced MITOMAP with a Global mtDNA Mutational Phylogeny." *Nucleic Acids Research* 35 (January 1, 2007): D823-D828.

▶ Other Resources

MITOMAP

A Human Mitchondrial Genome Database
http://www.mitomap.org/

National Cancer Institute

Cancer Genetics
http://www.cancer.gov/cancertopics/prevention-genetics-causes/genetics

See also Breast cancers; Cancer biology; Cytogenetics; Genetics of cancer; Germ-cell tumors; Molecular oncology.

▶ *MLH1* gene

Category: Cancer biology

Also known as: MutL homolog 1, colon cancer nonpolyposis type 2 (E. coli); HNPCC; FCC2; HNPCC2; mutL (E. coli) homolog 1 (colon cancer, nonpolyposis type 2)

Definition: The *MLH1* gene encodes a protein that is involved in deoxyribonucleic acid (DNA) mismatch repair.

Normal cellular function: When a cell divides, it must replicate its genetic material, which is contained within the DNA. During DNA replication, errors can be made that need to be corrected. The DNA mismatch repair machinery recognizes the errors that are made and recruits other proteins to repair the errors. If errors are not corrected, mutations are made that could affect the production or function of important proteins.

Relevance to cancer: *MLH1* and *MSH2*, another gene that is part of the DNA mismatch repair machinery, are the two genes most frequently mutated in hereditary nonpolyposis colorectal cancer (HNPCC). Inheriting mutations in either *MLH1* or *MSH2* predisposes patients to developing colorectal, stomach, ovarian, and biliary duct cancers. Mutations in DNA mismatch repair genes are also present in 10 to 20 percent of sporadic (noninherited) cancers.

Defects in mismatch repair proteins are correlated with tumors that show microsatellite instability (MSI). Microsatellites are regions of the genome that contain highly repetitive DNA sequences that are more likely to generate errors during DNA replication. If the DNA mismatch repair machinery does not correct these errors, this can lead to further mutations within the genome that may promote tumor formation and progression.

Diagnostic and genetic testing: There are a number of tests that can identify people with inherited mutations in mismatch repair genes as well as characterize the levels of these proteins in tumor cells, both of which have important clinical implications. DNA sequencing tests are currently available for both *MLH1* and *MSH2*, the two mismatch repair genes that are most commonly mutated in cancer. In addition to mutations in the genes themselves, other types of chromosome modifications can alter levels at which these proteins produced by these genes are expressed within the cells. Therefore, immunohistochemical analysis of tissue samples can be used to detect how much of the mismatch repair proteins are being produced.

Clinical implications: Because mutations in *MLH1* or *MSH2* significantly increase the risk of developing cancer, patients carrying these mutations should undergo frequent screening for colon and endometrial cancer. In addition, levels of MLH1 and MSH2 protein within tumor cells can be prognostic indicators, since differential protein levels are associated with differences in cancer progression, recurrence, and treatment response. For example, one study found that cells lacking MLH1 protein were more resistant to DNA damage-inducing chemotherapy than cells that contain MLH1.

Lindsay Lewellyn, B.S.

See also Ashkenazi Jews and cancer; Bethesda criteria; Cancer biology; Family history and risk assessment; Genetics of cancer; Hereditary cancer syndromes; *MSH* genes; Turcot syndrome.

▶ Mohs surgery

Category: Procedures
Also known as: Mohs micrographic surgery

Definition: Mohs surgery is a surgical technique for precisely excising malignant cutaneous tumors. It was developed in the 1930's by Dr. Fredric Mohs. In 1969, Dr. Mohs reported the use of the technique for excising basal cell carcinomas and squamous cell carcinomas and claimed a five-year cure rate of 100 percent. Subsequent data and studies led to the validation of the technique within the surgical community. Mohs surgery is now commonly used for the resection of malignant and nonmalignant tumors in cosmetically sensitive areas such as the face and neck, hands, and genitalia.

Cancers treated: Basal cell carcinomas, squamous cell carcinomas

Why performed: With Mohs surgery, the tumor can be surgically excised with precision, maintaining the best surgical and cosmetic outcome. Accurate tumor margin assessment and high cure rates are achievable with this technique. In addition, Mohs surgery allows the patient to be spared the unnecessary removal of normal tissues, ultimately providing a more functional and cosmetically optimal outcome.

Patient preparation: The patient is screened for allergies to numbing medicines such as lidocaine. The surgical site is prepped in a sterile fashion. Local anesthesia is typically used, and the patient's wound is covered between surgical stages.

Steps of the procedure: Mohs surgery is typically performed under local anesthesia by a dermatologist trained in the procedure in an outpatient setting. The procedure typically takes between two and four hours and is generally very well tolerated, with a low incidence of post-surgical complications.

During the procedure, the tumor, along with a small area of clinically normal-appearing skin around the tumor, is excised. The tissue is then immediately processed by a histology technician, and the margins are evaluated by the surgeon. Mohs micrographic diagrams are used to map out the tissue for the histology technician and the surgeon. If the microscopic margins are positive, then their precise locations are noted on the Mohs map and tissue is resected only from that area. This process is repeated in stages until the entire tumor is removed and clear margins are seen.

Following the complete resection of the tumor, the defect is either closed immediately using various surgical repair techniques or allowed to close by secondary intention. The type of closure depends on the type of defect and the preference of the surgeon.

After the procedure: The patient should be provided with thorough wound care instructions before discharge.

Risks: The risks of Mohs surgery include allergy to the numbing medication, scarring, pain, and infection.

Results: The procedure ideally results in the complete clearing of the tumor in question. The patient should be counseled that recurrence is always a possibility.

Sarah Kasprowicz, M.D.

See also Basal cell carcinomas; Bowen disease; Dermatofibrosarcoma protuberans (DFSP); Dermatology oncology; Penile cancer; Squamous cell carcinomas.

▶ Molecular oncology

Category: Medical specialties
Also known as: Molecular biology of cancer

Definition: Molecular oncology is a field in which physicians and researchers study and address the molecular basis for development and metastasis of cancer.

Subspecialties: Medical oncology, molecular genetics, molecular virology

Cancers treated: Most forms of neoplastic disease, including neoplasms of tissues and organs, such as brain, breast, gastrointestinal, and lung cancers, as well as leukemias and lymphomas

Training and certification: Molecular oncology is primarily an area of research rather than a medical specialty. Development of expertise in the field may involve either predoctoral or postdoctoral training. Predoctoral training involves development of a research project addressing a question in molecular oncology and the ensuing research that will ultimately result in the doctoral degree. Postdoctoral training involves advanced research carried out following the receipt of a doctorate. Postdoctorates train, or in a sense apprentice, under the auspices of an expert in the molecular field at a university or medical school.

Some medical programs provide concurrent training in both research and as clinical training. The end result, usually in a three- to four-year doctor of medicine (M.D.) and doctor of philsophy (Ph.D.) program, is that the individual earns both a medical degree and a doctorate. Applicants for such programs have completed an undergraduate program at an accredited university.

Certification in a clinical specialty may be established following completion of a terminal degree. The specialty reflects the clinical interest of the individual and may be in fields such as hematology, immunology, pediatrics, or medical microbiology. Interests in the molecular mechanisms underlying cancer can result in research within the field of specialty.

Services and procedures performed: The main aim of molecular oncology is to conduct research into the underlying cause of cancer. Most cancers have a basis in the disruption of regulation of cell division. However, as specific genetic defects may result in cancer development, molecular oncologists may work with the physician in charge or with the cancer team in diagnosis of the disease and to provide recommendations on the best course of treatment. For example, pathology samples obtained from a patient with leukemia may be analyzed to determine whether any obvious chromosomal abnormality is present.

Microscopic analysis of chromosomes may provide evidence for a particular form of leukemia or lymphoma but does not directly address the molecular mechanism underlying the disease. To do this, the molecular oncologist would carry out research to understand the disruption of regulation of the cell cycle and the progression by which the cell ultimately undergoes cell division. Defects may involve any of the steps in regulation, including overproduction of growth factors or other oncogene factors, or mutations involving receptors or signal mechanisms within the cell.

Analysis of the type of surface proteins found on cancer cells may provide clues as to the course of treatment. For example, certain forms of breast cancer develop or are characterized by estrogen receptors on the surface of cells. The molecular oncologist, as part of the medical team, may recommend the use of estrogen analogs or inhibitors as one course of treatment for the disease.

Although the cause of most forms of breast cancer is unknown, approximately 5 to 10 percent of such malignancies have a genetic basis and are associated with mutations in one of two specific genes: *BRCA1* and *BRCA2*. Areas of molecular oncology address the molecular basis by which mutations in these genes produce a high risk for cancer. Screening of women for the presence of these genes may allow for early intervention or monitoring in hopes of either preventing the disease or catching it at an early stage in women at risk.

Related specialties and subspecialties: Hematology is the clinical field addressing disorders of the blood, including leukemias and lymphomas. Although some forms of such cancers may be associated with infectious agents—for example, viruses are known to be the etiological agents for certain T cell lymphomas and Burkitt lymphoma—in general blood cancers are the result of molecular disorders that disrupt normal regulation of cell division. Hematologists who research such disorders are trained in molecular biology or biochemistry.

Pediatric oncology is a specialty dealing with cancers in children. Physicians in this area with an interest in research into the molecular basis for such diseases have undergone advanced training in the molecular field. Much the same may be said of researchers in cancer relevant to any field of specialty: The medical degree establishes the specialty of interest, while further training is carried out for research into the molecular or biochemical basis of cancer.

Richard Adler, Ph.D.

▶ For Further Information

Pecorino, Lauren. *Molecular Biology of Cancer*. 2d ed. New York: Oxford University Press, 2008.

Pelengaris, Stella, and Michael Khan. *The Molecular Biology of Cancer*. Malden, Mass.: Blackwell, 2006.

Tannock, Ian, et al. *The Basic Science of Oncology*. Columbus, Ohio: McGraw-Hill, 2005.

Weinberg, Robert. *Molecular Biology of Cancer*. New York: Garland Science, 2006.

▶ Organizations and Professional Societies

American Association for Cancer Research
http://www.aacr.org
615 Chestnut Street, 17th Floor
Philadelphia, PA 19106

American Society for Biochemistry and Molecular Biology
http://www.asbmb.org
9650 Rockville Pike
Bethesda, MD 20814-3996

American Society of Gene Therapy
http://www.asgt.org
555 East Wells Street, Suite 1100
Milwaukee, WI 53202

▶ Other Resources

National Center of Competence in Research in Molecular Oncology
http://www.nccr-oncology.ch

National Foundation for Cancer Research
http://www.nfcr.org

See also Blood cancers; Cancer biology; Cytogenetics; Cytology; Hematologic oncology; Pathology; Pediatric oncology and hematology; Sputum cytology; Viral oncology.

▶ Moles

Category: Diseases, symptoms, and conditions
Also known as: Nevi (singular, nevus or naevus)

Related conditions: Common acquired nevi (acquired in early decades of life), congenital nevi (acquired at birth), freckles, seborrheic keratoses, lentigos (age spots), dysplastic nevi, melanoma, basal cell carcinoma, squamous cell carcinoma

Definition: Moles, or nevi, are clustered melanocytes or nevus cells that appear on the skin, usually brown in color. Melanocytes are cells in the skin that produce the pigment called melanin that protects human skin from the damage of ultraviolet (UV) rays in sunlight.

Risk factors: Although almost everyone has moles, some factors may increase the risk of moles. People with lighter skin and with freckles have a slightly greater risk of developing melanoma. Exposure to ultraviolet rays from the sun can increase the number of moles, and the more moles a person has, the greater the risk of developing melanoma. Damage to the melanocyte deoxyribonucleic acid (DNA) can cause a mole to become cancerous. Lowered immune systems such as those in persons with the human immunodeficiency virus (HIV) or who have had an organ transplant can increase development of moles.

Etiology and the disease process: Nevus cells (melanocytes) are normally localized in the basal layer of the skin (epidermis). A mole of itself is not dangerous and remains a stable part of the skin unless it becomes damaged and then can change into cancer.

Within sunlight are two types of invisible rays: infrared radiation (the sun's heat) and ultraviolet radiation (ultraviolet light). Ultraviolet (UV) light is necessary for plants to live and generate energy. However, UV light can also cause sunburn, aging, and, under the right conditions, skin cancer. UV rays are further differentiated into UVA, UVB, and UVC. Studies are investigating UVA, once thought to be harmless, as a possible cause of skin cancer. Researchers believe that damaged melanocytes may reproduce in an uncontrolled and abnormal way, possibly causing melanoma, one dangerous form of skin cancer. The exact mechanisms by which skin cancer or malignant moles occur is still unclear.

Incidence: Most people have some form of moles, depending on their age, sun exposure, and genetic makeup. Usually people have few moles as an infant or child but may develop moles from puberty to the age of thirty. Often after that time, moles begin to disappear so that older adults may have fewer moles. White adults have an average of twenty-five or fewer moles, but an average person can have ten to forty moles over a lifetime, with a risk of 1:100 turning into a malignant melanoma. With lifestyle changes and more exposure to sunlight, this number can increase.

The number of moles a person has is determined by genetics and exposure to sunlight. Moles are more common on parts of the body that are exposed to sunlight. Some evidence points to a role by the immune system in developing moles because they tend to develop in people with depressed immune systems such those infected with HIV and those who have had organ transplants.

Studies suggest that malignant nevi such as melanoma arise from preexisting moles. If this proves true, the more moles a person has, the higher the incidence of malignant nevi. The percentage of persons with melanoma has increased 100 percent (doubled) in the past thirty years.

Symptoms: Moles come in various colors and shapes. Some are brown and others are pink. Some are yellow, dark blue, or black. Moles can be flat or raised.

Most moles are harmless but people should monitor their moles for changes in color, size, and texture, and for the development of asymmetrical or irregular borders. A benign or noncancerous mole will remain stable in size, color, and shape for years. During pregnancy or puberty, moles may naturally change in color and size, becoming darker and larger.

When a mole bleeds, itches, enlarges, turns multipigmented, or evolves with irregular edges, the patient should see a dermatologist, as this mole may need testing for cancer.

Screening and diagnosis: Health care providers can check their patients' moles during routine physicals or checkups. Also, people can check their own moles periodically. One way to check moles for signs of melanoma is called the

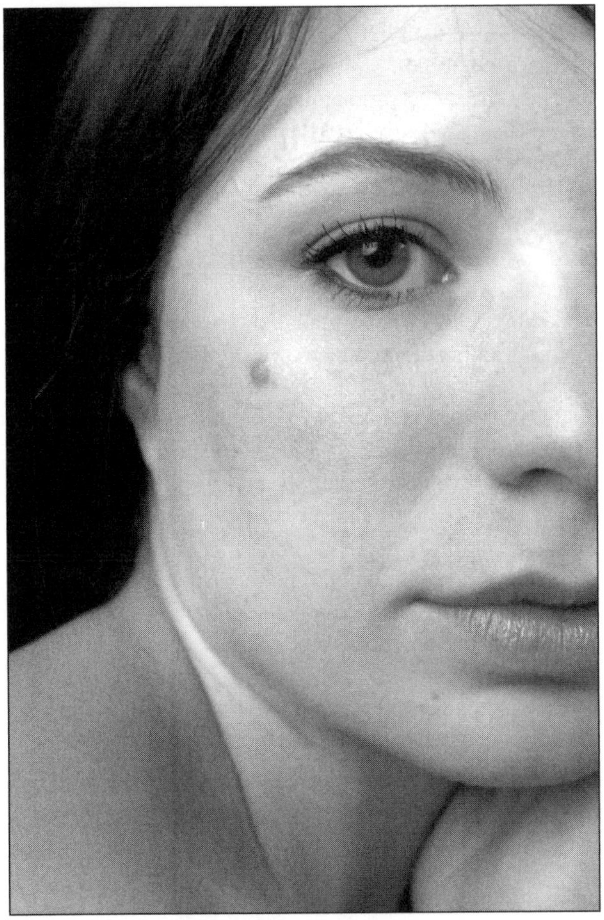

While most moles, like the one on this young woman's face, are harmless, they should be watched for changes in size, color, or shape that could possibly indicate the beginning of cancer. (©James Blinn/Dreamstime.com)

ABCDs of melanomas. "A" stands for asymmetry and indicates that the halves of a single mole should be checked to see if they are different or asymmetrical; a normal mole has identical halves. "B" means to look at the borders or edges of the mole to see if they are irregular; usually a noncancerous mole has regular distinct edges. "C" means that moles should be examined for color that varies within a single mole; ordinary moles are one color, not multipigmented. "D" is a reminder that the diameter of the mole should not exceed the size of a pencil eraser.

If changes appear in the mole, the patient should see a dermatologist who can provide more in-depth testing or removal of the mole. Some symptoms that may need evaluation are bleeding, itching, or an unusual change. The eyes alone cannot diagnosis a malignant mole. The dermatologist will biopsy or excise the mole for the pathologist to inspect. If the mole is malignant, the pathologist can provide a series of tests called staging. These tests may indicate whether the cancer has spread beyond the original site.

Treatment and therapy: Generally nevi require no treatment unless they change into a cancerous mole. However, sometimes they occur in an uncomfortable place and may be surgically removed. Failure to remove such a mole may result in bleeding from irritation.

When a mole is found to be cancerous, the mole, along with some surrounding tissue, is surgically removed.

Prognosis, prevention, and outcomes: Most moles are harmless and are just part of everyday life. However, there are known risk factors that increase the incidence of moles, and some can cause adverse changes in the structure of the moles, leading to malignancies. People at high risk for melanoma should be vigilant for changes in their moles.

Although some exposure to sunlight is healthful because it supplies the body with vitamin D, intense exposure to UV rays—such as tanning—puts people at risk. Sunburn experienced years earlier can still bring about changes in the skin that can precipitate a malignant mole. Young people often will not see the effects of overexposure to the sun's rays until years later, so they may not feel motivated to change their behavior. To decrease the risk of moles as well as the conversion of moles to cancer, people should use sun protection such as sunglasses, sunscreen, long-sleeved garments, and hats.

Robert W. Koch, D.N.S., R.N.

▶ For Further Information

Barnhill, Raymond, Michael Piepkorn, and Klaus Busam. *Pathology of Melanocytic Nevi and Malignant Melanoma*. 2d ed. New York: Springer, 2006.

Hearing, Vincent J., and Stanley P. L. Leong, eds. *From Melanocytes to Melanoma: The Progression to Malignancy*. Totowa, N.J.: Humana Press, 2006.

Poole, Catherine M., and Dupont Guerry IV. *Melanoma: Prevention, Detection, and Treatment*. 2d ed. New Haven, Conn.: Yale University Press, 2005.

Schofield, Jill R., and William A. Robinson. *What You Really Need to Know About Moles and Melanoma*. Baltimore: Johns Hopkins University Press, 2000.

▶ Other Resources

American Academy of Dermatology

Moles

http://www.aad.org/public/publications/pamphlets/common_moles.html

American Cancer Society
http://www.cancer.org

Medline Plus
Moles
http://www.nlm.nih.gov/medlineplus/moles.html

See also ABCD; Basal cell carcinomas; Carney complex; Chordomas; Choriocarcinomas; Craniosynostosis; Dermatology oncology; Dysplastic nevus syndrome; Gestational trophoblastic tumors (GTTs); Hereditary cancer syndromes; Human chorionic gonadotropin (HCG); Hydatidiform mole; Melanomas; Premalignancies; Sjögren syndrome; Skin cancers; Squamous cell carcinomas; Ultraviolet radiation and related exposures.

▶ Monoclonal antibodies

Category: Chemotherapy and other drugs

Definition: Monoclonal antibodies are antibodies that recognize only one antigen and that are mass-produced in the laboratory from a single clone of a B cell, the type of immune system cell that makes antibodies.

Cancers treated: Lymphoma, leukemia, breast cancer, head and neck cancers, colorectal cancer, lung cancer

Subclasses of this group: Murine (composed entirely of mouse sequences), chimeric (composed of approximately one-third mouse and two-thirds human sequences), humanized (composed of at least 90 percent human sequences), and human (antibodies that are fully human in composition)

Delivery routes: As a result of their molecular size and susceptibility to enzymatic digestion in the gut if administered orally, monoclonal antibodies must usually be administered by intravenous (IV) infusion.

How these drugs work: Antibodies are proteins that bind to a specific site, or epitope, on a specific target molecule. In response to infection or immunization with a foreign agent, the immune system generates many different antibodies that bind to the foreign molecules. This pool of polyclonal antibodies contains a mixture of different antibody molecules, each of which binds to a specific epitope. Isolation of a single antibody from a polyclonal antibody pool would yield a highly specific molecular tool with the ability to bind to a single epitope. Georges Köhler, César Milstein, and Niels Kaj Jerne invented the process of producing monoclonal antibodies in 1975 and shared the 1984 Nobel Prize in Physiology or Medicine for their discovery. Since then, monoclonal antibodies have become an important tool in biological research and in medicine.

The process of producing monoclonal antibodies involves fusing an individual B cell, which produces a single antibody with a single specificity but which has a finite life span, with a long-lived myeloma tumor cell. The B cell is taken from the spleen or lymph nodes of an animal that has been challenged with the antigen of interest. The combination of the B cell and the myeloma cell produces a hybridoma cell, a kind of perpetual antibody-producing factory. The hybridoma cell produces the single specific antibody and can be grown in culture indefinitely, allowing the production of large amounts of the monoclonal antibodies. Monoclonal antibodies are potentially more effective than conventional drugs in treating cancer, since conventional drugs attack not only cancer cells but also normal cells. Monoclonal antibodies attach only to the specific target molecule. Since monoclonal antibodies are specific for a particular antigen, one designed to bind to ovarian cancer cells, for instance, will not bind to colorectal cancer cells.

The first monoclonal antibodies were made from mouse B cells. When administered into humans, mouse antibodies are recognized by the human immune system as foreign (because they are from a different species) and can elicit an immune response against them, causing allergic-type reactions. Researchers have since learned how to replace some portions of the mouse antibody sequences with human antibody sequences. The application of genetic engineering techniques has allowed the production of chimeric, humanized, and, more recently, fully human monoclonal antibodies.

An antibody molecule is composed of two heavy polypeptide chains and two light polypeptide chains. Both heavy and light chains are composed of a region that varies from antibody to antibody, the variable region, and a constant region that is conserved. By combining human sequences for the constant region with murine sequences for portions of the variable region, the amount of murine sequence can be decreased. Depending on how much murine sequence is left, the result is either a chimeric (with approximately one-third murine and two-thirds human sequence) or a humanized (with at least 90 percent human sequence) monoclonal antibody. Genetically engineered mice strains are now available that contain a large portion of human deoxyribonucleic acid (DNA) that codes for the antibody heavy and light chains, with the mouse's own heavy and light chain genes inactivated. Using these mice to produce B cells for the construction of hybridomas allows the generation of fully human antibodies, which are likely to be safer and may be more effective than the previous generation of monoclonal antibodies.

Common Monoclonal Antibodies

Drug	*Brands*	*Subclass*	*Delivery Mode*	*Cancers Treated*
Alemtuzumab	Campath	Humanized	IV	Chronic lymphocytic leukemia
Bevacizumab	Avastin	Humanized	IV	Lung cancer, colorectal cancer
Cetuximab	Erbitux	Chimeric	IV	Head and neck cancers, colorectal cancer
Epratuzumab	LymphoCide	Humanized	IV	B-cell leukemia
Gemtuzumab ozogamicin	Mylotarg	Humanized	IV	Acute myelogenous leukemia
Ibritumomab tiuxetan	Zevalin	Murine	IV	B-cell lymphoma
Lym-1	Oncolym	Murine	IV	Lymphoma
Panitumumab	Vectibix	Human	IV	Colorectal cancer
Rituximab	Rituxan	Chimeric	IV	B-cell lymphoma
Tositumomab	Bexxar	Murine	IV	B-cell lymphoma
Trastuzumab	Herceptin	Humanized	IV	Breast cancer

One potential treatment for cancer involves using monoclonal antibodies that bind only to a cancer cell-specific component of interest and induce an immunological response against the target cancer cell (referred to as "naked" monoclonal antibodies). Monoclonal antibodies can also be designed for the delivery of another (nonspecific) agent, such as a toxin, radioisotope, or cytokine, to the cancer cell for the purpose of killing it (referred to as "conjugated" monoclonal antibodies).

Some naked monoclonal antibodies bind to cancer cells and exert their action by marking the cells to help the body's immune system destroy them. Rituxan (rituximab) and Campath (alemtuzumab) are examples of this type of monoclonal antibody. Rituximab binds to the CD20 antigen, a protein found on B cells, and is used to treat B-cell non-Hodgkin lymphoma. Alemtuzumab binds to the CD52 antigen, another protein present on B and T cells, and is used to treat some patients with B-cell chronic lymphocytic leukemia.

Some naked monoclonal antibodies bind to functional parts of cancer cells or other cells that help cancer cells grow and act by interfering with the cancer cells' ability to grow. Herceptin (trastuzumab), Erbitux (cetuximab), and Avastin (bevacizumab) are examples of this type of monoclonal antibody. Trastuzumab binds to the HER2/neu protein, a protein present in large numbers on tumor cells in some cancers that, when activated, helps these cells grow. Trastuzumab acts by inactivating these proteins. It is used to treat some breast cancers. Cetuximab binds to the epidermal growth factor receptor (EGFR) protein, which when present in high levels on cancer cells helps them grow. Cetuximab blocks the activation of EGFR and is used to treat some advanced colorectal cancers and some head and neck cancers. Bevacizumab binds to the vascular endothelial growth factor (VEGF), a protein that cancer cells produce to attract the new blood vessels they need for growth. Bevacizumab prevents VEGF from functioning and is used to treat some colorectal, lung, and breast cancers.

Some of these monoclonal antibodies have been used in cancer treatment for many years. At first they were used mainly after other treatments had failed, but as more studies have been done the trend is to use them earlier in the course of cancer treatment.

Conjugated monoclonal antibodies (also called "tagged" or "loaded" monoclonal antibodies) are attached to anticancer (chemotherapy) drugs, toxins, or radioactive substances and used as vehicles to deliver these toxic agents directly to cancer cells. Radiolabeled monoclonal antibodies are attached to radioactive substances; treatment with such agents is called radioimmunotherapy. Chemolabeled monoclonal antibodies are attached to anticancer drugs, and immunotoxins are monoclonal antibodies attached to toxins. Zevalin (ibritumomab tiuxetan) and Bexxar (tositumomab) are examples of radiolabeled monoclonal antibodies. Both bind to an antigen on cancerous B lymphocytes and are used to treat some B cell non-Hodgkin lymphomas. Mylotarg (gentuzumab ozogamicin) is an example of an immunotoxin. It contains the toxin calicheamicin attached to a monoclonal antibody that binds to the CD33, a protein antigen present on most leukemia cells, and is used to treat some acute myelogenous leukemias.

Clinical trials of monoclonal antibody therapy are in progress for patients with almost every type of cancer. As more cancer-associated antigens have been identified and studied, it has been possible for researchers to make monoclonal antibodies against more types of cancer.

Side effects: Antibodies that contain murine sequences can be recognized by the human immune system as foreign, causing systemic inflammatory effects such as fever, chills, weakness, headaches, nausea, vomiting, and diarrhea. Some monoclonal antibodies also have side effects associated with the antigen that they target. For example, some monoclonal antibodies can affect the bone marrow's ability to produce blood cells, which can result in an increased risk of bleeding or infection in some patients.

Jill Ferguson, Ph.D.

▶ For Further Information

George, Andrew J. T., and Catherine E. Urch, eds. *Diagnostic and Therapeutic Antibodies*. Totowa, N.J.: Humana Press, 2000.

Melero, I., et al. "Immunostimulatory Monoclonal Antibodies for Cancer Therapy." *Nature Reviews Cancer* 7 (2007): 95-106.

Reichert, J. M., and V. E. Valge-Archer. "Development Trends for Monoclonal Antibody Cancer Therapeutics." *Nature Reviews Drug Discovery* 6 (2007): 349-356.

Zafir-Lavie, I., Y. Michaeli, and Y. Reiter. "Novel Antibodies as Anticancer Agents." *Oncogene* 28 (2007): 3714-3733.

▶ Other Resources

Access Excellence
Monoclonal Antibody Technology: The Basics
http://www.accessexcellence.org/RC/AB/IE/Monoclonal_Antibody.html

American Cancer Society
Monoclonal Antibodies
http://www.cancer.org/docroot/ETO/content/ETO_1_4X_Monoclonal_Antibody_Therapy_Passive_Immunotherapy.asp

Lymphoma Information Network
Monoclonal Antibody Therapy
http://www.lymphomainfo.net/therapy/immunotherapy/mab.html

See also Biological therapy; CA 15-3 test; CA 19-9 test; CA 27-29 test; Carcinoembryonic antigen antibody (CEA) test; Carcinomas; Chemotherapy; Chronic lymphocytic leukemia (CLL); Colorectal cancer; Flow cytometry; Immunotherapy; Non-Hodgkin lymphoma; Oral and oropharyngeal cancers; Polyps; Radiation oncology; Radiopharmaceuticals; Receptor analysis; Richter syndrome.

▶ Motion sickness devices

Category: Complementary and alternative therapies
Also known as: ReliefBand, Sea-Band stimulators, BioBands

Definition: Nausea relief wristbands are economical devices that may decrease the nausea associated with cancer treatments such as chemotherapy and radiation therapy. Though these devices are not scientifically proven effective, many patients report relief of nausea when wearing a relief band on the wrist.

Delivery routes: Motion sickness relief bands are worn on the wrist and are available over the counter at pharmacies and drugstores.

Cancers treated: One common and disturbing side effect of cancer treatments, such as chemotherapy or radiation, is nausea and vomiting. These therapies are used as treatment for nearly all cancers.

Why used: Cancer patients who are receiving chemotherapy may feel a queasy feeling in the stomach (nausea), which can trigger vomiting, the forceful elimination of food or contents from the stomach. An estimated 70 to 89 percent of chemotherapy patients have this side effect. As many as 50 percent of cancer patients delay therapy because of fear of nausea and vomiting. Cancer patients who are receiving radiation therapy may experience a similar feeling of nausea that can lead to vomiting. Successful cancer treatment with chemotherapy or radiation depends on the patient's ability to tolerate this side effect.

How these bands work: These bands are usually made of a soft, elastic material that clings to the wrist. When a cancer patient puts on a motion sickness relief band, a small bead embedded in the band applies acupressure by pressing down on the neiguan, or P6, acupressure point. When this point on the median nerves of the inner wrist is stimulated, the trigger for nausea is suppressed.

Risks and results: Acupressure wristbands offer a cost-efficient and drug-free way to manage nausea and vomiting during cancer treatment. The therapy is safe for all ages, from children to older adults, as well as for pregnant and nursing women. The only risk is that they will not work for all people. However, the cost to try this therapy is minimal and does not require a doctor's prescription.

Marylane Wade Koch, M.S.N., R.N.

See also Acupuncture and acupressure for cancer patients; Adjuvant therapy; Chemotherapy; Cobalt 60 radiation; Complementary and alternative therapies; Nausea and vomiting.

▶ *MSH* genes

Category: Cancer biology
Also known as: MSH—MutS homolog 2, colon cancer, nonpolyposis type 1 (E. coli); HNPCC; HNPCC1; MSH3—mutS homolog 3 (E. coli); DUP; divergent upstream protein; mismatch repair protein 1; MRP1; MSH4—mutS homolog 4 (E. coli); MSH5—mutS homolog 5 (E. coli); MSH6—mutS homolog 6 (E. coli); GTBP

Definition: *MSH* genes are a class of genes that are normally involved in deoxyribonucleic acid (DNA) mismatch repair but can be mutated in many types of cancer.

Normal cellular function: DNA mismatch repair is the process whereby errors in DNA replication are recognized and repaired by proteins in the cell. If the mismatch repair machinery is defective, either by mutation of the genes encoding the proteins or by altering the expression levels of the proteins, errors are no longer repaired.

Relevance to cancer: Cells that contain defects in DNA mismatch repair show mutation rates that are one hundred to one thousand times higher than normal cells. Most mutations may not have negative effects, but if mutations are made in genes required to regulate cell growth and proliferation, this can lead to cancer. A readout of this increased mutation rate is microsatellite instability (MSI). Microsatellites are repetitive DNA sequences that are prone to replication errors, and cells that are defective in mismatch repair show variability in the length of these sequences.

One of the genes in this class, *MSH2*, is among the most frequently mutated genes in hereditary nonpolyposis colorectal cancer (HNPCC). Inheriting a mutation in this gene causes a genetic predisposition to cancer. In addition, *MSH* genes are often mutated in noninherited forms of cancer such as skin cancer and ovarian cancer. Other *MSH* genes—*MSH3* and *MSH6*—are also mutated in cancer, but at a lower frequency than *MSH2*.

Diagnostic and genetic testing: A number of tests are available to monitor the status of the mismatch repair machinery, which can provide diagnostic and prognostic information. DNA sequencing of the *MSH2* gene can be done to look for mutations that can predispose patients to cancer. Protein levels can be measured by immunohistochemical analysis of tissue samples, and tests to monitor the MSI status of tumor cells can also be performed.

Clinical implications: Because they strongly predispose people to developing cancer, patients carrying mutations in mismatch repair genes should undergo frequent colonoscopy as well as screenings for endometrial cancers. In addition, levels of mismatch repair proteins as well as MSI status can be strong predictors of tumor progression and prognosis. For example, although tumors that show high MSI tend to be aggressive, the outcome is usually favorable. Further, cells defective in mismatch repair have been shown to be less sensitive to platinum-based chemotherapy as well as methylating agents, which both work by inducing DNA damage.

Lindsay Lewellyn, B.S.

See also Ashkenazi Jews and cancer; Cancer biology; Family history and risk assessment; Genetics of cancer; Hereditary cancer syndromes; *MLH1* gene.

▶ Mucinous carcinomas

Category: Diseases, symptoms, and conditions
Also known as: Colloid carcinomas, mucinous adenocarcinomas, adenocystic carcinomas, mucoepidermoid carcinomas, gelatinous carcinomas

Related conditions: Breast cancers, ductal carcinoma in situ, colon cancer, pancreatic cancer, eyelid cancer

Definition: Mucinous carcinoma is a type of invasive duct cancer that occurs most frequently in the breast (MCB), although it has also been reported in the colon and pancreas. Primary mucinous carcinoma of the skin (MCS) is recognized as a rare variant of a sweat gland tumor.

Risk factors: Age is the only recognized risk factor. The average age at diagnosis is sixty-seven for mucinous carcinoma of the breast and sixty-three for mucinous carcinoma of the skin.

Etiology and the disease process: In all cases, the distinguishing feature is a type of mucus production called mucin. Poorly differentiated cancer cells are often completely surrounded by mucin in these tumors. The cancer spreads into the normal tissue surrounding it, although the mucin itself does not generally cause major problems.

Incidence: Mucinous carcinoma of the breast is a relatively rare form that accounts for about 3 percent of all breast cancer diagnoses. It occurs most frequently in women in their sixties. Mucinous carcinoma of the skin can originate at any location on the body, although the eyelid has been reported as the most commonly affected area (41 percent of cases). There is a slight preponderance of affected males.

Symptoms: Mucinous carcinoma of the breast is usually detected as medium to large size tumors that can be felt. They are usually highly estrogen dependent and only rarely spread to local lymph nodes. Mucinous carcinoma of the skin lesions are painless gray or red nodules measuring 0.5 to 7 centimeters in diameter.

Screening and diagnosis: Core needle biopsy (of the breast version) and skin biopsy (of the skin version) are usually very effective diagnostic tools. Tumor identification is most often straightforward, since the tumor cell morphology and mucin production are so characteristic of this type of cancer.

Treatment and therapy: Treatment of mucinous carcinoma of the breast generally includes some combination of surgery, chemotherapy, and radiation therapy. Since lymph node involvement is rare, surgery can often be conservative (lumpectomy). Standard treatment for mucinous carcinoma of the skin is wide local excision.

Prognosis, prevention, and outcomes: Mucinous carcinoma of the breast has a much better prognosis than other invasive ductal breast carcinomas because it is associated with a low risk of axillary metastases. A ten-year survival rate of more than 90 percent has been reported. Mucinous carcinoma of the skin lesions have a propensity for local recurrence and regional spread, although distant metastases are rare. One study of one hundred cases of primary mucinous carcinoma of the skin reported 29.4 percent local recurrences, 9.6 percent metastases, and an overall mortality rate of 2 percent.

Jeffrey A. Knight, Ph.D.

See also Adenocarcinomas; Adenoid cystic carcinoma (ACC); Breast cancers; Carcinomas; Colorectal cancer; Ductal carcinoma in situ (DCIS); Eyelid cancer; Pancreatic cancers.

▶ Mucosa-associated lymphoid tissue (MALT) lymphomas

Category: Diseases, symptoms, and conditions
Also known as: Extranodal lymphoma, MALT lymphomas, MALTomas

Related conditions: Indolent non-Hodgkin lymphoma (NHL), marginal zone B-cell lymphomas

Definition: Mucosa-associated lymphoid tissue (MALT) lymphomas are a form of non-Hodgkin lymphoma frequently involving the MALT of the stomach and the gastrointestinal tract, usually as a result of *Helicobacter pylori* infection. They are solid tumors that originate from B cells in the marginal zone of the MALT.

Disorders Linked to *H. pylori* Infection

- Stomach ulcers
- Duodenal ulcers
- Gastric cancer
- MALT lymphomas
- Possibly pancreatic cancer
- Possibly cardiovascular disease

Source: National Cancer Institute

Risk factors: Gastric MALT lymphoma is frequently associated (72 to 98 percent) with the presence of *H. pylori*. The causes of MALT lymphoma in other parts of the body are unknown. In general, the incidence of non-Hodgkin lymphoma is two to three times higher among individuals with relatives who developed non-Hodgkin lymphoma, indicating familial clusters. In addition, a compromised immune system is a major risk factor for non-Hodgkin lymphoma development.

Etiology and the disease process: MALT lymphoma starts in mucosa-associated lymphoid tissue, which is lymphatic tissue, such as the stomach, thyroid gland, and lungs. Virtually any mucosal site can be afflicted; however, colorectal involvement of MALT lymphoma is rare. MALT lymphoma is a cancer of the B-cell lymphocytes. It belongs to the group of marginal zone B-cell lymphomas. Marginal zone lymphoma can be either nodal or extranodal. In particular, MALT lymphoma is an extranodal marginal zone B-cell lymphoma.

Incidence: MALT lymphoma is a relatively rare form of non-Hodgkin lymphoma. Most cases, approximately two out of three, of MALT lymphoma affecting the stomach are caused by infection with *H. pylori*. The disease is more common in people over sixty, but it may occur at any age from early adulthood to old age. MALT lymphoma is slightly more common in women than in men. Ethnicity may play a role in geographic differences among non-Hodgkin lymphoma incidence rates. In particular, gastric lymphomas have the highest recorded incidence in northern Italy.

Symptoms: The most common symptoms experienced by those with MALT lymphomas range from no symptoms to occult or gross gastrointestinal symptoms. Regardless of organ of origin, all MALT lymphomas appear to have similar clinical, pathological, and molecular features.

The symptoms exhibited depend on the site for MALT lymphoma. MALT lymphoma in the stomach may cause indigestion, bleeding into the stomach, weight loss, loss of appetite, and tiredness.

Screening and diagnosis: The initial diagnosis of MALT lymphoma is typically made by esophagogastroduodenoscopy (EGD), or upper endoscopy, which is a flexible tube passed down the gullet and into the stomach. Endoscopy is used to obtain photographs of the stomach, and a small sample of cells is extracted for assessment (biopsy). Tests for *H. pylori* are also common when gastrointestinal MALT lymphomas are suspected.

Staging is based on how extensively the cancer has spread throughout and beyond the lymphatic system, which areas are affected, and whether constitutional symptoms, such as fever, night sweats, or weight loss, are present.

The staging of MALT lymphoma is essential for precise prognosis and to develop an effective treatment plan. The Ann Arbor Staging System is the most widely used system for non-Hodgkin lymphoma.

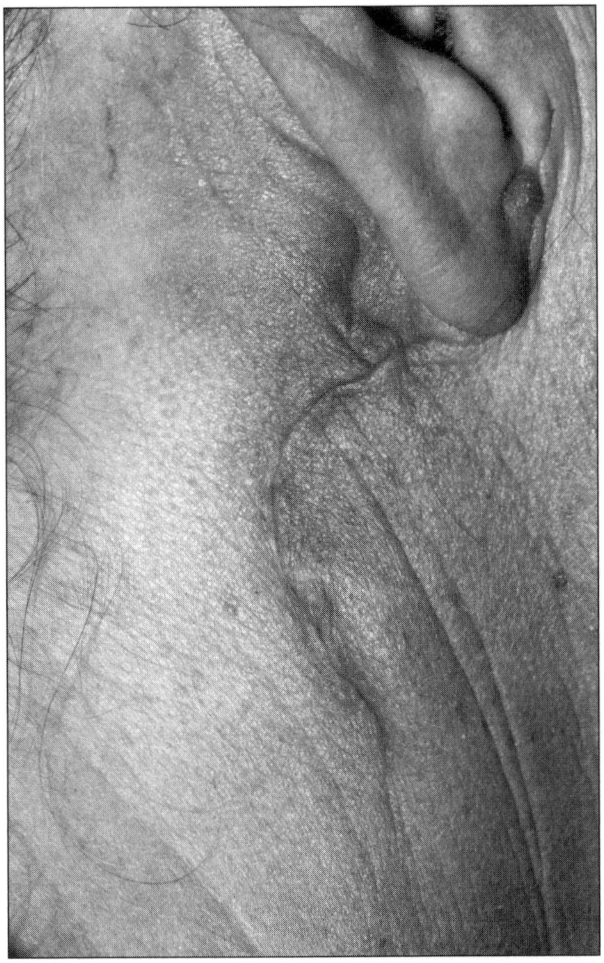

A scar on the neck of a woman marks where a MALT lymphoma was removed from her salivary gland. (Dr. P. Marazzi/Photo Researchers, Inc.)

Treatment and therapy: When bacteria are present in the tumor tissue, biological therapy, such as intensive antibiotic treatment, often leads to a complete remission of the lymphoma. Approximately 70 to 80 percent of patients will have a complete regression of malignancy with antibiotic treatment of *H. pylori* when MALT lymphoma is limited to the stomach. If antibiotics do not clear MALT lymphomas or the disease spreads, other treatments are given, including radiotherapy, surgery, or chemotherapy.

Some MALT lymphomas grow very slowly, especially if the site of origin is other than the stomach, and may not cause any problems for many years. In this case, treatment may not be needed immediately, and active monitoring is used instead.

For MALT lymphoma affecting the lung or the bowel, the typical treatment is chemotherapy. Low-grade MALT lymphoma may transform into high-grade lymphoma, in which case it requires more intensive chemotherapy.

MALT lymphoma may be removed during a surgical operation. If the lymphoma is affecting the stomach, total gastrectomy may be needed, which involves the removal of all of the stomach, along with the lower part of the gullet. The gullet is then joined directly to the small intestine. New treatments for MALT lymphoma are being researched.

If patients have been treated for a lymphoma affecting the stomach, typically they will undergo regular follow-up endoscopies and biopsies of the stomach to look for signs of recurrence. Other tests may be used for people whose MALT lymphoma affects areas apart from the stomach.

Side effects of non-Hodgkin lymphoma management may also vary depending on what part of the body is affected and the treatment used. The side effects of biological therapy are most often flulike symptoms, and external radiation to the abdomen may cause nausea, vomiting, and diarrhea.

Prognosis, prevention, and outcomes: The International Prognostic Index is the most widely used prognostic system for non-Hodgkin lymphoma, and it was designed to further clarify lymphoma staging. Paradoxically, in a significant number of cases, aggressive lymphomas can be cured by chemotherapy, while indolent non-Hodgkin lymphomas generally cannot be cured. Approximately 40 percent of indolent malignancies transform into high-grade aggressive lymphomas, and the cure potential of the transformed lymphoma is less favorable than that of aggressive lymphomas without transformation.

Anita Nagypál, Ph.D.

▶ For Further Information

Ferreri, A. J., et al. "Therapeutic Management of Ocular Adnexal MALT Lymphoma." *Expert Opinion on Pharmacotherapy* 8, no. 8 (June, 2007): 1073-1083.

Firat, Y., A. Kizilay, G. Sogutlu, and B. Mizrak. "Primary Mucosa-Associated Lymphoid Tissue Lymphoma of Hypopharynx." *Journal of Craniofacial Surgery* 18, no. 5 (September, 2007): 1189-1193.

Magrath, Ian T., ed. *The Non-Hodgkin's Lymphomas.* New York: Oxford University Press, 1997.

Roh, Jong-Lyel, Jooryung Huh, and Cheolwon. Suh. "Primary Non-Hodgkin's Lymphomas of the Major Salivary Glands." *Journal of Surgical Oncology* 97, no. 1 (October 10, 2007): 35-39.

Troch, M., et al. "Does MALT Lymphoma of the Lung Require Immediate Treatment? An Analysis of Eleven Untreated Cases with Long-Term Follow-Up." *Anticancer Research* 27, no. 5B (September/October, 2007): 3633-3637.

▶ Other Resources

Lymphoma Information Network
Mucosa-Associated Lymphatic Tissue Lymphomas
http://www.lymphomainfo.net/nhl/types/malt.html

Lymphomation.org
MALT Lymphomas
http://www.lymphomation.org/type-malt.htm

See also *Helicobacter pylori*; Lymphomas; Non-Hodgkin lymphoma.

▶ Mucositis

Category: Diseases, symptoms, and conditions
Also known as: Oral mucositis, gastrointestinal mucositis

Related conditions: In extreme cases, bacteremia and sepsis

Definition: Mucositis is ulceration in the mouth (oral mucositis) and esophagus, intestines, and anus (gastrointestinal mucositis) as a side effect of radiation or chemotherapy for cancer.

Risk factors: Mucositis is directly related to therapeutic radiation and chemotherapy. There may be genetic factors causing some people to be more sensitive or resistant to cellular damage following therapy.

Etiology and the disease process: Radiation and chemotherapy kill cancer cells but can also damage normal tissue in the gastrointestinal tract. Endothelial cells, which make up the capillaries under the skin, and fibroblast cells, which build connective tissue, are the most sensitive to therapeutic damage. These cells produce important growth factors that maintain the epithelial cells on the surface lining of the gastrointestinal tract. Because of cell death and inflammation, ulcers form along the gastrointestinal tract.

Incidence: Up to 100 percent of patients who receive high-dose radiation treatment will develop some level of mucositis.

Symptoms: Redness of the skin resulting from capiltary congestion (erythema) and swelling are early symptoms. More advanced cases develop ulcers in the mouth and intestines a few days following cancer treatment. Patients may also experience diarrhea, nausea and vomiting, a drop in blood volume (hypovolemia), dry mouth, change of taste, and loss of appetite. Ulcers can become infected, and infection can spread to the blood (bacteremia). Patients often stop eating because of the pain. Severe complications may lead to death due to blood infection (sepsis), electrolyte imbalances, and malnutrition.

Screening and diagnosis: Mucositis is diagnosed by clinical observation of symptoms according to different grades established by the World Health Organization:
- Grade 0: No symptoms
- Grade 1: Erythema
- Grade 2: Erythema, ulcers, can eat solid food
- Grade 3: Ulcers, liquid-only diet
- Grade 4: Ulcers, assisted (parenteral) feeding necessary

Treatment and therapy: After therapy ends, mucositis will resolve without treatment. While mucositis persists, palliative treatment is given, including narcotics for pain, antibiotics for infections, and assisted feeding.

Research on drugs to treat mucositis is ongoing. One drug, palifermin (Kepivance), is approved by the Food and Drug Administration for treating oral mucositis. Palifermin is related to a hormone that stimulates epithelial cells. Given before radiation therapy, palifermin strengthens and protects the oral epithelium, making it much more resistant to developing mucositis.

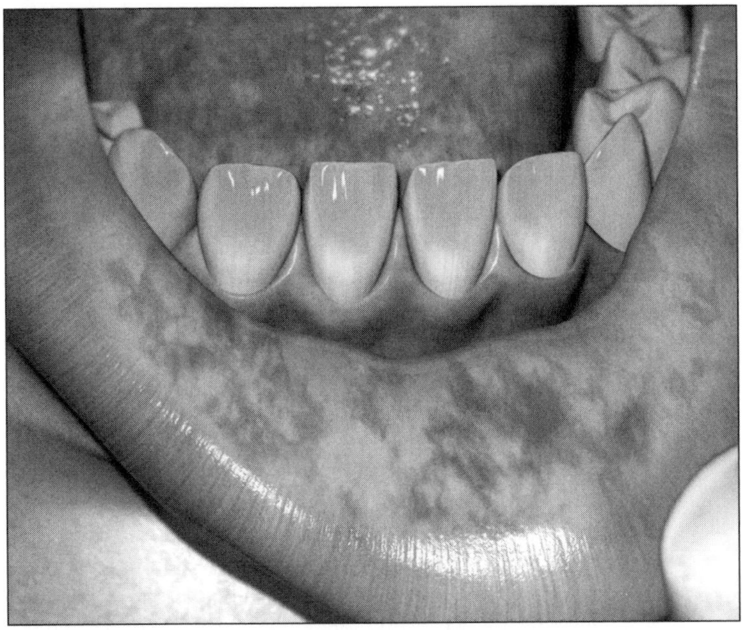

Inflammatory mucositis in the mouth, developed in response to radiation treatment of another part of the head. (©XVIVO LLC/Phototake—All rights reserved)

Prognosis, prevention, and outcomes: Most patients recover from mucositis, though a small percentage of patients die from complications. Cancer therapy is often reduced or stopped because of mucositis, which may compromise cancer care.

Christopher Pung, B.S., C.L.Sp. (CG)

See also Chemotherapy; External beam radiation therapy (EBRT); Fatigue; Gastrointestinal complications of cancer treatment; Intensity-modulated radiation therapy (IMRT); Radiation therapies; Side effects; Stomatitis.

▶ Multiple endocrine neoplasia type 1 (MEN 1)

Category: Diseases, symptoms, and conditions
Also known as: Wermer syndrome

Related conditions: Hyperparathyroidism, pituitary tumor, pancreatic tumor, duodenal tumor

Definition: Multiple endocrine neoplasia type 1 (MEN 1) is a hereditary tumor syndrome characterized by endocrine and nonendocrine tumors, most of which are benign. The characteristic findings include tumors of the parathyroid glands, pituitary gland, pancreas, and duodenum (part of the small intestine). Neuroendocrine tumors (nerve-cell tumors that may produce hormones) in the pancreas and duodenum are the main cause of tumor-related death. The severity varies within families and between families.

Risk factors: Because MEN 1 is hereditary, the main risk factor is having a family history of this disorder. Each child of a person with MEN 1 has a 50 percent chance of inheriting the disorder.

Etiology and the disease process: The underlying genetic cause of MEN 1 is a mutation, or a genetic change, in the *MEN1* gene. *MEN1* is a tumor-suppressor gene, and the protein it encodes helps stop uncontrolled cell growth and proliferation.

Usually, each person has two normal copies of the *MEN1* gene. A mutation in one copy of the gene is sufficient to cause MEN 1, which is why this condition is referred to as autosomal dominant (autosomal means the *MEN1* gene is located on one of the twenty-two pairs of autosomes, which are the nonsex chromosomes). An affected person has a *MEN1* gene mutation from the time of conception in the womb; however, symptoms of the disease may not manifest until later in life. Most mutations are inherited from a parent, but new mutations do occur.

Incidence: Approximately 0.2 to 2 per 100,000 people have MEN 1.

Symptoms: Parathyroid tumors can cause high calcium levels in the blood, nausea, fatigue, muscle pains, constipation, abdominal pain, kidney stones, and bone fractures. Symptoms of pituitary tumors vary depending on the type of hormone being made by the tumor. Tumors of the pancreas and duodenum cause many different symptoms depending on the tumor type.

Screening and diagnosis: Physicians diagnose MEN 1 in a person with an endocrine tumor in two of the three tissue systems usually affected in this syndrome: parathyroid glands, pancreas, and pituitary gland. Because MEN 1 is caused by mutations in the *MEN1* gene, genetic testing can be used to confirm a suspected diagnosis or to test a family member who is at risk for the disease but has no symptoms.

Treatment and therapy: A combination of surgery and medication may be used to treat MEN 1 tumors.

Prognosis, prevention, and outcomes: Because MEN 1 is a genetic condition, its manifestations cannot currently be prevented. However, physicians recommend monitoring that includes blood testing for hormone levels and imaging of the head and abdomen.

Abbie L. Abboud, M.S., C.G.C.

See also Duodenal carcinomas; Endocrine cancers; Endocrinology oncology; Family history and risk assessment; Gastrinomas; Histamine 2 antagonists; Human growth factors and tumor growth; Islet cell tumors; Multiple endocrine neoplasia type 2 (MEN 2); Neuroendocrine tumors; Pancreatic cancers; Parathyroid cancer; Pheochromocytomas; Pituitary tumors; Thyroid cancer; Zollinger-Ellison syndrome.

▶ Multiple endocrine neoplasia type 2 (MEN 2)

Category: Diseases, symptoms, and conditions
Also known as: MEN 2, MEN 2A, MEN 2B, Sipple syndrome, mucosal neuroma syndrome, familial medullary thyroid carcinoma

Related conditions: Medullary thyroid carcinoma, pheochromocytoma, parathyroid hyperplasia or adenoma, mucosal neuromas of the lips and tongue, gastrointestinal ganglioneuromas

Definition: Multiple endocrine neoplasia type 2 (MEN 2) is a hereditary cancer syndrome that affects the endocrine glands, which produce hormones in the body. MEN 2 is subclassified into three types: MEN 2A, MEN 2B, and familial medullary thyroid carcinoma (FMTC). All three types are associated with medullary thyroid cancer (MTC, a tumor that grows from the C cells in the thyroid gland). MEN 2A and MEN 2B are also associated with pheochromocytoma (an adrenal gland tumor that releases stress hormones). MEN 2A carries an increased risk for parathyroid hyperplasia (in which the parathyroid glands become enlarged and produce too much parathyroid hormone) or parathyroid adenoma (a benign tumor), both of which cause hyperparathyroidism (increased secretion of parathyroid hormone). MEN 2B is associated with mucosal neuromas (tumors growing from a nerve) of the lips and tongue, gastrointestinal ganglioneuromas (benign growths in the intestines), and characteristic facial appearance (a slender face, with prominent, bumpy lips). The disease findings and the severity of the syndrome vary within families and between families.

Risk factors: Because MEN 2 is hereditary, the main risk factor is having a family history of this syndrome. Each child of a person with MEN 2 has a 50 percent chance of inheriting the disease.

Etiology and the disease process: The underlying genetic cause of MEN 2 is a mutation, or a genetic change, in the *RET* gene. *RET* is a proto-oncogene, which means that it normally functions in cell growth and differentiation. Mutations in *RET* cause it to become an active oncogene, turning normal cells into cancer cells.

Usually, each person has two normal copies of the *RET* gene. A mutation in one copy of the gene is sufficient to cause MEN 2, which is why this condition is referred to as autosomal dominant (autosomal means the *RET* gene is located on one of the twenty-two pairs of autosomes—the nonsex chromosomes). A person with MEN 2 has a *RET* gene mutation from the time of conception in the womb; however, symptoms of the disease may not manifest until later in life. Most mutations are inherited from a parent, but new mutations do occur. The age of onset for medullary thyroid cancer is usually early childhood in MEN 2B, early adulthood in MEN 2A, and middle age in familial medullary thyroid carcinoma.

Mutations in different parts of the *RET* gene lead to the three subtypes of MEN 2. Nearly all cases of MEN 2B are caused by one specific mutation. Certain mutations are associated with a higher incidence of pheochromocytoma and hyperparathyroidism.

Incidence: Approximately 1 in 30,000 people has MEN 2.

Symptoms: Symptoms of medullary thyroid cancer may include a thyroid nodule (lump on the throat) and enlarged lymph nodes in the neck. Pheochromocytomas release catecholamines (stress hormones) that can cause dangerously high blood pressure levels. Hyperparathyroidism can cause high calcium levels in the blood, nausea, fatigue, muscle pains, constipation, abdominal pain, kidney stones, and bone fractures. In MEN 2B, gastrointestinal ganglioneuromas can cause constipation or megacolon (abnormally large colon).

Screening and diagnosis: The criteria to diagnose MEN 2 are different depending on the subtype. MEN 2A is diagnosed by the presence of two or more endocrine tumors (in one person or in close blood relatives). MEN 2B is diagnosed in a person with mucosal neuromas on the lips and tongue, medullary thyroid cancer, and, in some cases, pheochromocytoma. Familial medullary thyroid carcinoma is diagnosed in families with four or more cases of medullary thyroid cancer without any other findings of MEN 2. Tools used to check for disease include a blood test to

Relative Survival Rates for Medullary Thyroid Carcinoma, 1988-2001

		Survival Rates (%)					
Stage	*Cases Diagnosed (%)*	*1-Year*	*2-Year*	*3-Year*	*5-Year*	*8-Year*	*10-Year*
Stage II	42.5	97.5	94.5	89.6	89.6	86.3	77.1
Stage III	43.8	100.0	95.4	89.8	82.6	82.3	82.3

Source: Data from L. A. G. Ries et al., eds., *Cancer Survival Among Adults: U.S. SEER Program, 1988-2001—Patient and Tumor Characteristics*, NIH Pub. No. 07-6215 (Bethesda, Md.: National Cancer Institute, 2007)

Note: So few cases were diagnosed at Stages I and IV that percentages and relative survival rates were not meaningful.

measure levels of calcitonin (a hormone produced by medullary thyroid cancer) and urine testing to check for catecholamines and metanephrines released by pheochromocytomas. Blood and urine testing may also be done to assess for hyperparathyroidism.

Because MEN 2 is caused by mutations in the *RET* gene, genetic testing is a valuable tool to confirm a suspected diagnosis or to test a family member who is at risk for the disease but has no symptoms. Genetic testing detects *RET* gene mutations in approximately 95 percent of families with MEN 2A and MEN 2B and in approximately 88 percent of families with familial medullary thyroid carcinoma.

Treatment and therapy: The only way to cure medullary thyroid cancer is to remove the thyroid gland (thyroidectomy) at a young age. A patient who has had a thyroidectomy must take thyroid hormone replacement therapy. Because the risk for cancer is so high, removing the thyroid gland is recommended for people who have a *RET* mutation, even if they do not yet have cancer. Surgery to remove the adrenal gland is necessary to treat patients with pheochromocytoma. Sometimes pheochromocytomas occur in both adrenal glands. All or some of the four parathyroid glands may be removed to treat hyperparathyroidism.

Prognosis, prevention, and outcomes: Because MEN 2 is a genetic condition, its manifestations cannot be prevented. However, monitoring of individuals who are at risk for the disease based on their family history or who are known to have a *RET* gene mutation can detect problems early and lead to more effective treatment and better outcomes. Such monitoring includes yearly blood testing for calcitonin levels, yearly blood pressure checks, and yearly urine testing for catecholamines and metanephrines. The medical team caring for patients decides the age at which monitoring should start.

Abbie L. Abboud, M.S., C.G.C.

▶ For Further Information

Gertner, M. E., and E. Kebebew. "Multiple Endocrine Neoplasia Type 2." *Current Treatment Options in Oncology* 5 (2004): 315-325.

Gimm, O. "Multiple Endocrine Neoplasia Type 2: Clinical Aspects." *Frontiers of Hormone Research* 28 (2001): 103-130.

Ponder, B. A. J. "Multiple Endocrine Neoplasia Type 2." In *The Metabolic and Molecular Bases of Inherited Disease*, edited by Charles R. Scriver, Arthur L. Beaudet, David Valle, and William S. Sly. 8th ed. New York: McGraw-Hill, 2001.

▶ Other Resources

American Cancer Society
http://www.cancer.org

Genetics Home Reference
Multiple Endocrine Neoplasia
http://ghr.nlm.nih.gov/condition=multipleendocrineneoplasia

See also Endocrine cancers; Endocrinology oncology; Family history and risk assessment; Gastrinomas; Genetics of cancer; Histamine 2 antagonists; Human growth factors and tumor growth; Islet cell tumors; Multiple endocrine neoplasia type 1 (MEN 1); Neuroendocrine tumors; Parathyroid cancer; Pheochromocytomas; Pituitary tumors; Thyroid cancer; Zollinger-Ellison syndrome.

▶ Multiple myeloma

Category: Diseases, symptoms, and conditions
Also known as: MM, myeloma, plasma cell myeloma, cancer of the bone marrow

Related conditions: Multiple gammopathy of undetermined significance (MGUS), smoldering myeloma, indolent myeloma

Definition: Multiple myeloma is a cancer involving several clusters of cancerous plasma cells (a type of white blood cell found in the bone marrow that produces immunoglobulins to fight infection) in various bones of the body.

Risk factors: No one is sure what causes multiple myeloma. People who have been exposed to agricultural and other chemicals such as Agent Orange, some types of radiation, and some viruses appear to be more susceptible to multiple myeloma. People with multiple myeloma are usually diagnosed in their fifties and sixties. The disease is identified more often in men than in women and more often in African Americans than in members of other ethnic groups. Scientists have not been able to associate multiple myeloma with a genetic trait, but research suggests that chromosome 13 may be incomplete or entirely missing in myeloma cells.

Patients with a condition known as multiple gammopathy of undetermined significance (MGUS) have a relatively large amount of immunoglobulin protein (the M-protein) present in their blood. MGUS itself is benign, but about 16 percent of individuals with the condition eventually exhibit symptoms of multiple myeloma. Patients with smoldering or indolent myeloma, often a precursor disease, exhibit higher levels of calcium and kidney dysfunction, anemia, and bone disease.

Etiology and the disease process: Multiple myeloma occurs when abnormal plasma cells in the bone marrow multiply, accumulate, and overtake the healthy plasma cells. As the plasma cells circulate in the bloodstream, they often settle in other bones and interfere with the body's ability to produce normal antibodies, which leads to difficulty fighting infections.

Incidence: Approximately 53,000 Americans have multiple myeloma. Slightly fewer than 20,000 Americans were expected to be diagnosed with multiple myeloma in 2007. Using statistics gathered from 2002 to 2004, the National Cancer Institute estimates that 0.61 percent (1 in 165) of men and women born today will be diagnosed with multiple myeloma at some time during their lifetime.

Incidence of Multiple Myeloma per 100,000 People, by Gender

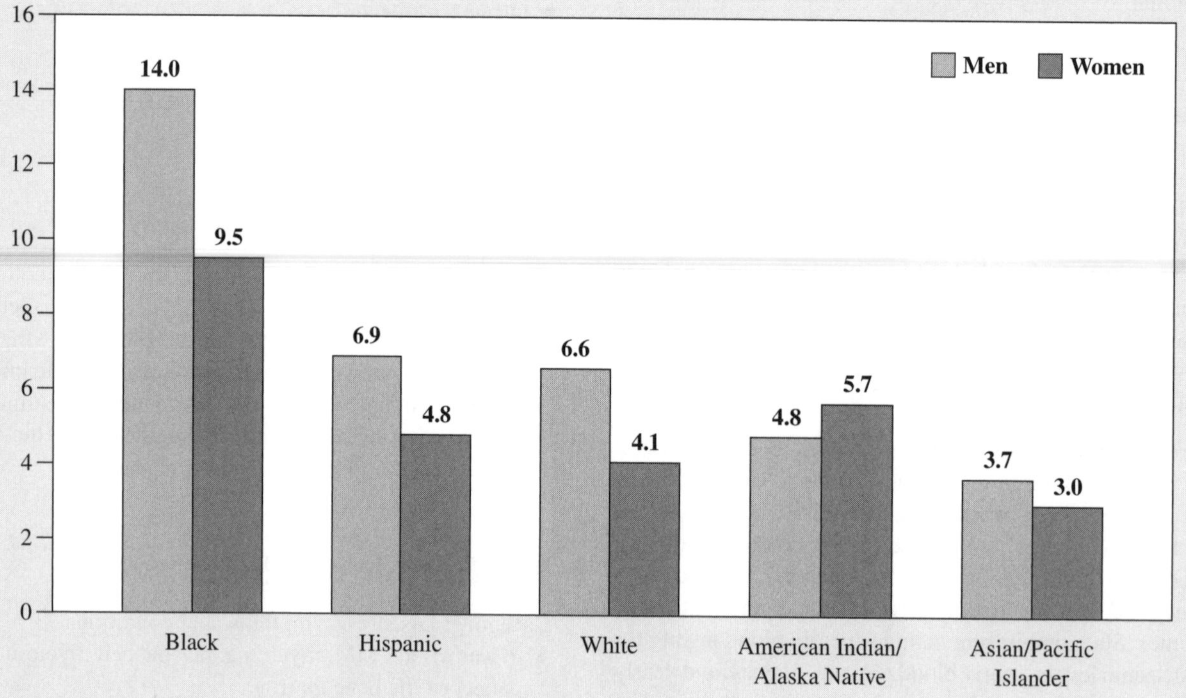

Source: Data from National Cancer Institute, Surveillance Epidemiology and End Results, Cancer Stat Fact Sheets, 2008
Note: Based on cases diagnosed in 2000-2004

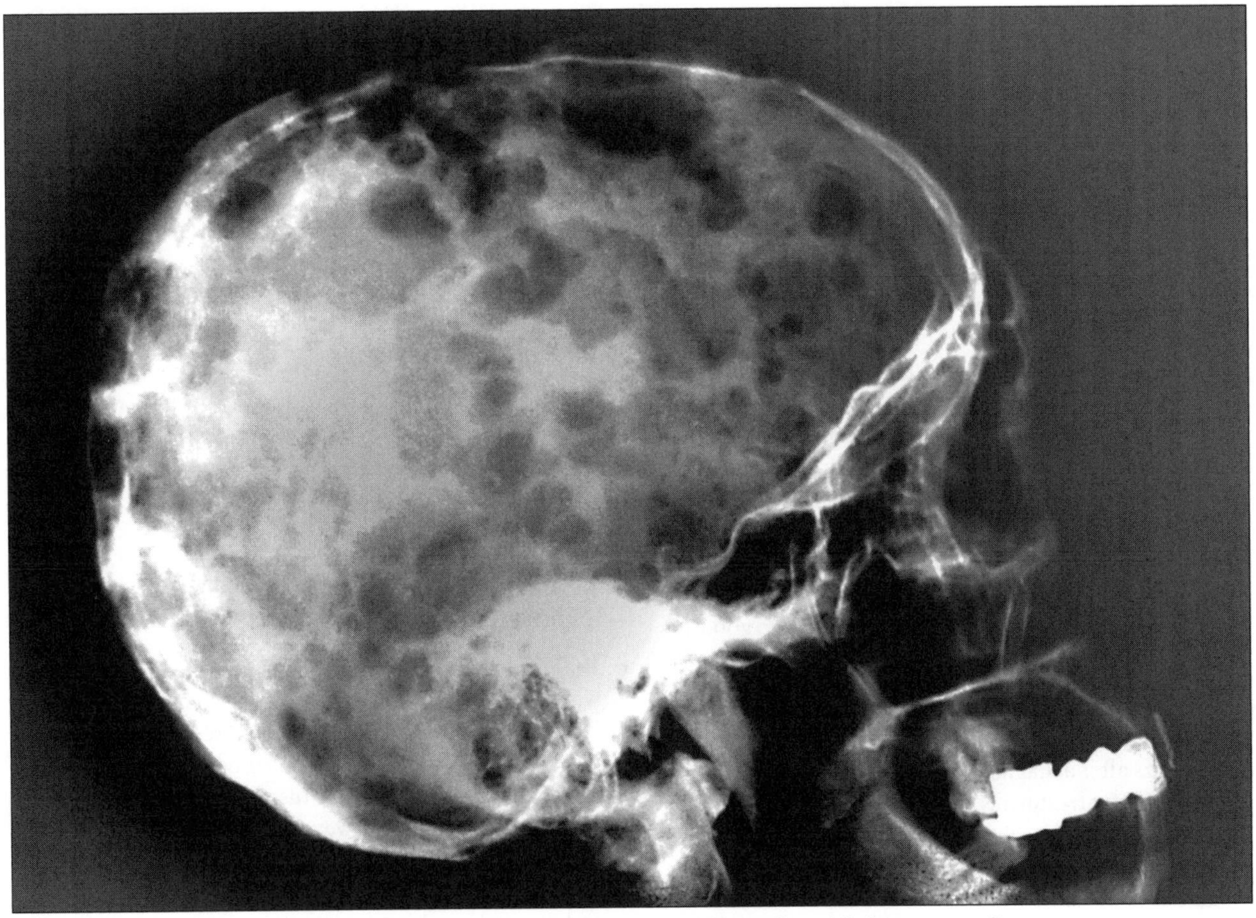

Multiple myeloma in the bone marrow. (©ISM/Phototake—All rights reserved)

Symptoms: The early stages of multiple myeloma may be uneventful and indistinct from other maladies. Multiple myeloma is often marked by successive infections, weight loss, fatigue or weakness, broken bones, or bone pain, most commonly in the ribs or back.

Screening and diagnosis: Kidney problems are often the first indication that something is wrong. High levels of protein in the blood can cause kidney damage, and high levels of calcium may indicate the beginning or presence of kidney problems. Symptoms of kidney problems include greater thirst and urine production, a loss of appetite, fatigue, muscle weakness, restlessness, confusion or an inability to concentrate, constipation, and nausea and vomiting. An accurate diagnosis requires consideration of the patient's history and symptoms, a complete physical, and an evaluation of laboratory results.

A diagnosis of multiple myeloma requires blood tests to determine the amount of calcium and plasma cells in the blood and the patient's degree of anemia. Technologists will look for the presence of M-protein, beta-2 microglobulin (β2M), and other proteins in a blood sample and for the presence of the Bence-Jones protein (a type of M-protein) in the urine. Additional testing will include imaging studies—X rays, computed tomography (CT) scans, or magnetic resonance imaging (MRI) studies—to examine whether bone cavities exist and whether they might be caused by a tumor. This is followed by taking a tissue sample from a large bone to examine whether myeloma cells are present in the marrow.

Most clinicians use the International Staging System to categorize multiple myeloma using the following criteria:

- Stage I: Serum β2M less than 3.5 milligrams/deciliter (mg/dl) and serum albumin greater than or equal to 3.5 grams/deciliter (g/dl)
- Stage II: Serum β2M less than 3.5 mg/dl and albumin less than 3.5 g/dl or serum β2M 3.5 to 5.5 mg/dl
- Stage III: Serum β2M greater than 5.5 mg/dl

Higher serum β2M levels and lower serum albumin levels usually indicate active or advanced disease. Increased values of C-reactive protein and serum lactate dehydrogenase also may indicate active disease.

Treatment and therapy: There is no cure for multiple myeloma, but several treatment options exist and new options are being developed. The aim of most therapy is to ease a patient's symptoms and slow the progression of disease, relieve pain and discomfort, and stabilize the immune system and metabolic functions. Various combination therapies are being used to combat multiple myeloma. These include dexamethasone, either alone or in combination with thalidomide or melphalan; melphalan plus prednisone; a combination drug known as VAD (vincristine/doxorubicin/dexamethasone); and bortezomib, either alone or in combination with other drugs such as dexamethasone, lenalidomide, or doxorubicin liposomal (Doxil). Additional therapies include the use of cyclophosphamide or etoposide. Each drug combination has advantages and disadvantages, and not all drug combinations work well in all patients. Some patients have had extremely good results using these drugs, and many have experienced disease remission.

Prognosis, prevention, and outcomes: Most patients live many years after a diagnosis of multiple myeloma. Physicians may offer treatments for bone pain, infections, anemia, and fatigue or weakness, which are considered to be the most common body effects associated with multiple myeloma.

Terry A. Anderson, B.S.

▶ For Further Information

Anderson, Kenneth C., and Irene Ghobrial, eds. *Multiple Myeloma*. New York: Informa Healthcare, 2007.

Brian, G., M., et al. "International Uniform Response Criteria for Multiple Myeloma." *Leukemia* 20, no. 9 (2006): 1467.

Dominik, D., et al. "Multiple Myeloma: A Review of the Epidemiologic Literature." *International Journal of Cancer* 120, suppl. 12 (2007): 40-61.

▶ Other Resources

International Myeloma Foundation
http://www.myeloma.org

Multiple Myeloma Research Foundation
http://www.multiplemyeloma.org

See also African Americans and cancer; Agent Orange; Amyloidosis; Angiogenesis inhibitors; Bisphosphonates; Blood cancers; Bone cancers; Bone marrow aspiration and biopsy; Bone marrow transplantation (BMT); Bone pain; Curcumin; Hair dye; Hematologic oncology; Hemolytic anemia; Hepatitis C virus (HCV); Hypercalcemia; Immunoelectrophoresis (IEP); Interferon; Malignant fibrous histiocytoma (MFH); Melphalan; Motion sickness devices; Myeloma; Myelosuppression; Proteasome inhibitors; Protein electrophoresis; Spinal axis tumors; Waldenström macroglobulinemia (WM).

▶ Mustard gas

Category: Carcinogens and suspected carcinogens
RoC status: Known human carcinogen since 1980
Also known as: HD, senfgas, sulfur mustard, blister gas, s-lost, lost, Kampfstoff LOST, yellow cross liquid, yperite

Related cancers: Cancers of the larynx, pharynx, upper respiratory tract, and lungs

Definition: Mustard gas is a member of the sulfur mustards, which are blister-inducing agents (vesicants). Mustard gas is actually a liquid at room temperature that is clear to yellow or brown in color and is either odorless or smells like garlic, onions, or mustard. Mustard gas was originally introduced as a chemical weapon during World War I and has been used throughout the world since then. It is a powerful irritant that damages the eyes and respiratory tract and causes large blisters on exposed skin.

Exposure routes: Inhalation and dermal contact

Where found: Used during chemical warfare attacks and in research laboratories.

At risk: Military personnel or civilians exposed to mustard gas during chemical warfare attacks, workers who manufacture it, and people who live near stockpiles of it or come into contact with unexploded ordnances loaded with it

Etiology and symptoms of associated cancers: Because mustard gas often has no odor, people are unaware that they have been exposed to it until the onset of symptoms, which usually begin two to twenty-four hours after exposure. Symptoms include redness, itching, yellow blistering of the skin, pain, swelling and tearing of the eyes, runny nose, sneezing, hoarseness, shortness of breath, sinus pain, bloody nose, cough, abdominal pain, diarrhea, fever, nausea, and vomiting. More severe exposures can cause second-to-third-degree burns of the skin, light sensitivity in the eyes or severe pain and blindness, chronic respiratory disease, and death.

Mustard gas is an alkylating agent that chemically alters

the nitrogenous bases in deoxyribonucleic acid (DNA). Alkylation of DNA damages it and generates mutations but can also cause chromosome breakage. Mustard-gas-induced mutations cause either cell death or transformation into a tumor cell. Therefore, mustard gas is a confirmed carcinogen in humans and animals, and exposure to it increases a person's risk for respiratory and lung cancer.

Some 25 percent of all people who get lung cancer show no symptoms, but normally, the symptoms include cough, shortness of breath, wheezing, chest pain, and coughing up blood (hemoptysis). Nonspecific symptoms include weight loss, weakness, fatigue, depression, and mood changes. The spread of the cancer decreases lung capacity, and patients die because they are unable to inspire sufficient quantities of oxygen.

History: During World War I, the German army first used mustard gas in July, 1917, against British soldiers near the Belgian city of Ypres. Since then, mustard gas has been used globally, but sporadically, in modern warfare.

Epidemiological studies from the 1970's and 1980's established that soldiers and production workers exposed to mustard gas for longer periods of time showed an increased risk of respiratory cancers.

The Geneva Protocol of 1925, which was modified and extended the Chemical Weapons Convention of 1993, prohibits the development, production, and stockpiling of chemical weapons, which includes mustard gas.

Michael A. Buratovich, Ph.D.

See also Alkylating agents in chemotherapy; Carcinogens, known; Chemotherapy; Laryngeal cancer; Lung cancers; Melphalan; Nasal cavity and paranasal sinus cancers; Oral and oropharyngeal cancers.

▶ Mutagenesis and cancer

Category: Cancer biology

Definition: Mutagenesis is the generation of changes or mutations in the genetic material of a cell. Normally, the cells in the body maintain a critical balance between cell growth and proliferation and cell death. This balance is maintained by the action of a number of different cellular mechanisms. When mutations are made that affect the ability of a cell to maintain this balance, it can begin to proliferate uncontrollably, leading to tumor formation and ultimately cancer. Mutations can be inherited or acquired over the lifetime of an individual. In addition, certain types of cancer cells show a characteristic increased rate of mutation, known as a mutator phenotype.

Mutagenesis and cancer formation: In normal cells, the processes of cell proliferation and cell death are tightly controlled by multiple redundant mechanisms. Therefore, multiple mutations are required to transform a normal cell into a cancer cell. Although the specific genes that are mutated in different tumors are highly variable, there is a common theme to the types of mutations that promote tumor formation. In general, mutations are likely to occur in two types of genes—proto-oncogenes and tumor-suppressor genes.

A proto-oncogene is a gene that normally promotes cell growth, differentiation, and proliferation. When a proto-oncogene undergoes a mutation that promotes tumor cell formation, it is known as an oncogene. Oncogenic mutations are considered to be dominant, which means that mutation of a single copy of the gene is sufficient to confer an increased risk of tumor formation. Conversion from a proto-oncogene into an oncogene can occur by a number of different mechanisms, most of which ultimately lead to increased levels of activity of the encoded protein. For example, mutations within the coding sequence of the gene can change the structure of the protein to increase its activity or disrupt its ability to be properly regulated. Mutations outside of the coding region of the gene can affect the expression of the protein, leading to increased levels within the cell.

The first identified oncogene, the protein kinase Src, was discovered in 1970 from a chicken retrovirus. In normal, nontumor cells, c-src is an enzyme that acts within a number of different signaling pathways to promote cell proliferation, cell survival, initiation of protein translation, metabolism, cell adhesion, and motility. The oncogenic form of the protein, v-src, contains a mutation that abolishes a regulatory site on the protein, leading to its constitutive activation. Cells that contain the oncogenic form of Src are able to grow in the absence of cell proliferation signals as well as without being anchored down. These properties give transformed cells a selective growth advantage over normal, nontransformed cells, which can ultimately lead to uncontrolled growth and tumor formation.

The other common type of mutation found in cancer cells occurs within tumor-suppressor genes. In normal cells, tumor-suppressor genes are involved in negatively regulating cell growth and proliferation. These genes produce proteins that prevent cells from dividing when there is deoxyribonucleic acid (DNA) damage, if the cell division apparatus is compromised, and in the absence of growth signals. Mutations in tumor-suppressor genes are characterized as recessive, since both copies of the gene must be mutated. One of the most common mutations found in human cancers is within the tumor-suppressor gene *TP53*. When a cell experiences damage or stress, *TP53* normally acts to suppress cell growth and proliferation, and if the damage is severe enough, promote cell death. Mutation of both copies of the *TP53* gene allows cells to survive and proliferate even in the presence of DNA damage.

Multiple mutations in proto-oncogenes and tumor-suppressor genes are required to transform a normal cell into a cancer cell. This idea was made famous by Alfred Knudson in 1971, who showed that the incidence of tumor formation was consistent with two mutational "hits." For example, mutation of *TP53* alone is not sufficient to induce tumor formation, since this mutation only effectively disengages the brake put on cell growth. This mutation does, however, confer on the cell a selective advantage, which will most likely cause it to produce more daughter cells than its neighbors that do not contain the mutation. Over time, progeny of this original mutant cell may accumulate an oncogenic mutation that will allow it to grow and proliferate even more and potentially form a tumor. Additional mutations can then occur that allow the cells to better survive in the harsh tumor environment, which contains very low levels of oxygen and nutrients, as well as to allow the cell to metastasize into other regions of the body.

Inherited mutations: One way to acquire a mutation is to inherit it from parents. Cells in the body contain two copies of each gene—one inherited from each parent. Inheriting a mutated copy of a gene, such as a tumor suppressor, from one parent can strongly predispose a person to developing cancer. Normally, a cell must undergo mutation of both copies of a tumor-suppressor gene to abolish its function. However, if a person inherits a mutation in one copy of the gene, then the amount of time that it takes to inactivate the remaining copy of the gene is much less. Therefore, patients with inherited mutations often show increased risk and decreased age of onset of cancer. For example, inheriting one mutant copy of the *TP53* tumor-suppressor gene often leads to Li-Fraumeni syndrome. Li-Fraumeni syndrome strongly predisposes a patient to developing cancer, which usually shows a very early age of onset, as well as formation of multiple tumors throughout the life of the individual.

For example, *BRCA1* is a tumor-suppressor gene encoding a protein whose normal function is to repair damaged DNA. Inheriting a mutation in *BRCA1* significantly increases a woman's risk of developing breast or ovarian cancer. This is because defects in *BRCA1* function lead to the accumulation of additional mutations in the genome.

Acquired mutations: In addition to inheriting mutations, an individual can acquire changes in the genetic material over his or her lifetime. Each time a cell in the body divides, it must faithfully replicate its genetic material, which is contained in the DNA. If the DNA is not correctly replicated, then mutations can arise, which, if left uncorrected, will be passed on to all of the daughter cells that descend from that cell. Because mutations are made each time the genome is replicated, the rate of mutation within a cell depends on the fidelity of the machinery that recognizes and repairs these mutations.

In addition to acquiring unrepaired mutations that may occur each time a cell replicates its genetic material, genes can become mutated because of exposure to different mutagenic agents that originate from within the cell as well as toxins originating from the environment. By-products of cellular metabolism such as reactive forms of oxygen can cause DNA mutation. Chemical carcinogens, ionizing radiation, and viruses are all environmental agents that can generate mutations.

Mutagenesis in cancer cells: Cancer cells often show rates of mutation that are significantly higher than those in normal cells. This can be due to mutations in genes that are normally involved in the identification and repair of mutations. Normally, if a mutation occurs in the DNA, either during replication or as a result of another type of damage, it is recognized by a set of proteins that first signal to the cell to stop dividing and then recruit other proteins to repair the damage. If the damage is too severe, then the cell will undergo programmed cell death, or apoptosis. If DNA damage is not correctly identified and repaired, then this could lead to increased rates of mutation, ultimately leading to the accumulation of multiple genetic "hits" and development of cancer.

Over time, the likelihood that mutations will occur in proto-oncogenes or tumor-suppressor genes increases. Genetic testing is available to detect mutations in some of these commonly mutated genes, and knowledge of specific mutational status can provide important insight into prognosis and treatment.

Lindsay Lewellyn, B.S.

▶ For Further Information

Hanahan, Douglas, and Robert A. Weinberg."The Hallmarks of Cancer." *Cell* 100 (2000): 57-70.

Knudson, Alfred G. "Two Genetic Hits (More or Less) to Cancer." *Nature Reviews Cancer* 2 (November 1, 2001): 157-162.

Sarasin, Alain. "An Overview of the Mechanisms of Mutagenesis and Carcinogenesis." *Mutation Research* 544 (2003): 99-106.

▶ Other Resources

Gene Tests
http://www.geneclinics.org

Human Genome Project Information
http://www.ornl.gov/sci/techresources/Human_Genome/home.shtml

National Human Genome Research Institute
http://www.genome.gov

See also Antioxidants; Ashkenazi Jews and cancer; Bioflavonoids; Cancer biology; Carcinogens, known; Carcinogens, reasonably anticipated; Chromosomes and cancer; Free radicals; Gene therapy; Genetic testing; Genetics of cancer; Herbs as antioxidants; Hereditary cancer syndromes; Oncogenes; Proto-oncogenes and carcinogenesis; Tumor-suppressor genes.

▶ Myasthenia gravis

Category: Diseases, symptoms, and conditions
Also known as: Familial myasthenia gravis, neonatal myasthenia gravis, congenital myasthenia gravis, juvenile myasthenia gravis

Related conditions: Autoimmune disorders, thymomas

Definition: The term "myasthenia gravis" comes from Latin and Greek meaning grave (severe) muscle weakness; this describes the condition very well. Although there are several forms of myasthenia gravis, the most common is a chronic autoimmune neuromuscular condition in which there is sporadic, severe weakness of the voluntary muscles of the body, especially those of the face and throat.

Risk factors: Most cases of myasthenia gravis appear to be sporadic (caused by unknown factors). An elevated risk has been noted for women between the ages of twenty and forty with family history of the disease, drug ingestion, or other autoimmune disorders. Myasthenia gravis is inherited in about 5 percent of all cases, associated with specific immune system alleles (HLA-B8 and DR3).

Etiology and the disease process: In myasthenia gravis, the body produces antibodies that attack its own proteins (an autoimmune response). With the exception of drug-induced myasthenia gravis (D-penicillamine ingestion, for example), there is no known causative agent or pathogen that accounts for onset of the disease, which can be quite sudden. As with other cancers, the body's regulatory mechanisms are not operating properly, in this case allowing antibody-producing cells that should be screened out to continue being produced.

In most cases of myasthenia gravis, the antibodies produced are directed against the acetylcholine (ACh) receptor. Receptors are proteins on the cell membrane that bind to a particular class of compounds, thus triggering the cell to perform some function or action. Acetylcholine receptors are present in the motor end plate of voluntary muscles, where they are stimulated by nerves. An electrical impulse in a nerve causes acetylcholine to be released; it binds with the receptor on the muscle cell, allowing sodium and calcium to move into the cell and stimulating it to contract. The acetylcholine is then broken down by the enzyme cholinesterase (so hyperstimulation does not occur) and recycled within the nerve cell. If antibodies to the receptor are present, they bind to the receptor first, so that very little acetylcholine can bind. Thus, sodium and calcium influx is limited, and muscle contraction is limited or nonexistent. In some cases, antibodies may actually destroy the receptors on the muscle cell membranes altogether, leaving muscles unable to contract even in the presence of a strong nerve signal.

The antibodies against acetylcholine receptors are produced by B cells, circulating white blood cells (leukocytes). B cells are activated by T-helper cells, which develop within the thymus. Therefore, myasthenia gravis is often associated with thymoma (tumor of the thymus), although the exact mechanism of this association is not clearly understood.

A second form of antibody in some patients develops against the receptor protein muscle-specific kinase (MuSK), required for formation of the nerve-muscle junction during early development. The result is an incomplete junction, making it harder for acetylcholine to span the gap and stimulate the muscle.

Incidence: The overall U.S. incidence is listed at 20 cases per 100,000 population, although many authors report it to be much higher. The discrepancy comes from the difficulty of diagnosis from initial symptoms. All ethnic groups and genders are susceptible, but there is a difference in age distribution. Generally this disease is seen in women under the age of forty, and in men and women between the ages of fifty and seventy. However, it can strike at any age including at birth (neonatal myasthenia gravis, congenital myasthenia gravis) or in children (juvenile myasthenia gravis). About 15 percent of those who contract myasthenia gravis have a thymoma.

Symptoms: The primary symptom of myasthenia gravis is muscle weakness, especially those muscles that control

Drugs to Be Avoided by People with Myasthenia Gravis

MG-Causing Drugs
- Alpha-interferon
- Botulinum toxin
- D-Penicillamine

Drugs That Increase Muscle Weakness
- Antibiotics: particularly aminoglycosides, ciprofloxacin, telithromycin
- Beta-blockers: propranolo, timolol maleate eyedrops
- Calcium channel blockers
- Iodinated contrast agents (for X rays)
- Neuromuscular blocking agents: succinylcholine and vecuronium; only anaesthesiologists familiar with MG should use these
- Quinine, quinidine, procainamide

Source: Myasthenia Gravis Foundation of America

eye and eyelid movement, chewing, talking, facial expression, and swallowing. This weakness usually increases during periods of muscle activity and decreases with periods of rest.

Screening and diagnosis: Myasthenia gravis can be difficult to diagnose. The symptoms can be subtle and hard to distinguish from other neurological disorders. A thorough physical exam is the first step in diagnosis, including various tests aimed at muscle fatigability (keeping arms stretched forward for sixty seconds or looking at the feet for sixty seconds while lying on the back). Blood tests can help to identify specific acetylcholine antibodies but may be negative (due to sensitivity of the assay) in up to 50 percent of cases, especially in the early stages. Repetitive nerve stimulation (with electrical impulses) can be used to measure fatigability, as can single fiber electromyography, a sensitive test that records the electrical impulse in muscle fibers.

Classification (staging) of myasthenia gravis is as follows:

- Stage I: Eye muscle weakness or ptosis of any severity; no other evidence of muscle weakness
- Stage II: Eye muscle weakness of any severity; mild weakness of other muscles
- Stage III: Eye muscle weakness of any severity: moderate weakness of other muscles
- Stage IV: Eye muscle weakness of any severity: severe weakness of other muscles
- Stage V: Severe weakness leading to intubation of the airway

Treatment and therapy: Myasthenia gravis is generally controlled through medication. The medications have two purposes: lessening muscle weakness and reducing the autoimmune response. Cholinesterase inhibitors (such as neostigmine and pyridostigmine) allow the acetylcholine to remain near the receptor for a longer period of time, thus increasing the chance that it will bind. Immunosuppresive drugs (such as prednisone, cyclosporine, or azathioprine) help reduce the antibody formation but may take weeks or months to show effects. For patients in a critical state, plasmapheresis may also be used to remove circulating antibodies from the bloodstream.

Patients experiencing myasthenia gravis caused by a thymoma may have the thymoma surgically removed (thymomectomy) to prevent possible spread of cancer in the event the thymoma is cancerous; most thymomas, however, are benign.

Prognosis, prevention, and outcomes: With proper treatment, patients have a normal life expectancy. However, those with malignant thymoma may experience rapid decline. Quality of life varies quite markedly, but myasthenia gravis is not a progressive disease, and therefore, some lifestyle changes can lessen the symptoms in some individuals. In some patients, symptoms come and go; for some the symptoms decrease after three to five years of treatment.

Kerry L. Cheesman, Ph.D.

▶ For Further Information

Baron-Faust, Rita, and Jill P Buyon. *The Autoimmune Connection: Essential Information for Women on Diagnosis, Treatment, and Getting on with Life*. Chicago: Contemporary Books, 2003.

Keesey, John Carl. *Myasthenia Gravis: An Illustrated History*. Roseville, Calif.: Publishers Design Group, 2002.

National Institutes of Health. *Understanding Autoimmune Diseases*. NIH Publication 98-4273. Bethesda, Md.: Author, 1998.

_______. *Understanding the Immune System: How It Works*. NIH Publication 03-5423. Bethesda, Md.: Author, 2003.

_______. *Questions and Answers About Autoimmunity*. NIH Publication 02-4858. Bethesda, Md.: Author, 2002.

Shannon, Joyce Brennfleck, ed. *Movement Disorders Sourcebook: Basic Consumer Health Information About Neurological Movement Disorders*. Detroit: Omnigraphics, 2003.

Vincent, Angela, and Camilla Buckley. "Myasthenia Gravis and Other Antibody-Associated Neurological Diseases." In *The Autoimmune Diseases*, edited by Noel R. Rose and Ian R. Mackay. Boston: Elsevier/Academic Press, 2006.

▶ Other Resources

American Cancer Society
http://www.cancer.org

Myasthenia Gravis Foundation of America
http://www.myasthenia.org

National Institute of Neurological Disorders and Stroke
NINDS Myasthenia Gravis Information Page
http://www.ninds.nih.gov/disorders/myasthenia_gravis/myasthenia_gravis.htm

See also Lambert-Eaton myasthenic syndrome (LEMS); Mediastinal tumors; Mediastinoscopy; Surgical biopsies; Thymomas; Thymus cancer.

▶ *MYC* oncogene

Category: Cancer biology
Also known as: *c-Myc*, v-myc myelocytomatosis viral oncogene homolog (avian)

Definition: First identified in humans based on its homology to the chicken viral oncogene (*v-myc*), *MYC* belongs to a family of *MYC* genes that codes for a transcription factor containing the basic-helix-loop-helix Leucine zipper (bHLH/LZ) domain. The MYC protein binds to the enhancer box (E-box) sequence and activates the expression of a larger number of genes. By modifying the expression of its target genes, *MYC* is able to activate numerous biological effects. It affects cell proliferation (downregulates *CDKN1A*, or *p21*), regulates cell growth (upregulates *TP53*), induces apoptosis (upregulates *BCL2*), and regulates differentiation (downregulates *C/EBPA*).

Role in cancer biology: The role of *MYC* in influencing critical aspects of the cell cycle machinery makes it a centerpiece and key to the enigma of cancer biology. In normal cells, *MYC* expression is under tight regulation, with the gene being expressed only in actively dividing cells. In contrast, genetic aberrations result in the uncontrolled expression of *MYC* in cancer cells. Aberrant expression of *MYC* plays a significant role in a wide variety of human cancers: 80 percent of breast cancers, 70 percent of colon cancers, 90 percent of gynecological cancers, 50 percent of hepatocellular carcinomas, and a variety of hematological tumors possessing abnormal *MYC* signatures. An estimated 100,000 cancer deaths per year in the United States are associated with changes in the *MYC* gene or its expression. The clinical significance of *MYC* gene alterations in human cancers is best illustrated by the amplification of *MYCN* (*N-myc*) in neuroblastoma and the translocation of *MYC* from its normal position on chromosome 8 to chromosome 14 in Burkitt lymphoma.

Inhibiting *MYC*: Experimental evidence shows that inhibiting *MYC* significantly halts tumor cell growth and proliferation; consequently *MYC* is an attractive target for cancer therapy. Another advantage of *MYC* as a therapeutic target is the fact that it is downstream of multiple converging signaling pathways that are affected by mutations in a number of genes in different cancer types. Major advances in drug development aimed at eliminating *MYC* include targeting it by antisense mitochondrial ribonucleic acid (mRNA) and deoxyribonucleic acid (DNA) oligonucleotides, triple-helix-forming oligonucleotides, ribozymes, porphyrins, and small interfering RNA (siRNA). Inhibition of *MYC* can be achieved with many of these approaches; however, for increased clinical efficacy it is probable that intervention, possibly in combination with traditional chemotherapy, will be necessary.

Banalata Sen, Ph.D.

See also Burkitt lymphoma; Cancer biology; Free radicals; Gene therapy; Genetics of cancer; Oncogenes; Protooncogenes and carcinogenesis; Tumor markers; Tumor-suppressor genes.

▶ Mycosis fungoides

Category: Diseases, symptoms, and conditions
Also known as: Cutaneous T-cell lymphoma (CTCL), cutaneous lymphoma, MF

Related conditions: Sézary syndrome (SS), lymphomatoid papulosis, cutaneous anaplastic large-cell lymphoma, adult T-cell leukemia/lymphoma, peripheral T-cell lymphoma, lymphomatoid granulomatosis, granulomatous slack skin disease, pagetoid reticulosis

Definition: Mycosis fungoides (MF) is the most common type of cutaneous T-cell lymphoma (CTCL). Mycosis fungoides was named after the mushroom-like skin tumors that were noted in the first patient diagnosed with the condition. A low-grade lymphoma that primarily affects the skin, it generally has a slow course and often remains confined to the skin. Over time, in only about 10 percent of the cases, it does slowly progress to the lymph nodes and internal organs such as the liver, lungs, and bone marrow.

The cutaneous T-cell lymphomas are a group of rare skin cancers that includes Sézary syndrome, lymphomatoid papulosis, cutaneous anaplastic large-cell lymphoma, adult T-cell leukemia/lymphoma, peripheral T-cell lymphoma, lymphomatoid granulomatosis, granulomatous slack skin disease, and pagetoid reticulosis.

Risk factors: The cause of mycosis fungoides is unknown. There is no supportive research indicating that this is a hereditary disease. Exposure to Agent Orange may be a risk factor for developing mycosis fungoides for veterans of the Vietnam War, but no direct cause-effect relationship has been established.

Etiology and the disease process: Mycosis fungoides is a special variant of lymphoma with major involvement of the skin as well as hilar and mediastinal lymphadenopathy. It is associated with reticular nodular pulmonary lesions and is often complicated by pneumonias, primarily caused by *Staphlococcus aureus* or *Pseudomonas aeruginosa*. The condition is not contagious. It is not an infection, and there are no infectious agents known to cause the disease. There has been research investigating the role of viruses, but the results are inconclusive.

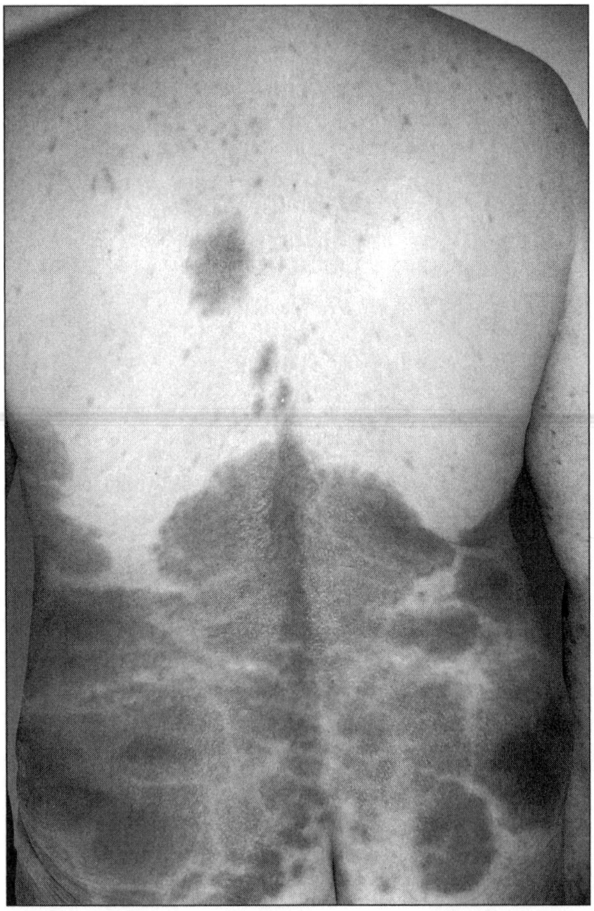

Mycosis fungoides on a patient's back. (©ISM/Phototake—All rights reserved)

Incidence: In the United states, approximately 1,000 new cases of mycosis fungoides occur per year. It affects men twice as often as women and is more common in blacks than in whites. Mycosis fungoides can begin at any age, but the most common age is fifty years old.

Symptoms: Mycosis fungoides progresses through four stages, which are defined by the skin symptoms, including the patch phase, skin tumors phase, skin redness stage, and lymph node stage, where mycosis fungoides begins to spread or metastasize, usually first to the lymph nodes, then to the liver, lungs, or bone marrow.

Screening and diagnosis: Typically there are about six years from the onset of symptoms to the diagnosis of mycosis fungoides. Confusion with other conditions is common. A sample of the skin known as a skin biopsy is usually performed. Other laboratory tests can be done to determine the progression of the cancer. There is no cure for mycosis fungoides, so long-term survival depends on early diagnosis and treatment.

Treatment and therapy: Treatments are directed at either the skin or the entire body (systemic therapy). Skin-directed treatments include ultraviolet light (psoralen and ultraviolet A, or PUVA, UVB, narrow-band UVB), topical steroids, topical chemotherapies (nitrogen mustard, carmustine), topical retinoids, local radiation to single lesions, or total skin electron beam (TSEB). Systemic treatments include oral retinoids, photopheresis, photochemotherapy (also known as PUVA), fusion proteins, interferon, systemic chemotherapy (most commonly cyclophosphamide, doxorubicin, vincristine, and prednisone), and orphan drugs such as bexarotene (Targretin). These treatments may be prescribed alone or in combination.

Prognosis, prevention, and outcomes: The course of mycosis fungoides is unpredictable, as some patients will progress slowly, some will progess rapidly, and some will not progress at all. Most patients will experience only skin symptoms, without serious complications. About 10 percent will experience progressive disease with lymph node involvement or spread to the liver, lungs, or bone marrow.

Many patients live normal lives while they treat their disease, and some are able to remain in remission for long periods of time. Although there is no known cure for mycosis fungoides, research has indicated that patients diagnosed with early-stage mycosis fungoides (which is 70 to 80 percent of patients) will have a normal life expectancy.

Debra B. Kessler, M.D., Ph.D.

▶ **For Further Information**

Dummer, R. "Future Perspectives in the Treatment of Cutaneous T-cell Lymphoma (CTCL)." *Seminars in Oncology* 33, no. 1 (2006): S33-S36.

Girardi, M., P. W. Heald, and L. D. Wilson. "The Pathogenesis of Mycosis Fungoides." *The New England Journal of Medicine* 350, no. 19 (2004): 1978-1988.

Kumar, Vinay, et al., eds. *Robbins and Cotran Pathologic Basis of Disease*. Philadelphia: Elsevier Saunders, 2005.

▶ **Other Resources**

Cutaneous Lymphoma Foundation
http://www.clfoundation.org/

The Skin Site
Mycosis fungoides
http://www.skinsite.com/info_mycosis_fungoides.htm

See also Agent Orange; Cutaneous T-cell lymphoma (CTCL); Lymphomas; Sézary syndrome; Skin cancers.

▶ Myelodysplastic syndromes

Category: Diseases, symptoms, and conditions
Also known as: Myelodysplasia

Related conditions: Acute myeloid leukemia

Definition: Myelodysplastic syndromes characterize a range of hematological disorders in which the bone marrow stem cells either do not mature into red or white blood cells or do not function properly. This lack of healthy blood cells can lead to life-threatening conditions.

Risk factors: No one is certain what causes myelodysplastic syndromes. Most researchers believe that a variety of factors will lead to different myelodysplastic syndrome subtypes, but no one has been able to pinpoint what causes their onset. Scientists believe that prior therapy for cancer and exposure to environmental toxins places individuals at great risk for myelodysplastic syndromes. The cancer-treatment drugs chlorambucil, mechlorethamine, and procarbazine are all toxic to the bone marrow and seem to lead to the onset of myelodysplastic syndromes later in life. This is particularly true when these drugs are used in combination with certain forms of radiation therapy.

People who have been exposed to benzene and ionizing radiation appear to be susceptible to myelodysplastic syndromes. Benzene is found in gasoline, detergents, furniture polish, and cigarette smoke. Some researchers believe that a connection can be made between myelodysplastic syndromes and people who have had long-term exposure to certain agricultural chemicals and heavy metals.

Other risk factors for myelodysplastic syndromes include the congenital disorders Fanconi anemia and Down syndrome. People who smoke cigarettes, which contain benzene and other cancer-causing substances, are also more likely to be at risk for myelodysplastic syndromes.

Etiology and the disease process: Myelodysplastic syndromes rarely occur in people younger than the age of sixty, although they are appearing more often in children and adults who survive chemotherapy regimens for cancer treatment. Myelodysplasia is diagnosed more often in men than women, but there appears to be no association with ethnicity. Scientists have not been able to associate myelodysplastic syndromes with a genetic trait.

Secondary myelodysplastic syndromes most often appear after treatment for acute lymphocytic leukemia, Hodgkin disease, and non-Hodgkin lymphoma, but they can also arise after chemotherapy for cancer of the breast, lung, testis, or intestinal tract, and after treatment for some autoimmune diseases.

Incidence: Approximately 10,000 to 15,000 Americans are diagnosed with myelodysplastic syndromes each year. This number may be rising as the number of those who survive cancer treatment increases. Approximately 80 to 90 percent of those who receive a myelodysplastic syndrome diagnosis are the age of sixty and older.

Symptoms: The early stages of myelodysplastic syndromes may be uneventful and indistinct from other diseases. Myelodysplastic syndromes are often marked by anemia, which leads to shortness of breath and fatigue during light exertion. Other symptoms may include unusually pale skin, easy bleeding or bruising, tiny red spots (petechiae) just beneath the skin, weight loss, and frequent infections. About 20 percent of patients with myelodysplastic syndromes exhibit infections or bleeding, and about 20 percent of patients have no symptoms and are diagnosed during routine blood tests.

Screening and diagnosis: A complete blood count will help determine the number of platelets, red and white blood cells, and hemoglobin levels in red cells. A peripheral blood smear may help determine the shape, size, and appearance of blood cells. Myelodysplastic syndromes are usually diagnosed after other diseases, such as leukemia, have been excluded. Bone marrow tests will help confirm a diagnosis of myelodysplastic syndrome. These include aspiration and biopsy to obtain bone and marrow tissues, which are then analyzed using cytochemistry, flow cytometry, immunocytochemistry, and cytogenetic profiles.

Some physicians use the French-American-British (FAB) system to classify myelodysplastic syndromes into five subtypes. In the 1990's, the World Health Organization expanded the FAB into seven subtypes on the basis of circulating blood counts or changes in the bone marrow. These subtypes are refractory anemia, refractory anemia with ringed sideroblasts, refractory cytopenia with multilineage dysplasia, refractory cytopenia with multilineage dysplasia and ringed sideroblasts, refractory anemia with excess blasts (types 1 and 2), unclassified myelodysplastic syndromes, and myelodysplastic syndromes associated with isolated del(5q) chromosome abnormality.

Physicians use the International Prognostic Scoring System to assess a patient's health. Although the system is not a precise science, it uses three factors—the percentage of blasts in the bone marrow, an assessment of the number of cell types in the circulating blood (cytopenia), and an assessment of cellular chromosomal abnormalities—each of which is assigned a score to determine a patient's degree of health.

Treatment and therapy: Most patients require a transfusion of red blood cells to help relieve anemia. Drugs such as darbepoetin and erythropoietin may help the body produce more red blood cells and thus reduce the need for transfusions.

The U.S. Food and Drug Administration has approved two drugs specifically for the treatment of myelodysplastic syndromes. Azacitidine (approved May 19, 2004) and decitabine (approved May 2, 2006) are administered to stimulate blast cells to mature into healthy blood cells, but the pharmaceuticals are ineffective in some people and may cause additional problems.

The only potential cure for myelodysplastic syndromes is allogeneic (donor) stem cell transplantation, but few patients are eligible for the procedure because it poses high risks.

Prognosis, prevention, and outcomes: Patients with fewer bone marrow blasts and a greater number of cells in the blood and better cytogenetic profiles may demonstrate a longer median survival time, whereas patients with more blasts, fewer blood cells, and chromosome 7 abnormalities have a shorter survival time.

Terry A. Anderson, B.S.

▶ For Further Information

Deeg, H. J., et al. *Hematologic Malignancies: Myelodysplastic Syndromes*. New York: Springer, 2006.

Hellstr-Lindberg, E., and L. Malcovati. "Supportive Care, Growth Factors, and New Therapies in Myelodysplastic Syndromes." *Blood Reviews* 22, no. 2 (March, 2008): 75-91.

▶ Other Resources

Aplastic Anemia & MDS International Foundation
http://www.aamds.org/aplastic

Myelodysplastic Syndromes Foundation
http://www.mds-foundation.org

See also Acute myelocytic leukemia (AML); Anemia; Benzene; Blood cancers; Cigarettes and cigars; Down syndrome and leukemia; Fanconi anemia; 5Q minus syndrome; Ionizing radiation; Leukemias; Leukopenia; Myelosuppression; Neutropenia; Premalignancies.

▶ Myelofibrosis

Category: Diseases, symptoms, and conditions
Also known as: Agnogenic myeloid metaplasia, idiopathic myelofibrosis, aleukemic megakaryocytic myelosis, leukoerythroblastosis

Related conditions: Myeloproliferative disorders, including polycythemia rubra vera (increased numbers of red blood cells) and essential thrombocytosis (overproduction of platelets in the bone marrow)

Definition: Myelofibrosis is a disorder that disrupts the normal production of blood cells, leading to scarring of the bone marrow.

Risk factors: Myelofibrosis is most common in patients over fifty years old. Exposure to radiation, benzene, or radioactive thorium dioxide (a chemical used during some radiology procedures) also increases one's risk. There may also be an association between myelofibrosis and certain autoimmune diseases (in which the body attacks its own cells), leukemias and lymphomas, and other myeloproliferative disorders.

Etiology and the disease process: Hematopoiesis is the process of making blood cells. It begins in the bone marrow with a hematopoietic stem cell that can develop into specialized blood cells, including red blood cells (which transport oxygen), white blood cells (which are involved in the immune system), and platelets (which form clots).

Myelofibrosis develops when the genetic material in a single hematopoietic stem cell changes or acquires a mutation, and then begins to replicate and affect normal blood cell production. Approximately 50 percent of patients with myelofibrosis have stem cells with mutations in the *JAK* kinase gene; mutations in the *GATA-1* and *MPL* genes are less common. Mutated stem cells may affect cellular proliferation, survival, and immune responses. They may also stimulate fibroblast cells, causing them to secrete collagen that can build up scar tissue in the bone marrow. Cytokines (signals secreted from cells to affect activity of other cells), including transforming growth factor-beta (TGF-β), basic fibroblast growth factor, and platelet-derived growth factor (PDGF), may also induce bone marrow scarring.

The accumulation of scar tissue may displace normal blood cells being produced within the marrow. Therefore, blood cell production may begin to occur in other parts of the body, most often the spleen and liver. However, blood cell production in those tissues is not as efficient and increases organ size. Severe anemia (a lack of red blood cells) can also occur, leading to weakness and fatigue. The abnormal hematopoietic stem cells can also spread to other organs in the body and form tumors (primarily in the adrenals, kidneys, lymph nodes, breasts, and lungs).

Incidence: Myelofibrosis is rare, with an incidence rate ranging from 0.3 to 1.5 cases per 100,000 people. Among clonal hematologic disorders, myelofibrosis is the least prevalent.

Symptoms: In the early stages, myelofibrosis does not cause any symptoms. However, as normal blood cell production becomes more affected, multiple signs may arise, including tiredness, weakness, shortness of breath, an enlarged liver or spleen, easy bruising and bleeding, fever, frequent infections, and bone pain.

Screening and diagnosis: Screening for myelofibrosis includes blood tests to determine the number of red blood cells and their shape, because low numbers and teardrop-shaped cells indicate myelofibrosis. To examine enlargement of the liver and spleen, physical exams, as well as imaging tests (ultrasounds, magnetic resonance imaging, and computed tomography scans) may be performed.

A bone marrow biopsy, in which a needle is used to withdraw the bone marrow from the hip bone, may be done to confirm a diagnosis. The harvested bone marrow cells can be viewed under a microscope to examine signs of scarring and the types and number of cells within the marrow.

The following criteria for staging have been accepted by the World Health Organization:

- A1: No other myeloproliferative disorders
- A2: Early clinical stage, with slight anemia and slight enlargement of the spleen
- A3: Intermediate clinical stage, with moderate anemia, teardrop-shaped red blood cells, enlargement of the spleen, and no other symptoms
- A4: Advanced clinical stage, severe anemia, and one or more other symptoms

Treatment and therapy: There are many treatment options for myelofibrosis symptoms. Blood transfusions may improve anemia. Androgen (a hormone) or thalidomide (a drug) in combination with corticosterioids may increase red blood cell production. Hydroxyurea, a chemotherapeutic agent, can shrink enlarged spleens and may reduce bone marrow scarring. Radiation and interferon-alpha not only reduce spleen size but also may alleviate bone pain. When other treatments do not work, the spleen may be surgically removed in a process known as a splenectomy.

The only way to cure myelofibrosis is through a stem cell transplant in which the patient, after being treated with high-dose chemotherapy to kill the diseased cells, is provided with healthy blood stem cells from a donor. Because this is an intensive procedure, patients must be healthy enough to undergo the process and numerous side effects may occur.

Prognosis, prevention, and outcomes: The mean survival time from diagnosis ranges from 3.5 to 5.5 years. Patients with severe anemia, certain symptoms (weight loss, fatigue, night sweats, and fever), and those older than the age of sixty-five tend to have poorer mean survival rates. In approximately 15 percent of patients, myelofibrosis can progress to acute lymphocytic leukemia or lymphoma, which can be fatal.

There are no known ways to prevent myelofibrosis. To alleviate or prevent symptoms of anemia, the diet should include nutrients that promote blood formation, such as iron, folic acid, and vitamin B_{12}.

Elizabeth A. Manning, Ph.D.

▶ For Further Information

Hennessy, B. T., et al. "New Approaches in the Treatment of Myelofibrosis." *Cancer* 103, no. 1 (January 1, 2005): 32-43.

Spivak, J. L., et al. "Chronic Myeloproliferative Disorders." *Hematology/The Education Program of the American Society of Hematology* (2003): 200-224.

Tefferi, A. "The Forgotten Myeloproliferative Disorder: Myeloid Metaplasia." *Oncologist* 8, no. 3 (2003): 225-231.

Tefferi, A., and D. G. Gilliland. "Oncogenes in Myeloproliferative Disorders." *Cell Cycle* 6, no. 5 (March 1, 2007): 550-566.

▶ **Other Resources**

MayoClinic.com
Myelofibrosis
http://www.mayoclinic.com/health/myelofibrosis/DS00886

MedlinePlus
Primary Myelofibrosis
http://www.nlm.nih.gov/medlineplus/ency/article/000531.htm

See also Anemia; Chronic myeloid leukemia (CML); Myeloproliferative disorders; Polycythemia vera.

▶ Myeloma

Category: Diseases, symptoms, and conditions
Also known as: Multiple myeloma, plasma cell myeloma

Related conditions: Non-Hodgkin lymphoma, other blood cancers

Definition: Myeloma is a cancer of the plasma cells found in the bone marrow. Plasma cells produce antibodies, which fight infection. In myeloma, abnormal plasma cells in the bone marrow overproduce monoclonal immunoglobulins. Multiple myeloma occurs when there are multiple bones affected.

Risk factors: As nearly all cases of multiple myeloma are diagnosed in adults over the age of forty, age is considered the most significant risk factor. It is thought, however, that myeloma is the result of several unknown factors working together.

Etiology and the disease process: The definitive cause of myeloma has not been determined. However, as age is its primary risk factor, potential causes include age-related factors such as long-term exposure to carcinogens, toxins, genetic variations, and decreased immune response.

Incidence: Myeloma is most commonly found in African Americans and occurs more frequently in women. Multiple myeloma is the second most common type of blood cancer (non-Hodgkin lymphoma is the first). Approximately 16,000 new cases are diagnosed each year. The average age of diagnosis is sixty-eight, and very few cases are diagnosed in people under the age of forty.

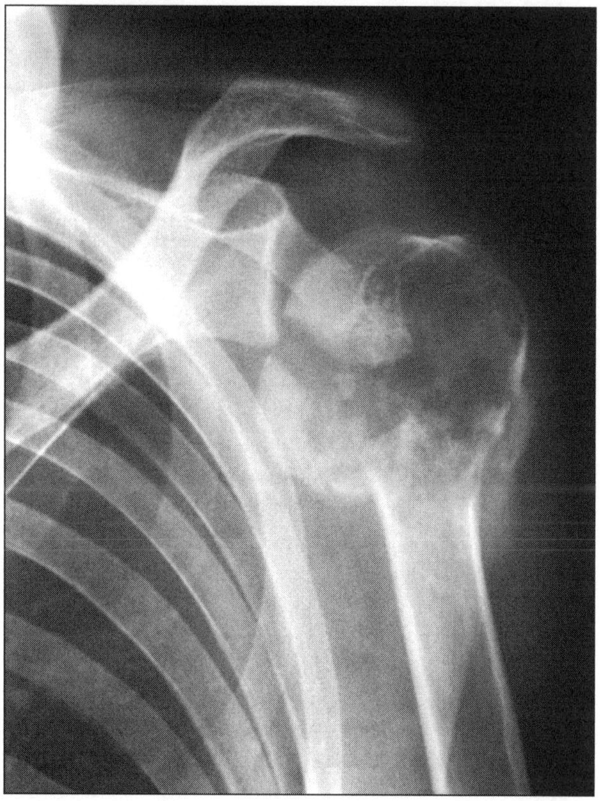

Myeloma in the head of the humerus. (CNRI/Photo Researchers, Inc.)

Symptoms: A common symptom is back pain, often accompanied by bone pain of the pelvis, ribs, and neck. Patients with myeloma have also reported excessive fatigue, iron deficiency, decreased immunity (frequent colds or sickness), a decrease in appetite, constipation, "pins and needles" in the feet and legs, and abnormal bleeding of the nose or gums.

Screening and diagnosis: There is no standard screening for myeloma; however, patients considered at risk and exhibiting symptoms should see a hematologist (a doctor who specializes in blood disorders) and have a series of tests performed to determine a diagnosis. Blood tests, urinalysis, X rays, bone scans, and bone marrow biopsy are typically performed.

There are two systems for staging myeloma: the Durie-Salmon Staging System and the International Staging System.

Treatment and therapy: Treatment for myeloma, like that for most cancers, depends on the stage of disease. Patients are often treated with chemotherapy and radiation, as well as additional therapies to target plasma cells.

Prognosis, prevention, and outcomes: Prognosis for myeloma depends on the stage at which the patient is diagnosed and the patient's overall health. While myeloma is not curable, it can be treated and managed. Most patients survive for at least one year following diagnosis, while at least half survive an additional five years and twenty out of every hundred patients diagnosed live an additional ten years.

Anna Perez, M.Sc.

See also African Americans and cancer; Aging and cancer; Blood cancers; Bone cancers; Immunotherapy; Lactate dehydrogenase (LDH) test; Leukapharesis; Multiple myeloma; Non-Hodgkin lymphoma; Stem cell transplantation; Thrombocytopenia; Umbilical cord blood transplantation.

▶ Myeloproliferative disorders

Category: Diseases, symptoms, and conditions
Also known as: Blood cancers, chronic granulocytic leukemia, chronic myeloid leukemia, agnogenic myeloid metaplasia, primary myelofibrosis, myelosclerosis with myeloid metaplasia, idiopathic myelofibrosis, essential thrombocytosis

Related conditions: Leukemia

Definition: Myeloproliferative disorders are a group of slow-growing blood cancers, in which the bone marrow produces too many red blood cells, white blood cells, or platelets. All myeloproliferative disorders arise from an overproduction of one or more types of blood cells.

Risk factors: The reason for the abnormal increase in blood cells is not well understood. Genetics and environmental factors such as overexposure to radiation may be risk factors for some of these malignancies. Some types of myeloproliferative disorders have been associated with familial clusters; one such case is marked by a mutation of the erythropoeitin receptor.

Etiology and the disease process: No obvious etiology exists for myeloproliferative disorders. These malignancies begin in the bone marrow when a greater than normal number of stem cells develop into one or more types of blood cells. Normally, the bone marrow makes stem cells that develop into mature blood cells. There are three types of mature blood cells. Red blood cells are mature blood cells that carry oxygen and other materials to all tissues of the body. White blood cells are mature blood cells that fight infection and disease. Platelets are mature blood cells that help prevent bleeding by causing blood to clot. The type of myeloproliferative disorder is based on which kind of mature blood cells are overproduced. Usually one type of blood cell is affected more than the others. The disorders get worse as the number of blood cells increase. There are six types of chronic myeloproliferative disorders:

- Chronic myelogenous leukemia (CML) is a slowly progressing disease of overproduction of white blood cells but not lymphocytes in the bone marrow. CML is also called chronic granulocytic leukemia and chronic myeloid leukemia.
- Polycythemia vera is a disease in which too many red blood cells are produced in the bone marrow and blood, causing the blood to thicken. In polycythemia vera, the number of white blood cells and platelets may also increase. The spleen is often enlarged as the extra blood cells may collect in it. Patients with polycythemia vera may also have bleeding problems and are at high risk for blood clotting.
- Chronic idiopathic myelofibrosis is a progressive, chronic disease in which the bone marrow is replaced by fibrous tissue, and blood is made in the liver and the spleen instead of in the bone marrow. The hallmark of this disease is an enlarged spleen. Chronic idiopathic myelofibrosis causes progressive anemia and is also called agnogenic myeloid metaplasia, primary myelofibrosis, myelosclerosis with myeloid metaplasia, and idiopathic myelofibrosis.
- Essential thrombocythemia is an increased number of thrombocytes (platelets) in the blood. The cause of this malignancy is not known. It is also called essential thrombocytosis.
- Chronic neutrophilic leukemia is a disease in which neutrophils, a type of white blood cell, are found in excess in the blood. The excess neutrophils in chronic neutrophilic leukemia may cause the spleen and liver to become enlarged. This disorder may not progress for years, or it may develop quickly into acute leukemia.
- Chronic eosinophilic leukemia is a disease in which eosinophils, a type of white blood cell, are found in the tissues, bone marrow, and blood. Similar to chronic neutrophilic leukemia, chronic eosinophilic leukemia may stay the same for years, or it may develop quickly into acute leukemia.

Incidence: Myeloproliferative disorders typically occur later in life. The prevalence of these diseases is low (approximately 5 per 1 million people), and they occur more commonly in men and women of East European Jewish ancestry compared with other populations. Men are more likely than women to develop polycythemia vera, primary myelofibrosis, and CML. However, women are 1.5 times more likely than men to develop essential thrombocytosis.

Symptoms: Many individuals with myeloproliferative disorders have no symptoms when their physicians first make the diagnosis. However, as the hematocrit or platelet count increases, most patients develop symptoms including headache, blurred vision, plethora (excess of body fluid), elevated white blood cell count, and hematocrit. A sign that is common to all myeloproliferative disorders, except of essential thrombocytosis, is an enlarged spleen, which may cause abdominal pain. Other signs of myeloproliferative disorders often include fatigue, difficulty breathing, intense itching after bathing in warm water, stomach aches, purple spots or patches on the skin, nosebleeds, gum or stomach bleeding, blood in the urine, throbbing and burning pain in the skin, high blood pressure, and blockage of blood vessels. Blockage of blood vessels may cause heart disease, stroke, or tissue death of the extremities.

As the disorders progress, patients may also develop cerebrovascular events, such as thrombosis. Thrombosis in small blood vessels may lead to serious events, such as cyanosis, erythromelalgia (painful vessel dilation in the extremities), ulceration, or gangrene (tissue death) in the fingers or toes. Thrombosis in larger vessels may lead to myocardial infarction, deep-vein thrombosis, transient ischemic attacks, and stroke.

Screening and diagnosis: Many of the myeloproliferative disorders are discovered by primary care physicians on routine blood tests. There is no standard staging system for chronic myeloproliferative disorders. Complete blood count is necessary for proper diagnosis, which includes the number of red blood cells and platelets, the number and type of white blood cells, the amount of hemoglobin (the protein that carries oxygen) in the red blood cells, and what portion of the blood sample is made up of red blood cells. Bone marrow aspiration and biopsy via inserting a hollow needle into the hip bone or breastbone is used to look for signs of blood cancer. In addition, cytogenetic analysis is often done to look for certain changes in the chromosomes.

Treatment and therapy: Treatment is based on the type of myeloproliferative disorder. Ten types of standard treatment are used: watchful waiting (monitoring a patient's condition), phlebotomy (removal of blood), platelet apheresis (removal of platelets from the blood), transfusion therapy, chemotherapy, radiation therapy, other drug therapy, surgery, splenectomy (removal the spleen), and biological therapy.

Unfortunately, there are no known cures for most myeloproliferative disorders. However, there are treatments available that help alleviate symptoms and prevent complications associated with the disorders. The method used to alleviate symptoms depends on the type of myeloproliferative disorder. For polycythemia vera, phlebotomy is used to lower red blood cell count. In essential thrombocytosis and primary myelofibrosis, symptoms are treated with medications. Medications such as interferon may also improve survival rates of certain myeloproliferative disorders.

When enlargement of the spleen becomes painful, a surgeon may perform a splenectomy to alleviate pain. Replacing the abnormal stem cells in the bone marrow with healthy stem cells may also help control the disorder. Bone marrow transplant is ideal for most patients with CML.

Prognosis, prevention, and outcomes: Though myeloproliferative disorders are serious, they are most often slow to develop; therefore, patients with these conditions often live for many years after diagnosis. Some complications of myeloproliferative disorders include enlargement of the spleen and liver, gout, anemia, bleeding, kidney or liver failure, heart attacks or stroke, and infection. In particular, CML can transform into acute leukemia.

The survival rates of those with myeloproliferative disorders depend on the type of disorder and symptoms. For example, the median survival rate for those with polycythemia vera is more than ten years with treatment. The major causes of death in untreated polycythemia vera patients are thrombosis and hemorrhage. Primary myelofibrosis and CML may be fatal within three to six years after diagnosis. However, if CML transforms into acute leukemia, the median survival rate may be only three months. Patients with other types of myeloproliferative disorders can live longer, especially when diagnosed early. Specifically, patients with primary thrombocythemia may have a normal life expectancy, and patients with polycythemia vera have a survival rate of between ten and twenty years.

Anita Nagypál, Ph.D.

▶ For Further Information

Hoffman, R., et al. *Hematology: Basic Principles and Practice*. 3d ed. New York: Churchill Livingstone, 2000.

Michiels, J. J., et al. "The 2001 World Health Organization and Updated European Clinical and Pathological Criteria for the Diagnosis, Classification, and Staging of the Philadelphia Chromosome-Negative Chronic Myeloproliferative Disorders." *Seminars in Thrombosis and Hemostasis* 32 (June, 2006): 307-340.

Talarico, L. D. "Myeloproliferative Disorders: A Practical Review." *Patient Care* 30 (1998): 37-57.

Yavorkovsky, L. L., and P. Cook. "Classifying Chronic Myelomonocytic Leukemia." *Journal of Clinical Oncology* 19 (2001): 3790-3792.

▶ Other Resources

The Leukemia and Lymphoma Society
Myeloproliferative Disorders
http://www.leukemia-lymphoma.org/all_page.adp?item_id=311829

National Cancer Institute
Myeloproliferative Disorders
http://www.cancer.gov/cancertopics/types/myeloproliferative

National Cancer Institute
http://www.cancer.gov/cancertopics/pdq/treatment/myeloproliferative/patient

See also Acute myelocytic leukemia (AML); Blood cancers; Chronic myeloid leukemia (CML); Cyclophosphamide; Hypercoagulation disorders; Leukemias; Melphalan; Myelofibrosis; Polycythemia vera.

▶ Myelosuppression

Category: Diseases, symptoms, and conditions
Also known as: Bone-marrow suppression, pancytopenia

Related conditions: Anemia, neutropenia, leukopenia, thrombocytopenia

Definition: Myelosuppression is a condition in which bone marrow function is decreased, with fewer than normal numbers of red blood cells, white blood cells, and platelets. Complete loss of bone-marrow function is called myeloablation.

Risk factors: Risk factors include having had chemotherapy, radiation therapy, or bone marrow or stem cell transplants, and having myelodysplastic syndromes.

Etiology and the disease process: Chemotherapy and radiation therapy for cancer destroy the rapidly dividing cancer cells as well as other rapidly dividing cells, or hematopoietic stem cells. As with anemia, leukopenia, and thrombocytopenia, hematopoietic stem cells are damaged by drugs used in chemotherapy or by radiation therapy. Cell counts often return to baseline values when treatment is stopped, reduced, or delayed.

Incidence: Nearly all patients who are being treated for cancer experience myelosuppression at some point and to some degree.

Symptoms: Depending on which cell line is involved, patients may feel weak, short of breath, and tired (anemia); may be susceptible to infections and have fevers (leukopenia); or may bruise and bleed easily (thrombocytopenia).

Screening and diagnosis: For routine monitoring during cancer therapy, myelosuppression is generally measured through blood tests. Anemia would be suspected with a red blood cell count less than 3.5×10^9 per liter in women and less than 4.3×10^9 per liter in men; leukopenia would be suspected with a white blood cell count less than 1.0 to 2.0×10^9 per liter; and thrombocytopenia would be suspected with a platelet count less than 200×10^9 per liter. Sometimes aspiration or core needle biopsy of the bone marrow is done to aid in the diagnosis of leukemia, lymphomas, and multiple myelomas, diseases associated with severe myelosuppression.

Treatment and therapy: Treatment for myelosuppression depends on which cell line is involved. Simply stopping or reducing the amount of chemotherapeutic drugs or radiation therapy given may relieve the myelosuppression. Anemia may be treated with red blood cell transfusions, steroids, supplements, or erythropoiesis-stimulating proteins such as epoetin alfa (Procrit, Epogen) or darbepoetin alfa (Aranesp). Leukopenia may be treated with hematopoietic growth factors such as filgrastim (Neupogen), pegfilgrastim (Neulasta), and sargramostim (Leukine). Thrombocytopenia may be treated with platelet transfusions or with a recombinant form of interleukin (oprelvekin, or Neumega).

Prognosis, prevention, and outcomes: Left untreated, myelosuppression can impair a patient's quality of life, increase the need for hospitalization and transfusions of red blood cells or platelets or both, increase the need for intravenous anti-infectives, and increase risk of bleeding and infections. Use of hematopoietic, erythropoietic, and thrombocyte growth factors and transfusions is routine in supportive cancer treatment.

MaryAnn Foote, M.S., Ph.D.

See also Anemia; Chemotherapy; External beam radiation therapy (EBRT); Leukopenia; Neutropenia; Radiation therapies; Thrombocytopenia.

▶ 2-Naphthylamine

Category: Carcinogens and suspected carcinogens
RoC status: Known human carcinogen since 1980
Also known as: 2-Aminonaphthalene, beta-naphthylamine

Related cancers: Bladder cancer

Definition: 2-Naphthylamine, an aromatic amine, is a yellowish crystalline solid that turns purplish-red in air and has an ammoniacal odor.

Exposure routes: For the general public, exposure to 2-naphthylamine comes from inhalation of emissions from burning organic matter that contains nitrogen. Two primary sources are coal furnaces and tobacco smoke. Occupational exposure occurs through inhalation by laboratory personnel doing research with 2-naphthylamine.

Where found: 2-Naphthylamine is used only in laboratory research. It is still found in some dyes and rubber compounds that were manufactured before 1974. It is a by-product of tobacco smoke and coal burning and is an impurity found in commercially produced 1-naphthylamine.

At risk: Scientists and laboratory technicians who work where 2-naphthylamine is used in research as a catalyst or an antioxidant have a high risk for 2-naphthylamine contamination. Because 2-naphthylamine is generated in tobacco smoke, people who smoke are at high risk for contamination. The general public is at risk for contamination from secondhand tobacco smoke and from the burning of organic matter that contains nitrogen, such as coal.

Etiology and symptoms of associated cancers: When 2-naphthylamine is metabolized, it can be activated by liver enzymes to form adducts with blood-serum proteins, such as hemoglobin. In some cases, 2-naphthylamine can undergo additional metabolism to form reactive compounds that are transported to the bladder, where they bind to deoxyribonucleic acid (DNA) molecules. In experimental laboratory animals, 2-naphthylamine DNA adducts have been found in the bladder and in the liver. In laboratory tests on cultured human cells, 2-naphthylamine caused genetic damage that involved DNA strand breaks, changes in chromosome structure or number, addition or deletion of chromosomes, and cell transformation.

History: 2-Naphthylamine was commercially produced in the United States from the early 1920's until the early 1970's. It was used in the production of sulfonic acids, red-dye stuffs, and agrochemicals, and as a catalyst and an antioxidant in the vulcanization of rubber. After the International Agency for Research on Cancer (IARC) showed its link to the increased risk of bladder cancer, its commercial production was banned in the early 1970's. There are still a few companies in the United States that manufacture 2-naphthylamine for use in laboratory research. The last time it was imported into the United States in any significant amount was in 1967.

Alvin K. Benson, Ph.D.

See also Bladder cancer; Carcinogens, known; Carcinogens, reasonably anticipated; Cigarettes and cigars; Occupational exposures and cancer.

▶ Nasal cavity and paranasal sinus cancers

Category: Diseases, symptoms, and conditions
Also known as: Nose cancers, sinus cancers

Related conditions: Lymphoma, melanoma, hemangiopericytoma, osteosarcoma, chondrosarcoma, adenosarcoma, squamous cell carcinoma

Definition: Nasal cavity and paranasal sinus cancers are cancers that arise in the paranasal sinuses or the nose. Many types of cancer can originate in the paranasal sinuses and nose. These include squamous cell carcinoma, adenocarcinoma, adenoid cystic carcinoma, lymphomas, chondrosarcoma, osteosarcoma, hemangiopericytoma, malignant melanoma, and esthesioneuroblastoma, as well as metastatic lesions from cancers of the kidney, lung, and breast.

Squamous cell carcinomas arise from the epithelial (skin) cells of the sinuses and are the most common type of paranasal sinus tumor. Adenocarcinoma tends to arise in the mucus-producing glands of the upper nasal cavity. This type of nasal cavity cancer is most common in woodworkers and people working with toxic chemicals and substances. Adenoid cystic carcinomas arise out of the salivary gland tissue and have a tendency to migrate to nearby nerve tissue. These tumors are slow growing but often metastasize to distant organs. Lymphomas arise from the cells of the lymph nodes and exhibit ulceration and necrosis (tissue death) of the lymph tissue in the nasal cavity or paranasal sinuses. Chondrosarcomas are rare in the nose and sinuses and arise out of the connective tissue. Osteosarcomas are cancers of the facial bones. Hemangiopericytomas are tumors of blood vessels. They are quite rare in the nose and sinuses. Malignant melanomas arise out of the epithelial tissue of the nasal septum and the lateral nasal wall. They appear to be more common in smokers and metastasize early. Esthesioneuroblastomas arise out of the sensory epithelial cells that control olfaction (smelling) and are quite rare.

Risk factors: The primary risk factor for nasal and paranasal sinus cancer is smoking. Occupational exposure to inhaled toxic substances can also put a person at risk for developing sinus cancer. These substances include dusts from wood, textiles, and leather; glues; formaldehyde; solvents; nickel and chromium dust; mustard gas; isopropyl alcohol; and radium. It is thought that heavy air pollution could lead to nasal and paranasal sinus cancers. These types of cancers do not appear to be hereditary.

Etiology and the disease process: Nasal cavity and paranasal sinus cancers develop in the walls of the nose or the walls of the six sinuses. Each side of the face has a maxillary, ethmoid, and sphenoid sinus. The paranasal sinuses are actually spaces that exist within the nasal and facial bones. Cancer occurs when a single cell mutates and grows uncontrollably. This tumor tends to invade nearby structures, which causes the symptoms of this type of cancer.

Incidence: Cancers of the nasal and paranasal sinuses are considered rare. Each year, only about 2,000 people in the United States develop one of these cancers. They are more common in men than in women. These cancers occur more frequently in countries other than the United States, such as Japan and South Africa.

Symptoms: The symptoms of nasal and paranasal sinus cancers are much like those of chronic sinus disease. They include blocked sinuses, decreased sense of smell, frequent sinus headaches, purulent drainage from the nose, facial swelling, epistaxis (bleeding from the nose), and frequent infections. Some patients will experience more definitive symptoms, such as a growth or mass on the nose, face, or soft palate; a lump inside the nose; numbness in areas of the face or head; loosening, pain, or numbness of the teeth; continuous tearing of the eyes; trouble opening the mouth; and swelling of the eyes.

Screening and diagnosis: No routine screening is performed for nasal or paranasal sinus cancers, because of their rarity. Diagnosis is achieved by physical examination, nasal endoscopy, computed tomography (CT) scan of the nose and sinuses, or magnetic resonance imaging (MRI) of the sinuses and orbits. If there is a visible mass, it is biopsied (a slice of tissue is removed for microscopic examination) to determine whether it is cancer, and if so, what type of cancer.

Only esthesioneuroblastomas and cancers of the maxillary sinuses, nasal cavity, and ethmoid sinuses are staged. The sinus cancers are staged using the American Joint Committee on Cancer (AJCC) staging system. This system uses the TNM (tumor/lymph node/metastasis) groupings. For esthesioneuroblastomas, the staging can be performed using one of two systems: the Kadish system or the UCLA system. Since esthesioneuroblastomas are extremely rare, these staging systems will not be discussed.

For cancers of the maxillary sinus, the stages are as follows:

- Stage 0 (T0, N0, M0): The cancer is confined to the epithelium and still resembles normal tissue.
- Stage I (T1, N0, M0): The cancer is confined to the nasal mucosa and has not spread to other sinuses or invaded the bones of the nose.
- Stage II (T2, N0, M0): The cancer has invaded the bones of the maxillary sinus, excluding the posterior wall. These bones include the hard palate and the opening into the maxillary sinus. The cancer has not spread beyond the maxillary sinus.
- Stage III (T1-3, N0-1, M0): The cancer has invaded the posterior wall of the maxillary sinus or has grown through the other bones of the sinus into the skin, the eye socket, or the ethmoid sinus. It may have metastasized to a single lymph node on the same side as the tumor. The involved node is a maximum of 3 centimeters (cm) in width.
- Stage IV (T1-4, any N, M0-1): The cancer has spread to the eye, the skull, the nasopharynx, or the sphenoid and frontal sinuses. There may be lymph node involvement. For a tumor to be Stage IV, there must be more than one node involved, nodes of greater than 3 cm, or involvement of nodes on the side opposite the tumor. Any maxillary cancer that has metastasized to other organs is Stage IV.

The stages for nasal cavity and ethmoid cancers are as follows:

- Stage 0 (T0, N0, M0): The cancer is confined to the epithelium and is very early stage.
- Stage 1 (T1, N0, M0): The cancer is localized to either the nasal cavity or the ethmoid sinus and its bones. There is no presence of lymph node involvement or metastases.
- Stage II (T2, N0, M0): The cancer has invaded another cavity close to the tumor, but there is no lymph node involvement or metastases.
- Stage III (T1-3, N0-1, M0): Either the cancer has invaded other structures, such as the eye socket, the palate, or the maxillary sinus, and there is no lymph node involvement or metastases, or it has invaded those structures, and one lymph node is involved. This node is a maximum of 3 cm.

- Stage IV (any T, any N, M0-1): The cancer has invaded other structures, such as the eye, skull, or the sphenoid or frontal sinuses, or the cancer has spread to two or more lymph nodes and these nodes are larger than 3 cm, or the cancer has spread to distant organs.

Treatment and therapy: Nasal cavity and paranasal cancers are treated with a combination of surgical resection of the tumor, radiation therapy, and chemotherapy. The actual surgical procedure performed will depend on the location of the tumor, the stage of the tumor, and whether it can be removed en block (as one piece of tissue). Cancer cells can be left in the surgical site if the tumor is incised (cut into).

Stage I and II cancers can be treated with computer-aided transnasal endoscopic surgery, which is performed using an endoscope that is inserted into the nostrils and then into the sinuses. Other surgical procedures used for tumors that remain within the nasal cavity are sublabial (under the upper lip) or lateral rhinotomy (incision along one side of the nose) approaches. Surgical procedures for Stage III and IV tumors may include midfacial degloving (separating the skin, subcutaneous tissue, nerves and tendons from the facial bones), orbital exenteration (removal of the eye and orbital bones), or craniofacial resections. After the latter surgical procedures, it may be necessary to perform grafts of skin or fascia (fibrous connective tissue that separates body structures) and to insert dental, orbital, or other prostheses to reconstruct the face. Tumors that have metastasized to the brain, the spinal column, and the optic nerve, and into the cavernous sinus (bilateral large venous blood vessels that drain blood from the dura mater that covers the brain) are generally considered inoperable.

Radiation therapy may be performed before or after surgery, and it may be applied internally or externally. Radiation therapy before surgery can decrease the size of the tumor and simplify tumor resection. If radiation therapy is performed after surgery, it is used to destroy any tumor cells that remain. Radiation therapy may be applied by an external beam or by radioactive objects placed within the nasal cavity, such as seeds, wires, or catheters. For radiation administered by an external beam, a mask is created to position the head precisely. Radiation beams must be carefully aimed to prevent radiation exposure of the thyroid and pituitary glands. Research is being performed on developing medications that can sensitize tumors to radiation.

Nasal cavity and paranasal sinus cancers can be treated with chemotherapy either before or after surgery. Chemotherapy before surgery is performed to decrease the size of the tumor so that surgical removal is easier. Chemotherapy administered after surgery is intended to destroy any remaining cancer cells. Traditional chemotherapy drugs include cisplatin and 5-fluorouracil for paranasal sinus cancers. Vincristine (Oncovin), cyclophosphamide (Cytoxan), doxorubicin (Adriamycin), and cisplatin are used to treat esthesioneuroblastomas. Epidermal growth factor receptor (EGFR) inhibitor drugs are also being used to treat nasal cavity and paranasal sinus cancers. These drugs interfere with the growth and division of tumor cells by inhibiting a hormone that encourages their growth. Some EGFR drugs being used are cetuximab (Erbitux), gefitinib (Iressa), and erlotinib (Tarceva). Genetic therapy is being explored and drugs tested against tumors with mutations of the *TP53* (also known as *p53*) tumor-suppressor gene.

Prognosis, prevention, and outcomes: Prognosis depends on the stage and location of the tumor and the age and condition of the patient. People with Stage I and II cancers of the nasal cavity and the paranasal sinuses often have full recovery after their treatments. For people with Stage III and IV cancers, full recovery is less likely. These patients, if they are cured, may be left with disfiguring facial changes due to surgery and radiation therapy. People who are elderly or in poor general health are less likely to survive Stage III and IV cancers.

Nasal cavity and paranasal sinus cancers cannot be prevented. There are many cases with no known cause. However, avoiding risk factors can decrease the likelihood of developing one of these cancers.

The outcome of a nasal cavity or paranasal sinus cancer depends on the type of tumor and the tissue from which it arises, the size of the tumor, and whether it has metastasized. Some types, like melanoma, are rapidly fatal. Other types grow slowly and may be resected successfully. The more extensive the tumor, the more likely it is that it will affect the cranial nerves and the sense of smell. More advanced tumors are quite likely to cause facial deformity as well as interference with tasting, smelling, and vision. Damage to the cranial nerves by surgery can affect the ability to open, close, and move the eyes; chew and swallow; and to change facial expressions.

Christine M. Carroll, R.N., B.S.N., M.B.A.

▶ For Further Information

Carper, Elise, Kenneth Hu, and Elena Kuzin. *One Hundred Questions and Answers About Head and Neck Cancer*. Sudbury, Mass.: Jones and Barlett, 2008.

Genden, Eric M., and Mark A. Varvares, eds. *Head and Neck Cancer: An Evidence-Based Team Approach*. New York: Thieme, 2008.

Petruzelli, Guy, ed. *Practical Head and Neck Oncology*. San Diego: Plural, 2008.

▶ Other Resources

American Cancer Society
Detailed Guide: Nasal Cavity and Paranasal Cancer
http://www.cancer.org/docroot/CRI/content/CRI_2_4_1X_What_is_nasal_cavity_and_paranasal_cancer.asp?sitearea=

American Rhinologic Society
An Introduction to Nasal Endoscopy
http://american-rhinologic.org/patientinfo.introendoscopy.phtml

National Cancer Institute
Paranasal Sinus and Nasal Cavity Cancer Treatment
http://www.cancer.gov/cancertopics/pdq/treatment/paranasalsinus

See also Air pollution; Bone cancers; Cigarettes and cigars; Head and neck cancers; Lymphomas; Melanomas; Occupational exposures and cancer; Sarcomas, soft-tissue; Squamous cell carcinomas; Tobacco-related cancers.

▶ National Cancer Institute (NCI)

Category: Organizations

Definition: The National Cancer Institute (NCI) is a United States government organization dedicated to reducing the burden of cancer through research into prevention and treatment of the disease. It is part of the National Institutes of Health (NIH), under the Department of Health and Human Services.

History: Recognizing the growing toll of cancer on the United States and the world, Congress enacted the National Cancer Institute Act on August 5, 1937. The act created the NCI and directed it to conduct research into the causes of cancer, ways it might be prevented, and means of diagnosing and treating cancer patients. The institute was also directed to aid and coordinate the research of other cancer research organizations and promote education and training related to the disease. By 1939, a research team was assembled through a merger of Harvard University's Office of Cancer Investigations and a pharmacology division within the National Institutes of Health.

In 1940 the NCI published the first issue of the *Journal of the National Cancer Institute*. It was the first major venue in the world to publish scientific papers exclusively related to cancer. Although ownership of the journal was fully transferred to Oxford University Press in 2001, it remains a peer-reviewed and highly respected source of new information about cancer research.

To promote clinical trials of new cancer treatments, the NCI established the Clinical Trials Cooperative Group Program in 1955. Within three years, the program had established 17 cooperative groups, consisting of various cancer centers, researchers, and physicians, each coordinated to investigate different methods of treating cancer. By 2007, more than 1,700 institutions were involved with the program and more than 22,000 patients were participating in trials each year.

In 1971 the National Cancer Act reinvigorated the National Cancer Institute. At the time, cancer was the second leading cause of death in the United States and President Richard M. Nixon vowed to change that. The act provided the institute with greater authority to coordinate national cancer activities, a significant increase in funding, and a new research facility at Fort Detrick in Frederick, Maryland, where a biological warfare laboratory was converted for cancer research purposes.

By the late 1970's, the institute began to recognize the potential of information services in the fight against cancer. In 1976, it established the Cancer Information Service, which provides information about cancer to patients and the public through a national phone service (1-800-4-CANCER) and various print publications. A year later, it established the first electronic registry of cancer clinical trials. This registry, known as CLINPROT, would be the first service available through the institute's Physician Data Query (PDQ). PDQ is available through the institute's Web site, and in 2007 CLINPROT contained abstracts of more thab 16,000 clinical trials.

In 1991 the institute's Surveillance Epidemiology and End Results (SEER) program showed a decline in the rate of deaths caused by cancer for the first time. In 2003 the program recorded the first decline in the actual number of deaths. In 2006 the U.S. Food and Drug Administration approved a vaccine that was created using technology developed by the institute. By fighting human papillomavirus (HPV), this vaccine (marketed as Gardasil) may reduce incidence of cervical cancer by as much as 70 percent.

Internal research: Research carried out within the National Cancer Institute is performed by either the Center for Cancer Research (CCR) or the Division of Cancer Epidemiology and Genetics at one of the two institute campuses. The main campus is within the National Institutes of Health, located in Bethesda, Maryland. The second campus is within the Fort Detrick Army Garrison. The NCI also maintains an Advanced Technology Center at the National Institute of Standards and Technology. A combined total of about 3,200 people work in these centers, alongside about 300 principal investigators.

The goal of the Center for Cancer Research is to discover better options for preventing, detecting, diagnosing, and treating cancer. Through close collaboration between basic scientific investigations and applied clinical trials, the center has found that cancer research can proceed more rapidly than was traditionally possible. By rapidly deploying innovative techniques and technologies to the scientific community, the center has made major contributions to the field.

Support of external research, education, and training: In addition to the research carried out within the governmental organization, the National Cancer Institute provides funding to private research organizations, universities, hospitals, and training facilities to further the goal of reducing the burden of cancer. In 2007 the institute anticipated an investment of more than $2 billion in about five thousand research project grants. Organizations that receive these grants must first submit a detailed grant proposal that demonstrates how their research will further the goals of the NCI and maintain safety for participants. All grant proposals are peer-reviewed and carefully scrutinized by the institute. By providing educational assistance in the form of fellowships, internships, grants, and loan repayment programs, the institute also aids both predoctoral and postdoctoral students in their pursuit of education.

Robert Bockstiegel, B.S.

▶ For Further Information

Epstein, Samuel S. *Cancer-Gate: How to Win the Losing Cancer War*. Amityville, N.Y.: Baywood, 2005.

Jeffries, Lee P., ed. *Leading Topics in Cancer Research*. New York: Nova Science, 2007.

Martakis, Ignatius K., ed. *Cancer Research at the Leading Edge*. New York: Nova Science, 2007.

Pereira, Larissa S., ed. *Cancer Research Perspectives*. New York: Nova Science, 2008.

United States Department of Health and Human Services, National Institutes of Health. *The NCI Strategic Plan for Leading the Nation to Eliminate the Suffering and Death Due to Cancer*. Washington, D.C.: National Cancer Institute, 2006.

▶ Other Resources

Association of American Cancer Institutes
http://www.aaci-cancer.org

National Cancer Institute
http://www.cancer.gov

See also American Association for Cancer Research (AACR); American Cancer Society (ACS); American Institute for Cancer Research (AICR); Cancer education; Dana-Farber Cancer Institute; Duke Comprehensive Cancer Center; Fox Chase Cancer Center; Fred Hutchinson Cancer Research Center; Jonsson Comprehensive Cancer Center (JCCC); M. D. Anderson Cancer Center; Mayo Clinic Cancer Center; Memorial Sloan-Kettering Cancer Center; National Science Foundation (NSF); Prevent Cancer Foundation; Robert H. Lurie Cancer Center.

▶ National Science Foundation (NSF)

Category: Organizations

Definition: The National Science Foundation (NSF) is a United States government organization dedicated to advancing scientific progress and promoting the health, welfare, and security of the nation by providing federal funding and support to scientific research.

History: After World War II, many U.S. scientists and politicians recognized the need for sustained government support of basic scientific research if the United States was to maintain its new role as a global leader. One engineer and scientist named Vannevar Bush, then head of the wartime Office of Scientific Research and Development, was particularly instrumental in advocating for the creation of a new government agency. Bush's 1945 report to the president, entitled "Science—The Endless Frontier," has been called the blueprint for the National Science Foundation. Five years after the report was presented, on May 10, 1950, President Harry S. Truman signed the act, which created the NSF.

After the Soviet launch of Sputnik, U.S. interest in funding science grew, and in 1958 the National Science Foundation's budget was significantly increased. With a larger budget, however, came greater congressional oversight. In 1968 the Daddario-Kennedy amendment to the NSF charter was passed, forcing the foundation to get annual authorization of its spending from both the House and the Senate. The act also authorized the foundation to fund applied science in addition to its usual support for basic science.

During the following three decades, the NSF continued to expand its budget as Congress and the nation increasingly recognized the value of investment in scientific research.

As the budget grew, so did the number of grants awarded. During the 1970's, the foundation provided as few as six thousand grants, but by the 1990's that number grew to more than ten thousand. Funding for graduate students also increased, and by the 1990's almost thirty-four thousand graduate students were receiving federal support.

By 2006 the National Science Foundation's budget had grown to approximately $5.6 billion. It is the primary source of all federal funding for many of the nonmedical sciences and provides nearly half of all the federal support for academic nonmedical basic research. More than two hundred Nobel laureates have been funded by the foundation.

Organization: The National Science Foundation is organized into two main parts: the Office of the Director and the National Science Board. Working under the director are all of the directorates for the various scientific divisions as well as several offices that provide support services. The director and all of the directorates and offices that work under the director are responsible for deciding which proposals will be funded. The twenty-four-member National Science Board provides oversight, establishes strategic policy, and approves new programs or particularly large grants. The director and members of the board serve six-year terms. They are appointed by the president of the United States and approved by the Senate.

The funding process: In 2007 the National Science Foundation received more than forty-thousand grant proposals. To decide which proposals are worthy of funding, it must be determined which proposed research projects would best serve the goals of the foundation. To do this, the foundation has developed a process that begins with its staff's participation in workshops, conferences, and symposia. By attending these gatherings, they keep in constant contact with the scientific community and identify possible areas for achievement.

The NSF next publishes a solicitation for proposals to serve a specific need or to achieve a specific goal. Scientific researchers and engineers respond by submitting detailed proposals that describe their idea, request a specific amount of funding, and describe how that funding will be used. The foundation also accepts proposals that are not a response to a solicitation.

Then the NSF assembles a panel of independent reviewers made up of experts in the field. For example, if a proposal seeks funding to conduct research into a new technique for studying ozone depletion, the foundation finds prominent environmental scientists. More than fifty thousand experts participate in review panels each year. These panels usually review numerous proposals at one time and confidentially decide which proposals would best advance the goals of the foundation. This process is known as merit review. Once a proposal is accepted, the NSF will then provide funding and periodically review the progress of the research.

Cancer research: The National Science Foundation does not directly fund medical research, since medical research is usually funded by other parts of the federal government, such as the National Institutes of Health. However, much of the research funded by the NSF does have applications within the medical field. Discoveries made using foundation funding are published in scientific journals and made available for scientists involved with cancer research. Often a discovery in one field will aid discovery in another. For example, in 1993 William Fenical, a foundation-funded researcher at the Scripps Institution of Oceanography in La Jolla, California, discovered a type of coral that possesses a chemical called eleutherobin. This chemical, it was discovered, binds to cellular microtubules and can prevent division of cancer cells. Like many other anticancer drugs being tested, this chemical was discovered through funding research in a completely different field.

Robert Bockstiegel, B.S.

▶ For Further Information

Jeffries, Lee P., ed. *Leading Topics in Cancer Research.* New York: Nova Science, 2007.

Martakis, Ignatius K., ed. *Cancer Research at the Leading Edge*. New York: Nova Science, 2007.

National Science Foundation. *Overcoming the Past, Focusing on the Future*. Arlington, Va.: Author, 2003.

Pereira, Larissa S., ed. *Cancer Research Perspectives.* New York: Nova Science, 2008.

▶ Other Resources

Association of American Cancer Institutes
http://www.aaci-cancer.org

National Science Foundation
http://www.nsf.gov

See also American Association for Cancer Research (AACR); American Cancer Society (ACS); American Institute for Cancer Research (AICR); Dana-Farber Cancer Institute; Duke Comprehensive Cancer Center; Fox Chase Cancer Center; Fred Hutchinson Cancer Research Center; Jonsson Comprehensive Cancer Center (JCCC); M. D. Anderson Cancer Center; Mayo Clinic Cancer Center; Memorial Sloan-Kettering Cancer Center; National Cancer Institute (NCI); Prevent Cancer Foundation; Robert H. Lurie Cancer Center.

▶ Native North Americans and cancer

Category: Social and personal issues
Also known as: American Indians, Native Americans, First Nations

Definition: Native North Americans are a widely dispersed group of people made up of individuals from hundreds of different tribes throughout the contiguous United States and Alaska. According to the National Institutes of Health, cancer is the second leading cause of death among individuals of American Indian and Native Alaskan descent.

Description of the population: According to the 2000 census, there were 2,475,956 individuals in the United States who identified themselves as being of American Indian or Native Alaskan descent. This included 1,233,982 men and 1,241,974 women. In 2000, 138,439 of these individuals were the age of sixty-five or older, or about 5.6 percent of the Native American and Alaskan Native population. In comparison, about 12.4 percent of the general American population were age sixty-five or older in 2000.

The median household income as reported by the 2000 census of individuals who identified themselves as American Indian or Alaskan Native was $30,599 compared with a median household income of $41,994 for the American population in general. At that time, 607,734 people, or about 25 percent of American Indians and Native Alaskans, lived below the poverty line, compared with about 12 percent of the American population in general.

There are 569 different American Indian and Native Alaskan tribes that are officially recognized by the United States government. American Indians and Native Alaskans speak more than three hundred different languages. Many of these individuals live on reservations, especially in the southwestern states such as Arizona and New Mexico. In total, American Indians live on nearly three hundred reservations throughout the United States, although more than half of those of American Indian or Native Alaskan heritage do not live on reservations.

Incidence, death, and survival statistics: According to the United States Centers for Disease Control, in 2002 cancer was the second most common cause of death among American Indians and Native Alaskans. In 2002, 2,467 individuals self-reporting as American Indians died of cancer, accounting for about 20 percent of the total 12,415 deaths of individuals from that heritage group. For American Indian children between the ages of five and nine, cancer was the second leading cause of death, following unintentional injuries. For American Indians of both sexes between the ages of forty-five and fifty-four, cancer was the leading cause of death, as it also was for those aged fifty-five to sixty-four and those aged sixty-five to seventy-four. For American Indians over the age of eighty-five, cancer was the second leading cause of death, following heart disease.

The rates of colon and rectal cancer among Native Alaskans are higher than the rates of the same cancers among Americans who are of European heritage. Native American women who have been diagnosed with cervical cancer have a poorer prognosis than women of many other heritages.

The history of the relationship between American Indians and Alaskan tribes and the United States federal government is complex and filled with problems. The result of centuries of interaction between the U.S. government and the many Native Alaskan and American Indian tribes is that the tribes have been recognized as sovereign entities. However, they are also entitled to health care and other services provided by the federal government. The Indian Health Service is a division of the federal government charged with providing health services to many American Indians and Alaskan Natives. It is a department of the U.S. Department of Health and Human Services and was founded in 1955. As of 2005 the Indian Health Service either provided service for, or covered the cost of health services for, about 1.5 million total individuals. The Indian Health Service operates mainly on recognized reservations, which means that many individuals of American Indian and Native Alaskan descent may not have access to available services because many such individuals do not live in or around reservations.

Risk statistics: There are many problems that may contribute to people of American Indian and Native Alaskan descent not getting preventive health care and medical screenings that lead to early diagnosis of cancer. Many Native Alaskans and American Indians live in remote areas away from large cities where cancer centers and hospitals are often located. This can cause individuals to delay seeking treatment and to not have access to regular comprehensive medical care.

Not receiving comprehensive medical care on a regular basis, including general health care and routine screenings for diseases such as cancer, is generally linked to negative health outcomes. When cancer is not detected early, it is less likely to be have a positive outcome. Many Native Alaskans and American Indians do not report receiving regular medical care and screenings that can lead to early diagnosis. According to a 2004 survey sponsored by the

Kaiser Family Foundation and published in the *American Journal of Public Health*, 26 percent of American Indians and Native Alaskans reported that they had not visited a medical doctor within the last year, compared with 20 percent of people of European heritage.

Some of this dissatisfaction doubtless relates to the historic relationship between Native Americans and the Indian Health Service. Perception of the quality and effectiveness of health care services is lower among American Indians and Native Alaskans than among individuals of European descent. Some 16 percent of American Indian and Native Alaskans who sought care reported that they were not satisfied with the quality and care of the medical services that they received, compared with only 10 percent of people of European descent who reported dissatisfaction. An even larger disparity was found relating to provider communication. Some 26 percent of American Indians and Native Alaskans reported poor communication with their health care provider, compared with 17 percent of those of European descent.

Lack of insurance coverage is another barrier to prevention and early diagnosis, as well as a barrier to receiving cancer care and treatment if cancer does develop. About 83 percent of Americans of European descent have access to health care through private coverage, usually through a job, while only 49 percent of American Indians and Native Alaskans have access to similar coverage. Although the Indian Health Service does provide services to many uninsured individuals, it is not available to all of them. About 35 percent of American Indians and Native Alaskans are not insured.

Because a disproportionate percentage of Native Alaskans and American Indians have incomes below the poverty line, many individuals have increased cancer risks that are tied to poverty. People who live in poverty are more likely to smoke, which is a significant risk factor for many types of cancer. Individuals who live in poverty are less likely to have a well-balanced diet rich in fruits, vegetables, and whole grains, which is believed to help reduce the risk of cancer. Poor diets and concomitant obesity have historically been exacerbated by the unhealthy commodity foods provided by the U.S. government.

Perspective and prospects: Many Native Alaskan and American Indian individuals have different perceptions of Western medicine, medical practitioners, and medical technology. Medical practitioners who are going to work with Native Alaskan or American Indian populations may benefit from cultural awareness training. Improving doctor-patient communication, relationships, and trust can be an important building block toward more positive cancer outcomes in this population. Individuals who have a positive relationship with their health care provider are more likely to seek screenings and early treatment, which can drastically improve cancer outcomes.

Although there are many barriers to prevention, early diagnosis, and effective treatment of cancer among Native Alaskans and American Indians, the outlook is improving. Many different groups and foundations have sponsored research into the health disparities faced by minorities in the United States as well as research and educational outreach programs designed specifically to help American Indians and Native Alaskans. Organizations such as the Native American Cancer Research group dedicate time and resources to providing education to American Indians about cancer, help organize research into genetic patterns of cancer inheritance among American Indians, and provide other cancer support services aimed specifically at helping reduce the incidence and mortality of cancer among the American Indian community.

Helen Davidson, B.A.

▶ For Further Information

Duran, Eduardo. *Healing the Soul Wound: Counseling with American Indians and Other Native Peoples*. New York: Teachers College Press, 2006.

LaVeist, Thomas A. *Minority Populations and Health: An Introduction to Health Disparities in the United States*. San Francisco: Jossey-Bass, 2005.

Metrosa, Elene V., ed. *Racial and Ethnic Disparities in Health and Health Care*. New York: Nova Science, 2006.

▶ Other Resources

National Cancer Institute
Surveillance Research: Overview of Native American Initiatives
http://surveillance.cancer.gov/disparities/native

Native American Cancer Research
http://www.natamcancer.org

Native American Cancer Research Partnership
http://nacrp.web.arizona.edu

See also Complementary and alternative therapies; Ethnicity and cancer; Financial issues; Geography and cancer; Insurance; Poverty and cancer; Prayer and cancer support; Psychosocial aspects of cancer.

▶ Nausea and vomiting

Category: Diseases, symptoms, and conditions
Also known as: Emesis, retching, heaving, gagging, being sick to the stomach, seasickness, throwing up, butterflies in the stomach, dry heaves

Related conditions: Chemotherapy, radiation therapy, food poisoning, morning sickness during pregnancy, inner ear syndrome, infections

Definition: Nausea is the uneasy sensation that one is about to vomit, expelling stomach contents or undigested food through the mouth. Nausea can sometimes result in dry heaves when the stomach is empty.

Risk factors: Because nausea and vomiting are symptoms of many disorders as well as cancer therapies, the risk depends on the individual patient's medical condition and circumstances.

Etiology and the disease process: Nausea and vomiting are not diseases but symptoms—a sign that something is wrong within the body. Nausea and vomiting are complex body functions coordinated by the vomiting center in the brain stem of the body's central nervous system. Retching usually occurs after nausea and before vomiting as the body prepares to expel the stomach contents.

Nausea and vomiting can occur as a reaction to many prompts, including overeating, ingesting too much alcohol or sugar, infection, viruses, inner ear disorders, irritation of the throat or stomach lining, food poisoning from contaminated food or fluids, migraine headaches, unpleasant smells or sights, stress, severe anxiety or emotional circumstances, medications, or treatments for cancer. A person experiencing a heart attack, appendicitis, or head injury with increased pressure on the brain may have nausea and vomiting. Determining the cause is critical to finding the appropriate treatment and correcting the problem.

Cancer patients may experience nausea and vomiting for several reasons. Cancer treatments such as chemotherapy can affect patients by causing side effects of nausea and vomiting. Not all chemotherapy causes nausea and vomiting. The level of nausea that chemotherapy induces can range from low to severe. Factors such as the amount of the drug used or the route of administration can affect the incidence of nausea and vomiting. The characteristics of the person receiving chemotherapy—age, gender, or history of motion sickness—can influence the occurrence of nausea and vomiting. Sometimes nausea and vomiting will happen when patients enter an environment in which they have received chemotherapy because of odors or a mental association with the setting (anticipatory nausea and vomiting).

Cancer patients may have nausea and vomiting as an extension of their disease. The tumor may have spread to the gastrointestinal tract, the liver, or the brain. Also, high-dose radiation treatments given for certain types of cancer can cause nausea and vomiting in the hours following therapy. Other causes for nausea and vomiting in cancer patients include bowel obstructions, infections, anxiety, and certain medicines.

Usually the side effects of treatment can be controlled with medication, but if they are uncontrolled, they can result in serious metabolic dysfunction or anxiety and depression for the cancer patient and family.

Incidence: Almost every person will experience nausea and vomiting at some stage of life for various reasons. Approximately 50 percent of all cancer patients have nausea and vomiting during their treatment or as their disease progresses. Some sources estimate that as many as 7 or 8 out of 10 (70 to 80 percent) cancer patients have some nausea and vomiting.

Symptoms: Nausea produces a queasy feeling in the stomach and increased salivation in the mouth. Sometimes a stomachache or headache will occur before the nausea occurs. The person may experience dizziness, a fast heart rate, skin temperature changes (either feeling chilled or hot and flushed), and difficulty swallowing with nausea. Retching usually precedes vomiting as the body prepares to push out the stomach contents. However, sometimes vomiting occurs without nausea. Loss of fluids and electrolytes can leave the patient feeling drained and fatigued.

Screening and diagnosis: The severity, duration, and frequency of nausea and vomiting will determine the need for further assessment and intervention by the health care provider. The key to screening and diagnosing nausea and vomiting is finding the underlying cause. Patients should review any health conditions they have that might contribute to nausea and vomiting such as migraine headaches or pregnancy (morning sickness).

Health care providers can prepare cancer patients for the likely possibility of nausea and vomiting during their treatment process. The degree to which nausea and vomiting affects the patient depends on many factors. Extension of cancer with metastatic disease to vital organs can increase the incidence of nausea and vomiting.

Treatment and therapy: Nausea and vomiting do not necessarily need treatment unless they continue for extended periods of time, as can occur with several types of radiation and chemotherapy. The first approach to treatment is to determine the cause. If the cause can be defined and treated successfully, the nausea and vomiting will subside.

Sometimes a simple breath of fresh air can resolve the problem. Some people successfully use ginger ale, cola, or crackers to decrease the nausea. Vomiting will immediately relieve nausea but nausea may return. Simple nausea and vomiting usually respond to limiting the intake of food and fluids. Gradually patients may take clear liquids, then small amounts of dry toast or crackers. If this is well tolerated without more nausea and vomiting, patients can return to a regular diet.

If the nausea and vomiting continue uncontrolled, further examination is necessary to remove or treat the cause. Over time, patients with uncontrolled nausea and vomiting will become dehydrated and may suffer an electrolyte imbalance. Patients with continuous nausea and vomiting may need antiemetics, medications that suppress these symptoms. If severe dehydration has occurred, patients may need to be given intravenous fluids by a health care provider. Dehydration and electrolyte imbalance can be serious and can even be life-threatening.

Alternative or complementary therapies may help control or minimize nausea and vomiting. Nonpharmacologic therapies include biofeedback, guided imagery, attentional distraction, massage, and hypnosis. Behavior therapy such as desensitization may be useful for anticipatory nausea and vomiting. Ginger, an herb used to decrease nausea and vomiting, can be used in food or taken in capsules. Acupressure may help some patients. Dietary approaches such as eating food with minimal smell (either cold or at room temperature) while having chemotherapy may decrease nausea and vomiting. Avoiding certain types of foods, such as high-fat, spicy, or salty foods, helps some patients.

Prognosis, prevention, and outcomes: Most people experience uncomplicated nausea and vomiting at some time in their lives but can regain their health through addressing the cause and allowing the body time to heal. However, a health care provider should be notified if people have nausea and vomiting that continue for longer than forty-eight hours, experience extreme dizziness, vomit blood, or are unable to retain fluids within twenty-four hours.

If people have begun taking a new medication before the onset of nausea and vomiting, they should notify their health care provider to possibly change the drug. People should consult a health care provider when they have yellowing of the skin or eyes, difficulty swallowing, mental confusion, dehydration and extreme thirst, trouble with urination, or constant or sharp pain in the chest or lower abdomen. Certain conditions when accompanied by nausea and vomiting may indicate a medical emergency, such

Medicines Used to Treat Nausea in Cancer Patients

Drug	*Use*
Aprepitant	Used for acute and delayed nausea and vomiting
Aexamethasone	Corticosteroid, given orally and intravenously; used alone or in combination
Aiphenhydramine	Antihistamine, used for low-risk chemotherapy or when other antiemetics have failed; used in combination and also to reduce side effects from other antiemetics
Aolasetron, granisetron, ondansetron	New antiemetics, given orally or intravenously
Aronabinol, nabilone	Tetrahydrocannabinol (THC) is main ingredient; used when other antiemetics have failed
Haloperidol	Tranquilizer, used when other antiemetics have failed; used in combination
Lorazepam, alprazolam	Anxiety drugs; generally used in combination
Metoclopramide	Used for low-risk chemotherapy or when other antiemetics have failed; used alone or in combination
Olanzapine	Used when other antiemetics fail
Palonosetron	Used for acute and delayed nausea and vomiting; given intravenously
Prochlorperazine	Used for low-risk chemotherapy or when other antiemetics have failed; used alone or in combination
Promethazine	Used when other antiemetics have failed

Source: National Comprehensive Cancer Network

as diabetic shock, severe headache, consistent chest pain, difficulty breathing, profuse sweating, or exposure to a known allergen.

At least half of all cancer patients will experience some nausea and vomiting at some point in their disease process. Using antiemetics or complementary therapies such as relaxation, massage, or meditation can sometimes produce a better outcome to the nausea and vomiting resulting from chemotherapy or radiation therapy. Education and knowledge can go a long way in helping patients help themselves.

Robert W. Koch, D.N.S., R.N.

▶ For Further Information

Anderson, Greg. *Cancer: Fifty Essential Things to Do*. New York: Penguin Books, 1999.

Donnerer, Josef, ed. *Antiemetic Therapy*. New York: Karger, 2003.

Lyss, Alan P., and Humberto M. Fagundes. *Chemotherapy and Radiation for Dummies*. Hoboken, N.J.: Wiley, 2005.

Tonato, M., ed. *Antiemetics in the Supportive Care of Cancer Patients*. New York: Springer, 1996.

▶ Other Resources

American Cancer Society

What Can I Do About Nausea and Vomiting?
http://www.cancer.org/docroot/MBC/content/MBC_2_2X_What_Can_I_Do_About_Nausea_and_Vomiting.asp?sitearea=MBC

National Cancer Institute

Nausea and Vomiting
http://www.cancer.gov/cancertopics/pdq/supportivecare/nausea/patient

National Comprehensive Cancer Network

Nausea and Vomiting Treatment Guidelines for Patients with Cancer
http://www.nccn.org/patients/patient_gls/_english/_nausea_and_vomiting/contents.asp

See also Acupuncture and acupressure for cancer patients; Adjuvant therapy; Antinausea medications; Cachexia; Chemotherapy; Complementary and alternative therapies; External beam radiation therapy (EBRT); Gastrointestinal complications of cancer treatment; Ginseng, panax; Living with cancer; Medical marijuana; Motion sickness devices; Nutrition and cancer treatment; Radiation therapies; Side effects; Taste alteration; Weight loss.

▶ Needle biopsies

Category: Procedures

Also known as: Fine needle biopsy, core needle biopsy, stereotactic (exact) biopsy, Mammotome biopsy, Advanced Breast Biopsy Instrumentation (ABBI)

Definition: A needle biopsy is a procedure in which a sample of body tissue is extracted by using a hollow needle or a similar instrument. There are two types of needle biopsies: fine needle biopsy and core needle biopsy.

In fine needle biopsy, a thin needle attached to a syringe is used to extract the tissue samples. In core needle biopsy, a wide-gauge needle or a special biopsy instrument, such as a Mammotome or ABBI, is used. The Mammotome and ABBI are used only to perform a breast biopsy. The core needle ranges from 0.25 to 1 centimeter in diameter. It has a special cutting edge and a spring-loaded device that suctions out the tissue samples. The Mammotome suctions in breast tissue and then cuts it with a rotating blade. The ABBI extracts a cylinder of breast tissue about the size of the tumor.

Cancers diagnosed: Breast, lung, prostate, kidney, thyroid, musculoskeletal, liver, heart, and skin cancers

Why performed: Needle biopsies are performed in order to obtain samples of tissue from a tumor or growth that is suspected of being cancer. Needle biopsies are considered less invasive than surgical biopsies and often can be performed as an outpatient procedure.

Patient preparation: The patient preparation will depend on the tissue that is being sampled, the risk of the procedure, and the type of facility where the biopsy is to be performed. If a core needle biopsy is carried out in a physician's office, then ultrasonic guidance is used to localize the tumor, unless it is palpable. If it is palpable, then no radiologic guidance is required.

Needle biopsies that require the use of fluoroscopy, computed tomography (CT), magnetic resonance imaging (MRI), or mammography to localize the tumor or that are considered high risk are performed in an outpatient surgical center. Patient preparation may include a preoperative physical examination, blood work, and possibly an electrocardiogram (EKG). The patient needs to fast for two to four hours before the procedure.

Occasionally, high-risk biopsy procedures require that the patient be admitted to the hospital for the biopsy and then stay overnight for monitoring. In this instance, patient preparation would require a preoperative physical examination, blood work, and an EKG. Also, the patient would need to fast after midnight the day of the biopsy.

Steps of the procedure: The patient is positioned so that the area to be biopsied is exposed. This area is then scrubbed and disinfected. A local anesthetic is injected into the biopsy area. If the tumor is not palpable, then radiologic imaging is used to localize the tumor and to follow the progress of the needle into the tissue. This is called stereotactic localization.

For a fine needle biopsy, the surgeon inserts the needle into the tumor and aspirates small samples of tissue. The needle is repositioned several times so that multiple tissue samples can be taken.

Unless the tumor is superficial, for core needle biopsy, a small incision (0.25 inch in length) is made into the tissue. The core needle is then inserted into the tumor through the incision. Multiple tissue samples are taken.

For core needle, Mammotome, and ABBI biopsies of the breast, the patient is positioned on her stomach with a single breast hanging through a hole in a specially designed table. This procedure uses either mammography or ultrasound guidance to localize the breast tumor. For MRI guidance, the patient is positioned on her stomach and both breasts are hanging pendent. The biopsy is performed on the hanging breast.

After the procedure: If an incision was made, then either a suture (stitch) or an adhesive paper (Steri-Strip) is applied to close the edges of the incision. A sterile dressing is applied over the biopsy site. For some biopsies, a pressure dressing is applied after the biopsy procedure. Usually, the patient is monitored for at least one hour after the biopsy.

The patient can remove the dressing in one to two days and should avoid vigorous physical exercise or heavy lifting for two weeks after a biopsy.

Once a needle biopsy has healed, including Mammotome and ABBI, the patient is unlikely to have a scar from the procedure.

Risks: The liver and the kidney are highly vascular (have many blood vessels) and thus are at high risk of bleeding following biopsies. Lung biopsies carry a risk for causing collapse of a portion of the lung (pneumothorax). Other risks of needle biopsy are nerve damage and infection.

Results: The biopsied tissue is sent to a cytologist or a pathologist to be examined under a microscope. A cytologist examines the cells from a fine needle biopsy, in which the specimens consist of aspirated cells. A pathologist examines the samples from core needle biopsies, which consist of cores of tissue. This tissue must be sliced thinly and applied to a slide for examination.

The surgeon will receive a pathology report that describes the cells of the tumor. It will discuss the size, shape, and activity of the cells and their nuclei, comparing them with normal cells. The report states whether the tumor is cancer and, if so, the type of cancer cells present within the tumor.

Christine M. Carroll, R.N., B.S.N., M.B.A.

▶ **For Further Information**

DeVita, Vincent, Jr., Samuel Hellman, Steven A. Rosenberg, et al., eds. *Cancer: Principles and Practice of Oncology*. 7th ed. Philadelphia: Lippincott Williams & Wilkins, 2005.

McPhee, Stephen J., Maxine A. Papadakis, and Lawrence M. Tierney, eds. *Current Medical Diagnosis and Treatment 2008*. New York: McGraw-Hill Medical, 2007.

Rosen, Paul Peter, and Syed A. Hoda. *Breast Pathology: Diagnosis by Needle Core Biopsy*. 2d ed. Philadelphia: Lippincott Williams & Wilkins, 2006.

Yang, Grace, Chia-yu Hsu, and Liang-Che Tao. *Transabdominal Fine-Needle Aspiration Biopsy: A Colour*

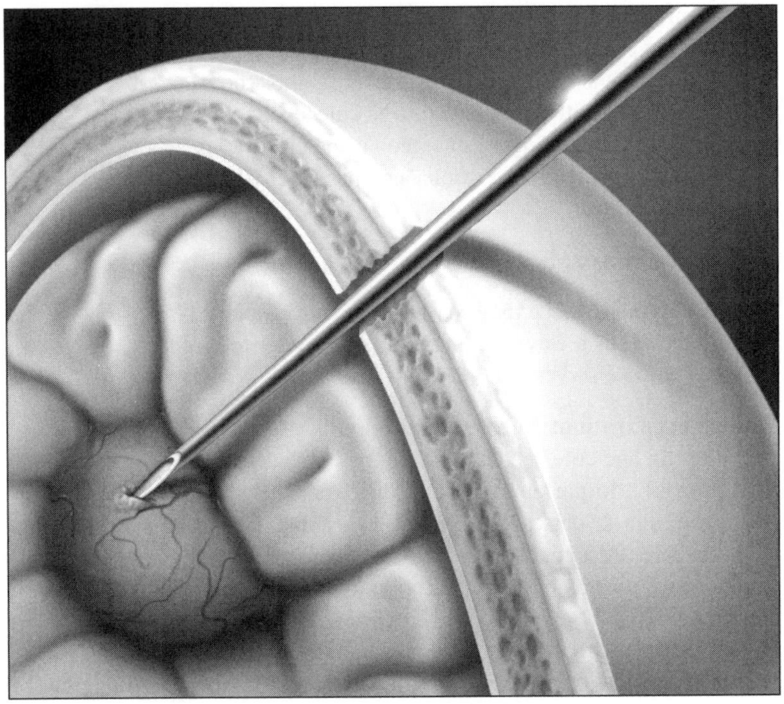

Needle biopsy of the brain. (Custom Medical Stock Photo)

Atlas and Monograph. 2d ed. Hackensack, N.J.: World Scientific, 2007.

▶ Other Resources

Radiology Info
Needle Biopsy of Lung Nodules
Http://www.radiologyinfo.org/en/info.cfm?pg=nlungbiop&bhcp=1

WebMD
Breast Biopsy
http://www.webmd.com/breast-cancer/guide/breast-biopsy

See also Biopsy; Bone marrow aspiration and biopsy; Computed tomography (CT)-guided biopsy; Core needle biopsy; Liver biopsy; Needle localization; Pathology; Pleural biopsy; Sentinel lymph node (SLN) biopsy and mapping; Stereotactic needle biopsy; Surgical biopsies; Wire localization.

▶ Needle localization

Category: Procedures
Also known as: Wire localization, stereotactic (exact) localization

Definition: Needle localization is a procedure that is used to mark a nonpalpable mass (one that cannot be felt) prior to biopsy (removal of a piece of tissue). It is most commonly associated with breast biopsies. Needle localization is performed by a radiologist or surgeon using ultrasound, mammography, or magnetic resonance imaging (MRI) to view the tumor.

Cancers diagnosed: Breast cancer

Why performed: Since the breast mass is not palpable, the surgeon needs a way to find the tumor in order to biopsy it. The wire serves as a marker for the tumor.

Patient preparation: Needle localization is associated with surgical and core needle breast biopsy. Usually, this procedure is performed in a radiology office or a breast biopsy room. For a surgical biopsy, within a month before the procedure, the patient has a preoperative physical examination, routine blood work, and possibly an electrocardiogram (EKG). Also, she will have to fast after midnight the day of the procedure. For core needle biopsy, the patient needs to fast only for two to three hours before the procedure.

Steps of the procedure: First, the mass is localized. When ultrasound is used, the transducer (used to transmit and receive sound waves) is held to the side of the mass while the needle is inserted. With mammography, it is necessary to use special mammography plates with a screen or a small door in them, so that the needle can be inserted while the breast is compressed. MRI imaging requires the use of a special attachment through which the needle can be inserted.

A local anesthetic is injected over the tumor. Either a thin wire or a needle is then inserted into the tumor. The position of the wire or needle is verified with the radiologic imaging being used.

After the procedure: The biopsy is performed either in an operating room (for a surgical biopsy) or in the biopsy room (for a core needle biopsy). The wire or needle is removed with the breast tumor.

Risks: There is a slight risk of bleeding or infection after this procedure.

Results: The surgeon is able to localize the nonpalpable breast tumor by the presence of the wire and then to remove it. Pathology will be performed on the tissue sample to determine whether it is cancerous.

Christine M. Carroll, R.N., B.S.N., M.B.A.

▶ For Further Information

Rosen, Paul Peter, and Syed A. Hoda. *Breast Pathology: Diagnosis by Needle Core Biopsy*. 2d ed. Philadelphia: Lippincott Williams & Wilkins, 2006.

Rubin, Eva, and Jean F. Simpson. *Breast Specimen Radiography: Needle Localization and Radiographic Pathologic Correlation*. Philadelphia: Lippincott-Raven, 1998.

▶ Other Resources

eMedicine
Breast Needle Localization
http://www.emedicine.com/Radio/topic911.htm

WebMD
Breast Biopsy
http://www.webmd.com/breast-cancer/guide/breast-biopsy

See also Biopsy; Breast ultrasound; Magnetic resonance imaging (MRI); Mammography; Needle biopsies; Stereotactic needle biopsy; Ultrasound tests; Wire localization.

▶ Nephroblastomas

Category: Diseases, symptoms, and conditions
Also known as: Wilms' tumors

Related conditions: Beckwith-Wiedemann syndrome, WAGR complex (Wilms' tumor aniridia-genitourinary anomalies-mental retardation), Denys-Drash syndrome

Definition: Nephroblastomas are the most common malignant kidney tumors of early childhood.

Risk factors: Nephroblastomas may arise sporadically (in otherwise healthy children) or can be inherited. A nephroblastoma is sometimes linked to birth defects such as aniridia (absence of the iris), hemihypertrophy (enlargement of one side of the body), and genitourinary abnormalities. Birth defect syndromes associated with nephroblastoma include Beckwith-Wiedemann syndrome (tongue and internal organ enlargement and omphalocele), WAGR syndrome (Wilms' tumor aniridia-genitourinary anomalies-mental retardation), and Denys-Drash syndrome (Wilms' tumor, kidney disease, and pseudohermaphroditism). Children aged seven and younger are at highest risk, although older children and adults are occasionally affected. No gender or racial predilection exists.

Etiology and the disease process: There is compelling evidence that genetic factors (two mutational events involving the inactivation of tumor-suppressor genes) may be responsible for tumor development. As a result, primitive embryonic cells of the kidney fail to develop and instead multiply to form a tumor.

Incidence: Annually, 450 to 500 children in the United States are diagnosed with a nephroblastoma, with 24 percent of these cases forming part of a developmental defect syndrome.

Symptoms: Most patients have a painless abdominal mass, usually an incidental finding by the doctor or the parent. Some complain of abdominal pain, bloody urine, nausea and vomiting, anorexia, weight loss, and constipation.

Screening and diagnosis: Lab tests, a thorough family medical history, and diagnostic imaging—ultrasound, chest X ray, computed tomography (CT) scan, and magnetic resonance imaging (MRI)—will help determine the extent of tumor spread. Surgical tumor removal and tissue sampling will confirm the diagnosis. Tumor staging helps establish the treatment plan:

- Stage I: Tumor confined to the kidney, completely resectable
- Stage II: Tumor metastasis to local surrounding area, completely resectable
- Stage III: Tumor metastasis to surrounding area, not completely resectable
- Stage IV: Tumor metastasis to distant organs (lungs, liver, and brain)
- Stage V: Tumor present in both kidneys

Treatment and therapy: Treatment consists of a combination of surgery, chemotherapy, and radiotherapy. Surgery can be partial, complete, or radical nephrectomy (surgical removal of the kidney). The drugs dactinomycin, doxorubicin, vincristine, and cyclophosphamide are used for chemotherapy. Radiotherapy is usually confined to Stage III and IV nephroblastoma.

Prognosis, prevention, and outcomes: The prognosis is good, with an overall survival rate of 90 percent. Outcomes for nephroblastoma patients have vastly improved since the 1970's, thanks to concerted efforts by the National Wilms' Tumor Study Group (NWTSG) and the International Society of Pediatric Oncology (SIOP).

Ophelia Panganiban, B.S.

See also Beckwith-Wiedemann syndrome (BWS); Denys-Drash syndrome and cancer; Pediatric oncology and hematology; Wilms' tumor; Wilms' tumor aniridia-genitourinary anomalies-mental retardation (WAGR) syndrome and cancer.

▶ Nephrostomy

Category: Procedures
Also known as: Percutaneous nephrostomy (PCN), nephropyelostomy

Definition: Nephrostomy is a procedure in which an opening is made and a nephrostomy tube (catheter) is placed into the kidney to drain urine to outside the body. Urine is collected into a bag attached to the nephrostomy tube. The procedure is done either through a surgical incision or percutaneously (through the skin).

Cancers treated: Ovarian, cervical, colon, and other cancers of the pelvic area

Why performed: Tumors may cause a blockage of one or both of the ureters, the tubes that normally carry urine from the kidneys to the bladder. The blockage causes a backup of urine into the kidneys, creating a great risk of infection and kidney damage that cannot be repaired. The insertion of nephrostomy tubes prevents the backup of urine.

Nephrostomy tubes may also be placed during a diagnostic procedure called an antegrade pyelogram, which is done to determine the location of the blockage. In some cases, the nephrostomy tubes are inserted to allow the placement of anticancer drugs directly into the kidney. Nephrostomy tubes are also used for other conditions that affect the urinary tract.

Patient preparation: Nephrostomy is usually performed on hospitalized patients. Some patients may have the procedure done without admission to a hospital. Preparation for the procedure may vary depending on the patient's condition, the physician's practice, and the facility. Generally, the patient must not have anything to eat or drink for four to eight hours before the procedure. The physician may ask the patient to temporarily stop or adjust the dose of some medications, including aspirin, blood thinners, and diabetes medications. Laboratory tests such as a complete blood count (CBC), coagulation tests, urinalysis, and urine culture for bacteria may be done before the procedure. The physician discusses the procedure, including the type of local anesthetic used, sedation, risks, and aftercare. The patient gives the physician permission to perform the procedure by reading and signing a consent form. Before signing the form, the patient may ask the physician questions to clarify anything that the doctor has said or any part of the consent form that the patient does not understand.

Steps of the procedure: An intravenous (IV) line is inserted, usually in the patient's arm or hand, to provide fluids, antibiotics, pain medication, and sedation. Nephrostomy is generally performed in the interventional radiology department by an interventional radiologist or urologist. The patient lies on the stomach and remains awake, although medication is given that may cause drowsiness. Monitoring of blood pressure, heart rate, and oxygen level is done throughout the procedure. Imaging procedures such as ultrasound, computed tomography (CT), or fluoroscopy are used to visualize the area. These procedures are done before and during insertion of the nephrostomy tube to guide the physician in placing the tube.

The site where the tube will be inserted is sterilized. A medication such as lidocaine (Xylocaine) is given to numb the skin and tissues. A small incision is made, and a needle is inserted into the kidney. Contrast dye is injected for visualization, and the nephrostomy tube is inserted. The needle is removed. A dressing is placed over the site, and the nephrostomy tube is connected to a drainage bag. The tube site is on the right or left side of the back near the waistline, depending on which kidney is blocked. If both kidneys are blocked, then the physician will insert tubes for each kidney.

After the procedure: The patient is taken to the recovery room or back to the hospital room. A nurse will monitor the patient for any changes in blood pressure, heart rate, or breathing. The nurse monitors the urine output by measuring the urine collected in the bag. The bag may be attached to the patient's leg by use of straps that are provided. Before discharge, the physician and/or a nurse will give the patient instructions on caring for the nephrostomy site, emptying the bag, monitoring the urine output, and noting signs of complications. Patients may need others to assist them in caring for the site and emptying the bag once they are home. In addition to the urine drained through the nephrostomy tube, the patient will still need to urinate. If only one tube is placed but the other kidney works normally, then the urine from that kidney still passes into the bladder. If nephrostomy tubes are placed in both kidneys, then there may still be drainage of some urine into the bladder.

Risks: The risks of nephrostomy include bleeding, infection, blood clots in the nephrostomy tube or bladder, and dislodgement of the nephrostomy tube.

Results: The placement of nephrostomy tubes will alleviate the backup of urine in the kidneys or allow treatment to be given. Although their use is normally for a short time, in some cases the blockage cannot be removed and the nephrostomy tubes remain in use permanently. In these cases, the tubes are replaced periodically.

Wanda E. Clark, M.T. (ASCP)

▶ For Further Information

Berman, Joel. *Understanding Surgery: A Comprehensive Guide for Every Family*. Wellesley, Mass.: Branden Books. 2001.

Nurse's Five-Minute Consult: Treatments. Philadelphia: Lippincott Williams & Wilkins, 2007.

▶ Other Resources

National Institutes of Health

Caring for Your Nephrostomy Tube
http://clinicalcenter.nih.gov/ccc/patient_education/pepubs/percneph.pdf

See also Cervical cancer; Kidney cancer; Ovarian cancers; Renal pelvis tumors; Urinary system cancers; Urologic oncology; Urostomy.

Neuroblastomas

Category: Diseases, symptoms, and conditions
Also known as: Childhood autonomic nervous system tumors

Related conditions: Ganglioneuroblastomas, ganglioneuromas

Definition: Neuroblastomas are cancers, most often found in infants and young children, that grow from primitive, embryonic nerve cells. Two-thirds of tumors begin in the adrenal glands or the sympathetic nervous system ganglia, with growth in the abdomen. The remaining third of neuroblastomas grow in the chest, neck, or pelvis, but all evolve from sympathetic nervous system ganglia.

Risk factors: Heredity may play a role in some neuroblastomas and is the only known risk factor. Infants with the familial form of neuroblastoma usually have a parent or someone in the family who had a neuroblastoma as an infant, and familial cases are usually diagnosed before one year of age. When familial neuroblastoma develops, there may be two or more tumors in various organs in the body. It is necessary to differentiate metastasis from multiorgan familial neuroblastoma.

Etiology and the disease process: There is no known cause of neuroblastoma other than heredity, which is involved in only 1 to 2 percent of cases. Neuroblastoma may form before birth and is occasionally found by fetal ultrasound. Most tumors develop before five years of age. Tumors are generally found only as the cancer grows and causes symptoms by pressing on organs. The tumor has usually metastasized by the time of diagnosis, and metastasis to the bone is common. Most tumors are fast growing, but in rare cases, the tumor cells may die spontaneously (apoptosis), and the tumor disappears. Occasionally, the tumor cells may quit dividing and become normal ganglia. This causes the tumor to become a ganglioneuroma, which is benign.

Incidence: The incidence rate of neuroblastoma in children under one year of age is 35 per million, decreasing to 1 per million between ten and fifteen years of age. Neuroblastoma is slightly more common in boys than in girls, with a ratio of 5:4. Neuroblastoma accounts for 25 percent of cancers in children under one year of age and 7 percent of cancers in children under the age of fifteen.

Symptoms: Common symptoms of neuroblastoma include fatigue; diarrhea; a swollen abdomen; difficulty breathing as the tumor gets larger or spreads to the chest area; dark circles under the eyes; pale or flushed, red skin; excessive sweating; bone pain or tenderness; rapid pulse; high blood pressure; poorly controlled movement of the extremities; or paralysis. Symptoms depend on the site of the tumor, and parents may notice or feel a mass in the abdomen, chest, or neck.

Screening and diagnosis: There is no screening test for neuroblastoma. If a family has a history of neuroblastoma, it is important to tell the pediatrician at the first visit. Parents should take note of any unusual lumps, swellings, or changes in bowel or bladder patterns, as the symptoms ofneuroblastoma often manifest in this manner. The diagnosis of neuroblastoma begins with a careful physical examination, as masses may be palpated (felt) in the abdomen, chest, or neck. A twenty-four-hour urine test, blood work, and cytogenetic analysis to look for changes in chromosomes are done. A bone marrow aspiration or biopsy specimen may also undergo cytogenetic analysis and pathology review. Imaging (X-ray) studies may include ordinary X rays, computed tomography (CT) scans, ultra-

Possible Causative Factors for Neuroblastoma

Studies have looked at these factors as possible causes for neuroblastoma, but so far the results have been inconclusive or contradictory.

Pregnancy-Related Factors
- Previous miscarriage (higher risk per one study, lower per another)
- Fertility drug use before pregnancy
- Alcohol use during pregnancy
- Smoking during pregnancy (higher risk per one study, lower per another)
- Taking certain medications during pregnancy: amphetamines, diuretics, tranquilizers, muscle relaxants, vaginal anti-infection drugs

Paternal Factors
- Father's exposure to electromagnetic fields, pesticides, dust, rubber, paint, radiation

Birth-Related Factors
- Birth defects
- Low birth weight

Source: L. A. G. Ries et al., eds., *Cancer Incidence and Survival Among Children and Adolescents: United States SEER Program, 1975-1995*, NIH Pub. No. 99-4649 (Bethesda, Md.: National Cancer Institute, SEER Program, 1999)

sound, a magnetic resonance imaging (MRI) scan, and a positron emission tomography (PET) scan.

Once a diagnosis is made, staging neuroblastoma is important to determine the treatment needed. The first step is to determine if the tumor has spread to other parts of the body. Additional tests may be indicated, including lymph node biopsy or fine needle aspiration of fluid from a lymph node as well as imaging studies with dye injection or injection of a small amount of radioactive tracer material. Four stages are used to classify neuroblastoma: Stages I, IIA and IIB, III, and IV and IVS. The higher the stage, the more extensive the disease and its spread. Neuroblastomas are categorized as low risk, intermediate risk, and high risk based on stage, with treatment determined by risk group.

Treatment and therapy: Because neuroblastoma is rare, treatment in a clinical research trial is recommended by the National Cancer Institute. Treatment for neuroblastoma is multimodal, which means that surgery, radiation therapy, chemotherapy, and in rare instances watchful waiting may be used. The higher the risk group, the more aggressive the therapy. Surgery is the initial treatment of choice to remove as much of the tumor as possible and to biopsy lymph nodes. Radiation therapy may be used, especially if part of the tumor has been left behind after surgery or if distant metastases exist. Chemotherapy is used to kill any cells remaining after surgery or to attack cells that may have spread elsewhere in the body. Patients may be watched carefully until a change in their condition indicates the method of therapy. A team will make the best treatment decisions for the child based on staging, location of the tumor, and other factors.

Prognosis, prevention, and outcomes: The prognosis for neuroblastoma depends on the age of the child at diagnosis, the stage of the disease, the site of the tumor, the size of the tumor, and the type of tumor cells. Infants do better than older children. Low-risk group survival at five years is 95 percent, intermediate group survival is 85 to 90 percent, and high-risk group survival is approximately 30 percent. Neuroblastoma cannot be prevented.

Patricia Stanfill Edens, R.N., Ph.D., FACHE

▶ For Further Information

Maris, J. M., M. D. Hogarty, R. Bagatell, and S. I. Cohn. "Neuroblastoma." *Lancet* 369, no. 9579 (June 23, 2007): 2106-2120.

Nishimura, H., et al. "Proton-Beam Therapy for Olfactory Neuroblastoma." *International Journal of Radiation Oncology, Biology, Physics* 68, no. 3 (July 1, 2007): 758-762.

▶ Other Resources

American Cancer Society
http://www.cancer.org

National Cancer Institute
Neuroblastoma Treatment
http://www.cancer.gov/cancertopics/pdq/treatment/neuroblastoma/patient

See also Adrenal gland cancers; Beckwith-Wiedemann syndrome (BWS); Bone marrow transplantation (BMT); Brain and central nervous system cancers; Breast cancer in children and adolescents; Childhood cancers; Horner syndrome; *HRAS* gene testing; Mediastinal tumors; *MYC* oncogene; Nasal cavity and paranasal sinus cancers; Pediatric oncology and hematology; Stem cell transplantation; Syndrome of inappropriate antidiuretic hormone production (SIADH); Tumor markers; Umbilical cord blood transplantation.

▶ Neuroectodermal tumors

Category: Diseases, symptoms, and conditions
Also known as: Primitive neuroectodermal tumors (PNETs)

Related conditions: Medulloblastomas, peripheral neuroepitheliomas, central neuroblastomas, ependymoblastomas, Gorlin syndrome, nevoid basal cell carcinoma syndrome, Askin tumor (thoracopulmonary PNET), peripheral PNET/Ewing sarcoma family tumor (pPNET/ESFT), extraosseous Ewing sarcoma

Definition: Neuroectodermal tumors refer to a group of cancers that were formerly thought to have a common origin from the neuroectodermal tissue layer cell line (neural crest) in the embryo. Presently, they are classified according to cell differentiation. They possess embryonic cell characteristics of brain (neuronal), neuronal support (glial), or mesenchymal cells depending on the degree of differentiation assumed. Neuroectodermal tumors may arise from bone or soft tissue (peripheral Ewing sarcoma family tumor, pPNET/ESFT), or neurons in the peripheral or central nervous system (medulloblastomas; infratentorial PNET, or iPNET; supratentorial PNET, or sPNET). Medulloblastomas represent the prototype neuroectodermal tumor.

Risk factors: Neuroectodermal tumors have risk factors associated with alterations in the patient's genome as a sporadic mutation, as part of a syndrome, or as a result of environmental exposure to a mutagen. Syndromes associated with the risk of developing iPNET include multiple-tumor, autosomal dominant diseases such as Gorlin syndrome, Turcot syndrome, and Li-Fraumeni syndrome. Exposure of children to pesticides, particularly organophosphates, has been implicated in several studies as an environmental risk factor for the subsequent development of PNET. Organophosphates have been associated in at least one study with a mutation in the *PON1*(-108T) allele, which is responsible for expression of the organophosphate detoxification pathway (cytochrome P450/paraoxonase) in the liver.

Etiology and the disease process: The genesis of neuroectodermal tumors is associated with chromosomal changes. The most common chromosomal aberration seen in medulloblastomas is deletion of the short arm of chromosome 17 (17p13.3), seen in as many as 30 to 40 percent of medulloblastoma cases. Other gene aberrations associated with medulloblastomas may involve the *TP53*, *PAX*, and sonic hedgehog (*SHH*) genes and the tumor-suppression region *RASSF1A*, among others. The Ewing sarcoma family tumor (ESFT) is associated with the translocation t(11;22)(q24;q12), expressing the *EWS-FLI1* fusion protein modulator.

Incidence: The Swedish Cancer Registry reported that medulloblastomas represented 21 percent of all primary pediatric brain malignancies. The incidence of all neuroectodermal tumors is highest in children, with 0.5 medulloblastoma cases per 100,000 per year reported in the United States. Medulloblastomas represent the most common solid malignant brain tumor found in children (30 percent), with the incidence decreasing to only 1 percent of brain tumors found during adulthood. The majority of medulloblastomas occur in the cerebellum, below the tentorium (extension of the protective tissue covering the brain); only 4 percent of neuroectodermal tumors occur above the tentorium (midbrain, cerebral cortex). Neuroectodermal tumors outside the central nervous system occur in 1 percent of all sarcomas found.

Symptoms: More often than not, the more common signs and symptoms relate to obstruction of cerebrospinal fluid (CSF) flow and subsequent pressure buildup and tissue compression. Symptoms of increased pressure include nausea, vomiting, morning headache, and vision changes. Brain stem compression or encroachment can manifest as irritability, lethargy, and decreased social interaction. Cerebellar signs of involvement include frequent loss of balance. Physical examination findings may include papilledema (swelling of both optic nerves); abnormal eye movements; gaze, gait, and limb incoordination; deficits in affected cranial nerves, especially those going to the throat, mouth, shoulders, and tongue; and an increase in head circumference in babies less than two years old. In other sites, neuroectodermal tumors such as pPNET/ESFT can manifest as localized bone pain, a soft-tissue mass located along the middle of long bones with fever and weight loss.

Screening and diagnosis: The final diagnosis of a neuroectodermal tumor is mainly pathological, when a tissue sample is examined microscopically and with immunohistochemistry (tests determining cell markers). However, the neuroanatomical location of the tumor as suggested by clinical history, physical examination, and neuroimaging tests such as magnetic resonance imaging (MRI) can suggest a medulloblastoma. Alternatively, a computed tomography (CT) scan may reveal the tumor but has significantly less resolution than an MRI. There are no screening tests available for neuroectodermal tumors. X rays and CT of the affected limb may reveal signs of simultaneous bone destruction and remodeling ("sunburst sign") and a periosteal reaction (disruption in the continuity of the outer bone) as well as bone infiltration. X rays and CT of the chest should also be done to find metastases.

Treatment and therapy: Treatment of a neuroectodermal tumor irrespective of location includes surgical removal, radiation therapy, and chemotherapy. Surgical removal must be able to extract the entire primary tumor and probable areas of spread, and restore normal cerebral spinal fluid circulation. The latter may be achieved with the addition of a device diverting excess cerebral spinal fluid to the abdominal cavity (ventriculoperitoneal shunt). For other neuroectodermal tumors outside the nervous system, the same therapeutic principles apply. In children with limb involvement, amputation may be done because of the stunting effect of therapeutic radiation levels on growth plates.

Prognosis, prevention, and outcomes: The prognosis of neuroectodermal tumors after therapy completion is good. Five-year survival rates for central nervous system tumors approach 75 percent with aggressive surgical removal, radiotherapy, and chemotherapy. pPNET/ESFT exhibits similar survival rates with the same treatment, as opposed to radiotherapy and chemotherapy alone (50 percent). Prevention of recurrence includes interval imaging and "second look" surgeries when residual disease is present.

Aldo C. Dumlao, M.D.

▶ For Further Information

Eiser, Christine. *Children with Cancer: The Quality of Life*. Mahwah, N.J.: Lawrence Erlbaum Associates, 2004.

Pagé, Michel. *Tumor Targeting in Cancer Therapy*. Totowa, N.J.: Humana Press, 2004.

Parker, James N., and Philip M. Parker, eds. *The Official Parent's Sourcebook of Ewing's Family of Tumors*. San Diego, Calif.: Icon Health, 2002.

▶ **Other Resources**

National Cancer Institute

Childhood Supratentorial Primative Neuroectodermal Tumors and Pineoblastoma
http://www.cancer.gov/cancertopics/pdq/treatment/childSPNET

WebMd

Primitive Neuroectodermal Tumors of the Central Nervous System
http://www.emedicine.com/NEURO/topic326.htm

See also Brain and central nervous system cancers; Ewing sarcoma; Medulloblastomas; Pineoblastomas.

▶ Neuroendocrine tumors

Category: Diseases, symptoms, and conditions
Also known as: NET

Related conditions: Multiple endocrine neoplasia (MEN) type 1 (Wermer syndrome), MEN type 2A (Sipple syndrome), MEN type 2B, carcinoid tumors, islet cell tumors, pheochromocytomas, thyroid carcinomas (medullary), parathyroid carcinomas, Zollinger-Ellison syndrome (gastrinoma), prolactinomas, Cushing syndrome, small-cell lung carcinomas

Definition: Neuroendocrine tumors are a group of rare tumors affecting organs that originate embryologically from the neural crest, the layer that gives rise to the brain, spinal cord, peripheral nerves, and endocrine glands (organs that secrete hormones). These tumors mostly arise from hormone-secreting tissues; however, some tumors may not secrete hormones at all.

Neuroendocrine tumors may be classified as functional or nonfunctional, or hereditary or nonhereditary. The hereditary MEN syndromes consist of two main variants, MEN 1 and MEN 2. MEN 1 has pituitary, parathyroid, and pancreas involvement. MEN 2A manifests as medullary thyroid cancer (MTC), pheochromocytoma (adrenal medulla tumor), and parathyroid hyperplasia. MEN 2B is essentially type 2A without parathyroid involvement and with the addition of mucosal neuromas and gut ganglioneuromas with a Marfanoid body habitus. Isolated medullary thyroid cancer may also be familial but less aggressive compared to MEN-associated variants of the disease. The nonhereditary tumors include pheochromocytoma, carcinoid tumors, islet cell, small-cell, and nonfamilial medullary thyroid carcinomas.

Risk factors: Although most cases involving a single organ are more sporadic, the most prominent risk factor for the development of neuroendocrine tumors is a genetic predisposition. The MEN syndromes are autosomal dominant, implying that every generation has an afflicted individual, with a 50 percent probability of offspring inheriting the disease. Exposure to leuprolide acetate and medroxyprogesterone acetate in female rats was associated with a higher incidence of pancreatic islet cell tumors.

Etiology and the disease process: The genetic etiology of the heritable as well as most sporadic cases of somatic (mature, differentiated cells) cell mutations in parathyroid adenomas, gastrinomas, insulinomas, and bronchial carcinoids most commonly originates from *MEN1* tumor-suppressor gene mutations, with the *RET* proto-oncogene implicated in sporadic medullary thyroid carcinoma cases. MEN 1 originates from one of two etiologies: a mutation within the embryonic crest cell or inactivation of the tumor-suppressor gene *MEN 1*, located on the long arm of chromosome 11 (11q13). In MEN 2A, MEN 2B, and familial medullary thyroid carcinoma, the origin is believed to be a mutation in the *RET* proto-oncogene, located on the long arm of chromosome 10 (10q11.2). Gastrinomas originate from HER2/neu (human epidermal growth factor receptor 2/neu) proto-oncogene.

Incidence: The overall occurrence of neuroendocrine tumors is extremely rare, accounting for only 0.5 percent of all malignant cancers. However, an increase in the number of cases of these tumors has been observed. The gastrointestinal tract has the highest incidence of neuroendocrine tumors, accounting for 62 to 67 percent of all primary tumors, followed by the lungs (22 to 27 percent) in one study conducted in the Netherlands.

Symptoms: The symptoms associated with neuroendocrine tumors vary widely and are often insidious in onset. Tumors may be found during the course of an unrelated imaging study. Some neuroendocrine tumors are related to location rather than the disease entities they mimic. For example, pancreatic tumors may manifest as poorly controlled diabetes in glucagonoma and somatostatinoma; pituitary tumors as amenorrhea in prolactinomas, unintentional skin darkening, high blood pressure, and psychosis in Cushing disease; sudden episodes of high blood pressure, cold sweats, and palpitations in pheochromocytomas;

or as a plethora of unrelated signs and symptoms such as flushing, abdominal cramps, diarrhea, or new-onset heart murmur in carcinoid tumors.

Both nonfunctioning tumors and bulky functioning tumors can compress or infiltrate surrounding tissue or structures and cause obstructive symptoms.

Screening and diagnosis: Diagnosis of neuroendocrine tumors is often difficult and missed because of misleading disease symptoms. Medullary thyroid cancer, especially when a family history is present, should initiate a comprehensive search for high calcitonin, blood and urine calcium (medullary thyroid, parathyroid), adrenocorticotropic hormone (ACTH), growth hormone, thyroid-stimulating hormone (TSH), prolactin levels (pituitary), and twenty-four-hour urine metanephrine (adrenal medulla) levels as well as computed tomography (CT) or magnetic resonance imaging (MRI) of the head, neck, chest, and abdomen, as appropriate, to look for primary as well as metastatic sites. Insulin-to-glucose ratios, chromogranin A, gastrin levels, octreoscans, endoscopy, and CT and MRI imaging studies are useful for aiding in pancreatic tumor diagnosis.

Although neuroendocrine tumors have a clear genetic etiology, genetic testing for *RET* is reserved for patients presenting with medullary thyroid cancer.

Treatment and therapy: Treatment of neuroendocrine tumors includes surgical removal, radiation therapy, and chemotherapy and is highly dependent on the tumor location and type. Precautions should be taken to stabilize the patient preoperatively for many functioning tumors. Control of blood pressure, high glucose levels, electrolyte imbalances, and gastrin excess are essential. Surgery must be able to remove the entire primary tumor and, if needed, structures susceptible to infiltration. For islet cell tumors, chemotherapy with streptozocin, doxorubicin, and 5-fluorouracil (5-FU) alone or in combination have proved beneficial (54 to 69 percent response rate).

Prognosis, prevention, and outcomes: Most cases of neuroendocrine tumors have a good prognosis with radical surgery, chemotherapy, or radiotherapy. Metastatic disease at the time of diagnosis implies a poor prognosis. Gastrinomas in particular have poorer prognosis, as 60 percent are malignant; associated with MEN 1 syndrome, they have a better prognosis than gastrinoma alone. Medullary thyroid cancer and MEN 2 have a five-year survival rate of 90 percent, attributable to early treatment of medullary thyroid cancer. Observation for recurrence is needed, through periodic clinical examinations, laboratory tests for tumor markers, and CT and MRI. Genetic counseling and testing are helpful in individuals with a strong family history of neuroendocrine tumors.

Aldo C. Dumlao, M.D.

▶ For Further Information

Clark, Orlo H. *Endocrine Tumors*. Hamilton, Ont.: BC Decker, 2003.

Fossel, Michael B. *Cells, Aging, and Human Disease*. New York: Oxford University Press, 2004.

Kelloff, Gary, Ernest T. Hawk, and Caroline C. Sigman. *Cancer Chemoprevention*. Totowa, N.J.: Humana Press, 2005.

▶ Other Resources

American Cancer Society

Detailed Guide: Gastrointestinal Carcinoid Tumors
http://www.cancer.org/docroot/CRI/content/CRI_2_4_1X_What_are_gastrointestinal_carcinoid_tumors_14.asp

Dana-Farber Cancer Institute

Neuroendocrine Tumors
http://research.dfci.harvard.edu/neuroendocrine/

See also Cushing syndrome and cancer; Endocrine cancers; Lung cancers; Multiple endocrine neoplasia type 1 (MEN 1); Multiple endocrine neoplasia type 2 (MEN 2); Parathyroid cancer; Pheochromocytomas; Thyroid cancer; Von Hippel-Lindau (VHL) disease; Zollinger-Ellison syndrome.

▶ Neurofibromatosis type 1 (NF1)

Category: Diseases, symptoms, and conditions
Also known as: von Recklinghausen's neurofibromatosis, von Recklinghausen disease

Related conditions: Neurofibromas, iris Lisch nodules, optic gliomas, café-au-lait spots, freckling, learning disabilities, bone complications such as scoliosis or bone overgrowth

Definition: Neurofibromatosis type 1 (NF1) is a hereditary disorder of the nervous system that affects growth and development of nerve cell tissues. This disorder is associated with neurofibromas (bumplike tumors under the skin or elsewhere in the body that develop anywhere along a nerve), café-au-lait spots (flat spots on the skin that are darker than the surrounding area), freckling in places not exposed to the sun (such as the armpit and groin), eye developments such as optic glioma (a tumor growing on the nerve to the eye) and Lisch nodules (harmless growths on the colored part of the eye), and bone problems such as scoliosis (curvature of the spine) or bone overgrowth. Up to 10 percent of affected individuals have malignant peripheral nerve sheath tumors (tumors that form along the protective covering around nerves located outside the brain and spinal cord), which are the most common malignant tumors associated with NF1. Although rare, malignant brain tumors do occur. Fewer than 1 percent of people with NF1 have pheochromocytomas (adrenal gland tumors that release stress hormones) that cause dangerously high blood pressure. Approximately half of individuals with NF1 have a learning disability, although it is usually mild. The severity of the disorder varies within families, between families, and even within an individual at different times during life.

Risk factors: Because NF1 is hereditary, the main risk factor is having a family history of this disorder. Each child of a person with NF1 has a 50 percent chance of inheriting the disorder.

Etiology and the disease process: The underlying genetic cause of NF1 is a mutation, or a genetic change, in the *NF1* gene. The purpose of the protein made by the *NF1* gene is not fully understood, but it most likely helps stop uncontrolled cell growth and proliferation. Mutations in the *NF1* gene either prevent the protein from being made or cause the protein to be made incorrectly, and the multistep process of tumorigenesis (formation or production of tumors) is left unchecked.

Usually, each person has two normal copies of the *NF1* gene. A mutation in one copy of the gene is sufficient to cause NF1, which is why this condition is referred to as autosomal dominant (autosomal means the *NF1* gene is located on one of the twenty-two pairs of autosomes, which are the nonsex chromosomes). An affected person has an *NF1* gene mutation from the time of conception; however, symptoms of the disease may be present at birth or not manifest until later in life. Nearly all individuals with NF1 have signs and symptoms of the disorder by the end of childhood. The average life expectancy of affected individuals is reduced about fifteen years.

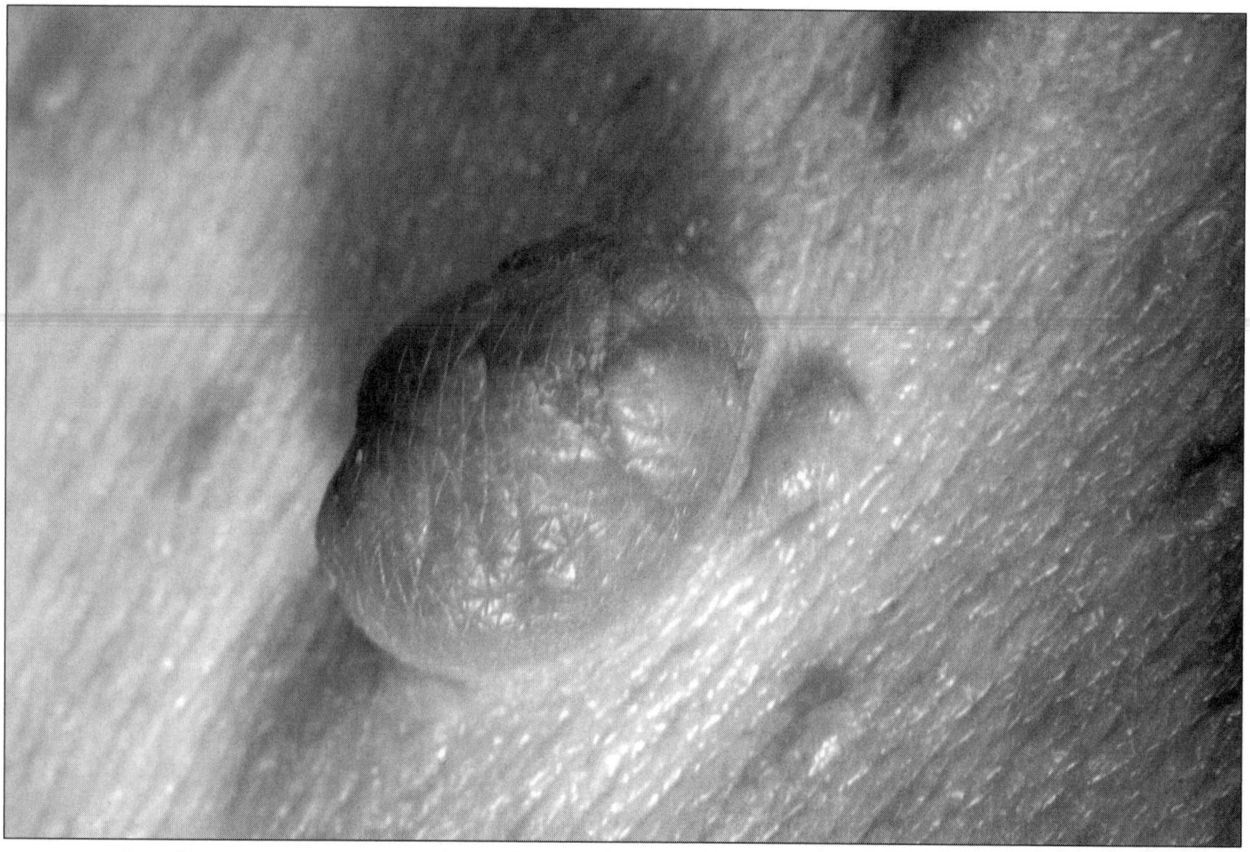

Neurofibromas are one symptom of neurofibromatosis type 1. (Biophoto Associates/Photo Researchers, Inc.)

Incidence: Approximately 1 in 3,000 people has NF1, which makes it one of the most common dominantly inherited genetic disorders. Nearly half of people with NF1 inherit the disorder from a parent. The other 50 percent have a new gene mutation, meaning the mutation occurred for the first time in those individuals.

Symptoms: Symptoms vary and are usually mild to moderate and not life-threatening. Adults with NF1 may have anywhere from a few neurofibromas to hundreds or thousands, and these tumors—which continue to develop throughout life—can affect any organ in the body. Neurofibromas can cause pain and disfigurement and, more rarely, cause problems with organ function. Malignant peripheral nerve sheath tumors can cause pain, numbness, or paralysis. Optic gliomas can lead to blindness. Of the learning disabilities observed in more than half of people with NF1, visual-spatial performance and attention deficits are the most common.

Screening and diagnosis: Doctors diagnose NF1 based on certain criteria, which include having two or more of the following: six or more café-au-lait spots, two or more neurofibromas or one plexiform neurofibroma (weblike neurofibroma that entwines surrounding tissues), freckling in the armpit or groin, optic glioma, two or more Lisch nodules, an unusual bone complication, or a first-degree relative (parent, sibling, or child) with NF1.

Because NF1 is caused by mutations in the *NF1* gene, genetic testing can be used to confirm a suspected diagnosis. However, diagnostic genetic testing is rarely needed because doctors can easily diagnose the disease based on clinical findings. Genetic testing detects more than 95 percent of *NF1* gene mutations in individuals who have been clinically diagnosed by a physician.

Treatment and therapy: The main focus of treatment for NF1 is controlling symptoms. Surgery can be performed to treat bone malformations or to remove tumors that cause pain or disfigurement. In the case of malignancy, the tumor is surgically removed if possible, and the patient may also have adjuvant chemotherapy and radiotherapy.

Prognosis, prevention, and outcomes: The way neurofibromatosis affects a person over a lifetime varies widely. Because NF1 is a genetic condition, its manifestations cannot be prevented. However, physicians recommend that individuals with NF1 have monitoring that includes a yearly physical examination, a yearly ophthalmologic examination (eye exam) for children (less frequently for adults), regular blood pressure checks, and regular assessment of development for children.

Abbie L. Abboud, M.S., C.G.C.

▶ For Further Information

Ferner, R. E. "Neurofibromatosis 1." *European Journal of Human Genetics*. 15 (2007): 131-138.

Korf, Bruce R., and Allan E. Rubenstein. *Neurofibromatosis: A Handbook for Patients, Families, and Health Care Professionals*. New York: Thieme Medical, 2005.

Tonsgard, J. H. "Clinical Manifestations and Management of Neurofibromatosis Type 1." *Seminars in Pediatric Neurology* 13 (2006): 2-7.

▶ Other Resources

Children's Tumor Foundation: Ending Neurofibromatosis Through Research
http://www.ctf.org

Neurofibromatosis, Inc
http://www.nfinc.org

See also Acoustic neuromas; Astrocytomas; Ependymomas; Fibrosarcomas, soft-tissue; Gastrointestinal stromal tumors (GISTs); Gliomas; Mediastinal tumors; Medulloblastomas; Meningiomas; Pheochromocytomas; Sarcomas, soft-tissue; Schwannoma tumors; Spinal axis tumors.

▶ Neurologic oncology

Category: Medical specialties
Also known as: Neuro-oncology

Definition: Neurologic oncology is a specialty practice involving the study and treatment of cancers of the brain and the peripheral and central nervous systems. Physicians who practice in this field are known as neuro-oncologists. It is a branch of medicine that studies tumors in an effort to understand their evolution, diagnosis, treatment, and prevention. The discipline of neurologic oncology has developed steadily since the 1980's as advances in understanding of epidemiology, cellular and molecular biology, genetics, immunology, and radiobiology have come together to increase knowledge of the process of oncogenesis.

Cancers treated: Brain, spine, and peripheral and central nervous system cancers

Training and certification: The practice of neurologic oncology requires training and experience in two essential areas: neurology or neurosurgery to properly diagnose and assess patients based on expert knowledge of nervous system function and oncology—as it pertains to central nervous system (CNS) involvement and generic oncologic management principles—for competence in the use of chemotherapeutic agents and related measures. Although no official or regulated prerequisites have been established for neuro-oncologists, all physicians practicing neurologic oncology have graduate medical degrees. Most physicians practicing neuro-oncology have backgrounds in neurology, neurosurgery, radiology/radiation oncology, or internal medicine/medical oncology. The specialty of neurology generally requires the completion of a minimum four-year residency program; the specialty of neurosurgery requires completion of a seven-year residency program. Radiologists complete a four-year residency program. Physicians trained in internal medicine complete a three-year residency program. After successful completion of a residency program, the physician assumes a fellowship in neurologic oncology for an additional two to three years, depending on whether the individual plans to engage in research and academic activities or in treating patients with brain, spinal cord, or CNS cancers. Prior board certification by the American Board of Medical Specialties (ABMS) is recommended but not required. The ABMS has twenty-four member specialty boards that certify their members through written and oral examinations and continuing education programs. Many of the physicians who study neurologic oncology have already been board certified in their original fields of study.

Services and procedures performed: Neuro-oncologists provide therapy for primary and metastatic tumors of the brain, spine, and the peripheral and central nervous systems. Tumors are diagnosed using modern neuroimaging techniques such as positron emission tomography (PET) and functional magnetic resonance imaging (MRI) to facilitate diagnostic biopsies and appropriate treatment. The imaging studies are usually interpreted with the assistance of a neuroradiologist.

Treatment may include chemotherapy, radiation therapy (conventional, brachytherapy, or radiosurgery), neurosurgery, or a combination of these treatments. Whenever possible, and especially in the case of rapidly growing, aggressive disease, neurosurgical resection of the tumor is the treatment of choice, usually followed by chemotherapy, radiotherapy, or both. In the case of inoperable cancers, a combination of chemotherapy and radiotherapy may be the treatment of choice. Chemotherapy involves the use of chemical compounds that are toxic to malignant cells. Traditional chemotherapeutic agents include carmustine (BCNU, or BiCNU), lomustine (CCNU, or CeeNU), and a combination of procarbazine, CCNU, and vincristine known as PCV.

Chemotherapy may be administered orally (for example, temozolomide, or Temodar, a relatively new agent, may be taken in tablet form), intravenously (most agents), or through direct surgical implantation of a chemotherapeutic wafer, usually placed in the tumor cavity after resection. Chemotherapy is typically performed in stages over time. Conventional radiotherapy alone or in combination with chemotherapy, surgery, or both may also be administered.

Radiotherapy uses high-energy external X rays, gamma rays, or charged particles (electron or proton beams) to damage important biological molecules in tumor cells. If enough damage is done to the chromosomes of a cell, cell death (or apoptosis) will occur. Radiotherapy is generally administered at regular intervals over a several-week course. Brachytherapy is a type of radiotherapy in which radioactive material (most often iridium-192), usually in the form of a tiny pellet or seed, is inserted inside or next to the tumor. Brachytherapy is commonly used to treat localized cancer. Radiosurgery is a variation of radiotherapy that uses highly focused gamma rays to kill cancerous cells; radiosurgery is performed in a single session.

Neurosurgery is the incision and excision of cancerous tissue. Tumors may be completely resected or partially resected, depending on their location and accessibility. The tumor may be approached via an open surgical procedure such as a craniotomy or via an endoscopic approach such as a transnasal (through the nose) route. A relatively new, but U.S. Food and Drug Administration-approved, technique is convection-enhanced delivery, which involves the implantation of a catheter into the tumor and slow infusion of a chemotherapeutic agent into the brain or tumor. Convection-enhanced delivery relies on a small, continuous gradient of pressure to infuse the chemotherapeutic agent up to several centimeters from the site of infusion.

Related specialties and subspecialties: The primary care physician is often the source of the referral to the neuro-oncologist and thus may remain involved in some way with the patient's care. Other comorbidities may necessitate the primary physician's continued involvement as well as that of other physicians outside the general field of neurologic oncology. For the purposes of cancer treatment, the practice of neurologic oncology involves the cooperation of a multidisciplinary team, which, depending on the course of treatment chosen, may include neuro-oncology nurse specialists, medical oncologists, neurologists, neurosurgeons, radiation oncologists, neuroradiologists, neuropathologists, neuroanesthesiologists and pain management personnel, rehabilitative and cognitive physicians, neuropsychologists and psychiatrists, palliative care specialists, and hospice care providers. All team members will have expertise in a neuro-related or oncologic specialty. If the treatment chosen does not involve surgery, the need for the participation of a neurosurgeon and neuropathologists will most likely be mitigated. Ideally if the course of treatment is successful, it will not be necessary for the palliative care specialists and hospice workers to play their roles.

Keller Kaufman-Fox, B.A.

▶ For Further Information

Ali-Osman, Francis, ed. *Brain Tumors*. Totowa, N.J.: Humana Press, 2003.

Lawson, C. H., et al. "Interstitial Chemotherapy for Malignant Gliomas: The Johns Hopkins Experience." *Journal of Neuro-Oncology* 83 (2007): 61-70.

McAllister, L. D., J. H. Ward, S. F. Schulman, and L. M. DeAngelis. *Practical Neuro-Oncology: A Guide to Patient Care*. 5th ed. Boston: Butterworth-Heinemann, 2001.

Strother, D. R., et al. "Tumors of the Central Nervous System." In *Principles and Practice of Pediatric Oncology*, edited by P. A. Pizzo and D. G. Poplack. 4th ed. Philadelphia: Lippincott Williams & Wilkins, 2002.

▶ Organizations and Professional Societies

American Brain Tumor Association
http://www.abta.org
2720 River Road, Suite 146
Des Plaines, IL 60018

Brain Tumor Society
http://www.tbts.org
124 Watertown Street, Suite 3H
Watertown, MA 02472-2500

National Brain Tumor Foundation
http://www.braintumor.org
22 Battery Street, Suite 612
San Francisco, CA 94111-5520

Society for Neuro-Oncology
http://www.soc-neuro-onc.org
4617 Birch Street
Bellaire, TX 77401-5509

▶ Other Resources

American Association of Neurological Surgeons
http://www.tumorsection.org

National Institute of Neurological Disorders and Stroke
NINDS Brain and Spinal Tumors Information Page
http://www.ninds.nih.gov/disorders/brainandspinaltumors/

See also Astrocytomas; Brain and central nervous system cancers; Gliomas; Meningiomas; Pediatric oncology and hematology.

▶ Neutropenia

Category: Diseases, symptoms, and conditions
Also known as: Agranulocytosis, granulocytopenia

Related conditions: Leukopenia, aplastic anemia, myelodysplastic syndromes

Definition: Neutropenia is a decreased number of circulating neutrophils, which are the most abundant type of white blood cell and are an essential component of the immune response to infections, especially bacterial or fungal infections. Neutrophils are the first to respond to an infection, ingesting the microorganisms and killing them, thus preventing an infection or lessening its severity. A patient who has a significantly reduced number of neutrophils is at increased risk for infection.

Normal total white blood cell counts range from 5,000 to 10,000 cells per cubic millimeter (mm^3) of blood, with neutrophils making up 50 to 70 percent of the circulating white blood cells. Therefore, the normal absolute number of neutrophils is about 2,500 to 7,000 neutrophils/mm^3 of blood. People are considered to have neutropenia when levels drop below 500 neutrophils/mm^3 of blood.

Risk factors: Because most chemotherapeutic agents work to kill fast-growing cells, including neutrophils, almost all cancer patients are at risk for neutropenia. Radiation therapy for cancer treatment can also cause neutropenia. Other factors, including age, nutritional status, and previous exposure to chemotherapy or radiation, increase the risk of neutropenia in someone undergoing chemotherapy or radiation therapy. Patients with hematologic cancers, such as leukemias or lymphomas, are also at increased risk for neutropenia.

Etiology and the disease process: Four main circumstances lead to neutropenia: prolonged, severe infection; decreased survival of neutrophils; abnormal distribution of neutrophils to a body site; and decreased production of neutrophils. In the case of cancer patients, the problem is decreased production. Most anticancer drugs work to disrupt the growth of cancer cells, which tend to grow very quickly. These drugs target cell components involved in cell division and deoxyribonucleic acid (DNA) synthesis. As a result, other fast-growing cells in the body may also be affected by the drugs. This includes the cells of the bone marrow that are precursors to blood cells. Neutrophils are short-lived (surviving two to three days) in the body, with millions of new neutrophils released every minute from the bone marrow. Therefore, the bone marrow cells that are rapidly dividing to make new neutrophils are at high risk for damage from anticancer agents.

Radiation therapy can cause neutropenia if the targeted treatment area includes bones that contain productive marrow (not all marrow actively produces blood cells). Additionally, patients who need a bone marrow transplant must have the diseased bone marrow completely destroyed before the transplant.

Incidence: Chemotherapy is the most common cause of neutropenia, but its incidence among patients varies. Each drug and drug combination has been shown to cause neutropenia at a different rate. For example, the cisplatin/fluorouracil combination used to treat head and neck cancers has been shown to cause neutropenia in only 9 percent of patients. Cisplatin combined with gemcitabine to treat bladder cancer causes neutropenia in 71 percent of patients. The other risk factors, such as age, also contribute to the different incidence rates.

Symptoms: Because low neutrophil counts predispose patients to infection, the first symptom is usually fever, followed by symptoms specific to the infection, including a cough, a sore throat, bronchitis, sinusitis, pneumonia, gingivitis, sores around the mouth and anus, fatigue, and frequent or unusual infections.

Screening and diagnosis: A complete blood count (CBC) with differential tests for levels of the different types of cells in the blood can screen for neutropenia. The differential portion of the test tells the percentage of each type of white blood cell, including the percentage of neutrophils. From this, the absolute number of neutrophils/mm^3 can be calculated to determine if a patient is neutropenic and at risk for infection. Patients with borderline levels at 500 to 1,500 cells/mm^3 have a slight-to-moderate risk of infection, while patients with counts below 500 cells/mm^3 (neutropenic) have a severe risk of infection.

Treatment and therapy: The first priority of treatment is to address fever and underlying infection. Antibiotics or antifungals are necessary to treat the infection. The patient may also require granulocyte-macrophage colony-stimulating factor (GM-CSF) or granulocyte colony-stimulating factor (G-CSF). These drugs stimulate the bone marrow to increase production of neutrophils and are used following chemotherapy and following bone marrow transplantation. Additionally, changes in the chemotherapy regimen may be necessary. The physician may choose to lower the dose of medication, remove a drug from the regimen, or change the most harmful drug to a less toxic drug.

Prognosis, prevention, and outcomes: A neutropenic cancer patient who acquires an infection has a mortality rate of 4 to 30 percent. To prevent neutropenia in cancer patients receiving treatment, doctors can lower the dose of chemotherapy for patients who have a documented history of neutropenia. Doctors can also use colony-stimulating factors in patients at higher risk for neutropenia, such as when a treatment regimen is known to cause neutropenia in a high percentage (greater than 40 percent) of patients. Most cases of chemotherapy-induced neutropenia resolve within two weeks of discontinuing drug treatment.

Michelle L. Herdman, Ph.D.

▶ For Further Information

Beers, Mark H., ed. *The Merck Manual of Diagnosis and Therapy*. 18th ed. Whitehouse Station, N.J.: Merck, 2006.

Mosby's Drug Consult 2007. St. Louis: Mosby Elsevier, 2007.

Tisdale, James E., and Douglas A. Miller. *Drug-Induced Diseases: Prevention, Detection, and Management*. Bethesda, Md.: American Society of Health-System Pharmacists, 2005.

▶ Other Resources

American Cancer Society
http://www.cancer.org

Cancer Symptoms.org
Neutropenia
http://www.cancersymptoms.org/neutropenia/index.shtml

Neutropenia Support Association
http://www.neutropenia.ca/index.html

See also Aplastic anemia; Chemotherapy; Leukopenia; Myelodysplastic syndromes; Side effects.

▶ Nickel compounds and metallic nickel

Category: Carcinogens and suspected carcinogens
RoC status: Metallic nickel, reasonably anticipated human carcinogen since 1980; nickel compounds, known human carcinogens since 2002
Also known as: Ni

Definition: Nickel is a silvery white, hard, malleable, and ductile metal that forms complex compounds, most often with oxygen, sulfur, iron, and arsenic. Some nickel uptake is essential to humans but more concentrated amounts can be harmful. It remains unknown exactly which forms of nickel compounds are carcinogenic, but studies show that airborne and water-soluble compounds may be most associated with cancer risk, possibly because of greater exposure.

Because nickel is widely distributed in soils, water, air, detergents, tobacco, and food, everyone is exposed to varying levels of nickel and its compounds. Food, including vegetables and chocolates, often contains larger amounts of nickel, as does tobacco. Nickel fumes or contaminants released by tobacco smoking may cause an increased risk of respiratory cancers, including those of the nose, larynx, and lungs. Contaminant levels of nickel in humans have also been linked with birth defects, including heart disorders, and have been implicated in cancerous proliferation of breast cells.

In addition to being identified in the National Toxicology Program's *Report on Carinogens* as carcinogenic, nickel compounds are classified by the International Agency for Research on Cancer (IARC) as Group 1 compounds, which are "causally associated with cancer in humans." Metallic nickel is currently classified as a Group 2B compound, or "possibly carcinogenic to humans," but will most likely be changed to category A, a known human carcinogen. Nickel and its compounds have also been identified as hazardous air pollutants in the United States' Clean Air Act.

Related cancers: Nasal, throat, lung, breast, and prostate cancer

Exposure routes: Inhalation of nickel fumes from tobacco smoke and aerosols from burning of fossil fuels; ingestion of foods, especially chocolates and vegetables

Where found: Earth has a solid core of nickel but this is far within the interior. Most soils typically contain trace amounts, which can be absorbed in plants and ingested by animals, including humans. Soil nickel and nickel compounds may be leached into water systems or wind driven and carried as nickel-contaminated dust in the atmosphere. Small amounts of nickel and its compounds also occur in the world's oceans and seas, where organisms can absorb it. It is a contaminant in coal and oil and is emitted into the atmosphere by powerplants and incinerators. Nickel compounds are also found in jewelry, other metals, and in everyday household items such as detergents.

At risk: Everyone is at some risk. Workers in smelters that process ores containing nickel, in the electroplating industry, and in steel manufacturing are at risk of higher levels of exposure to nickel and its compounds. Smoking tobacco in all its forms also exposes heavy smokers to nickel contaminants that may increase the risk of cancer.

Etiology and symptoms of associated cancers: Nasal, throat, lung, breast, and prostate cancer are all related to inhalation or ingestion of nickel compounds and metallic nickel in excess amounts. Nasal, throat, and lung cancer can affect breathing, speaking, taste, and smell. Breast cancer can be present in the form of a subdermal lump that may be painful. Prostate cancer can cause severe pain, decrease urination flow, frequency, or strength, and inhibit ejaculation.

History: Nickel and its compounds are primarily used in the preparation of alloys of steel and other metal products. For example, addition of nickel to steel, copper, and other metals produces an alloy that is stronger and more resistant to heat and corrosion. Thus, nickel is important in gas turbines and rocket engines, where strength and resistance to high temperatures are factors. Nickel alloys are also used to manufacture propeller shafts of boats and piping in desalinization plants, where resistance to corrosion is important. Nickel is also used as a key ingredient in the manufacture of rechargeable nickel cadmium batteries, coinage, and in nickel plating of jewelry and other products. Nickel wire also continues to be in demand for some industrial purposes.

Nickel and its compounds are recognized and listed as carcinogenic substances, especially in occupations in which workers are routinely exposed to nickel fumes. The Environmental Protection Agency (EPA) formally determined that nickel and its compounds, especially nickel subsulfides, are human carcinogens in 1984, and in 1990 the International Agency for Research on Cancer also listed nickel as potentially carcinogenic. Further regulations are possible pending ongoing reviews at federal and state levels.

Dwight G. Smith, Ph.D.

See also Carcinogens, known; Carcinogens, reasonably anticipated; Head and neck cancers; Laryngeal cancer; Nasal cavity and paranasal sinus cancers; Occupational exposures and cancer; Salivary gland cancer.

▶ Night sweats

Category: Diseases, symptoms, and conditions
Also known as: Sleep hyperhydrosis

Related conditions: Menopause, obstructive sleep apnea, infection, low blood sugar, lymphoma and other cancers, certain medications

Definition: Night sweats are excessive nighttime sweating that causes the individual to wake up and may require the individual to bathe or change nightclothes.

Risk factors: There are some diseases and conditions that may be associated with an increased incidence of night sweats. Individuals who have obstructive sleep apnea, a disorder in which breathing is interrupted during sleep, are more likely to experience night sweats. Risk factors for sleep apnea, such as obesity, therefore may also be risk factors for night sweats. Women experiencing menopause are also more likely to experience night sweats.

Etiology and the disease process: Night sweats can be caused by a number of underlying diseases and conditions as well as by a simple excess of bedding or an overly warm room. Some of the most common medical causes of night sweats include the changing hormone balance that occurs during menopause, obstructive sleep apnea, infection, low blood sugar, cancer (especially lymphoma), and certain medications. Other causes can include infection with the human immunodeficiency virus (HIV), tuberculosis, hyperthyroidism, epilepsy, and head injury.

Incidence: There are very few significant scientific studies on the incidence of night sweats; however, they are believed to be very common. One study of night sweats found that 41 percent of the 2,267 patients who were studied reported night sweats. Many physicians report a significant percentage of individuals they see in their general practice complaining of night sweats.

Symptoms: The symptoms of night sweats are waking up in the night because of excessive sweating. Night sweats are considered mild if they wake sleepers, who then remove some or all bed coverings and may turn over the pillow to use the dry side. Night sweats that make sleepers feel the need to wash the sweat off their hands or faces are considered moderate. Night sweats are considered severe when the sweating is so excessive as to cause sleepers to change their clothes or to take a shower. Some people who experience night sweats also experience excessive sweating during the day.

Screening and diagnosis: The physician will typically take a history of the patient's night sweat experiences and perform a physical exam to see if any common causes of night sweats seem to be a likely cause. The physician may also ask a series of questions, which may involve travel history, to determine if the patient has been in any areas that increase the likelihood of becoming infected with a disease such as tuberculosis, or if there is a risk of infection with HIV. The doctor may also ask the patient's sleeping partner about symptoms of which the individual may be unaware, such as the loud snoring that often accompanies obstructive sleep apnea.

If these steps fail to determine why the night sweats are occurring, the doctor may order blood tests or additional screening procedures to test for other causes. The doctor will also ask the patient about other unusual symptoms, even those that do not seem to be related. Many diseases and conditions that can cause night sweats usually cause other symptoms as well. Types of cancer that cause night sweats are usually associated with unintentional weight loss and fever. Tuberculosis is also usually accompanied by weight loss, a cough, and a low-grade fever.

Treatment and therapy: Most night sweats are treated by trying to assess the underlying cause of the night sweats and treating that disease or condition, including a possible lymphoma. Resolving the underlying problem will usually eliminate the night sweats. However, while the underlying problem is being diagnosed and treated, or if no treatable underlying cause can be found, there are some techniques that may help relieve the symptoms.

Reducing the quantity of bedclothes or switching from heavy blankets made of insulating materials such as wool to lighter blankets made of fabrics such as cotton may help reduce the occurrence of night sweats or reduce their severity. Sleeping with a window open or a fan pointed toward the bed may also help to relieve the problem. Avoiding spicy food, excessive exercise before bedtime, alcohol, and tobacco may help to reduce the severity of night sweats.

Prognosis, prevention, and outcomes: Sleeping in a cool room without an excess of bedding may be able to help prevent some episodes of night sweats. The prognosis for most cases of night sweats is good. Treating the underlying cause if one can be found is usually effective at eliminating the night sweats. Night sweats can be extremely frustrating as they can lead to poor quality of sleep and increased drowsiness during the day. Treating night sweats successfully can lead to a better quality of sleep, as well as an increased quantity of sleep, which can improve mood and lead to a better quality of life overall.

Robert Bockstiegel, B.S.

▶ **For Further Information**

Freedman, Jeri. *Lymphoma: Current and Emerging Trends in Detection and Treatment.* New York: Rosen, 2006.

Souhami, Robert, and Jeffrey Tobias. *Cancer and Its Management.* 5th Edition. Malden, Mass.: Blackwell, 2005.

Yarbro, Connie Henke, Margaret Hansen Frogge, and Michelle Goodman, eds. *Cancer Symptom Management.* Sudbury, Mass.: Jones and Bartlett, 2004.

▶ **Other Resources**

MedicineNet.com

Eight Causes of Night Sweats
http://www.medicinenet.com/script/main/art.asp?articlekey=57394

Sleep Disorders Guide

Sleep Hyperhydrosis
http://www.sleepdisordersguide.com/topics/sleep-hyperhidrosis.html

See also Hormonal therapies; Hormone replacement therapy (HRT); Hot flashes; Hysterectomy; Lymphomas; Symptoms and cancer.

▶ Nijmegen breakage syndrome

Category: Diseases, symptoms, and conditions
Also known as: Berlin breakage syndrome, Seemanova syndrome II, ataxia telangiectasia variant V1

Related conditions: Bloom syndrome, Fanconi anemia, ataxia telangiectasia

Definition: Nijmegen breakage syndrome is a rare autosomal recessive condition that causes chromosomal instability, sensitivity to radiation, and increased incidence of malignant lymphomas.

Risk factors: A risk factor for Nijmegen breakage syndrome is the inheritance of a mutation in both copies of the *NBS1* gene.

Etiology and the disease process: The *NBS1* gene encodes the nibrin protein, which helps heal double-stranded breaks (DSBs) in deoxyribonucleic acid (DNA) molecules. Sometimes double-stranded breaks occur as a result of DNA-severing agents or as a normal physiological process during gamete and antibody production. Without the capacity to repair double-stranded breaks, cells are unable to repair damage to DNA, make antibodies to fight infections, or produce viable gametes.

Incidence: As of 2007, there were only 200 estimated cases of Nijmegen breakage syndrome worldwide.

Symptoms: Children born with Nijmegen breakage syndrome show microcephaly (small head), growth retardation, progressive mental retardation, and characteristic facial features (birdlike face, sloping forehead, and receding jaw). The immune system is unable to fight infections, and recurrent sinus, pulmonary, and ear infections are common. More than half of Nijmegen breakage syndrome patients also show skin pigmentation irregularities. At puberty, female Nijmegen breakage syndrome patients fail to experience sexual maturation. Their ovaries are small and poorly developed (premature ovarian failure). Finally Nijmegen breakage syndrome patients show increased tendencies to develop lymphomas.

Screening and diagnosis: Cytogenetic analyses, which isolate and view chromosomes from individual cells, show chromosomal instabilities that typically involve chromosomes 7 and 14. Immunologic testing shows an inability of immune cells to divide rapidly or properly synthesize antibodies in response to infections. Nijmegen breakage syndrome patients are also extremely sensitive to ionizing radiation or clastogens (substances that cause chromosome breaks). DNA sequencing of the *NBS1* gene should reveal loss-of-function mutations in this gene.

Treatment and therapy: Antibiotic treatments and intravenous administration of antibodies are used to treat recurrent infections that accompany immune system deficiency. Bone marrow transplants can permanently treat the immune system defects in children with Nijmegen breakage syndrome. Prepuberty female patients are treated with hormone replacement therapy to allow the development of secondary sexual characteristics and prevent osteoporosis. Cancer treatments in patients with Nijmegen breakage syndrome patients must avoid radiation and chemotherapeutic agents that damage DNA, since they can cause toxic complications.

Prognosis, prevention, and outcomes: Prophylactic antibiotics are prescribed to prevent recurring infections, and vitamin E supplements are recommended to ameliorate chromosome instability. The long-term prognosis for Nijmegen breakage syndrome patients is typically quite poor. Most patients die from aggressive malignancy or complications from infections.

Michael A. Buratovich, Ph.D.

See also Ataxia telangiectasia (AT); Childhood cancers; Chromosomes and cancer; Fanconi anemia.

▶ Nipple discharge

Category: Diseases, symptoms, and conditions
Also known as: Breast discharge

Related conditions: Galactorrhea, mastitis, papilloma, Paget disease of breast intraductal breast carcinoma

Definition: Nipple discharge refers to secretions from either one (unilateral) or both (bilateral) breasts. Discharge can be spontaneous or appear only when expressed through squeezing and "milking" the nipple, and it can be occasional or constant. It can be clear, milky, brown, green, yellow, pink, or deeply bloody.

Risk factors: Nipple discharge is more likely to be the result of underlying malignancy when it is a unilateral discharge, occurs in a woman past reproductive age, is associated with a mass, or contains blood. Older women with nipple discharge are much more likely to have a malignancy than younger women.

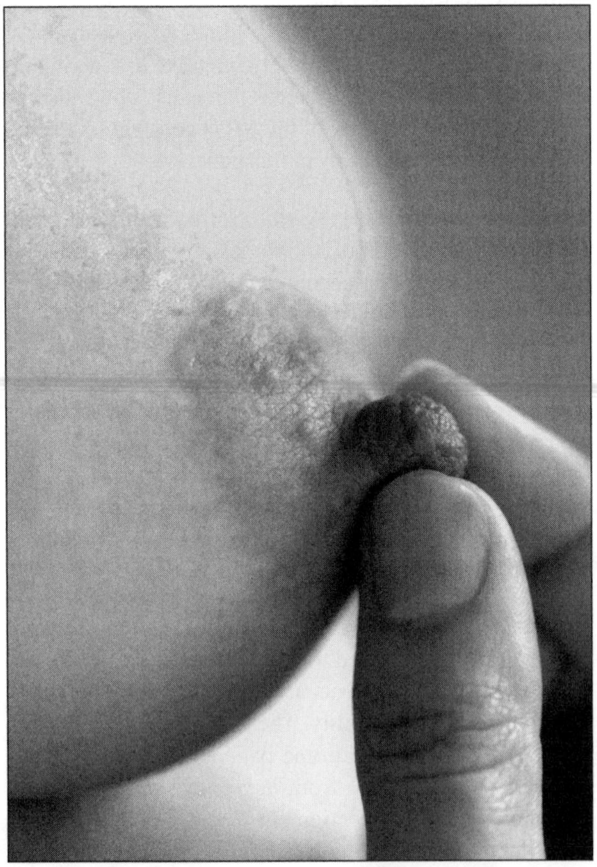

A woman examines her breasts, checking for possible signs of cancer, such as nipple secretions. (Phanie/Photo Researchers, Inc.)

Etiology and the disease process: High levels of the hormone prolactin can cause galactorrhea, which is a milky discharge. Galactorrhea is the most common nipple discharge. Medications that commonly cause galactorrhea include psychotropics, oral contraceptives, and antiemetics.

Incidence: Nipple discharge is very common and usually benign. As many as 80 percent of women are able to express fluid with manual manipulation. Although it is far more common in women, men may occasionally exhibit nipple discharge.

Symptoms: Discharge may be spontaneous or occur only with manual expression, or "milking," of the nipple. It may be a few drops of fluid or a continual leakage.

Screening and diagnosis: A clinical breast exam includes taking a history of breast nipple discharge and examination of the nipples with gentle squeezing to see if fluid is expressed. Milky fluid in breast-feeding women is of no concern as long as the woman does not have symptoms of infection (breast is painful to the touch, redness is present, milk has a foul odor or has changed color), and many women continue to express milk long after they stop breast-feeding. Other testing includes cytologic examination of the discharge, mammography, and ductoscopy.

Treatment and therapy: Often discharge will resolve if all stimulation of the breast is ceased; this means the woman must avoid the urge to check to see if the discharge is still occurring. Sometimes drugs that cause increased prolactin need to be adjusted, and any nipple discharge that is suspicious in terms of malignancy must be evaluated. Nipple discharge can also be a symptom of disorders in other hormone-producing glands, and those conditions may need to be treated.

Prognosis, prevention, and outcomes: Prognosis and outcomes depend on the type of discharge. Prevention can often be managed by decreasing medications that increase prolactin and avoiding a cycle of stimulation of the nipple.

Clair Kaplan, R.N., M.S.N., A.P.R.N. (WHNP), M.H.S., M.T. (ASCP)

See also Breast cancer in men; Breast cancer in pregnant women; Breast cancers; Clinical breast exam (CBE); Comedo carcinomas; Duct ectasia; Ductal carcinoma in situ (DCIS); Ductogram; Estrogen-receptor-sensitive breast cancer; HER2/neu protein; Invasive ductal carcinomas; Invasive lobular carcinomas; Lobular carcinoma in situ (LCIS); Mammography.

▶ Non-Hodgkin lymphoma

Category: Diseases, symptoms, and conditions
Also known as: Lymphoma, non-Hodgkin's lymphoma, NHL

Related conditions: Hodgkin disease, autoimmune disorders

Definition: Non-Hodgkin lymphoma describes a group of cancers that originate in the lymphatic system, a part of the immune system. This system, which fights disease and infection, consists of the lymph nodes, spleen, bone marrow, and other organs throughout the body. Non-Hodgkin lymphoma develops in white blood cells called lymphocytes, of which there are two main types: B cells and T cells. Most lymphomas (85 to 90 percent) start in B cells.

More than thirty types of non-Hodgkin lymphoma exist, with many subtypes. Non-Hodgkin lymphomas are classified by cell type; tumor size, shape, and pattern (nodular or diffuse); and growth rate (low grade, which are slow growing and indolent, and high grade, which are fast growing and aggressive). All lymphomas except Hodgkin disease are classified as non-Hodgkin lymphomas.

Risk factors: Some known and potential risk factors for non-Hodgkin lymphoma include age (over sixty); gender (more common in men); a compromised immune system (such as from drugs and other treatments or acquired immunodeficiency syndrome, AIDS); autoimmune disorders, such as rheumatoid arthritis and Sjögren syndrome; history of infection, such as with Epstein-Barr virus (increases risk of Burkitt lymphoma), *Helicobacter pylori*, and possibly hepatitis C virus; radiation exposure; and chemical exposure (such as pesticides and fertilizers).

Despite the list of known and suspected risk factors for non-Hodgkin lymphoma, most people diagnosed have no known risk factors, and many who have risk factors never develop the disease.

Etiology and the disease process: For most patients, the exact cause of non-Hodgkin lymphoma is unknown. One suspected cause is the activation of certain abnormal genes that allow uncontrollable lymphocyte division and growth. This uncontrolled growth causes lymph nodes and other lymphatic tissues to swell. Because lymphatic tissue is in various locations throughout the body, non-Hodgkin lymphoma can start almost anywhere and tends to be widespread, although slower growing types may be confined to one place. Typically, non-Hodgkin lymphoma begins in the lymph nodes and spreads to other parts of the lymphatic system. Occasionally, non-Hodgkin lymphoma also invades organs outside the lymphatic system, including the stomach, brain, and lungs.

Incidence: Non-Hodgkin lymphoma is the fifth most common type of cancer among adults, and its rapidly increasing incidence in the United States is primarily unexplained (rates have nearly doubled since the 1970's). According to the National Cancer Institute, in 2008, an estimated 66,120 non-Hodgkin lymphoma cases will be diagnosed and 19,160 deaths will be attributed to non-Hodgkin lymphoma. A person's risk of getting non-Hodgkin lymphoma is 1 in 50. The disease is more common among whites than African Americans or Asian Americans.

Non-Hodgkin lymphoma occurs in all age groups, but the risk of developing the disease increases with age (95 percent of cases occur in adults age forty and older). Some subtypes are more common in certain age groups. In children, non-Hodgkin lymphoma is most commonly diag-

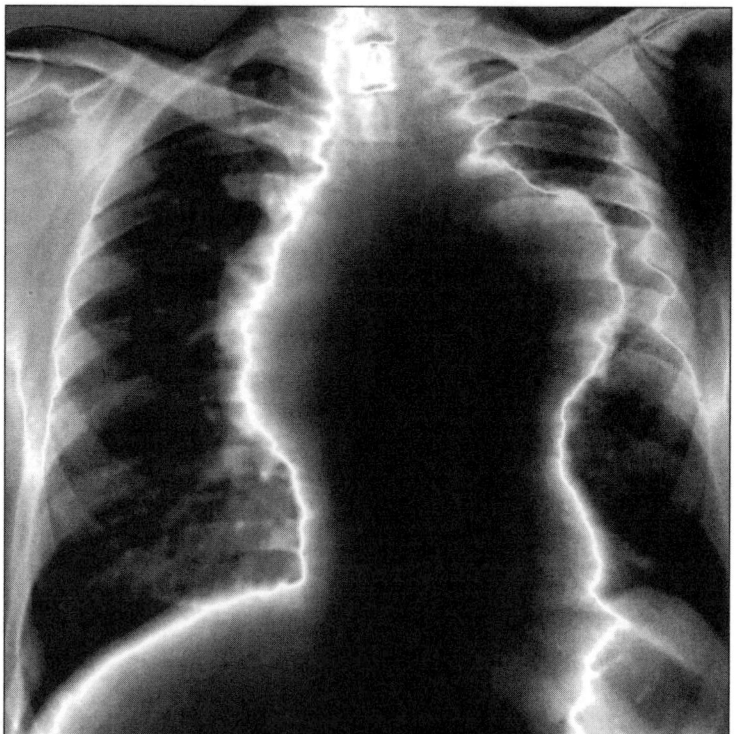

This patient with non-Hodgkin lymphoma has a swollen lymph node in the center of the chest.(Zephyr/Photo Researchers, Inc.)

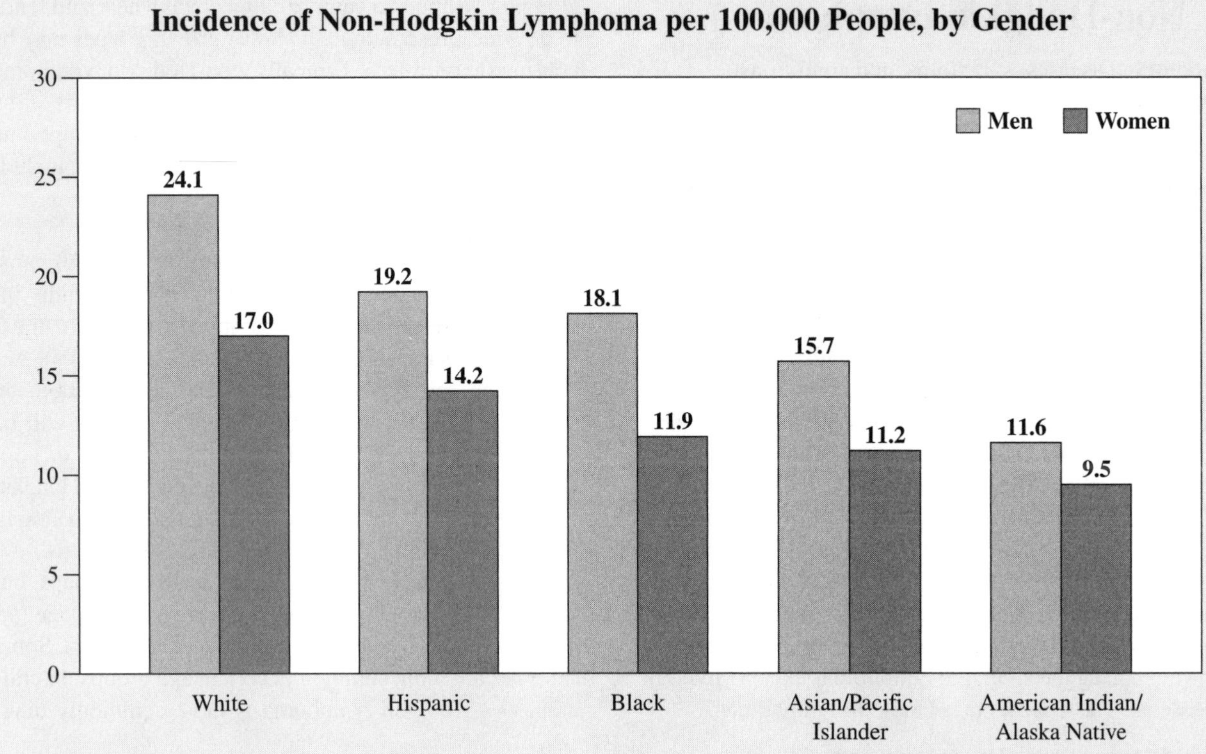

Source: Data from National Cancer Institute, Surveillance Epidemiology and End Results, Cancer Stat Fact Sheets, 2008
Note: Based on cases diagnosed in 2000-2004

nosed between the ages of seven and eleven, and some types of non-Hodgkin lymphoma are among the most common childhood cancers.

Symptoms: Symptoms vary depending on the area of the body in which the tumor originated and the areas to which the cancer has spread. Swollen, painless lymph nodes in the neck, underarms, stomach, or groin are commonly the only sign of non-Hodgkin lymphoma in early stages.

Generalized symptoms include fever, unexplained weight loss, fatigue, excessive sweating, night sweats, chills, easy bruising, itchiness, and unusual infections.

Tumors in the stomach can cause pain and swelling, which can lead to loss of appetite, constipation, nausea, and vomiting. Tumors in the thymus or chest lymph nodes can cause coughing and shortness of breath. Lymphoma of the brain can cause headaches, personality changes, and seizures.

Screening and diagnosis: Many tests are used to diagnose non-Hodgkin lymphoma and assess the spread of the disease. Diagnosis begins with a medical history and physical examination, which commonly focuses on the lymph nodes, liver, and spleen. Blood and urine tests may be performed to help rule out infections and other diseases that cause swollen nodes.

A biopsy is the best way to definitively diagnose lymphoma and determine the subtype.

Lymph node biopsy from the neck, armpits, or groin is most common. Bone marrow biopsy may be performed to establish whether the disease has spread.

Imaging tests such as X rays, magnetic resonance imaging, and computed tomography scanning may be used to detect the presence of non-Hodgkin lymphoma, determine the size of tumors, and determine the extent to which the cancer has spread.

Staging helps to determine treatment. A system commonly used to stage non-Hodgkin lymphoma is the Ann Arbor staging system. This system classifies lymphoma into four stages:

- Stage I: Lymphoma is limited to a single region, usually one lymph node or one lymph node region in the body.

- Stage II: Lymphoma involves two or more regions, usually an affected lymph node or lymphatic organ and a second affected area, that are next to each other and on the same side of the diaphragm.
- Stage III: Lymphoma has spread to both sides of the diaphragm.
- Stage IV: Widespread disease has affected nonlymphatic organs.

A lettering system is commonly used in combination with the stage to indicate the presence of symptoms. An "E" indicates involvement of organs outside the lymph system; a "B" indicates the presence of weight loss, night sweats, or unexplained fever; and an "A" indicates the absence of symptoms.

Treatment and therapy: Treatment of non-Hodgkin lymphoma depends on the type and stage of the disease, symptoms, and the patient's age and overall medical condition. Three main treatments are used: chemotherapy, radiation therapy (RT), and immunotherapy (also called biological therapy). Surgery is rarely used to treat the disease but may be used to relieve problems caused by non-Hodgkin lymphoma, such as bowel obstruction and spinal cord compression.

Chemotherapy is the primary treatment for non-Hodgkin lymphoma. It may be used alone or in combination with other treatments. Intermediate- and high-grade lymphomas and advanced low-grade lymphomas are commonly treated with multiple agents; single-drug therapy may be used for early-stage, low-grade disease. The exact medications, routes, doses, and duration of treatment depend on the stage and type of lymphoma. A common chemotherapy regimen for the initial treatment of non-Hodgkin lymphoma includes cyclophosphamide, doxorubicin, vincristine, and prednisone. Patients are usually treated on an outpatient basis unless problems arise.

Radiation therapy is used to kill or shrink cancer cells. In some cases of Stage I and II non-Hodgkin lymphoma, curative treatment with radiation therapy is possible. Sometimes, radiation therapy is used with chemotherapy to treat intermediate-grade tumors or tumors in specific sites, such as the brain. However, it is typically ineffective against more advanced lymphomas. Radiation therapy may also be used to ease symptoms.

Immunotherapy is an evolving treatment in which substances naturally made by the immune system are used to kill lymphoma cells or slow their growth. Investigational immunotherapies for non-Hodgkin lymphoma include monoclonal antibodies and interferons. Rituximab is a monoclonal antibody approved by the Food and Drug Administration for the treatment of B-cell non-Hodgkin lymphoma. It is commonly used in combination with chemotherapy. Some forms of radioimmunotherapy, in which monoclonal antibodies are attached to radioactive substances, are also used to treat non-Hodgkin lymphoma. Examples include ibritumomab and tositumomab. Because of their life-threatening side effects, these drugs are used only after other treatments have failed.

If non-Hodgkin lymphoma recurs, treatment with high-dose chemotherapy, total-body or total-lymph node irradiation, or bone marrow or stem cell transplantation may be necessary.

Prognosis, prevention, and outcomes: The one-year relative survival rate for non-Hodgkin lymphoma is 81 percent; five-year, 63 percent; and ten-year, 49 percent. Rates vary depending on the person, type of lymphoma, and stage of disease. As with most other cancers, the earlier the diagnosis, the greater the chances for successful treatment. Typically, the type of tissue involved is a better prognostic predictor than cancer stage.

The International Prognostic Index (IPI) is used to help predict lymphoma growth and patient response to treatment. Based on patient age, cancer stage and spread, patient function, and lactate dehydrogenase levels, the IPI is mainly used in patients with aggressive lymphomas.

Low-grade non-Hodgkin lymphomas tend to be advanced when diagnosed. Although they usually respond well to treatment, they may also recur. High-grade non-Hodgkin lymphomas sometimes require intensive chemotherapy. These lymphomas are often curable (some have 60 to 80 percent cure rates). However, if the cancer does not respond to chemotherapy, the disease can rapidly cause death.

Because most people who have non-Hodgkin lymphoma have no known risk factors and the cause of the cancer is unknown, prevention is elusive.

Jaime Stockslager Buss, M.S.P.H., ELS

▶ For Further Information

Adler, E. M. *Living with Lymphoma: A Patient's Guide*. Baltimore: Johns Hopkins University Press, 2005.

American Cancer Society and National Comprehensive Cancer Network. *Non-Hodgkin's Lymphoma Treatment Guidelines for Patients*. Atlanta: Author, 2005.

Holman, Peter, Jodi Garrett, and William Jansen. *One Hundred Questions and Answers About Lymphoma*. Sudbury, Mass.: Jones and Bartlett, 2004.

▶ Other Resources

Leukemia and Lymphoma Society
http://www.leukemia-lymphoma.org

Lymphoma Research Foundation
http://www.lymphoma.org

National Cancer Institute
http://www.cancer.gov

See also Agent Orange; Anthraquinones; Antimetabolites in chemotherapy; Azathioprine; Biological therapy; Blood cancers; Burkitt lymphoma; Childhood cancers; Cutaneous T-cell lymphoma (CTCL); Dioxins; Elderly and cancer; Epstein-Barr virus; Hair dye; *Helicobacter pylori*; Hepatitis C virus (HCV); HIV/AIDS-related cancers; Hodgkin disease; Immune response to cancer; Klinefelter syndrome and cancer; Lambert-Eaton myasthenic syndrome (LEMS); Lymphomas; Mantle cell lymphoma (MCL); Mucosa-associated lymphoid tissue (MALT) lymphomas; Myeloma; Oncogenic viruses; Pediatric oncology and hematology; Pesticides and the food chain; Primary central nervous system lymphomas; Radiopharmaceuticals; Richter syndrome; Simian virus 40; Splenectomy; Veterinary oncology; Virus-related cancers; Waldenström macroglobulinemia (WM).

▶ Nonsteroidal anti-inflammatory drugs (NSAIDs)

Category: Chemotherapy and other drugs
ATC code: M01A

Definition: Nonsteroidal anti-inflammatory drugs, or NSAIDs, are a large, heterogeneous group of medications intended to treat pain, fever, and inflammation.

Cancers treated: NSAIDs are used to treat all types of pain and discomfort associated with cancer, arthritis, gout, and dysmenorrhea (painful or difficult menstruation). They have an inhibitory effect on bone tumor growth and may promote centrally mediated analgesia.

Subclasses of this group: NSAIDs are weak organic acids. Subclasses include salicylates, propionic acids, pyrrolealkonic acid derivatives, phenylalkanones, indolic acids, pyrazolone derivatives, and phenyl-naphthyl-acetic acids.

Delivery routes: These drugs are generally administered orally as a suspension in a liquid or in capsule or tablet

Nonsteroidal Anti-inflammatory Drugs (NSAIDs)

Drug	*Brands*	*Subclass*	*Delivery Mode*
Aspirin	Anacin, Bayer, Excedrin, Bufferin	Acetylsalicylic acid	Oral
Celecoxib	Celebrex	Sulfonamide pyrazole	Oral
Diclofenac/misoprostol	Arthrotec	Carboxylic acid	Oral
Diclofenac sodium	Voltaren	Phenylacetic acid	Oral
Difunisal	Dolobid	Salicylic acid derivative	Oral, topical ointment
Etodolac	Lodine	Acetic acid derivative	Oral
Flurbiprofen	Ansaid	Difluoro-propionic acid	Oral
Ibuprofen	Motrin, Advil, Nuprin	Phenylpropionic acid	Oral, IV
Indomethacin	Indocin	Indole acetic acid	Oral, ophthalmic, epidural
Ketorolac	Toradol	Pyrrolizine-carboxylate	Oral, IV, intramuscular, ophthalmic
Meclofenamate sodium	Meclomen	Meclofenamic acid	Oral
Meloxicam	Mobic	Enolic acid	Oral
Nabumetone	Relafen	Naphthylalkanone (only nonacid NSAID)	Oral
Naproxen	Anaprox, Naprosyn, Aleve	Naphthylpropionic acid	Oral, topical, ophthalmic
Piroxicam	Feldene	Oxicam	Oral
Sulindac	Clinoril	Sulfinyl acetic acid	Oral
Tolmetin sodium	Tolectin	Pyrrolealkanoic acid	Oral

form. Certain drugs can be given intravenously, as an intramuscular injection, as a rectal suppository, as a topical ointment, or in an ophthalmic solution.

How these drugs work: NSAIDs inhibit cyclooxygenase enzyme activity, resulting in decreased synthesis of prostaglandins (hormones that produce inflammation and pain). Cyclooxygenase 2 (COX-2) inhibitors perform the same function but mediate the metabolic pathway by selectively blocking the COX-2 enzyme.

Side effects: Common complaints from NSAID use include headache, dizziness, gastrointestinal symptoms (nausea, stomach cramps, gastric ulceration, and diarrhea), tremor, insomnia, skin rash, and platelet dysfunction. An anaphylactic (allergic) response to a particular NSAID can present as hives, rash, intense itching, and respiratory difficulties. This condition can be life threatening, and immediate emergency treatment is required.

The COX-2 inhibitors Vioxx and Bextra were pulled from the U.S. market by the Food and Drug Administration (FDA) in the early 2000's. Over an extended period of use (more than eighteen months), they place patients at significantly increased risk for heart attack and stroke. Only Celebrex remains on the market, but with significant warnings attached to its use and potential risks.

John L. Zeller, M.D., Ph.D.

See also Breakthrough pain; Cyclooxygenase 2 (COX-2) inhibitors; Opioids; Pain management medications; Phenacetin.

▶ Nuclear medicine scan

Category: Procedures
Also known as: Radionuclide scan, positron emission tomography (PET) scan, single photon emission computed tomography (SPECT) imaging

Definition: A nuclear medicine scan detects electromagnetic radiation, usually gamma rays, emitted from an injected radioactive tracer than has been taken up by an organ in the body to be studied, with the goal of producing an image.

The most common radioisotope used is technetium 99m, known as the workhorse of nuclear medicine, whose gamma rays are absorbed by a sodium iodide crystal detector. Interaction of the gamma rays with the crystals results in production of a pulse of fluorescent light proportional in intensity to the energy of the gamma ray. The light is amplified and converted into an electrical signal by the photomultiplier tubes. The electrical signal is then fed to a computer, which analyzes the pulse height and generates an image of the distribution of the radiotracer in the body or organ under study. An array of these crystal detectors attached to a collimator, along with the photomultipliers and computer, is called a gamma camera. The gamma camera is used to scan the patient. The pattern of uptake of radiotracer in the organ or whole body under study varies depending on the disease process.

Multiple gamma cameras are sometimes used to generate a three-dimensional view of an organ; this particular type of nuclear medicine scan is called single photon emission computed tomography (SPECT) imaging.

The exceptions to the use of technetium in nuclear medicine scanning include gallium scanning, which uses gallium as the radionuclide; some thyroid imaging that uses radioactive iodine; indium-labeled white cell studies and cerebral perfusion scans; some cardiac imaging that uses thallium; the Schilling test, which uses cobalt-labeled vitamin B_{12}; and PET scanning, which uses antimatter or positron emission instead of a gamma emitter.

PET imaging utilizes fluorodeoxyglucose (FDG) labeled with F-18, a positron emitter. The F-18-labeled FDG is preferentially taken up by cancer cells because of their increased metabolic rate and therefore increased need for sugar compared to normal cells. The scanner used in PET imaging is not the gamma camera but a separate scanner based on coincidence detection of the annihilation photons resulting from positron decay. PET scanning is often combined with computed tomography (CT) performed at the same time.

Cancers diagnosed: All types of cancers, both primary and secondary (metastatic), can be diagnosed using nuclear medicine scans; for PET scans, the cancers more commonly diagnosed are lymphoma (Hodgkin and non-Hodgkin), esophageal cancer, lung cancer, head and neck cancers, colorectal cancer, pancreatic cancer, renal cancer, breast cancer, thyroid cancer, and melanoma.

Most cancers are identified as a result of their increased uptake of the radiotracer. Others are identified as a result of their lack of uptake, called photopenia, as can be seen in some liver tumors evaluated with HIDA or sulfur colloid. For HIDA scans, differentiation among primary hepatic tumors is performed because of increased uptake seen in focal nodular hyperplasia but not hepatic adenoma, which appears photopenic. In sulfur colloid liver-spleen scans, hepatic adenoma is again seen as a cold defect because of the lack of Kupffer cells (the phagocytic or "sweeper" cells in the liver that form part of the reticuloendothelial

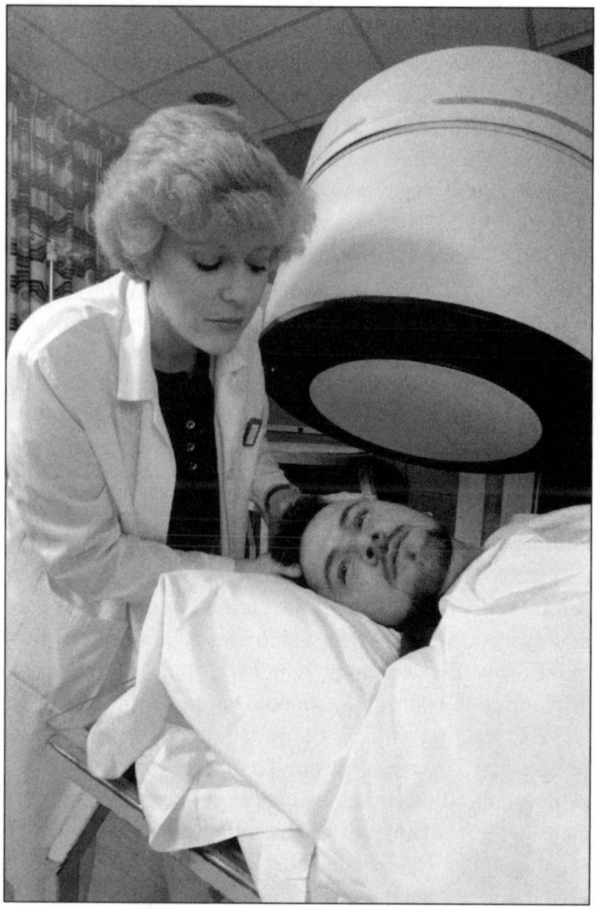

A patient undergoes a nuclear medicine scan. (Digital Stock)

system) compared with focal nodular hyperplasia, which has either normal or increased colloid uptake as a result of the presence of Kupffer cells. Macrophages in the spleen function similarly. A type of benign hepatic tumor known as a cavernous hemangioma is often diagnosed by increased uptake of radiotracer on red blood cell scans in a pattern that is virtually pathognomonic. For bone scans, metastatic disease from prostate and breast as well as osteosarcoma and osteiod osteoma are most commonly diagnosed as a result of increased radiotracer activity from osteoblastic activity of the cancer cells (that is, increased bone turnover caused by the cancer cells). Multiple myeloma, on the other hand, is photopenic on bone scans. For iodine scans, thyroid cancer of both primary and secondary types is identified because of the increased uptake of radioiodine. In some cases, such as thyroid cancer, the scan and the treatment can be combined using radioactive iodine. Carcinoid tumor and medullary carcinoma of the thyroid are diagnosed with somastatin receptor imaging called indium DTPA-labeled octreotide, and pheochromocytomas are diagnosed with iodine-labeled metaiodobenzylguanidine (MIBG).

Why performed: Nuclear medicine scans (bone scan, iodine scan, HIDA scan, red blood cell scan, sulfur colloid scan, octreotide scan, PET scan) are used to diagnose primary and secondary cancer. They are also used to diagnose various ailments depending on the type of scan, including but not limited to the following: acute and chronic cholecystitis and evaluation for postoperative leaks following cholecystectomy (HIDA or DISIDA scan); gastrointestinal bleeding (red blood cell pertechnetate scan); goiter, hypothyroidism versus hyperthyroidism, and evaluation for ectopic thyroid tissue (thyroid scan); hyperparathyroidism caused by parathyroid adenoma (parathyroid scan); Meckel's diverticulum (Meckel's pertechnetate scan); pernicious anemia and malabsorption as a result of sprue (Schilling test); testicular torsion, testicular trauma, orchitis, and epididymitis (testicular pertechnetate scan); bone fractures, Paget disease, prosthesis evaluation, reflex sympathetic dystrophy, bone infarction, and bone infection (bone scan); kidney obstruction, renal transplant rejection, and renal artery stenosis (renal scan); infectious and inflammatory disorders of the lungs, abdomen, pelvis, genitourinary tract, and bone, including acquired immunodeficiency syndrome (AIDS), sarcoidosis, and fever of unknown origin, among others (gallium scan); infection (indium-labeled white blood cells); cardiomyopathy-myocarditis and ejection fraction of the heart, often performed after doxorubicin chemotherapy for breast cancer (MUGA scan); coronary artery disease, coronary artery bypass graft surgery evaluation, valvular heart disease, and risk stratification following myocardial infarction (myocardial perfusion imaging, radionuclide ventriculography, cardiac SPECT, cardiac PET); pulmonary embolus (lung or V/Q scan); gastrointestinal bleeding, portal hypertension, and gastric emptying (sulfur colloid scan); normal pressure hydrocephalus, cerebral spinal fluid leaks, and surgical shunt patency (indium-labeled DTPA cisternography); evaluation for brain death (DTPA cerebral blood flow study); stroke (HMPAO cerebral perfusion imaging with SPECT); identification of seizure focus, evaluation for Alzheimer's disease versus other forms of dementia and depression, Parkinson's disease, and drug addiction (brain SPECT and brain PET).

Patient preparation: Patients are asked to fast at least four hours prior to most scans, especially DISIDA scans and PET scans. For thyroid imaging, patients should stop thyroid medication (synthroid) and avoid CT contrast intravenous dye for one month prior to the scan, as both synthroid and CT contrast dye will interfere with the scan results. Cisternography requires the injection of indium-labeled DTPA radiopharmaceutical into the lumbar subarachnoid space by lumbar puncture, also called spinal tap, prior to scanning. The Schilling test requires the patient to collect urine for twenty-four hours after injection of the radiotracer labeled vitamin B_{12}, and the urine is then evaluated. The patient also receives an intramuscular injection of nonlabeled vitamin B_{12} as part of the test, prior to the urine collection.

Steps of the procedure: The radioisotope is prepared by the technologist and injected into a peripheral vein by the radiologist or nuclear medicine physician. For white blood cell scans and some red blood cell scans, a small amount of blood is withdrawn from the patient and labeled with the radioisotope and is then reinjected prior to scanning. The patient is then placed on the back on a table under a gamma camera connected to a computer. Scan time is variable depending on the procedure but usually takes about one hour.

After the procedure: The scan is generated by the computer attached to the detector and read by the radiologist the same day. The patient will need to contact his or her doctor for the radiology report and for follow-up treatment.

Risks: Minor pain or bruising at the injection site may occur. If the patient is pregnant, then the scan should be avoided if possible, since the radiation dose, although small in most cases, is not negligible. Radioactive iodine should not be administered to a pregnant patient because of the risk to the fetus as the radioiodine crosses the placenta with significant exposure to the fetal thyroid, causing cretinism. Radioiodine is also excreted in human breast milk, and nursing should be stopped following diagnostic or therapeutic studies performed using radioiodine.

Results: The results of a nuclear medicine scan are dependent on the type of scan performed and the reason for the study. Their use in detecting tumors helps the cancer care team stage the cancer and develop a treatment plan.

Debra B. Kessler, M.D., Ph.D.

▶ For Further Information

Mettler, Fred A., Jr., and Milton J. Guiberteau. *Essentials of Nuclear Medicine Imaging*. 5th ed. Philadelphia: Saunders/Elsevier, 2006.

Sandler, Martin P., R. Edward Coleman, and James A. Patton, eds. *Diagnostic Nuclear Medicine*. 4th ed. Philadelphia: Lippincott Williams & Wilkins, 2003.

Wahl, Richard L., ed. *Principles and Practice of Positron Emission Tomography*. Philadelphia: Lippincott Williams & Wilkins, 2002.

See also Brain scan; Cold nodule; Gallium scan; Imaging tests; Positron emission tomography (PET); Radionuclide scan; Thyroid nuclear medicine scan; X-ray tests.

▶ Nutrition and cancer prevention

Category: Lifestyle and prevention

Definition: Everyday eating habits are increasingly associated with cancer incidence, prevention, and management. According to the National Cancer Institute, 80 percent of cancers are caused by environmental factors that are within people's control. It is estimated that the types of foods people eat directly cause 35 to 50 percent of environmental cancers. Studies show that diet and lifestyle changes can prevent and reduce the risk and recurrence of most cancers.

Epidemiology: As a rule, the human immune system is able to stop carcinogens from damaging cells within the body. However, sometimes cell deoxyribonucleic acid (DNA) is attacked and altered, causing cancer cells to begin to develop and multiply. Studies show that most cancers can be prevented through lifestyle choices (a healthful diet, avoidance of tobacco and excessive alcohol use, and adequate physical activity) and changes in the environment. Strong associations link diet to some cancers, but many other factors contribute as well. Genetics, infectious agents, some viruses, and exposure to radiation, chemicals, and some carcinogenic substances in the air, water, and soil also play a role. The American Cancer Society reported that 23.1 percent of deaths in the United States in 2004 were due to cancer.

Nutrition risk factors: Studies find populations that eat a diet rich in fatty foods, especially animal fats, have higher rates of cancer than populations that eat a plant-based diet high in whole grains, vegetables, fruits, and legumes. Increased death rates from breast, prostate, and colon cancers are associated with high-fat diets. Higher rates of cancer have also been linked with the consumption of low-fiber diets and excessive alcohol.

Being overweight or obese is also strongly linked with cancer. Overweight people are more likely to develop breast (postmenopausal women), colon, endometrial, esophageal, and kidney cancers. Obese individuals are also at risk for developing cervical, gallbladder, ovarian, pancreatic, thyroid, and colorectal cancers; Hodgkin disease; multiple myeloma; and aggressive forms of prostate cancer. These findings are of particular concern as westernized societies are experiencing increasing rates of obesity.

Excessive alcohol intake, defined as more than two drinks per day for men and more than one drink per day for women (one serving equals 5 ounces of wine, 12 ounces of beer, or 1.5 ounces of liquor), is clearly associated with cancers of the mouth, throat, larynx, esophagus, liver, and breast.

No known nutrition factors are associated with brain cancer, leukemia, and lymphoma. However, some cancers related to diet may result in secondary tumors or metastatic disease in these areas.

Research findings: A number of different food compounds, minerals, and vitamins are thought to protect against some cancers. Some of those that have become well known are antioxidants, carotenoids, and phytochemicals, substances or nutrients found in foods. Antioxidants include vitamins C and E and the mineral selenium; carotenoids include lycopene, lutein, and beta-carotene; and phytochemicals include a number of plant-based compounds, such as resveratrol (found in red wine), catechin (found in teas), and allium (found in garlic). The use of dietary supplements containing these substances has increased dramatically in the United States because of the popular belief that they prevent aging and illness.

Research shows that antioxidants, carotenoids, and phytochemicals do have some protective effects against free radicals, which are cell-damaging molecules arising from normal biological functions and the environment. Free radical cell destruction is believed to cause aging and many diseases in humans. However, although some studies show benefits from including antioxidants, carotenoids, and phytochemicals in the diet, other studies actually show that they cause harm. In two studies in which high doses of beta-carotene supplements were taken to prevent lung cancer, former cigarette smokers experienced increased lung cancer death. However, when beta-carotene was consumed via food sources (not supplements), cancer risk was reduced.

Coffee, aspartame, saccharin, and sugar have been suspected of causing cancer, but studies have not conclusively linked them to cancer. An increased cancer risk has been associated, however, with the consumption of highly salted, preserved, or smoked meats and those cooked at high temperatures (fried, broiled, and grilled). Many experts recommend limiting consumption of these types of meats.

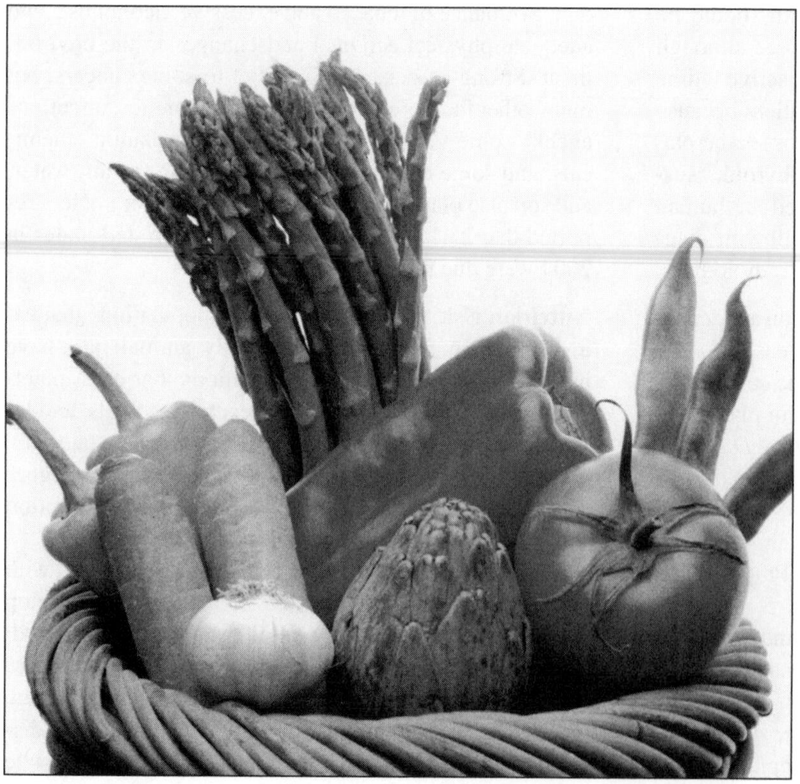

Vegetables are an important part of a cancer-prevention diet. (PhotoDisc)

Studies regarding concerns over the effects of bioengineered and irradiated foods, fish contaminated with mercury, food additives, fluoride in dental products and water, and pesticide residue on foods have not shown any increased risk for cancer. There is no evidence to date that distinguishes organic foods from conventional foods in terms of a cancer risk. However, some studies have shown that the phytochemical content of organic fruits and vegetables may be higher than that of conventionally grown crops. This finding leads some to think that this might convey some level of protection against cancer.

Soy, calcium, and vitamin D are thought by some to help prevent cancers. Soy is an excellent source of protein and phytochemicals, but very little data supports the premise that soy lowers the risk of cancer. Soy contains compounds called phytoestrogens (plant estrogens), which closely resemble the hormone estrogen and may actually increase the risk of estrogen-

A Healthful Diet

The U.S. Department of Agriculture, in its *Dietary Guidelines for Americans*, 2005, gave these broad guidelines for a diet that would be healthful for most Americans.

- Centers on fruits, vegetables, whole grains, nonfat or low-fat dairy products.
- Contains some lean meats, poultry, fish, beans, eggs, and nuts.
- Has minimal amounts of saturated fats, trans fats, cholesterol, salt, and added sugar.

responsive cancers, such as breast and endometrial cancers. It may also reduce the effectiveness of tamoxifen drug treatments. Therefore, some researchers recommend that soy foods and products containing soy isoflavones should be limited to two servings per day and that dietary soy supplements should be avoided. Patients taking tamoxifen should avoid all soy products. The connection between soy and cancer, however, remains unclear.

Calcium has been associated with a lower incidence of colorectal cancers, but there is also evidence that calcium supplements may increase prostate cancers, especially the aggressive form. Because of this, calcium recommendations remain at 1,000 milligrams per day for people between the ages of nineteen and fifty and 1,200 milligrams per day for people older than fifty. Nonfat or low-fat dairy sources of calcium and some leafy green vegetables are preferable to supplements as sources of calcium. Vitamin D is also increasingly thought to protect against colon, prostate, and breast cancer. The existing recommendations for intake of vitamin D, between 200 and 600 International Units (IU) daily, may not be sufficient to provide protection against cancers, especially for those living in northern climates, the elderly, people with dark skin, and exclusively breastfed babies. However, more research is needed before these recommendations can be changed. In the meantime, many researchers suggest exposing the skin (without sunscreen) to sunlight for 15 minutes every day and balancing the diet to include foods fortified with vitamin D.

Many more studies need to be done to verify diet and cancer connections, but the best way for people to lower their cancer risk appears to be eating a balanced, low-fat diet that includes a variety of fruits and vegetables daily.

Dietary recommendations: Research points to a number of dietary recommendations that should be followed to lower the risk for developing cancer or having it recur. The following recommendations are from the American Cancer Society:

- Maintain a healthy weight throughout life: People are advised to lose weight if they are overweight or obese, avoid excessive weight gain, and balance food intake with physical activity.
- Adopt a physically active lifestyle: Adults are advised to exercise at least 30 minutes a day (ideally 45 to 60 minutes a day), five or more days of the week. Children and adolescents are advised to exercise at least 60 minutes per day, five or more days per week.
- Eat a healthy diet, with an emphasis on plant sources: People are advised to eat five or more servings of vegetables and fruits every day, choose whole grains, and include legumes for protein. Also, they are to limit intake of processed and refined foods, sugars, red meat, and processed meats. A simple way to make sure the diet has the right emphasis is to fill one-fourth of the plate with a protein source, one-fourth with whole grains, and one-half with colorful vegetables. One serving of fruit is one-half cup of canned fruit, three-quarters cup of 100 percent juice, or a small to medium-sized piece of fresh fruit. One serving of vegetables is one-half cup of cooked or one cup of raw vegetables.
- Limit consumption of alcoholic beverages: Women should not exceed one drink per day, and men, two drinks per day.

Alice C. Richer, R.D., M.B.A., L.D.

▶ For Further Information

American Institute for Cancer Research. *Diet and Health Recommendations for Cancer Prevention: Healthy Living and Lower Cancer Risk.* Washington, D.C.: Author, 2006.

Awad, Atif B., and Peter G. Bradford, eds. *Nutrition and Cancer Prevention.* Boca Raton, Fla.: CRC, Taylor & Francis, 2006.

Kushi, Lawrence H., et al. "American Cancer Society Guidelines on Nutrition and Physical Activity for Cancer Prevention." *Cancer: A Cancer Journal for Clinicians* 56 (2006): 254-281.

McTiernan, Anne, ed. *Cancer Prevention and Management Through Exercise and Weight Control.* Boca Raton, Fla.: Taylor & Francis, 2006.

▶ Other Resources

American Institute of Cancer Research

Recommendations for Cancer Prevention

Http://www.aicr.org/site/PageServer?pagename=dc_home_guides

The Cancer Project
Cancer Prevention and Survival
http://www.cancerproject.org/survival/cancer_facts/factors.php

National Cancer Institute
Cancer Prevention Overview
http://www.cancer.gov/cancertopics/pdq/prevention/overview/healthprofessional

Prevent Cancer Foundation
http://www.preventcancer.org

See also Aflatoxins; Alcohol, alcoholism, and cancer; Antioxidants; Beta-carotene; Bioflavonoids; Calcium; Carotenoids; Cartilage supplements; Chemoprevention; Coenzyme Q10; Complementary and alternative therapies; Cruciferous vegetables; Dietary supplements; Fiber; Folic acid; Fruits; Garlic and allicin; Ginseng, panax; Green tea; Herbs as antioxidants; Indoles; Isoflavones; Lutein; Lycopene; Macrobiotic diet; Nutrition and cancer treatment; Obesity-associated cancers; Omega-3 fatty acids; Phytoestrogens; Poverty and cancer; Prevention; Resveratrol; Saw palmetto; Soy foods; Sun's soup; Wine and cancer.

▶ Nutrition and cancer treatment

Category: Lifestyle and prevention

Definition: Cancer treatments often affect people differently, and side effects can range from minor to severe. Eating well and following good nutrition habits before and during treatment help maintain strength, prevent body tis-

Effects of Cancer Treatments on Nutrition

Treatment	*Common Nutrition Problems*	*Nutrition-Related Side Effects*
Surgery	May slow digestion; affect proper function of mouth, throat, stomach; increase healing and recovery needs	• May be unable to eat normally and require liquid nutrition • Chewing, swallowing, digestion functions may be impaired
Radiation therapy	Affects healthy tissues and may affect digestive system	Head, neck, chest, breast cancer treatments may cause: • dry or sore mouth • difficulty swallowing • changes in food taste • dental problems • phlegm production Stomach or pelvis cancer treatments may cause: • nausea, vomiting • diarrhea • cramps, bloating
Chemotherapy	May affect the digestive system and desire or ability to eat	• nausea, vomiting • loss of appetite • diarrhea • constipation • sore mouth or throat • weight gain or loss • changes in food taste
Hormonal therapy	May affect ability and desire to eat	• nausea, vomiting • diarrhea • sore or dry mouth • severe weight loss • changes in food taste • fatigue, muscle aches, fever
Immunotherapy	May increase appetite and how the body handles fluid	• change in appetite • fluid retention

Tips for Managing Nutritional Side Effects of Treatment

Side Effect	*Suggestions for Managing Effect*
Constipation	• Eat high-fiber foods (whole grains, fresh fruits and vegetables) • Add unprocessed wheat bran to foods • Get daily exercise • Drink a hot beverage about one-half hour before usual time for bowel movement • Discuss fiber supplements with doctor
Diarrhea	• Avoid: beans, onions, strong spices greasy, fried, and fatty foods raw vegetables, fruits, nuts high-fiber vegetables (broccoli, corn, beans, cabbage, cauliflower, peas) alcohol dairy only if it increases diarrhea very cold or hot liquids/foods • Try: rice or noodles hot wheat cereal well-cooked eggs bananas pureed or soft-cooked vegetables canned/cooked fruits (no skin) white bread skinless chicken/turkey soft or ground beef fish mashed potatoes clear liquid diet during first 24 hours • Eat foods high in sodium and potassium (bananas, peaches, apricot nectar, potatoes)
Difficulty swallowing	• Take deep breaths before swallowing • Exhale or cough after swallowing • Try thick liquids or gelatin • Mash foods to thin or pureed consistency • Drink room-temperature fluids between meals • Use a straw or spoon to eat • Avoid very hot or cold foods • Work with a speech therapist on safe swallowing techniques
Dry mouth	• Avoid: salty or tart foods and beverages • Try: ice pops, sugar-free gum, hard candy, thick nectars sip water every few minutes • Discuss products that protect your mouth with doctor or dentist
Food aversion	• Avoid favorite foods until treatment over
Mouth or throat pain, tooth decay	• Avoid: citrus fruit and juices spicy and salty foods rough and dry foods hot spices alcohol • Try: bananas, applesauce, watermelon, canned fruits peach, pear, and apricot nectars cottage cheese, yogurt, and milkshakes mashed potatoes macaroni and cheese custards, puddings, gelatin scrambled eggs hot cooked cereals pureed or mashed vegetables and meats foods cooked until tender and then cut up or pureed stews and casseroles • Mix food with margarine, gravy, or sauces • Use a straw to drink liquids • Eat foods and drink liquids cold or at room temperature

(continued on page 866)

sue breakdown, rebuild tissues, defend against infection, cope with side effects, and make some treatments more effective.

Cancer treatments: There are five main treatments used to fight cancer: surgery, radiation therapy, chemotherapy, hormone therapy, and immunotherapy. Surgery is used to remove tumors and cancer cells that have not spread to surrounding body tissues. It is often combined with other treatment methods. After surgery, the protein content and number of calories in the diet need to be increased to assist in wound healing and the recovery process. Eating health-

Tips for Managing Nutritional Side Effects of Treatment *(continued)*

Side Effect	*Suggestions for Managing Effect*
Nausea	• Avoid: fatty, greasy, fried, spicy foods sweets (candy, cake, and so on) foods with strong odors or warm or strong-smelling rooms • Try: toast, crackers, pretzels yogurt sherbet, ice pops angel food cake canned fruits skinless chicken (baked or broiled) hot cooked cereals clear liquids (apple juice, broth) ice chips • Eat small amounts often and slowly • Sip cool or chilled liquids throughout the day, except at meals • Eat room temperature or cool foods • Do not eat favorite foods • Always sit upright when eating • Rest after meals for at least one hour • Eat dry toast or crackers before getting up if nauseated in the morning • Wear loose-fitting clothes • Do not eat 1-2 hours before treatment • Keep track of which foods cause nausea • Eat biggest meal of the day when hungry • Discuss antinausea medications with doctor
Taste changes	• Choose and eat foods that look and smell good • Try different foods • Marinate meats, fish, poultry, or try different spices • Try tart foods • Eat foods at room temperature • Maintain good oral hygiene
Vomiting	• Do not drink or eat while vomiting • Sit upright after vomiting for at least an hour • When feeling better, try small amounts of clear liquid, such as apple juice, flat ginger ale, or room temperature broth, drinking 1 teaspoon every 10 minutes as tolerated, gradually increasing to 2 tablespoons every 30 minutes • When able to tolerate clear liquids without vomiting, increase to full liquids (hot wheat cereal, ice cream, broth, gelatin, milk, custard, pudding, and so on)
Weight gain, fluid retention	• Avoid salty foods, add less salt to foods • Drink at least 3-4 glasses of water daily and when thirsty • Exercise as much as is realistic • Meet with a registered dietitian
Weight loss, poor appetite	• Maintain normal activities as much as possible • Do not hurry meals and stay calm when eating • Eat whenever hungry • Keep nutritious snacks available • Try new foods or restaurants • Eat favorite foods • Use candlelight or favorite music at mealtimes, or change timing of meals • Meet with a registered dietitian

fully following surgery also helps the patient feel better by maintaining strength, energy, and a stable weight while maintaining the body's stores of nutrients. Good nutrition is essential for the healing process, to decrease risk of infection, and to increase tolerance to side effects from other treatments used. Any surgery involving the gastrointestinal tract must be carefully monitored, as it can lead to malnutrition.

Radiation therapy directs radiation at the affected body area, preventing cancer cells from multiplying and spreading. Although healthy tissue is affected along with the cancer cells, it usually recovers after treatment ends. Radiation can be used alone or combined with other treatments. Treatments are usually given five days a week and last from two to nine weeks. Nutrition side effects depend on the length of treatment and the area to which the radiation is directed.

Chemotherapy requires the use of strong drugs to disrupt the cancer cells' ability to grow and multiply. Chemotherapy drugs are either taken orally or injected and may be used alone or combined with other treatments. Chemotherapy affects the entire body, not just the cancer site. As a result, healthy tissue is affected. The digestive tract is very susceptible to side effects from this treatment.

Hormone therapy uses drugs to block hormone production by the body. Hormones that influence the growth of some cancers, such as breast and prostate cancers, are targeted. Hormone therapy can also involve the removal of hormone-producing organs, which is thought to end or slow tumor growth by removing the source of the hormones on which these tumors thrive. Hormone therapy can affect the ability and desire to eat.

Immunotherapy, also called biological therapy, enlists the body's immune system to stimulate natural defenses to help fight the offending cancer. It can be used alone but is usually combined with other therapies. This type of therapy can affect fluid retention and may actually increase the appetite.

Nutrition suggestions during treatment: Eating a healthy diet is very important during treatment. This often requires that patients plan ahead, enlist the help of family and friends, and be ready to try different foods and preparation techniques. When experiencing nutrition-related side effects during active treatment, patients are advised to eat foods and liquids that are well tolerated. All patients undergoing treatment should be encouraged to drink plenty of fluids throughout the day and visit with a registered dietitian to ensure proper eating habits.

Alice C. Richer, R.D., M.B.A., L.D.

▶ For Further Information

Bloch, Abby, et al., eds. *Eating Well, Staying Well During and After Cancer*. Atlanta: American Cancer Society, 2004.

Elliott, Laura, Laura L. Molseed, and Paula Davis McCallum, eds. *The Clinical Guide to Oncology Nutrition*. 2d ed. Chicago: American Dietetic Association, 2006.

Keane, Maureen, and Daniella Chace. *What to Eat If You Have Cancer: Healing Foods That Boost Your Immune System*. 2d ed. New York: McGraw-Hill, 2007.

▶ Other Resources

American Cancer Society

Handling the Side Effects of Treatment

Http://www.cancer.org/docroot/MBC/MBC_6_1_what_to_do_about_side_effects.asp

American Institute of Cancer Research

Nutritional Effects of Cancer Treatment

Http://www.aicr.org/site/PageServer?pagename=dc_cr_treatment#nutrition

National Cancer Institute

Eating Hints for Cancer Patients: Before, During, and After Treatment

http://www.cancer.gov/cancertopics/eatinghints/page3

See also Anthraquinones; Antioxidants; Cancell; Carotenoids; Cartilage supplements; Coenzyme Q10; Complementary and alternative therapies; Curcumin; Delta-9-tetrahydrocannabinol; Dietary supplements; Electroporation therapy; Essiac; Gerson therapy; Ginseng, panax; Green tea; Herbs as antioxidants; Integrative oncology; Laetrile; Mistletoe; PC-SPES; Phenolics; Saw palmetto; Sun's soup.

▶ Obesity-associated cancers

Category: Diseases, symptoms, and conditions

Related conditions: Many types of cancer

Definition: Obesity is an increase in body weight through an accumulation of fat in the body such that people exceed their ideal weight (taking into account height, sex, age, and body build) by 20 percent or more. The National Institutes of Health define obesity as a body mass index of 30 and above; 40 and above is generally considered severely obese. (A BMI of lower than 18.5 is underweight, 18.5 to 24.9 is healthy, and greater than 25.0 is overweight.) Body mass index, which relates a person's height and weight, is calculated by multiplying the person's weight in pounds by 703, then dividing that number by the person's height in inches, squared.

Another important measurement that relates to obesity is a person's waist measurement. A woman with a waist measurement of more than 35 inches and a man with a measurement of more than 40 inches are considered to be at higher risk for disease. Even if a person's BMI falls within a healthy range, the risk of developing health problems is greater if body fat is concentrated mainly in the waist area.

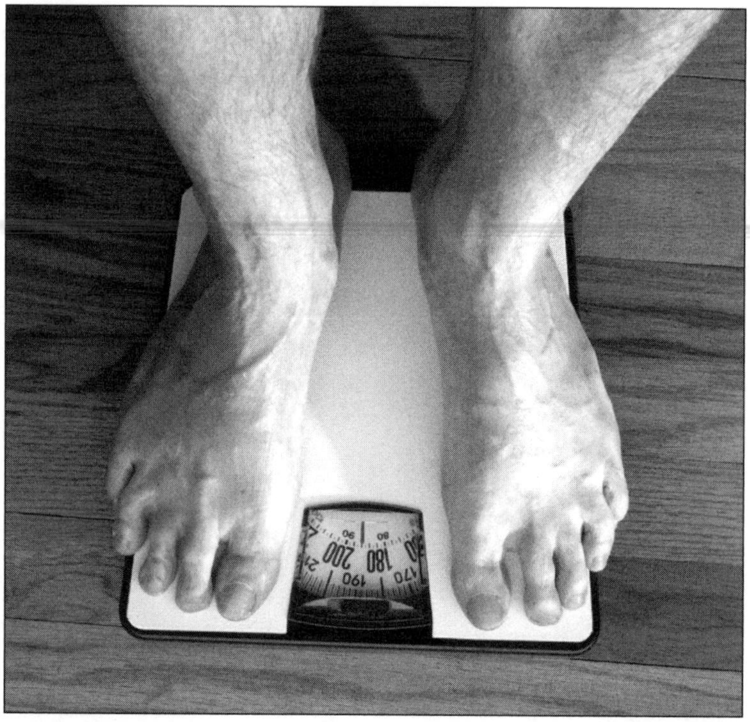

A body mass index of 30 or greater indicates obesity, a cancer risk factor. (PhotoDisc)

Obesity has long been connected with the risks of developing many disorders, including diabetes, arthritis, stroke, and respiratory and heart disease. Years of research have shown that obesity has a significant effect on the development of cancer and its prognosis after treatment. The cancers that are known to be affected by obesity include breast (postmenopausal), endometrial, ovarian, esophageal, colon, prostate, testicular, kidney, pancreatic, non-Hodgkin lymphoma, multiple myeloma, and gallbladder. Further research may find links to other cancers as well.

Risk factors: Obesity is primarily caused by poor diet (excessive intake of calories) and physical inactivity. Weight gain may be caused in part by the abundance of readily available high-calorie food choices and the lack of physical exertion in modern lives, psychological factors such as stress or depression, physical conditions such as hypothyroidism, and certain medications including migraine medications and antidepressants.

Etiology and the disease process: Many researchers have studied obesity and its relationship to an increased incidence of certain cancers. It is believed that fat cells in the body produce hormones and other substances that affect cell growth. Obese people have significantly increased levels of these compounds because of the increased number of fat cells, which can have potentially important effects on cellular growth and planned cellular death, perhaps allowing damaged cells to survive and grow into tumors. The roles of estrogen, insulin, insulin-like growth factor-1 and insulin-like growth factor-binding protein-3, leptin, and cytokines, as well as other substances and growth factors, are being examined for their relationship to obesity-associated cancers.

An example of these actions by fat tissue can be found in postmenopausal breast cancer, which is known to have a 50 percent incidence rate in obese women. Estrogen, important in the reproductive cycle, is produced by fat tissue in addition to being produced by the ovaries. After menopause, when the ovaries stop producing hormones, fat tissue becomes the most important estrogen source. In obese women, postmenopausal estrogen levels are 50 to 100 percent higher than in women who are not overweight or obese. As a result, estrogen-sensitive tissues in obese women are overexposed to estrogen stimulation, leading to a more rapid growth of estrogen-responsive

Body Mass Index

	Height (inches) BMI	58	59	60	61	62	63	64	65	66	67	68	69	70	71	72	73	74	75	76
		Weight (pounds)																		
Normal	19	91	94	97	100	104	107	110	114	118	121	125	128	132	136	140	144	148	152	156
Normal	20	96	99	102	106	109	113	116	120	124	127	131	135	139	143	147	151	155	160	164
Normal	21	100	104	107	111	115	118	122	126	130	134	138	142	146	150	154	159	163	168	172
Normal	22	105	109	112	116	120	124	128	132	136	140	144	149	153	157	162	166	171	176	180
Normal	23	110	114	118	122	126	130	134	138	142	146	151	155	160	165	169	174	179	184	189
Normal	24	115	119	123	127	131	135	140	144	148	153	158	162	167	172	177	182	186	192	197
Overweight	25	119	124	128	132	136	141	145	150	155	159	164	169	174	179	184	189	194	200	205
Overweight	26	124	128	133	137	142	146	151	156	161	166	171	176	181	186	191	197	202	208	213
Overweight	27	129	133	138	143	147	152	157	162	167	172	177	182	188	193	199	204	210	216	221
Overweight	28	134	138	143	148	153	158	163	168	173	178	184	189	195	200	206	212	218	224	230
Overweight	29	138	143	148	153	158	163	169	174	179	185	190	196	202	208	213	219	225	232	238
Obese	30	142	148	153	158	164	169	174	180	186	191	197	203	209	215	221	227	233	240	246
Obese	31	148	153	158	164	169	175	180	186	192	198	203	209	216	222	228	235	241	248	254
Obese	32	153	158	163	169	175	180	186	192	198	204	210	216	222	229	235	242	249	256	263
Obese	33	158	163	168	174	180	186	192	198	204	211	216	223	229	236	242	250	256	264	271
Obese	34	162	168	174	180	186	191	197	204	210	217	223	230	236	243	250	257	264	272	279
Obese	35	167	173	179	185	191	197	204	210	216	223	230	236	243	250	258	265	272	279	287
Obese	36	172	178	184	190	196	203	209	216	223	230	236	243	250	257	265	272	280	287	295
Obese	37	177	183	189	195	202	208	215	222	229	236	243	250	257	265	272	280	287	295	304
Obese	38	181	188	194	201	207	214	221	228	235	242	249	257	264	272	279	288	295	303	312
Obese	39	186	193	199	206	213	220	227	234	241	249	256	263	271	279	287	295	303	311	320
Extremely Obese	40	191	198	204	211	218	225	232	240	247	255	262	270	278	286	294	302	311	319	328
Extremely Obese	41	196	203	209	217	224	231	238	246	253	261	269	277	285	293	302	310	319	327	336
Extremely Obese	42	201	208	215	222	229	237	244	252	260	268	276	284	292	301	309	318	326	335	344
Extremely Obese	43	205	212	220	227	235	242	250	258	266	274	282	291	299	308	316	325	334	343	353
Extremely Obese	44	210	217	225	232	240	248	256	264	272	280	289	297	306	315	324	333	342	351	361
Extremely Obese	45	215	222	230	238	246	254	252	270	278	287	295	304	313	322	331	340	350	359	369
Extremely Obese	46	220	227	235	243	251	259	267	276	284	293	302	311	320	329	338	348	358	367	377
Extremely Obese	47	224	232	240	248	256	265	273	282	291	299	308	318	327	338	346	355	365	375	385
Extremely Obese	48	229	237	245	254	262	270	279	288	297	306	315	324	334	343	353	363	373	383	394
Extremely Obese	49	234	242	250	259	267	278	285	294	303	312	322	331	341	351	361	371	381	391	402

Source: National Heart, Lung, and Blood Institute

breast tumors. Researchers believe that the fat cells stimulate surges of hormones, insulin, proteins, and the other substances mentioned above that may, in turn, cause reactions that initiate uncontrollable growth among certain cell types.

Incidence: According to the American Cancer Society, the risk of cancer from obesity is similar to the risk from using tobacco. Obesity has reached epidemic proportions and affects the entire population, regardless of age, gender, race, or ethnicity. In the United States, obesity has been increasing at an alarming rate. In 1980, about 15 percent of adults were classified as obese; by 2004, that number had more than doubled to about 33 percent; and, between 1986 and 2000, the number of adults classified as severely obese had increased from about 1 in 200 to 1 in 50. Estimates from the Centers for Disease Control associate about 112,000 deaths per year with obesity.

Childhood obesity has been at the forefront of concern because of the staggering numbers of overweight children and the projected long-term health effects. From 1994 to 2000, the number of overweight children between the ages of two and five increased by more than 40 percent; overweight children aged six to eleven doubled in number between 1980 and 2002; and overweight adolescents aged twelve to nineteen more than tripled between 1980 and 2002. Overweight and obesity are most common among black and Mexican American women, with the same patterns seen for children and adolescents in these groups.

Studies have increasingly linked obesity and cancer. Many studies show that the greater the degree of obesity, the stronger the association with cancer. In one study of more than 900,000 adults, the death rates from all cancers combined were 52 percent higher in men and 62 percent higher in women who were classified as severely obese. In another study, obesity links were found in an estimated 51 percent of women and 14 percent of men with newly diagnosed cases of cancer. The studies also show a higher recurrence rate after radical prostatectomy for prostate cancer in obese men and an incidence rate of 50 percent and decreased survival rate in obese women with postmenopausal breast cancer.

By applying the current levels of overweight and obesity, Graham Colditz, a physician with the Harvard School of Public Health, estimated the number of cancer cases that could be avoided if no one were overweight or obese. His estimates of avoidable cancer cases included 49 percent of endometrial cancers, 39 percent of esophageal cancers, 31 percent of kidney cancers, 20 percent of non-Hodgkin lymphoma cases, 17 percent of multiple myeloma cases, 14 percent of pancreatic cancers, 14 percent of colon cancers, and 11 percent of breast cancers.

Symptoms: There are no symptoms that are specific to obesity-associated cancers.

Screening and diagnosis: Screening for obesity-associated cancers includes annual physical examinations to calculate BMI and take waist measurements as well as annual laboratory tests, such as serum lipid panel, fasting glucose level, and thyroid function tests. In addition, people can essentially screen themselves by monitoring their own weights. There are no specific tests for obesity-related cancers; testing is done when patients exhibit other symptoms. Staging is specific to the type of cancer that develops.

Treatment and therapy: Treatment for obesity-associated cancer is specific to the type of cancer. However, based on data obtained during various studies, patients must also reduce their weight to avoid the increased risk that obesity places on successful treatment. Patients must set weight-loss goals and obtain assistance from a registered dietitian or weight-loss program for in-depth counseling. Many reputable commercial and community programs exist for obesity treatment. Desirable programs should include diets that meet the United States recommended daily allowance for nutrients, exercise counseling, behavior modification, and provision for long-term maintenance.

The National Institutes of Health guidelines suggest nonpharmacologic treatment for six months and then consideration of medication if weight loss is unsatisfactory in those with a BMI greater than 30 or a BMI greater than 27 with associated risk factors. Patients with severe obesity (BMI greater than 40) may also be considered for gastric bypass or gastroplasty procedures.

Prognosis, prevention, and outcomes: Long-term maintenance of weight loss is extremely difficult. If the patient is not motivated, successful weight loss is unlikely. Obesity can be prevented by educating children and adults in healthy dietary habits and exercise requirements, but only if individuals choose to follow the guidelines and do not have physical causes for the excess weight. Weight reduction can have a significant impact on a person's risk for developing obesity-associated cancers.

Dorothy P. Terry, R.N.

▶ For Further Information

Calle, E. E., et al. "Overweight, Obesity, and Mortality from Cancer in a Prospectively Studied Cohort of U.S. Adults." *New England Journal of Medicine* 348, no. 17 (April 24, 2003): 1625-1638.

Giovannucci, E., and D. Michaud. "The Role of Obesity and Related Metabolic Disturbances in Cancers of the Colon, Prostate, and Pancreas." *Gastroenterology* 132 (May, 2007): 2208-2225.

Polednak, A. P. "Trends in Incidence Rates for Obesity-Associated Cancers in the U.S." *Cancer Detection and Prevention* 27 (2003): 415-421.

▶ Other Resources

American Cancer Society
http://www.cancer.org

National Cancer Institute
Obesity and Cancer: Questions and Answers
http://www.nci.nih.gov/cancertopics/factsheet/Risk/obesity

See also Appendix cancer; Bile duct cancer; Breast cancers; Cervical cancer; Comedo carcinomas; Craniopharyngiomas; Endometrial cancer; Gallbladder cancer; Gynecologic cancers; Hepatomegaly; Klinefelter syndrome and cancer; Leiomyosarcomas; Medulloblastomas; Nutrition and cancer prevention; Pancreatic cancers; Paraneoplastic syndromes; Rectal cancer; Risks for cancer; Stomach cancers; Urinary system cancers; Uterine cancer.

▶ Occupational exposures and cancer

Category: Social and personal issues

Definition: Cancers or malignancies can be partly or entirely caused by exposure to chemicals, physical agents, biological agents, or industrial processes at a person's place of work or in a person's occupation.

Related conditions: Cancers linked to occupational exposure include leukemia, lymphoma, and cancers of the lung, breast, bladder, skin, larynx, nose, throat, prostate, pancreas, liver, scrotum, and soft tissue.

Workers at risk: The International Agency for Research on Cancer (IARC) has identified fifty known and about one hundred suspected occupational carcinogens. Certain workplaces and jobs carry a greater risk of exposing workers to substances that may increase their chance of cancer. The workplace may be indoors, as with restaurant or factory workers, or outdoors, as with landscapers or construction workers. Because the effects of exposure to occupational toxins usually do not surface until years after exposure, linking the cancer to the workplace is sometimes difficult. However, one in five workers is exposed to and at an increased risk for cancer from toxins in the workplace.

The World Health Organization (WHO) reported that of the seven million deaths from cancer each year, about 40 percent could be prevented by dedicated efforts to reduce workplace toxins. Occupational cancer claims more lives (32 percent) than any other work-related disease (circulatory disease claims 26 percent) or even work accidents (17 percent). The incidence of occupational cancers is from 4 to 20 percent of all cancers but may be higher, as many go unreported. In the United States, each year about 20,000 people die of cancers attributed to occupational toxins and about 40,000 people are newly diagnosed with cancers due to occupational causes. Globally, an estimated 609,000 workers are affected yearly.

Lung cancer: Lung cancer has been linked to occupational exposure to numerous substances. Lung cancer, particularly mesothelioma, is high in people exposed to asbestos and can develop years after the exposure. If the person exposed to asbestos is a smoker, that person is 50 to 90 times more likely to be diagnosed with lung cancer compared with the average person. Asbestos has been used to strengthen the walls of buildings; as insulation for walls, boiler pipes, and steam pipes; and as soundproofing. In 1989, the United States Environmental Protection Agency (EPA) banned most asbestos-containing products. Although the ruling was overturned in a 1991 appeal, some asbestos-containing products remain prohibited, and all nonhistorical, or new, uses are banned. Therefore, automobile parts manufacturers still use asbestos in brake shoes and clutch linings. Some products contain substances that may be contamined with asbestos, such as vermiculite (in garden products) and talc (in crayons). Asbestos often is present in the ceiling or floor tiles in older buildings. Workers who remove asbestos-containing materials from old buildings need to use protective masks to avoid inhalation and cover their clothes so they do not take asbestos dust home with them. Other industries where employees can be exposed to asbestos are railroads, insulation factories, and shipbuilders.

Lung cancer risk is increased for people who work in places where they are exposed to secondhand smoke, such as bars, casinos, bowling alleys, or restaurants; tin miners and refining industry workers who are exposed to toxins such as arsenic, nickel, or chloromethyl ether; and quarrying, stone industry, and glass-manufacturing workers exposed to silica dust.

Radon, a natural radioactive gas that causes lung cancer, is present at harmful levels in one in fifteen homes by the EPA's estimate. Chemicals inhaled by painters, chemists, and printers increase their risk of lung cancer. Formaldehyde, a chemical used to disinfect surgical rooms and dialysis units and also found in carpet and furniture glues, diesel fumes, and embalming fluid, is believed to cause respiratory cancers.

Bladder cancer: Bladder cancer has been linked to exposure to dyes containing benzine and naphthylamine. IARC found a small increased risk of developing bladder cancer among barbers and male hairdressers. However, some cancer-causing coloring agents were removed from dyes in the 1970's, and the study was unable to determine if the risk was caused by past or present exposure to carcinogens. Employees who work with rubber, paint, or leathers may also be at greater risk of developing bladder cancer.

Skin cancer: Skin cancers such as melanomas are more common in workers who are exposed to the ultraviolet (UV) radiation from the sun. Workers at greater risk include construction workers, farmworkers, landscapers, roofers, and fishing boat workers. Asphalt and diphenyls as well as reflections from water, sand, concrete, snow, and any light-colored surface increase the harmful effects of UV rays.

Other cancers: Workers exposed to herbicides and pesticides have an increased risk of lymphomas. Farmers and others working with these chemicals demonstrate a higher

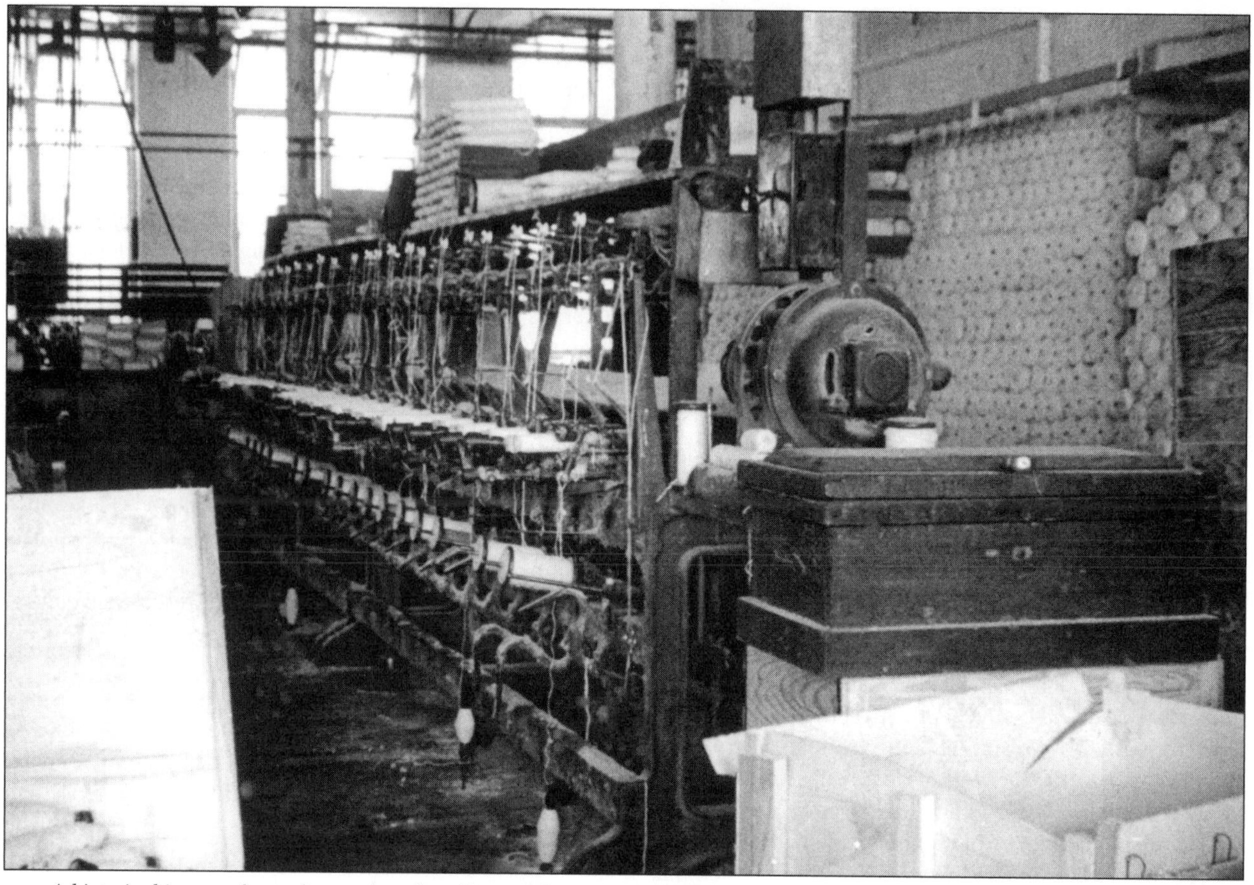

A historical image of an asbestos thread-making machine in an asbestos mill. (Centers for Disease Control and Prevention)

incidence of prostate cancer. Pancreatic cancer is associated with pesticides, dyes, and gasoline. Health care workers can be exposed to occupational toxins as well as body fluids that harbor hepatitis B and C viruses, which can cause liver cancer.

Prevention and policy: Occupational exposures to carcinogens can be limited and in many cases are preventable. Removing the risk or the toxin from the workplace is the primary way to prevent occupational cancer. When the carcinogen cannot be removed from the environment, as in the case of UV rays, workers can use protective clothing and sunscreens, and work practices can be altered to minimize exposure (such as providing a shady place for breaks and lunches). The WHO's Global Occupational Health Network offers the following steps to prevent occupational cancers:

- Develop regulations and an enforcement process for monitoring carcinogens in the workplace.
- Avoid use of known carcinogens in the workplace.
- Replace known toxins with safe substitutes.
- Educate workers about primary prevention of work-related cancers.
- Implement a health surveillance program for workers exposed to occupational toxins.

Several other approaches can decrease the risk of occupational cancer. These include testing of new chemicals before they are placed on the market, keeping hazardous toxins in an enclosed area with adequate ventilation, and using protective masks and clothing. Workers are advised to avoid smoking, as the incidence of occupational cancer increases with tobacco use. All workers must examine and weigh the risk that each occupation brings, as few jobs are risk-free, but some involve more exposure than others.

The prevention of occupational cancer is directly related to legislation as laws are needed to control the use of carcinogens and to provide workers with adequate protection from exposure. Legislators, politicians, lobbyists, unions, and grassroots occupational health groups have brought pressure on the various industries to introduce protective laws and stricter inspections.

Robert W. Koch, D.N.S., R.N.

▶ For Further Information

Blanc, Paul D. *How Everyday Products Make People Sick: Toxins at Home and in the Workplace*. Berkeley: University of California Press, 2007.

Bozzone, Donna M. *Causes of Cancer*. New York: Chelsea House, 2007.

Landrigan, Phillip J. "Prevention of Occupational Cancer." *CA Cancer Journal for Clinicians* 46 (1996): 67-69.

Raffle, P. B., et al., eds. *Hunter's Diseases of Occupations*. 8th ed. Boston: Arnold, 1994.

Rapp, Doris J. *Our Toxic World: A Wake Up Call*. New York: Environmental Medical Research Foundation, 2004.

Veys, C. A. "ABC of Work Related Disorders: Occupational Cancer." *British Medical Journal* 313 (1996): 615-619.

▶ Other Resources

Hazards Magazine
Occupational Cancer/Zero Cancer
http://www.hazards.org/cancer

National Institute for Occupational Safety and Health
http://www.cdc.gov/niosh

World Health Organization
Occupational Health
http://www.who.int/occupational_health

See also Agent Orange; 4-Aminobiphenyl; Arsenic compounds; Asbestos; Benzidine and dyes metabolized to benzidine; Beryllium and beryllium compounds; Bladder cancer; Blood cancers; Bone cancers; Breast cancer in men; 1,3-Butadiene; 1,4-Butanediol dimethanesulfonate; Cadmium and cadmium compounds; Cancer clusters; Cancer education; Carcinogens, known; Carcinogens, reasonably anticipated; Carcinomatosis; Case management; Chlorambucil; 1-(2-Chloroethyl)-3-(4-methylcyclohexyl)-1-nitrosourea (MeCCNU); Chromium hexavalent compounds; Coke oven emissions; Dioxins; Electromagnetic radiation; Epstein-Barr virus; Ethylene oxide; Formaldehyde; Head and neck cancers; Lung cancers; Lymphomas; Melanomas; Mesothelioma; 2-Naphthylamine; Nasal cavity and paranasal sinus cancers; Organochlorines (OCs); Pesticides and the food chain; Polycyclic aromatic hydrocarbons; Radon; Rehabilitation; *Report on Carcinogens* (RoC); Risks for cancer; Salivary gland cancer; Silica, crystalline; Surgical oncology; Ultraviolet radiation and related exposures; Urinary system cancers; Vinyl chloride; Wood dust.

▶ Occupational therapy

Category: Medical specialties

Definition: Occupational therapy is a medical specialty that helps patients function more successfully in their everyday lives. Occupational therapy is not limited to skills that are necessary for a job but rather can include any skills that are needed for daily living or participating in regular activities, which can range from work and school to hobbies. Occupational therapists can work with cancer patients during all periods of cancer treatment and afterward to help patients maintain participation in daily life and pleasurable activities, or to help patients return to their normal activities as completely as possible.

Subspecialties: Pediatric occupational therapy, geriatric occupational therapy, palliative occupational therapy

Cancers treated: All

Training and certification: Occupational therapists receive specialized training in a number of fields, including biology, physiology, behavioral science, and specific training in the skills necessary to assess patient needs and meet them effectively. Occupational therapists could be qualified with only a bachelor's degree until 2007, when the licensing requirements for all new occupational therapists were raised to completion of at least a master's degree.

In addition to education, occupational therapists must fill many other requirements to practice. They must successfully complete at least six months of closely monitored work in the field and must pass a national certification exam, administered by the National Board for Certification in Occupational Therapy. After passing the certification exam, occupational therapists must apply to be licensed in the state or territory in which they plan to practice. States and territories may have their own additional licensing requirements.

Because of the high cost of health care, many health care companies are encouraging licensed occupational therapists to delegate work to occupational therapy assistants and aides, who are paid less. Although the licensed occupational therapist oversees the treatment, much of the hands-on work can be done by the assistants and aides. Generally, an occupational therapist assistant must complete either an associate's degree in occupational therapy or a certification course. Occupational therapist aides do not usually have to complete a degree or certification program but may instead receive the majority of their training in occupational therapy while on the job.

Services and procedures performed: The occupational therapist provides different services and uses varying techniques according to the specific needs of the patient. The therapist starts by meeting with the patient and sometimes the patient's family to determine what the needs of the patient are. This may include gathering information about what kinds of activities the patient performed on a daily basis before the cancer diagnosis and what kinds of activities are most important to the patient to be able to participate in at present. These can include work, hobbies, or activities such as spending time with the family or coaching a children's softball team. Activities of daily living can be a primary concern for the occupational therapist and the patient. If there are activities such as eating, bathing, or dressing that the patient is unable to do without help, the therapist will gather information about these as well.

After gathering information about the patient's normal activities, the therapist can work with the patient to develop realistic goals. These goals will then enable the therapist to determine which therapeutic activities will be most effective. If treatment has not yet begun, the first therapies may focus on techniques that will help the patient get through treatment as successfully as possible, such as techniques for energy conservation.

If treatment has been completed successfully, the occupational therapist may focus on helping the patient regain old skills or adjust to any permanent changes resulting from the cancer and its treatment. The goals for this type of therapy may range from regaining the full function present before the cancer and treatment, to regaining the skills to allow a return to a job, to functioning in the most independent way possible. If the treatment was not successful, the occupational therapist may focus on palliative care and therapy intended to help the patient maintain independence and a range of desired skills and abilities for as long as possible.

The techniques used by occupational therapists to help cancer patients depend on a wide variety of factors such as the desired skills, the location in which the therapy is being performed, and the age of the patient. Much occupational therapy is done on an outpatient basis, although it is also provided in a hospital setting. Occupational therapy for children often focuses on play, sometimes even making skills useful for daily living into play activities. For adults, therapy may focus on practicing a skill, such as dressing. The occupational therapist can provide adaptive equip-

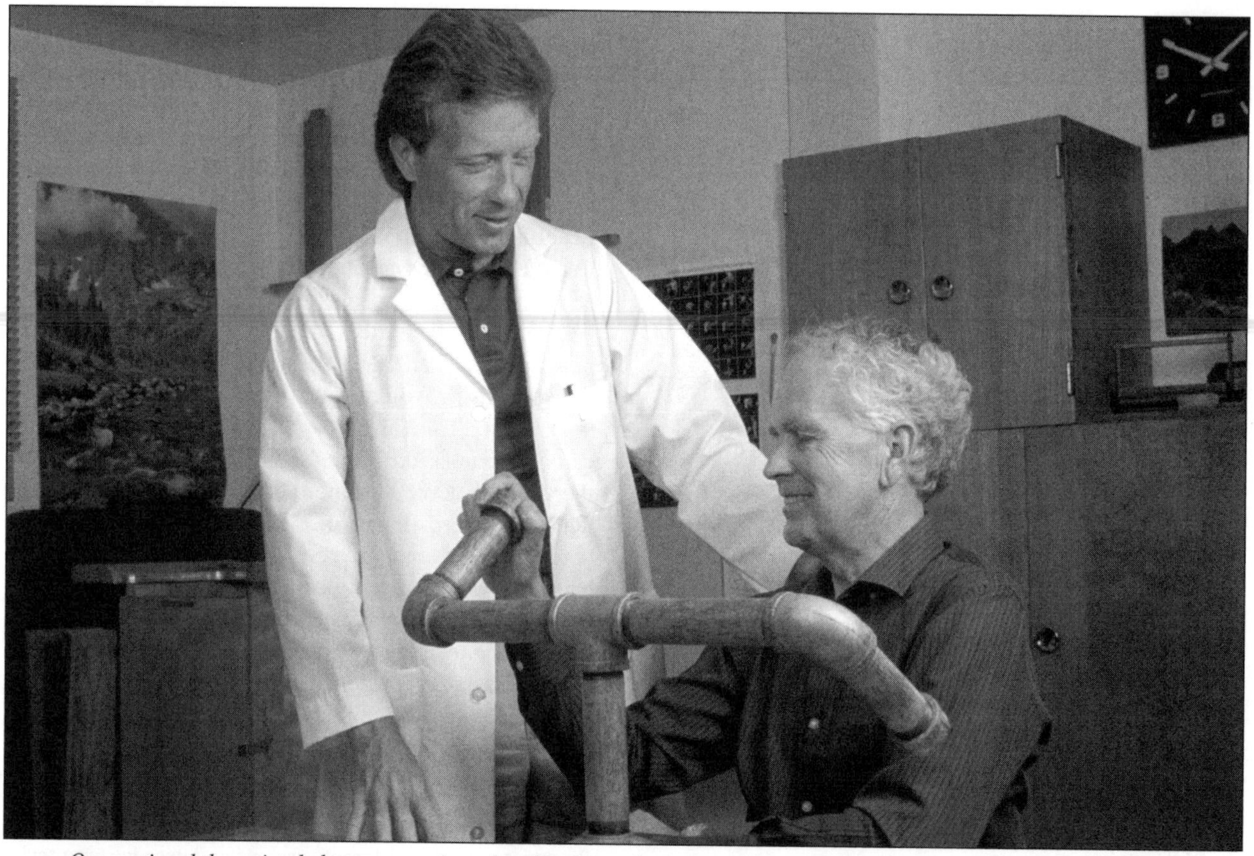

Occupational therapists help cancer patients function better during and after treatment. (Custom Medical Stock Photo)

ment, if it is available, to help with the needs of the patient and spends time helping the patient learn to use the equipment in the most effective way. Therapists may visit a workplace to help determine if adaptive equipment or a change of duties may help a patient return to work. In the home, an occupational therapist may be able to recommend changes to make it more comfortable for the patient or easier to negotiate effectively. Therapists can also help patients come up with productive alternatives for activities that may be especially difficult or can no longer be done, such as helping patients who can no longer drive find alternative modes of transportation.

Related specialties and subspecialties: The occupational therapist is one of many members of the health care team who help individuals with cancer have as positive an experience as possible during treatment and afterward. An integral part of this process is helping the individual perform as many of the activities that are normally a part of the daily routine as possible. Depending on the type of cancer and the procedures used to treat it, the other members of the health care team who will work with the occupational therapist to meet this goal will vary.

A physical therapist may work with the patient to increase muscle tone, flexibility, and balance. A speech therapist may work with the patient if speech and language abilities have been adversely affected by the cancer. If an amputation has been necessary, the prosthetisist works with the occupational therapist and the physical therapist to help choose the prosthetic that will best meet the patient's needs and to help the patient develop the skills to properly use it. Therapists who work with cancer patients may be involved in helping patients work through any emotional problems that are interfering with their ability to function as normally as possible. Of course, the patient's doctor and other members of the cancer care team will be involved to ensure that the treatment has the best possible outcome with the least negative effect on the patient's daily life.

Helen Davidson, B.A.

▶ For Further Information

Christiansen, Charles H., and Kathleen M. Matuska, eds. *Ways of Living: Adaptive Strategies for Special Needs*. Bethesda, Md.: American Occupational Therapy Association, 2004.

Cooper, Jill, ed. *Occupational Therapy in Oncology and Palliative Care*. Hoboken, N.J.: Whurr, 2006.

Marcil, William Matthew. *Occupational Therapy: What It Is and How It Works*. Clifton Park, N.Y.: Thomson Delmar, 2007.

Ross, Joanna. *Occupational Therapy and Vocational Rehabilitation*. Hoboken, N.J.: John Wiley and Sons, 2007.

Taylor, M. Clare. *Evidence-Based Practice for Occupational Therapists*. Malden, Mass.: Blackwell, 2007.

▶ Organizations and Professional Societies

American Occupational Therapy Association
http://www.aota.org
4720 Montgomery Lane
P.O. Box 31220
Bethesda, MD 20824-1220

National Board for Certification in Occupational Therapy
http://www.nbcot.org
12 South Summit Avenue, Suite 100
Gaithersburg, MD 20877-4150

National Cancer Institute
http://www.cancer.gov/
National Institutes of Health
Building 31, Room 11A48
31 Center Drive
Behesda, MD 20892-2590

▶ Other Resources

American Cancer Society
http://www.cancer.org

Occupational Therapist.com
http://www.occupationaltherapist.org

See also Aids and devices for cancer patients; Cancer care team; Cancer education; Cognitive effects of cancer and chemotherapy; Electrolarynx; Esophageal speech; Home health services; Insurance; Karnofsky performance status (KPS); Limb salvage; Living with cancer; Orthopedic surgery; Psychosocial aspects of cancer; Rehabilitation; Relationships; Transitional care.

▶ Oligodendrogliomas

Category: Diseases, symptoms, and conditions
Also known as: Glial brain tumors, OD

Related conditions: Elevated intracranial pressure, personality changes, neurological deficits

Definition: Oligodendrogliomas are a type of glial tumor arising in the brain in which the oligodendroglial cell is the predominant cell type. There are several kinds of glial

Relative Survival Rates of Adults with Oligodendroglioma by Race, 1988-2001

	Survival Rates (%)	
Years	*Whites*	*Blacks*
1	89.1	79.6
2	81.7	71.9
3	77.9	63.1
5	68.8	50.2
8	58.7	37.6
10	52.2	28.5

Source: Data from L. A. G. Ries et al., eds., *Cancer Survival Among Adults: U.S. SEER Program, 1988-2001—Patient and Tumor Characteristics*, NIH Pub. No. 07-6215 (Bethesda, Md.: National Cancer Institute, 2007)

cells in the central nervous system, but each functions in support of the nerve cells (neurons). The oligodendrocytes are glial cells that coat the axons in the central nervous system with an insulating membrane called myelin. Without myelin, the nerve impulses flowing down the axon lose efficiency.

The third most common of the glial neoplasms, oligodendrogliomas usually originate in the cerebral hemispheres (predominantly the frontal lobe) but on rare occasions can arise in the cerebellum, brain stem, and spinal cord. Although they are typically considered a rare neoplasm, newer diagnostic techniques such as genotyping indicate that the condition is more common than once thought.

Oligodendroglioma neoplasms often contain anaplastic cells, primitive, undifferentiated cells that are a distinguishing feature of emerging embryonic cells and are often seen in malignant neoplasms. Tumors with anaplastic cells are called anaplastic oligodendrogliomas.

Risk factors: There are no known causes or risk factors for oligodendroglioma. The problem occasionally clusters in some families, but this is unrelated to any mechanisms of inheritance. The disease strikes men about twice as often as women, with the risk equally distributed among the races. Although the median age of diagnosis is between forty and fifty years, oligodendroglioma can occur at any age. The anaplastic variant usually occurs between the ages of sixty and seventy. Children are less frequently affected, accounting for 6 percent of oligodendroglioma cases.

Etiology and the disease process: Oligodendrogliomas evolve from primitive precursor glioma cells. The tumor begins as a slow-growing, mixed tumor, combining elements of astrocytes (another type of glial cell), neurons, and oligodendroglial cells. The tumor consists of poorly defined anaplastic components, mature oligodendroglial cells, or a mixture of the two. It is impossible to predict how long it will take for patients to experience symptoms because although oligodendrogliomas usually grow quite slowly, they can quickly evolve into an aggressive malignancy and shorten the crisis point from upwards of thirty years to only a few months. When the neoplasm exhibits features of oligodendroglioma cells with astrocytic components, it is called oligoastrocytoma, but this is less common.

Incidence: Intracranial tumors are second only to stroke as the most common neurological cause of death. In the United States, the incidence of oligodendrogliomas compared with all intracranial tumors may be as high as 19 percent, and they may represent 20 to 54 percent of all gliomas. Oligodendrogliomas may account for 4 percent of all brain tumors, with an annual incidence in the United States of 0.3 per 100,000 people.

Symptoms: Symptoms depend on the size, location, invasiveness, and rate of growth of the tumor. Warning signs will vary but may include seizures, vomiting, fatigue, headache, numbness, pain, ataxia, paralysis, sensations of tingling or burning, hearing or vision deficits, and changes in temperature and taste sensitivity. The most common first symptom is a seizure, representing half of all patients.

Screening and diagnosis: Imaging studies and biopsy examination are central to a diagnosis of oligodendroglioma. Laboratory tests are useful only in excluding other causes and determining overall health. Magnetic resonance imaging (MRI) is performed with and without the radiocontrast medium gadolinium. Computed tomography (CT) scans are helpful in revealing some details missed in MRI studies, and sometimes immunohistochemical markers further help in establishing the diagnosis. However, ultimately, only biopsy will result in a definitive diagnosis. Following biopsy, most pathologists will simply grade oligodendrogliomas according to the presence or absence of anaplastic features.

Treatment and therapy: Treatment depends on the patient's symptoms and the location and nature of the tumor. As with most cancers, the three mainstays of treatment are chemotherapy, radiation, and surgery. Chemotherapy using a combination of procarbarazine, lomustine, and vincristine has been used in the earliest diagnosed stage of the tumor, but typically relapses occur between eighteen months and two years. Newer treatments in combination with radiation may prolong the time until relapse, but the classic treatment for oligodendroglioma remains surgical resection. Often, however, the tumor is poorly defined, making complete resection impossible. In the past, when surgery completely removed the tumor, further treatment was believed unnecessary. However, several years following total resection, almost all patients suffer recurrence of the tumor at the surgical site. Regardless of whether resection is complete or incomplete, typically no further treatment is given until relapse occurs. In the event of relapse, chemotherapy is the treatment of choice; radiation is reserved for patients not responding to chemotherapy.

Prognosis, prevention, and outcomes: The prognosis depends on the growth rate of the tumor, its location, and its pressure effects inside the cranium. Some specific prognostic indicators have been noted: Older age at the time of diagnosis, the presence of a neurological deficit, or a central location in a child's brain usually results in a shorter survival time. From the time of diagnosis, the median survival time ranges between three and seventeen years. Five-year survival rates range from 39 to 75 percent and ten-year rates from 19 to 59 percent, but ultimately all patients will die of the disease.

Richard S. Spira, D.V.M.

▶ For Further Information

Baumann, Nicole, and Danielle Pham-Dinh. "Biology of Oligodendrocyte and Myelin in the Mammalian Central Nervous System." *Physiological Reviews* 18, no. 2 (2001): 871-927.

Central Brain Tumor Registry of the United States. *Primary Brain Tumors in the United States: Statistical Report, 1992-1997*. Chicago: Author, 2000.

Ellis, T. L., V. W. Stieber, and R. C. Austin. "Oligodendroglioma." *Current Treatment Options in Oncology* 4, no. 6 (2003): 479-490.

Kleihus, P., and W. K. Cavenee. *Pathology and Genetics of Tumours of the Nervous System*. New York: Oxford University Press, 2000.

Mason, W. P. "Oligodendroglioma." *Current Treatment Options in Neurology* 7, no. 4 (July, 2005): 305-314.

Ohgaki, H., and P. Kleihues. "Population-Based Studies on Incidence, Survival Rates, and Genetic Alterations in Astrocytic and Oligodendroglial Gliomas." *Journal of Neuropatholy and Experimental Neurology* 64, no. 6 (June, 2005): 479-489.

Van den Bent, M. J. "Advances in the Biology and Treatment of Oligodendrogliomas." *Current Opinion in Neurology* 17, no. 6 (December, 2004): 675-680.

▶ Other Resources

The Brain Tumor Foundation
Tumor Types: Oligodendrogliomas
http://www.braintumorfoundation.org/Oligodendrogliomas.php

National Cancer Institute
Adult Brain Tumors Treatment
http://www.cancer.gov/cancertopics/pdq/treatment/adultbrain/Patient

See also Brain and central nervous system cancers; Carcinomatous meningitis; Gliomas; Meningeal carcinomatosis.

▶ Omega-3 fatty acids

Category: Lifestyle and prevention
Also known as: Polyunsaturated fatty acids (PUFAs)

Definition: Omega-3 fatty acids are essential polyunsaturated fats that must be obtained from food, particularly cold-water fish, fish oil, flaxseeds, soybeans, walnuts, green leafy vegetables, and canola oil. Three forms of omega-3 fatty acids exist: alpha-linolenic acid (ALA), eicosapentaenoic acid (EPA), and docosahexaenoic acid (DHA).

Cancers treated or prevented: Colon cancer, breast cancer, prostate cancer, pancreatic cancer

Delivery routes: Oral by food, capsule, or liquid

How this substance works: Omega-3 fatty acids are highly concentrated in the brain and appear to play an important role in cognitive and behavioral functions, as well as normal growth and development. Research indicates that these acids are important in numerous physiological functions, particularly muscle contraction and relaxation, movement of calcium and other material into and out of cells, regulation of blood clotting, and secretion of substances including hormones and digestive enzymes. They also play a role in controlling cell division and fertility, indicating their possible importance in protection against certain types of cancer. Omega-3 fatty acids seem to reduce inflammation and retard tumor growth. On the other hand, omega-6 fatty acids, which are found in sunflower oil, safflower oil, and most saturated fats and vegetable oils, promote inflammation and feed tumor growth. An appropriate balance between omega-3 and omega-6 fatty acids is necessary to promote good health.

Some research indicates that omega-3 fatty acids help

to prevent certain chronic diseases, including heart disease and some cancers. EPA appears to be important in cancer prevention by affecting the production of cytokines and the tumor necrosis factor (TNF). Other research indicates that omega-3 fatty acids may play an adverse role in treating some cancers. If the latter is true, then these acids still play an indirect role in cancer prevention if cold-water fish, such as salmon, halibut, and tuna, are substituted for red and processed meats, which are known to increase the risk of colon and prostate cancers.

Side effects: The consumption of omega-3 fatty acids and cancer incidence have had unfavorable associations in some case studies. One study on skin cancer and another on lung cancer showed that these fatty acids increased the risk for developing these cancers. A study on prostate cancer showed that ALA increased its risk, while EPA and DHA reduced the risk. More specific case studies need to be conducted in order to build a significant statistical database.

Alvin K. Benson, Ph.D.

See also Alopecia; Chemoprevention; Dietary supplements; Thyroid cancer.

▶ Ommaya reservoir

Category: Procedures
Also known as: Implanted intrathecal device, intraventricular device

Definition: An Ommaya reservoir is a device surgically placed under the scalp that allows administration of drugs, such as chemotherapy, directly into the cerebrospinal fluid (CSF), bypassing the blood-brain barrier. It may also be used to sample CSF.

Cancers treated: Brain and related nervous system lesions, any brain metastasis

Why performed: Blood vessels that provide blood to the brain filter out drugs and other substances, preventing them from reaching the brain and cerebrospinal fluid. This blood-brain barrier also blocks chemotherapy from reaching cancer cells in the brain and CSF. With the surgical placement of an Ommaya reservoir under the scalp, drugs may be delivered directly to tumors or metastases. In some cases, the Ommaya reservoir has been used to drain cystic lesions in the brain.

Patient preparation: The Ommaya reservoir, a small dome-shaped device with an attached tube, is placed by a neurosurgeon during surgery. The patient is under general anesthesia, so there is no pain. An area of the head is shaved and an incision is made in the skin. The tube, or catheter, is inserted through a small hole made in the skull and threaded into a hollow space, or ventricle, which holds CSF.

Steps of the procedure: After the surgical site heals, a physician or specially trained nurse may access the device to remove CSF or to administer chemotherapy or other drugs. This procedure may be done in the hospital or specialty outpatient clinic. Accessing the device is a sterile procedure. The skin over the device is cleansed, and then a sterile needle is used to pierce the dome and instill the chemotherapy or drug. The needle is withdrawn and pressure is applied to the needle site to control any bleeding.

After the procedure: The patient should report any symptoms such as headache, unusual sleepiness, stiff neck, nausea, and vomiting immediately. Any usual side effects of chemotherapy administration may occur. It is important to observe the area over the Ommaya reservoir for signs of infection, such as redness and warmth at the needle site. Patients may go home between treatments with the device in place and may continue normal activities.

Risks: The risks associated with an Ommaya reservoir are generally related to blockage of the tube or infection.

Results: The patient may expect that chemotherapy and other drugs reach the necessary site of action with minimum pain.

Patricia Stanfill Edens, R.N., Ph.D., FACHE

See also Chemotherapy; Infusion therapies; Medulloblastomas.

▶ Oncogenes

Category: Cancer biology; carcinogens and suspected carcinogens
Also known as: Proto-oncogenes

Related cancers: Leukemias, lymphomas, most sarcomas (of bone and muscle), carcinomas (of epithelial origin)

Exposure routes: Inherited as genetic information

Where found: Proto-oncogenes are genes found within the chromosomes of all eukaryotic (nucleated) cells and organisms.

At risk: Proto-oncogenes are universal among all eukaryotic cells and organisms, which include humans and all animals. Congenital mutations in some of these genes are associated with a significantly increased risk for certain cancers.

Definition: Oncogenes are variations of cellular proto-oncogenes that normally function in the regulation of cell division. Mutations in these genes may result in the cell becoming cancerous. The term "proto-oncogene" refers to the normal cell copy of the gene, while the term "oncogene" refers to a mutated, or activated, form of the same gene that results in disruption of cell regulation.

Most oncogenes have a three-letter name based on their initial identification or the type of cancer with which they were first found to be associated. For example, the *SRC* gene was first identified in the Rous sarcoma virus. The *RAS* oncogene was first identified as a gene in rat sarcomas.

Selected Oncogenes and Tumor-Suppressor Genes and Their Related Cancers

Gene	*Associated Cancers*
APC	Colorectal cancer
BCL2	B-cell lymphoma
BRC-ABL1	Chronic myelogenous leukemia
BRCA1, BRCA2	Breast, ovarian
EWSR1 (*EWS*)	Ewing sarcoma
HER2/neu (*ERBB2*)	Breast, ovarian
MLH1, MSH2	Colorectal
MYC (*c-myc*)	Burkitt lymphoma, others
MYCN (*N-myc*)	Neuroblastoma
RB1	Retinoblastoma, others
TP53 (*p53*)	Brain, skin, lung, head and neck

Source: American Cancer Society

Etiology and symptoms of associated cancers: More than one hundred proto-oncogenes have now been recognized in cells. Most are involved in regulating movement through the cell cycle (regulation of chromosome replication followed by cell division). The cell cycle is characterized as having four phases: G1, which regulates events leading to deoxyribonucleic acid (DNA) replication; S, in which cell chromosomes replicate; G2, which regulates events leading to cell division; and mitosis, the period in which the chromosomes separate and the cell divides. Each phase is regulated by specific enzymes, signals, and other molecules, as well as suppressors that prevent movement through the phase. Many of the regulatory proteins involved in these events are encoded by proto-oncogenes. Not all proto-oncogenes are expressed in every cell, and the type of cancer that potentially develops is related to the particular oncogene that has undergone a mutation.

Proto-oncogenes are subdivided into four categories, each of which represents a particular set of steps that regulate the cell cycle: growth factors, growth factor receptors, signal mechanisms, and tumor suppressors/regulators of apoptosis (cell death).

Growth factors are small proteins that bind specific cell surface receptors and set in motion events that will result in cell division. Overproduction of growth factors may result in repeated cell division, setting the stage for development of cancer. For example, the *PDGFB* (commonly known as *sis*) oncogene, originally isolated from the simian sarcoma virus, encodes one of the protein chains that make up the platelet-derived growth factor. PDGFB is secreted by platelets and binds receptors on certain fibroblast cells. Overproduction of PDGFB may induce uncontrolled cell division, resulting in a sarcoma.

Growth factor receptors are cell surface proteins that bind specific growth factors. Each cell type expresses a particular form or forms of receptors, and the ability of any growth factor to stimulate a cell depends on expression of these surface molecules. Some of these receptor proteins are actually enzymes that, when activated, begin a series of signals within the cell, resulting in cell division. Certain mutations in the genes that encode these receptors may, in effect, cause a "short circuit" in regulation, resulting in loss of control and continuous movement of the cell through the cell cycle.

One example of such a receptor mutation is that of the HER2/neu (also known as ERBB2) receptor protein expressed on certain breast cells. The HER2/neu protein is similar in its amino acid sequence to the human epidermal growth factor receptor molecule and is an example of a transmembrane enzyme that begins the signal transmission in the cell. A mutation in the *HER2/neu* proto-oncogene converts it into the *HER2/neu* oncogene (named for the neuroblastoma in which it was first identified). Overexpression of the HER2/neu protein is associated with the aggressive nature of certain forms of breast cancer. The basis for the chemotherapeutic action of Herceptin is its ability to inhibit the activity of the HER2/neu protein.

Signal mechanisms represent a series or cascade of enzymatic reactions that move the cell through the cell cycle and regulate cell division. At the molecular level, intermediates in this pathway are enzymes that activate DNA-binding proteins (DBPs), inducing gene expression. The *RAS* supergene family and the greater than one hundred proteins its members encode are examples of such inducers. RAS proteins are also called G proteins, reflecting their utilization of guanosine triphosphate (GTP) for their activity. Mutations in these genes may result in a continuous activating signal within the cell and uncontrolled cell division. Certain forms of colon and bladder cancers are the result of such mutations, and some forms of mutations are associated with mutations in the DNA-binding protein substrates for these RAS proteins. *RAS* gene mutations have been observed in nearly one-third of all cancers.

Tumor suppressors/regulators of apoptosis control steps at the end of the cell cycle. The proto-oncogenes that regulate apoptosis can either promote or inhibit cell death. The *BCL2* gene family produces proteins that are pro-apoptosis and anti-apoptosis (the *BCL2* gene itself inhibits apoptosis, and its overexpression has been implicated in cancers such as lymphoma). Proto-oncogenes and tumor suppressors provide the cell with the means not only to block division if chromosome replication is incomplete or if a mutation has occurred that could cause the cell to become cancerous but also to actually cause the cell to die. Tumor suppressors promote apoptosis and therefore are usually inactivated in cancers.

The first of the tumor suppressors to be discovered was the retinoblastoma RB1 protein, isolated in the 1980's. The RB1 protein regulates the steps that allow DNA replication to begin in the cell. The TP53 protein, named for its size, detects mutations that have occurred in DNA and induces repair of the DNA site or, if the mutation is too extensive, induces steps that culminate in the death of the cell.

As is true for other genes that regulate cell division, mutations in the genes associated with tumor suppression are associated with certain forms of cancer. For example, mutations in the *RB1* gene may predispose the person for retinoblastoma. Mutations in the *TP53* gene have been found in nearly 50 percent of all forms of cancer. The ability of oncogenic viruses such as hepatitis B, the etiological agent for hepatocarcinoma, or the human papillomavirus, the agent for cervical carcinoma, to initiate cancer is related to their abilities to inactivate tumor suppressors. At least two dozen types of tumor suppressors were identified in the first decade of the twenty-first century.

Mutations at these sites may be caused as a result of infection by certain viruses or by exposure to carcinogens, most of which are also mutagens, chemicals that induce DNA mutations. In some cases, the mutation is congenital, the individual having been born with that specific mutation. Childhood retinoblastoma, for example, results from congenital mutations in the *RB1* gene.

In some cases, it is not "simply" a point mutation in a proto-oncogene that leads to a cancer. Certain forms of the disease are known to result from chromosomal breaks and translocations, the movement of pieces of chromosomes from one site to another in the cell chromatin. The DNA in patients suffering from chronic myelogenous leukemia was found to possess a specific type of translocation. What became known as the Philadelphia chromosome is characterized by translocation of the *ABL1* oncogene, on chromosome 9, into the region of the *BCR* oncogene on chromosome 22. The combined gene product disrupts the normal signaling mechanism in these cells, resulting in uncontrolled cell division. Inhibition of this activity is the basis of action for at least one type of antileukemic drug, imatinib mesylate (Gleevec), lending further support to this mutation as being the actual cause of chronic myelogenous leukemia.

Cancer, however, generally is not the result of any individual mutation. The molecules previously described regulate cell division, The difference between a benign growth and a true malignancy is the result of accumulated mutations over time. For example, a malignancy would require not only a mutation in the signal pathway but also, at a minimum, additional mutations in tumor-suppressor genes or in steps that inhibit cell death.

History: The evidence for existence of oncogenes dates to the early history of retroviruses, viruses with genomes of ribonucleic acid (RNA), which are copied into DNA following infection and which were found to be etiological agents for some forms of cancer. In the late nineteenth century, leukemia in animals was demonstrated to be transmissible using extracts from cells. However, leukemia was not considered to be a true cancer at the time. It was only when Peyton Rous demonstrated in 1911 that solid tumors in chickens—sarcomas—could be transmitted using cell-free extracts that scientists began to believe cancer, at least in animals, was associated with infectious agents. Eventually what became known as the Rous sarcoma virus (RSV) was isolated and identified with this disease in chickens.

As an increasing number of such tumor viruses, in which RNA was shown to be the genetic material, were isolated by the 1950's, the question that followed was how these viruses could change, or transform, cells from normal to cancerous. In 1958 Howard M. Temin and Harry Rubin demonstrated that single virus particles could transform chicken cells. Further work by Temin indicated that it was possible to disrupt viral replication and transformation by adding inhibitors acting at the level of DNA. Temin proposed that such viruses act using a DNA intermediate and that they encode an enzyme that copies RNA into DNA, allowing what has become viral DNA to integrate into the cell chromosome. By the late 1960's Temin and David Baltimore independently discovered an enzyme, popularly known as reverse transcriptase, that carries out this function. Viruses that encode the enzyme have become known as retroviruses and include the RNA tumor viruses. Temin and Baltimore were each awarded the Nobel Prize in Physiology or Medicine in 1975.

The seemingly simplistic genetic structure of the RNA tumor viruses lent itself to determining which viral genes are associated with cancers. The discovery of a temperature-sensitive mutation in one of these genes led to the identification of the *SRC* gene in the Rous sarcoma virus, the first such oncogene to be discovered.

The *SRC* gene was shown to be required for transformation by the Rous sarcoma virus. However, strains of the virus that lacked that gene were found to replicate normally, suggesting the *SRC* gene was superfluous for the virus and may even have originated as genetic material extraneous to the virus. In 1976 J. Michael Bishop and Harold Varmus provided the answer. Creating DNA probes from transformation defective mutants of the Rous sarcoma virus, they found that normal avian cells contained cellular homologs of the viral *SRC* gene—that is, a cellular proto-oncogene. The proto-oncogene product of the gene was subsequently shown to be an enzyme critical in the signaling pathway that regulates cell division.

Through the 1980's, an increasing number of cellular proto-oncogenes were identified, and evidence for their association with cancers was increasingly demonstrated. When carcinogens were used to transform cells growing in laboratory cultures, mutations were found in proto-oncogenes carried by these cells. Indeed, the only difference found between proto-oncogenes in normal cells and oncogenes expressed in cancer cells was often a mutation at a single site. For example, the *RAS* oncogene found in cases of bladder cancer differed from its counterpart in a normal cell at only one amino acid position, suggesting the origin of the cancer was a mutation at that site. The *RAS* product, as was the *SRC* product described above, was shown to be involved in the signaling pathway within the cell.

Richard Adler, Ph.D.

▶ For Further Information

Bishop, J. Michael. *How to Win the Nobel Prize*. Cambridge, Mass.: Harvard University Press, 2003.

Coffin, John, et al. *Retroviruses*. Plainview, N.Y.: Cold Spring Harbor Laboratory Press, 1997.

Cooper, Geoffrey. *Oncogenes*. 2d ed. Sudbury, Mass.: Jones and Bartlett, 1995.

Pelengaris, Stella, and Michael Khan. *The Molecular Biology of Cancer*. Malden, Mass.: Blackwell, 2006.

Vogelstein, Bert, and Kenneth Kinzler. *The Genetic Basis of Human Cancer*. New York: McGraw-Hill, 2002.

▶ Other Resources

American Cancer Society
Oncogenes and Tumor Suppressor Genes
http://www.cancer.org/docroot/ETO/content/ETO_1_4x_oncogenes_and_tumor_suppressor_genes.asp

CancerQuest
Important Oncogenes
http://www.cancerquest.org/index.cfm?page=181

See also Angiogenesis; Ataxia telangiectasia (AT); Biological therapy; *BRAF* gene; Breast cancer in pregnant women; Breast cancers; Cancer biology; Carcinomas; Chromosomes and cancer; Craniosynostosis; Cytogenetics; Endocrine cancers; Free radicals; Gene therapy; Genetics of cancer; Giant cell tumors (GCTs); Hemangiosarcomas; HER2/neu protein; HIV/AIDS-related cancers; *HRAS* gene testing; Hypercalcemia; Mesothelioma; Mitochondrial DNA mutations; Monoclonal antibodies; Multiple endocrine neoplasia type 2 (MEN 2); Mutagenesis and cancer; *MYC* oncogene; Myelofibrosis; Neuroendocrine tumors; Oncogenic viruses; Parathyroid cancer; Proto-oncogenes and carcinogenesis; *RhoGD12* gene; *SCLC1* gene; Tumor-suppressor genes; Viral oncology; Virus-related cancers.

▶ Oncogenic viruses

Category: Carcinogens and suspected carcinogens
Also known as: Oncoviruses

Related cancers: Cancers of the cervix, skin, uterus, penis, nasopharynx, and liver; adenocarcinoma; Kaposi sarcoma; Burkitt lymphoma; non-Hodgkin lymphoma; adult T-cell leukemia

Definition: An oncogenic virus is a virus that infects normal cells, alters the cells' properties, and transforms them into cancer cells. Oncogenic viruses can cause cancer in a variety of animals, including humans. These viruses can have either deoxyribonucleic acid (DNA) or ribonucleic acid (RNA) as their genetic material.

Exposure routes: Sexual, blood-to-blood contact; exchange of bodily fluids

Where found: Ubiquitous

At risk: People who are in contact with others

Etiology and symptoms of associated cancers: Etiology depends on whether the genetic material is DNA or RNA. DNA viruses include the Epstein-Barr virus (EBV), human papillomavirus (HPV), human herpesvirus 8 (HHV-8), hepatitis B virus (HBV) and RNA viruses include the human T-cell lymphotropic viruses 1 and 2 (HTLV-1 and HTLV-2), hepatitis C virus (HCV), and the human immunodeficiency virus (HIV).

The Epstein-Barr virus (EBV), also known as human herpesvirus 4 (HHV-4), has been strongly linked to nasopharyngeal cancer and certain forms of Burkitt lymphoma that are endemic in central Africa. EBV is also suspected of causing some cases of Hodgkin disease. Human herpesvirus 8 (HHV-8) is linked to Kaposi sarcoma. The hepatitis B virus (HBV) is suspected of causing liver cancer, and adenoviruses are suspected of causing cancer of glandular epithelial tissues, a disease known as adenocarcinoma. Human papillomavirus (HPV) can cause various conditions from benign warts to malignant cancers such as carcinomas of the cervix, uterus, and penis. Some cancers of the lung, larynx, and esophagus may be related to HPV. Although there are more than one hundred recognized types of HPV, only a few are known to cause cancer.

Upon entering a cell, viral DNA may integrate into the host genome and express its viral genes, the oncogenes, which cause tumors. Sometimes the virus integrates next to a cellular gene and causes cancer by inducing an overexpression of that cellular gene.

The RNA viruses associated with human cancers are human T-cell lymphotropic viruses 1 and 2 (HTLV-1 and HTLV-2), which cause adult T-cell leukemia and hairy cell leukemia, respectively; the hepatitis C virus (HVC); and the human immunodeficiency virus (HIV), which is suspected of causing lymphomas.

When an RNA tumor virus enters the cell, a DNA copy of its RNA is made in a process known as reverse transcription. The DNA copy may integrate into the host genome and express the viral gene that causes cancer. Alternatively, the integrated DNA can cause cancer by inducing the overexpression of a cellular gene.

History: In 1911, Peyton Rous discovered that sarcomas in chickens were caused by viruses. By the late 1970's it had become clear that certain viruses also caused cancer in humans.

Charles L. Vigue, Ph.D.

See also Cancer biology; Oncogenes; Proto-oncogenes and carcinogenesis; Viral oncology; Virus-related cancers.

▶ Oncology

Category: Medical specialties
Also known as: Cancer medicine

Definition: Oncology is a word derived from the Greek word for lump. It is the medical specialty that studies tumors, focusing on their causes, their development, and means of treating them. Although tumors may be cancerous (malignant) or noncancerous (benign), oncologists are largely concerned with the malignant type because they are more life-threatening and present greater medical challenges than benign tumors.

Subspecialties: Biochemistry, radiology, radiation and cancer biology, radiation physics, chemotherapy, genetics, surgery, hematology

Cancers treated: All

Training and certification: Several subspecialties exist under the broad umbrella term "oncologist." Minimally, those pursuing oncological training and certification must possess a recognized medical degree or, in the case of oncological nurses, must be registered nurses.

Among the basic fields in which oncologists practice is surgical oncology, in which board-certified surgeons take special training in biopsy, tumor staging, and tumor resection or removal by surgical means. Another distinct field is pediatric oncology and hematology, in which board-certified pediatricians take special training that focuses on various malignancies frequently found in babies or in children. Medical oncology is a field that attracts internists who complete special oncological training. Yet another field is radiation oncology, which is staffed by radiologists who complete special training directed toward the radiological diagnosis and treatment of malignancies. Gynecological oncology is studied by board-certified gynecologists and obstetricians, while board-certified hematologists may continue their studies with an emphasis on cancers of the blood, such as leukemia.

Specific training in oncology usually involves a residency of two to four years, generally pursued at a recognized cancer center. Such training follows the residency in each candidate's special field, such as surgery, pediatrics, or radiology.

Certification is granted by such regulatory agencies as the Accreditation Council of Graduate Medical Education, the American Board of Radiology, and the American Board of Pediatrics. Specific oncological training may focus on clinical research, on the integration of oncological training with other medical specialties, on clinical practice, or on a combination of these activities.

Once physicians have received initial certification in their specific fields, they usually must renew this certification at regular intervals. Such renewals may require them to take refresher courses or to pass qualifying examinations in the field. Although it is seldom necessary to withhold the renewal of certification, practicing oncologists must keep abreast of their fields to assure themselves that they will qualify for recertification.

Services and procedures performed: Although cancer is the broad term used to describe the runaway proliferation of malignant cells within the body, this catch-all term is too broad to describe the many types of malignancies that oncologists encounter and are called on to treat. Cancer occurs when masses of tissue, termed neoplasms, behave abnormally, when their growth is out of control to the extent that it poses the possibility of spreading to other organs, a process know as metastasis.

Because a metastasized cancer is more difficult to control than one that is confined to a small area, physicians urge patients to seek immediate medical intervention if any sign of a malignancy is detected. Cancers caught in the early stages usually can be controlled and possibly eliminated through radiation, chemotherapy, surgery, or a combination of these procedures. Early detection is key to controlling and eliminating malignancies.

Oncologists in all subspecialties of oncology are fundamentally concerned with attempting to understand how normal cells mutate into malignant cells. Their research is concentrated on determining the process through which malignancies develop so that they can find means of thwarting such abnormal development.

As oncologists come to understand the process through which normal somatic cells are transformed into malignant cells, they are better equipped than ever before to deal with the inroads of cancer. As knowledge of the molecular biology of cancer proliferates, oncologists have been increasingly able to develop biochemical and genetic means of not only treating malignancies but also anticipating them in patients who are at risk genetically of developing cancer.

Certainly the most effective treatment of cancer is anticipatory and preventive. A family history of cancer may substantially increase the likelihood that a patient will eventually develop cancer, so oncologists can provide preventive treatment to lessen or eliminate such a possibility.

Cancer genes are essentially of two types. Dominant oncogenes, as they are called, are relatively rare. Of the more than thirty thousand human genes that have been identified, less than one hundred are oncogenes. Such genes increase the ability of cells to divide. When they grow uncontrolled in organisms, they result in both malignant and benign tumors. Anti-oncogenes are designed to suppress tumors. They sometimes undergo a mutation that thwarts the cell's ability to develop its means of suppressing such tumors.

Through mutation, dominant oncogenes and anti-oncogenes can both serve to cause the generation of cells that are difficult to control. Great progress has been made in understanding the basic molecular factors involved in the development of cancer, giving oncologists the tools, both genetic and biochemical, that they require to diagnose the behavior of neoplasms, or abnormal new cells, and to find ways to treat such cellular growth effectively.

With medical advances and an increased understanding of the role that genetics plays in cellular growth, oncologists have developed sophisticated means of treating abnormalities in the growth of cells, particularly of malignant cells. With the unraveling of some of the mysteries of how deoxyribonucleic acid (DNA) determines cellular growth, oncologists have come to realize that the four nucleotides found in cells (adenine, guanine, cytosine, and thymine) occur in various sequences and that they contain the genetic information required to comprehend the development and configuration of cellular organisms.

The genes provide cells with the information they need to develop the cellular sequence of amino acids needed to build the proteins, the building blocks, required for cells to develop and grow. Dominant oncogenes can distort the division of cells so that instead of an orderly production, a runaway production of cells takes place, resulting in tumors. Oncologists strive to understand the genetic activities of cells and to bring under control any cellular activity that thwarts or threatens the orderly production of cells and causes tumors to form.

Although the primary goal of oncologists is to evaluate malignancies and work either to eliminate them or to greatly reduce their size, an important secondary goal is to offer reassurance to patients and their families and to work assiduously to make patients as comfortable and pain-free as possible in the course of their treatment. Ongoing research in oncology has proliferated greatly in the twenty-first century. Oncologists necessarily strive to keep abreast of it. Whereas major surgery was often indicated for malignancies in the 1980's or 1990's, much treatment of comparable malignancies has become either noninvasive or minimally invasive.

Prolonged radiation therapy with all of its side effects has, in many cases, been replaced by much more benign procedures such as the implantation at the site of the malignancy of radioactive seeds that provide an uninterrupted but much reduced dose of radiation. Such procedures provide a constant bombardment of malignant cells with radiation but reduce substantially the side effects that accompany a more extensive radiological procedure. These means of treating malignancies often permit patients to engage quite normally in their day-to-day activities.

Related specialties and subspecialties: Initially, many of the patients who consult oncologists do so because they have been referred by internists or family physicians to whom they turned when symptoms begin to appear. Oncologists to whom such patients are referred generally keep in contact with the referring physician, who often continues to see such patients on a regular basis.

Most of the work oncologists do is highly collaborative. Ideally it is carried out at large medical centers staffed by specialists in each of the many subspecialties of oncology. Regardless of the site of a malignancy, a radiation oncologist is necessarily involved in helping determine the extent of radiological treatment and in plotting its course. Oncologists working together make diagnoses and determine the stage of a malignancy, with stages ranging from I to IV. The two higher numbers indicate a malignancy that has metastasized or spread to organs outside the original site of the growth.

Increasingly Stage IV malignancies, once considered death sentences, are being treated successfully. Some such growths have been eliminated altogether through radiation or chemotherapy, sometimes combined with surgical intervention. In such cases, the oncologist works closely with radiologists, physical oncologists, geneticists, and surgeons, all of whom have had special training in oncology, to determine an effective course of treatment that can result in eliminating or controlling the malignancy. Even in cases in which there is no cure, the quality and extent of a patient's life can be considerably enhanced by oncological treatments devised by various specialists in the field.

Cancers exist in so many forms that specialists from many fields, some only ancillary to the medical profession, may be called on to be involved in their treatment. As research increasingly indicates that diet may substantially affect the growth of cancer cells, nutritionists have become involved in working collaboratively with oncologists. Since 1911, when American pathologist Peyton Rous first detected an oncogenical virus in a malignant tumor that grew in a chicken, virologists have worked with oncologists to identify viruses that may be associated with cancer.

Oncologists may also refer patients and those close to them to mental health professionals and social workers to help them cope with the depression and uncertainties that frequently accompany diagnoses of cancer and their subsequent treatment. In cases that are clearly terminal, oncologists may help patients obtain hospice care so that they will be looked after either in their homes or in facilities that are less forbidding and less costly than hospitals.

R. Baird Shuman, Ph.D.

▶ For Further Information

De Vito, Vincent T., Samuel Hellman, and Steven A. Rosenberg, eds. *Cancer: Principles and Practice of Oncology*. Philadelphia: Lippincott Williams and Wilkins, 2005.

Langhorne, Martha E., Janet S. Fulton, and Shirley E. Otto, eds. *Oncological Nursing*. 5th ed. St. Louis: Mosby Elsevier, 2007.

Leibel, Steven A. *Textbook of Radiation Oncology*. 2d ed. Philadelphia: Saunders, 2004.

Pappas, Alberto S., ed. *Pediatric Bone and Soft Tissue Sarcomas*. New York: Springer, 2006.

Parker, Robert G. *Radiation Oncology for Cure and Palliation*. New York: Springer, 2003.

Pazdur, Richard, ed. *Medical Oncology: A Comprehensive Overview*. Huntington, N.Y.: PRR, 1995.

Pollock, Raphael E., ed. *Surgical Oncology*. Boston: Kluwer Academic Press, 1997.

Rizzo, Phillip A., and David G. Poplack, eds. *Principles and Practice of Pediatric Oncology*. Philadelphia: Lippincott Williams and Wilkins, 2002.

Tomlinson, Deborah, and Nancy E. Kline, eds. *Pediatric Oncology Nursing: Advanced Clinical Handbook*. New York: Springer, 2005.

Vasilev, Steven A., ed. *Perioperative and Supportive Care in Gynelogic Oncology: Evidence-Based Management*. New York: Wiley-Liss, 2000.

▶ Organizations and Professional Societies

American Board of Internal Medicine (ABIM)
http://www.abim.org
613 New York Ranch Road
Jackson, CA 95642

American Board of Obstetrics and Gynecology (ABOG)
http://www.abog.org
2915 Vine Street
Dallas Texas, 75204

American Board of Pediatrics (ABP)
https://www.abp.org/ABPWebSite/
111 Silver Cedar Road
Chapel Hill, NC 27514

American Board of Radiology (ABR)
http://www.theabr.org/index.htm
5441 East Williams Boulevard, Suite 200
Tucson, AZ 85711

American Board of Surgery (ABS)
http://www.absurgery.org
1617 John F. Kennedy Boulevard #860
Philadelphia, PA 19103

American Society for Therapeutic Radiology and Oncology (ASTRO)
http://www.astro.org
Post Office Box 631567
Baltimore, MD 21263

American Society of Clinical Oncology
http://www.asco.org
1900 Duke Street, Suite 200
Alexandria, VA 22314

▶ Other Resources

American Academy of Hospice and Palliative Medicine
http://www.aahpm.org

National Comprehensive Cancer Network
http://www.nccn.org

Oncology Nursing Society
http://www.ons.org

See also Dermatology oncology; Endocrinology oncology; Gastrointestinal oncology; Gynecologic oncology; Hematologic oncology; Immunocytochemistry and immunohistochemistry; Medical oncology; Molecular oncology; Neurologic oncology; Ophthalmic oncology; Pediatric oncology and hematology; Pharmacy oncology; Psycho-oncology; Radiation oncology; Surgical oncology; Urologic oncology; Veterinary oncology; Viral oncology.

▶ Oncology clinical nurse specialist

Category: Medical specialties
Also known as: Oncology nurse specialist, cancer nurse specialist, advanced practice oncology nurse specialist

Definition: An oncology clinical nurse specialist is a registered nurse who has a master's degree and extensive training to provide specialized consultation and care for cancer patients and families.

Subspecialties: The oncology nurse clinical specialist may choose to specialize in a particular cancer practice working with a selected population of patients. Examples of specialties include medical hematology oncology, hematology oncology, outpatient radiation, outpatient hematology oncology, outpatient pediatric oncology, and palliative care.

Cancers treated: Depends on area of specialty

Training and certification: The oncology clinical nurse specialist completes a bachelor's degree in nursing and a master's degree in nursing with appropriate clinical practicum from an accredited graduate nursing program. Education programs will vary, but the master's degree generally takes about two years to complete and requires at least five hundred hours of clinical practicum. Required courses for a master's degree vary from school to school. Courses included in these programs are advanced physiology and cancer pathophysiology, pharmacology, cancer genomics, epidemiology, disease and symptom management, palliative care, nursing research, nursing and medical ethics, public policy, leadership, health care financing, health program planning and evaluation, technology use, and advanced nursing concepts. Practicum hours are usually accrued in the nurse's chosen specialty.

Additional training and skills necessary to effectively practice in the role of oncology clinical nurse specialist include crisis management, in-depth knowledge of the chosen clinical cancer specialty, maturity to take responsibility for patients' lives, understanding of medical ethics, teaching proficiency, and expertise in interpersonal relations to work with the patient, caregivers, and multidisciplinary health care team. Oncology clinical nurse specialists must have valid nursing licenses issued by the boards of nursing in their states.

In some states, oncology clinical nurse specialists must also receive certification by successfully completing examinations in their specialty. In other states, attaining certification status is voluntary. Proficiency is validated through examination based on predetermined standards and given by a nongovernment agency. The Oncology Nursing Certification Corporation provides several different certifications for nurses working with cancer patients. The Advanced Oncology Certified Clinical Nurse Specialist (AOCNS) certification examination is available to professional nurses who hold a current, active license that is nonrestricted, have completed a master's degree or higher from an accredited school of nursing, and have completed a minimum of five hundred hours of supervised clinical practice in oncology nursing. Documentation of the supervised clinical practicum hours is required and verified before certification is granted. AOCNS certification is valid for four years. The AOCNS nurse can renew certification by earning 125 points (at least 75 in oncology nursing) through activities such as continued academic education, nursing continuing education, publication, precepting, presentation, or volunteer service.

Services and procedures performed: Oncology clinical nurse specialists can work in a variety of settings, including hospitals (acute care), clinics, long-term care or elder care homes, home care or hospice agencies, and private and joint practices. They can also work as consultants. The oncology clinical nurse specialist recognizes and values the expanding and evolving nature of cancer care and remains current with complex services, procedures, and treatments. The services and procedures performed depend on the setting and function of the nurse's specific role.

Some oncology clinical nurse specialists work as clinicians and provide direct care for patients and caregivers. They often work alongside other health care professionals such as physicians, nurses, and therapists to plan and evaluate patient care. These nurse specialists schedule and coordinate diagnostic and therapeutic procedures or tests for oncology patients. They will monitor the test results and revise the cancer patient's care plan based on individual and changing needs. At a cancer care clinic or oncology hospital unit, the oncology clinical nurse specialist may perform the initial admission assessment for new patients and develop the plan of care. This nurse will monitor the plan of care and make adjustments as indicated for the individual cancer patient. The nurse assists with discharge planning to include referrals for other community resources or establish follow-up appointments to physicians' offices or cancer care clinics.

Oncology clinical nurse specialists often function as teachers. In clinical settings, these nurses keep abreast of current research and new therapies. They use their expanded knowledge of cancer and cancer treatment to teach new concepts or treatment modalities to staff members and members of the multidisciplinary health care planning team. In the hospital cancer unit or cancer care clinic, oncology clinical nurse specialists help assess current staff education, develop new educational strategies, coordinate educational agendas, and revise teaching programs. Educational programs are provided as in-service programs or as clinical practicums. They serve as advisers to staff and other professionals. The goal of this education is to organize and implement an educational strategy that trains professional caregivers to provide the best possible cancer care for patients and their caregivers.

Cancer care education is critical for the cancer patient, family, and caregivers to live life to the fullest. The oncology clinical nurse specialist builds a relationship with the cancer patient and caregivers and provides individualized patient teaching. Cancer patients need accurate and up-to-date information about their disease and treatment options to make decisions about their care. The highly educated and informed oncology clinical nurse specialist is often the person who spends time with the patient and family, teaching them necessary components of self-care and disease management. Even after discharge from the hospital cancer care unit, the patient and caregivers may contact the oncology clinical nurse specialist with questions and concerns. The positive relationship developed during hospitalization often carries over to the home setting as the oncology clinical nurse specialist fills the role of consultant and educator.

Administrative functions are sometimes part of the services delivered by oncology clinical nurse specialists. They monitor the medication regimen of the cancer patient and suggest changes when needed for improved patient outcomes. Sometimes they manage the research protocol as primary investigator for grants and clinical studies. Oncology clinical nurse specialists are stewards in fiscal management of resources by keeping an eye on cancer care costs, noting where services can be delivered more efficiently.

Related specialties and subspecialties: Oncology clinical nurse specialists can work in a number of subspecialties depending on their interests and the positions available in the nurses' area. Roles are evolving and diverse, as the oncology nurse clinical specialist contributes many skills to the health care team. Some assume administrative roles and perform in high levels of leadership within the cancer care settings. For example, oncology clinical nurse specialists can become nurse managers over specialized hospital oncology units or serve as directors of community cancer care centers, or they might become health care administrators for managed care or insurance companies and consult with key decision makers about covered services for cancer care patients.

Oncology clinical nurse specialists can pursue further education and receive a doctorate degree in various academic fields. One example is the oncology clinical nurse specialist who completes a doctorate and enters the field of cancer research. Another nurse might earn a doctorate in nursing science or a doctorate in education and join a university graduate faculty to teach others to become oncology clinical nurse specialists. As faculty, these nurses can work as consultants and mentors to undergraduate nursing students to help them become proficient in cancer care. Some pursue additional education to function in the dual role of oncology clinical nurse specialist and nurse practitioner. Still others assume an entrepreneurial spirit and use their knowledge and skills in creative and innovative private and joint practice.

Marylane Wade Koch, M.S.N., R.N.

▶ For Further Information

Carper, E., and M. Hass. "Advanced Practice Nursing in Radiation Oncology." *Seminars in Oncology Nursing* 22, no. 4 (November, 2006): 203-211.

Skilbeck, J., and S. Payne. "Emotional Support and the Role of Clinical Nurse Specialists in Palliative Care." *Journal of Advanced Nursing* 43, no. 2 (September, 2003): 521-530.

Zuzelo, Patti R. *Clinical Nurse Specialist Handbook.* Sudbury, Mass.: Jones and Bartlett, 2007.

▶ Organizations and Professional Societies

National Association of Clinical Nurse Specialists
http://www.nacns.org
2090 Linglestown Road, Suite 107
Harrisburg, PA 17110

Oncology Nursing Certification Corporation
http://www.oncc.org/publications/options.shtml
125 Enterprise Drive
Pittsburgh, PA 15275

Oncology Nursing Society
http://www.ons.org
125 Enterprise Drive
Pittsburgh, PA 15275

See also Cancer care team; Counseling for cancer patients and survivors; Dermatology oncology; Endocrinology oncology; Ewing sarcoma; Gastrointestinal oncology; Gynecologic oncology; Hematologic oncology; Medical oncology; Neurologic oncology; Pediatric oncology and hematology; Radiation oncology.

▶ Oncology social worker

Category: Medical specialties
Also known as: Cancer social worker, certified social worker in health care, C-SWHC

Definition: Oncology social workers provide psychosocial support, emotional counseling, and referrals for cancer patients and their caregivers.

Subspecialties: Oncology social workers may support patients with diverse types of cancer or specialize in the care of patients with a certain type of cancer. An example is a social worker who is employed in a setting dedicated to women's cancers, such as breast, ovarian, or uterine cancers. Specialization may also be based on the age of the patients such as pediatric oncology.

Cancers treated: Depends on the social worker's specialization

Training and certification: An oncology social worker is a medical social worker with a master's in social work (MSW). This program generally requires two years of course study and about nine hundred hours of supervised clinical work. Classes include subjects such as human growth and development, social research, social policy, and methods of practice. Licensure varies from state to state. Oncology social workers receive cancer care training through continuing education, in-service education courses, and on-the-job training. Certification is voluntary through the National Association of Social Workers (certified social worker in health care, or C-SWHC).

Services and procedures performed: Oncology social workers serve a key role in the multidisciplinary cancer care team. They provide support and referral services tailored to the needs of cancer patients and caregivers. Oncology social workers are the liaison between the cancer patient and the health care system. They support the cancer patients as whole human beings with diverse roles in their daily lives.

Some of the support services oncology social workers can provide are as follows:

- Help the patient understand the cancer diagnosis and deal with the emotional aspects
- Provide case management and discharge planning
- Maximize insurance coverage
- Mobilize community services
- Access financial resources for equipment, medications, and support services
- Assist in applying for disability and social security benefits

• Make important referrals to community agencies and support groups

Related specialties and subspecialties: Oncology social workers practice in many settings. Hospitals that provide cancer care services usually employ oncology social workers. Freestanding cancer care centers, clinics, and oncology physician offices may provide oncology social workers for their patients and caregivers. Hospice services use oncology social workers in their residential or home care services. Nursing homes may contract with an oncology social worker to assist patients and families.

Marylane Wade Koch, M.S.N., R.N.

See also Cancer care team; Case management; Counseling for cancer patients and survivors; Family history and risk assessment; Gastrointestinal oncology; Hematologic oncology; Home health services; Medical oncology; Medicare and cancer; Oncology; Otolaryngology; Palliative treatment; Pediatric oncology and hematology; Psycho-oncology; Throat cancer; Transitional care.

▶ Oophorectomy

Category: Procedures
Also known as: Ovariotomy, ovariectomy, bilateral oophorectomy, preventive or prophylactic bilateral oophorectomy (PBO), prophylactic oophorectomy, laparoscopic oophorectomy

Definition: Oophorectomy is the surgical removal of both ovaries as a treatment for ovarian cancer or metastasized cancer. The two ovaries are the part of the female reproductive system that produces egg cells (ova) and releases hormones, including estrogen. Both ovaries may be removed as a preventive measure for women with a high risk of ovarian cancer or breast cancer. Oophorectomy may be used for patients with estrogen-sensitive breast cancer to prevent its recurrence.

Cancers treated: Ovarian cancer, metastasized cancer, preventive treatment for patients at high risk for ovarian or breast cancer, treatment for estrogen-sensitive breast cancer

Why performed: Both ovaries are removed with an oophorectomy to help treat ovarian cancer. Most ovarian cancers develop in the epithelial cells that cover the outside of the ovary. Ovarian cancer can also develop in the germ cells (the cells that produce eggs) or in the stromal cells (the cells inside of the ovary that produce estrogen and progesterone).

Ovarian cancer can spread to other parts of the body. Other parts of the female reproductive system such as the Fallopian tubes, which transport eggs to the uterus for fertilization, may be removed in a surgery termed a bilateral salpingo-oophorectomy. Oophorectomy is used to treat metastasized cancer that originated elsewhere in the body and has spread to the ovaries.

Women with the *BRCA1* or *BRCA2* gene mutations have a high risk for breast cancer and gynecologic cancer. A preventive bilateral oophorectomy (PBO) is used to remove both ovaries of women with a family history and high risk of ovarian cancer. A PBO is usually performed after a woman has experienced childbirth or at about the age of thirty-five. Research has shown that PBO does reduce the risk of ovarian cancer for high-risk women.

Research shows that PBO before the age of forty can significantly reduce the risk of breast cancer for women with the *BRCA1* or *BRCA2* gene mutations. Oophorectomy may also be used as a preventive treatment for premenopausal women with estrogen-sensitive breast cancer. Removing both ovaries removes the main source of estrogen in the body and can help to prevent estrogen-sensitive cancer cells from growing.

Patient preparation: Patients receive laboratory and blood tests prior to surgery. X rays or ultrasound images may be taken to help plan the procedure. Patients should eat a light dinner and not eat or drink after midnight on the day prior to the surgery. In some cases, preparations may be used to empty the colon.

Steps of the procedure: Oophorectomy for the treatment of cancer uses general anesthesia and an open surgical method. A vertical incision is made on the abdomen. The abdominal muscles are spread apart to allow the surgeon access to the ovaries. The vertical incision allows the surgeon to view the abdominal cavity for disease or cancer. After both ovaries are removed, the incision is closed and bandaged.

A horizontal incision may be used to remove both ovaries if cancer is not present. A horizontal incision is associated with less scarring and bleeding. A laparoscopic oophorectomy may also be used if cancer is not present, in cases of preventive surgery.

Laparoscopic oophorectomy is guided by images produced by a laparoscope, a narrow tube with a light, viewing instrument, and miniature camera. The laparoscope is inserted through small incisions in the abdomen. Surgical instruments are inserted through the laparoscope to remove the ovaries. Because laparoscopic surgery is minimally invasive and uses only small incisions, it is associated with less pain, less bleeding, fewer complications or infections, a shorter hospital stay, and a quicker recovery time.

After the procedure: The patient remains in the hospital for three to five days and returns to regular activity levels in about six weeks. Patients receiving open surgery may experience discomfort from having the abdominal muscles moved during the procedure. Patients receiving laparoscopic surgery may remain in the hospital for a night or two and resume regular activities sooner.

Patients who have both ovaries removed are no longer able to become pregnant and therefore experience "surgical menopause." Those without cancer may receive hormones to help ease the risk of medical complications and menopausal symptoms. Symptoms of menopause may be greater in women experiencing surgical menopause than in women with naturally occurring menopause.

Patients with ovarian cancer usually receive chemotherapy following oophorectomy. Chemotherapy uses medication, or a combination of medications, delivered over a period of time to help kill any remaining cancer cells. Radiation therapy is rarely used.

Risks: The surgical risks of oophorectomy include infection, bleeding, blood clots, and damage to other organs. Some women experience decreased sex drive and decreased orgasm. Bilateral oophorectomy increases the risk of cardiovascular disease, osteoporosis, and thyroid cancer. Hormone therapy can help reduce the risk.

Results: Normal results are removal of both ovaries without complications and no findings of cancer. Abnormal results include removal of both ovaries with findings of cancer, metastasized spread, or complications.

Mary Car-Blanchard, O.T.D., B.S.O.T.

▶ For Further Information

Fader, A. N., and R. G. Rose. "Role of Surgery in Ovarian Carcinoma." *Journal of Clinical Oncology* 25, no. 20 (July 10, 2007): 2873-2883.

Kauff, N. D., and R. R. Barakat. "Risk-Reducing Salpingo-oophorectomy in Patients with Germline Mutations in *BRCA1* or *BRCA2*." *Journal of Clinical Oncology* 25, no. 20 (July 10, 2007): 2921-2927.

Parker, W. H., et al. "Elective Oophorectomy in the Gynecological Patient: When Is It Desirable?" *Current Opinion in Obstetrics and Gynecology* 19, no. 4 (August, 2007): 350-354.

See also *BRCA1* and *BRCA2* genes; Breast cancers; Fallopian tube cancer; Gynecologic oncology; Hormonal therapies; Hot flashes; Hysterectomy; Hystero-oophorectomy; Salpingectomy and salpingo-oophorectomy.

▶ Ophthalmic oncology

Category: Medical specialties
Also known as: Cancer of the eyes

Definition: Ophthalmic oncology is a medical specialty that deals with the diagnosis and treatment of cancers of the eye.

Subspecialties: Ophthalmic oncologists often specialize in one particular type of cancer, such as retinoblastoma or intraocular melanoma.

Cancers treated: Intraocular melanoma (sometimes called uveal melanoma), primary intraocular lymphoma, retinoblastoma, medulloepithelioma

Training and certification: Training to be an ophthalmic oncologist requires many years of specialized medical training. After receiving a medical degree from an accredited school, ophthalmic oncologists then complete a residency program. This residency is usually in ophthalmology, although during this time the individual will also often receive training in surgery and oncology.

After successful completion of a residency program, the individual can apply to be board certified in ophthalmology. Board certification is a long and difficult process that requires at least one and one-half years to two years to complete. Candidates for board certification must apply to take the first test. Candidates whose applications are approved are allowed to take a five-hour written exam. Those candidates who pass are invited to take an extensive oral exam. Only after successful completion of all these steps is the candidate board certified. The individual must take extensive ongoing steps to retain board certification. Board certifications completed after 1992 must be renewed every ten years.

During the board-certification process and afterward, most ophthalmic oncologists complete one or more additional fellowships or other training programs. These fellowships last one or more years and provide the doctor additional training and expertise in the chosen field. Often these fellowships are very specialized.

Ophthalmic oncologists often receive training during their residencies, fellowships, training programs, or at other times in research and clinical trials. Research is continuously being conducted to develop new methods, procedures, and drugs to help with the diagnosis and treatment of cancers of the eye. Clinical trials are experiments designed to determine the effectiveness and safety of newly developed procedures, methods, drugs, and other treatments that have not yet been accepted into common practice. Individuals who have cancer may be asked by

The Anatomy of the Human Eye

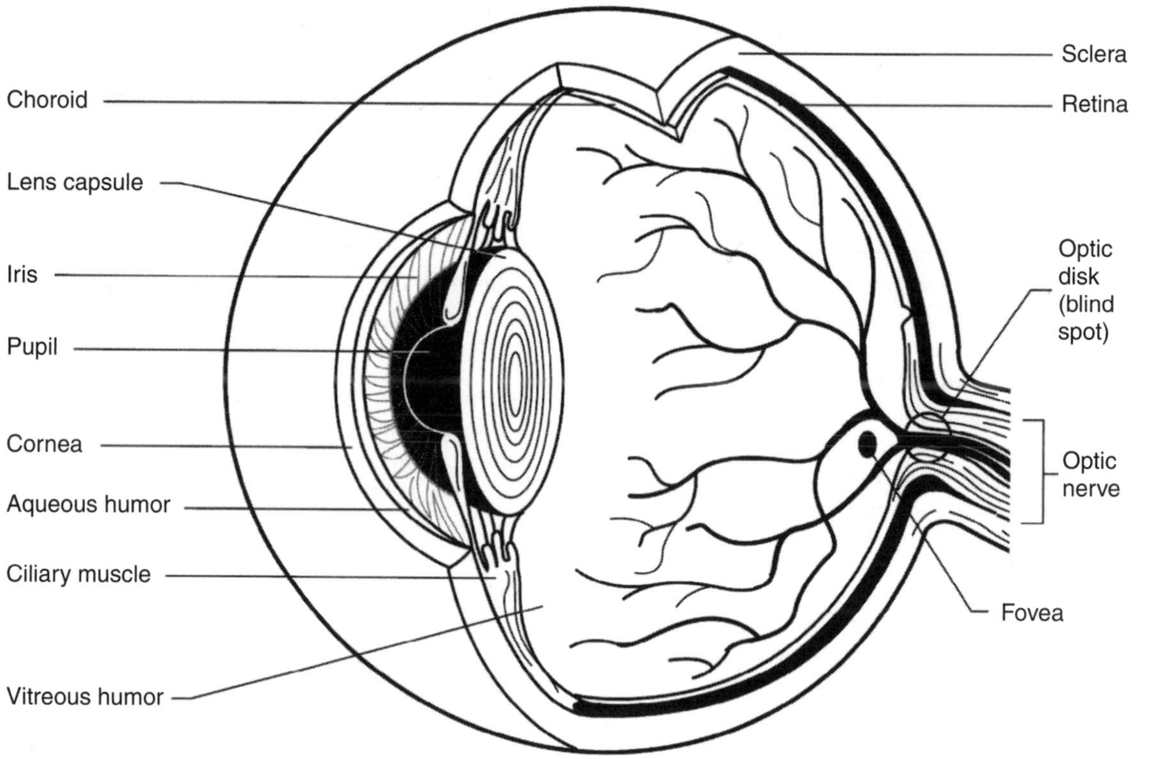

their oncologist or other doctor if they wish to participate in a clinical trial. Clinical trials have varying possible risks and benefits, and the decision of whether to participate should be discussed carefully with the cancer care team.

Services and procedures performed: Cancers of the eye are relatively rare. According to the American Cancer Society, about 2,340 people were likely to be newly diagnosed with primary eye cancer in 2007. Most of these eye cancers are intraocular melanomas. Many ophthalmic oncologists specialize in treating only one type of eye cancer or in a certain type of treatment.

Before ophthalmic oncologists can begin to treat an eye cancer, they must determine that the eye cancer does in fact exist and, if so, what type of cancer it is. A patient may be referred to an ophthalmic oncologist because of a suspicious finding during a routine vision screening or because of a visit to a primary care physician with symptoms that indicate a possible eye cancer.

To diagnose eye cancer, the ophthalmic oncologist will use a specialized tool called an ophthalmoscope that allows the doctor to look inside the patient's eye. The ophthalmic oncologist will look for any abnormalities inside the eye such as spots, discoloration of the pupil, or cloudiness of the gel inside the eye. The ophthalmic oncologist will also ask the patient about any signs or symptoms, such as pain, problems with vision, seeing flashes of light or floating spots that are not really there, or other abnormalities. The ophthalmic oncologist may also examine the eye to see if there are any problems such as the eyeball moving abnormally, bulging, or seeming out of place.

In many cases, further diagnostic procedures are necessary. In some cases a biopsy of the suspected tumor may be done, although this is often avoided if possible because performing a biopsy has some risk of damaging the eye. Technology such as an ultrasound, computed tomography (CT) scan or magnetic resonance imaging (MRI) may also be performed to help the ophthalmic oncologist get a better picture of the eye. Additional scans or tests may be done to determine if the cancer has spread outside the eye.

Once the cancer has been diagnosed, the ophthalmic oncologist will work with the patient and the health care team to develop a plan of treatment. The four main types of treatment for eye cancers are surgery, radiation therapy, laser therapy, and chemotherapy. New technologies and procedures are being developed all the time, and different treatments are appropriate for different types and stages of eye cancer.

Surgery is often the treatment of choice for eye cancers. During the procedure, the ophthalmic oncologist will remove the cancerous area. In some cases vision out of the affected eye will still be possible after the surgery, and in others it may be diminished or gone altogether. In very severe cases the best option may be to remove the cancerous eye completely and replace it with a prosthetic.

Radiation therapy and chemotherapy are used to treat many forms of eye cancer. Radiation therapy is targeted as specifically as possible so that it affects as little of the healthy area of the eye as possible. Chemotherapy is not specifically targeted to an area of the eye but instead is put into the blood intravenously or is given by mouth. The chemotherapy drugs then travel in the bloodstream to the eye.

The fourth type of treatment that some ophthalmic oncologists use is laser therapy. The laser may use infrared light or a high-energy light beam to kill the cancer cells. One positive aspect of laser therapies is that lasers can be focused into a very thin beam of light that allows a high degree of accuracy, generally affecting fewer of the surrounding cells than other treatment methods.

After the cancer has been successfully treated, many patients return regularly to see their ophthalmic oncologist to check for any side effects and to ensure that the cancer has not returned.

Related specialties and subspecialties: There are many doctors and other health care team members who assist or work closely with an ophthalmic oncologist. An ophthalmologist is a doctor who specializes in the diagnosis and treatment of eye diseases and conditions. This can include things as diverse as eye surgery or prescribing corrective lenses. It is important for people to visit an ophthalmologist regularly for vision screening and a general checkup of their eye health. It is during this kind of routine screening that many eye problems, including cancer of the eye, are first suspected or diagnosed.

There are many other members of the allied health professions who may be part of the cancer care team for someone with eye cancer. The specific individuals who will work with the ophthalmic oncologist will differ depending on the kind of cancer and the type of treatment. The team may include specialists in administering radiation or chemotherapy, nutritionists, medical technologists, and nurses specializing in the care and treatment of cancer patients. The ophthalmic oncologist may also be called on to be part of a larger oncology team involving oncologists who specialize in cancer of other areas of the body if the cancer has metastasized from another area of the body to the eye.

Helen Davidson, B.A.

▶ For Further Information

Albert, Daniel M., and Arthur Polans, eds. *Ocular Oncology*. New York: Marcel Dekker, 2003.

Denniston, Alastair K. O., and Phillip I. Murray. *Oxford Handbook of Ophthalmology*. New York: Oxford University Press, 2006.

Shields, Jerry A., and Carol L. Shields. *Intraocular Tumors: Atlas and Textbook,* 2d ed. Philadelphia: Lippincott Williams & Wilkins, 2008.

▶ Organizations and Professional Societies

American Board of Ophthalmology
http://www.abop.org/index1.asp
111 Presidential Boulevard, Suite 241
Bala Cynwyd, PA 19004-1075

International Council of Ophthalmology
http://www.icoph.org
945 Green Street
San Francisco, CA 94133

European Organization for Research and Treatment of Cancer
http://www.helsinki.fi/laak/silk/oog
Ophthalmic Oncology Group
Avenue Mounierlaan, 83/11
Brussel 1200 Bruxelles, Belgium

▶ Other Resources

Eye Cancer Network
http://eyecancer.com

Retinoblastoma International
http://www.retinoblastoma.net

See also Eye cancers; Eyelid cancer; Gonioscopy; Lacrimal gland tumors; Neurofibromatosis type 1 (NF1); Orbit tumors; Retinoblastomas; Rothmund-Thomson syndrome; Sjögren syndrome.

▶ Opioids

Category: Chemotherapy and other drugs
Also known as: Narcotics

Definition: Opioids are controlled drugs prescribed for the management of moderate to severe pain. Opioids include natural alkaloids (opiates) such as morphine and codeine, which are extracted from the seedpod of the poppy plant, as well as semisynthetic derivatives and fully synthetic forms.

ATC code: N02A

Cancers treated: Various

Subclasses of this group: Phenanthrenes, phenylpiperidines, diphenylheptanes, benzomorphans

Delivery routes: Oral administration is preferred because it is the least invasive and least costly route. If a patient has difficulty swallowing or suffers from nausea or vomiting, then other options may include rectal, transdermal, and transmucosal administration or injection under the skin or into the vein or spinal area. Patient-controlled access pumps that deliver opioids to these areas are also available. Opioids are produced in both long-acting and immediate-release forms and are often used with other pain medications for enhanced analgesia.

How these drugs work: Opioids mimic the body's natural painkillers (for example, endorphins) by binding to receptors on the surfaces of cells in the central nervous system and gastrointestinal tract. Full agonists, the largest group of opioids, stimulate the receptors, blocking the release of neurotransmitters and interfering with the transmission of pain signals to the brain. They also alter the perception of pain. Partial agonists produce weaker effects and may also block the analgesic action of other opioids.

Side effects: Adverse events are common across opioids and include sedation, nausea and vomiting, constipation, respiratory depression, dry mouth, itching, sexual dysfunction, and urinary retention. Because of the wealth of opioid receptor sites in the central nervous system, cognitive effects such as hallucinations, euphoria, and depression may also occur. Tolerance and physical dependence may develop, although psychological addiction is rarely associated with opioid use by cancer patients.

Judy Majewski, M.S.

See also Acupuncture and acupressure for cancer patients; Bone pain; Breakthrough pain; Brief Pain Inventory (BPI); Brompton cocktail; Cordotomy; Do-not-resuscitate (DNR) order; End-of-life care; Hospice care; Medical marijuana; Nonsteroidal anti-inflammatory drugs (NSAIDs); Pain management medications; Palliative treatment.

Common Opioids

Drug	*Brands*	*Subclass*	*Delivery Mode*
Codeine	Tylenol Codeine, Empirin	Phenanthrenes	Oral
Fentanyl	Actiq, Duragesic, Fentora, Sublimaze	Phenylpiperidines	Oral, transmucosal, buccal, transdermal
Hydrocodone	Vicodin, Vicodin ES, Norco, Lorcet, Anexsia	Phenanthrenes	Oral
Hydromorphone	Dilaudid, Hydrostat	Phenanthrenes	Oral, rectal, IV, subcutaneous
Levorphanol	Levo-Dromoran	Phenanthrenes	Oral, IV, subcutaneous
Methadone	Dolophine, Methadose	Diphenylheptanes	Oral, rectal, IV, subcutaneous
Morphine	MS Contin, Avinza, MSIR, Duramorph, Roxanol IR, Kadian, Oramorph SR	Phenanthrenes	Oral, IV, epidural, intrathecal, intraventricular
Oxycodone	Oxycontin, OxyIR, OxyNorm, Percocet, Percodan, Roxicodone	Phenanthrenes	Oral
Oxymorphone	Numorphan, Opana, Opana ER	Phenanthrenes	Oral, rectal, IV, subcutaneous

▶ Oral and maxillofacial surgery

Category: Procedures
Also known as: Mouth surgery, maxillectomy, laryngectomy, neck dissection

Definition: Oral surgery and maxillofacial surgery are general terms for surgery of the mouth (oral) and of the upper jaw and face (maxillofacial). Specially trained dentists, known as oral and maxillofacial surgeons, perform this type of surgery. Otorhinolaryngologists (ear, nose, and throat specialists) also perform certain oral and maxillofacial surgeries, as do cosmetic, or plastic, surgeons. Surgeons use oral and maxillofacial surgery to treat a wide range of injuries, defects, and diseases.

Cancers treated: Oral or mouth cancer, including cancer of the lips, mouth, gums, salivary glands, tongue, face, neck, jaws, and hard and soft palates (roof of the mouth)

Why performed: In treating cancer, doctors use oral and maxillofacial surgery most often to destroy or remove cancerous tumors. In some cases, doctors use oral and maxillofacial surgery to repair or reconstruct parts of the jaw and other boney structures of the face and throat to help patients speak or swallow better, or to restore a patient's appearance following surgery or an injury.

Patient preparation: What happens before oral and maxillofacial surgery to remove or destroy a tumor depends on its location. Patients who are undernourished because chewing or swallowing is difficult, owing to the site of the tumor, receive fluids intravenously to build up their strength before the operation. Generally, patients are instructed not to eat or drink anything eight hours before the procedure. Because various general and local anesthetics are used during the surgery, patients should inform their doctors of substances to which they are allergic. Surgeons sometimes perform oral and maxillofacial surgery in an operatory, so patients need to arrange for a ride home after the procedure. Nurses help hospital patients prepare for their surgery.

Steps of the procedure: Because tumors can develop in so many sites in the mouth and face, and because surgeons may either destroy or remove the tumor, surgical procedures vary widely. For example, surgeons remove early-stage tumors of the tongue with a laser instrument operated directly through the mouth. In cases where the cancer has spread to the neck lymph nodes, a common occurrence, surgeons remove the affected lymph nodes, a procedure know as a neck dissection. Following this primary surgery, surgeons may have to perform additional operations to restore normal function to the patient's neck, shoulder, or other nearby parts of the body. In some cases, surgeons perform secondary surgery to restore nerve function. In many cases, oral and maxillofacial surgery disfigures the patient's face or neck. When that happens, surgeons perform restorative, or reconstructive, surgery to restore the patient's appearance. Such secondary surgery includes the use of tissue flaps to restore soft tissue, skin grafts, bone grafts, and prostheses (metal or plastic parts to replace original body parts).

Whatever the type of surgery, patients receive, as needed, a combination of anesthetics, medicines that put the patient to sleep, relax the patient, and block pain.

After the procedure: Following surgery, care varies for each patient depending on the type of surgery and the location and extent of the cancer. Some patients may return home several hours after surgery. Others may have to stay in the hospital for several days. Postoperative care and rehabilitation may include additional surgery, speech therapy, dietary guidance, and psychological counseling.

Risks: The risks from oral and maxillofacial surgery include harmful reactions to anesthetics and medications, wound infection, excessive bleeding, and slow healing, which are common to most surgeries. More specifically, oral and maxillofacial surgery can adversely affect a variety of body functions, including speaking, chewing, swallowing, and controlling the flow of saliva. These risks depend on the size and location of the tumor. Sometimes when destroying or removing a tumor, surgeons destroy or remove surrounding tissue or structures in the mouth. In addition, some patients disfigured by oral and maxillofacial surgery experience psychological problems because of the change in their appearance. Coupled with a severe illness or aggressive treatment, a changed look creates mental and social problems for some patients.

Results: Typically, the earlier oral cancer is detected and treated, the better the chances of survival. When a tumor is destroyed or removed in the early stages of the cancer and the cancer has not spread, the five-year relative survival rate for patients is about 81 percent; the five-year relative survival rate for all stages of oral cancer is about 59 percent, according to the American Cancer Society. This does not mean, however, that five-year survivors are cancer-free or that the cancer will not reappear.

Wendell Anderson, B.A.

▶ For Further Information

Hupp, James R., Edward Ellis, and Myron R. Tucker. *Contemporary Oral and Maxillofacial Surgery.* 5th ed. Philadelphia: Elsevier Health Sciences, 2008.

Parker, James N., and Philip M. Parker, eds. *The Official Patient's Sourcebook on Lip and Oral Cavity Cancer.* San Diego, Calif.: Icon Health, 2005.

Wray, David, et al. eds. *Textbook of General and Oral Surgery.* New York: Churchill Livingstone, 2003.

▶ **Other Resources**

American Association of Oral and Maxillofacial Surgeons
http://www.aaoms.org

Oral Cancer Foundation
http://www.oralcancerfoundation.org

See also Cordectomy; Electrolarynx; Erythroplakia; Esophageal speech; Glossectomy; Laryngeal cancer; Laryngectomy; Oral and oropharyngeal cancers; Throat cancer.

▶ Oral and oropharyngeal cancers

Category: Diseases, symptoms, and conditions
Also known as: Mouth cancer, tongue cancer, salivary gland cancer, gum cancer, throat (instead of oropharyngeal) cancer

Related conditions: Neck cancer, esophageal cancer

Definition: Oral cancer is a collective term that encompasses cancers of the lips, mouth, tongue, gums, and salivary glands. Oral cancers mostly occur on the lips, tongue, or floor of the mouth but may also occur inside the cheeks, in the gums, or on the roof of the mouth. The oropharynx or throat is situated between the soft palate and the hyoid bone. The top of the oropharynx connects with the oral cavity and, further up, with the nasopharynx. The bottom of the oropharynx connects with the supraglottic larynx and the hypopharynx. The oropharynx consists of the base of the tongue (including the pharyngoepiglottic folds and the glossoepiglottic folds), the tonsillar region, the soft palate (including the uvula), and the pharyngeal walls. Practically all oral and oropharyngeal cancers are squamous cell carcinomas (SCCs), which refer to cancers that originate in squamous cells.

Because the lymphatic system is one of the major ways that tumors spread or metastasize to other organs, knowledge of the location of lymph nodes in this area is crucial for understanding oral and oropharyngeal cancer. The lymph nodes that supply the head and neck run parallel to the jugular veins and can be classified into five levels: Level I, which refers to the submental and submandibular lymph nodes; Level II, which includes the upper jugular lymph nodes; Level III, which refers to the mid-jugular lymph nodes; Level IV, containing the lower jugular lymph nodes; and Level V, which refers to the lymph nodes of the posterior triangle.

Risk factors: Risk factors include cigarette smoking, chewing tobacco, excessive alcohol intake, extensive exposure to ultraviolet light, denture irritation, leukoplakia (white spots on the tongue or inside the cheeks), erythroplakia (red patches inside the mouth that bleed readily when bruised), and infection with human papillomavirus (HPV). Infection with HPV has been linked to one in five oral cancers. One study conducted at the Johns Hopkins University concluded that HPV infection is a stronger risk factor for oropharyngeal squamous cell carcinoma than tobacco and alcohol use. Gastroesophageal reflux disease (GERD), in which stomach acids enter the esophagus and destroy the esophageal lining, also contributes to the risk of throat cancer.

Etiology and the disease process: Oral and oropharyngeal cancers appear to be caused by deoxyribonucleic acid (DNA) damage in the cells in the mouth and throat. This DNA damage can occur from exposure to too much ultraviolet light from the sun, or from cigarette smoking, tobacco chewing, or excessive alcohol intake. Most oral

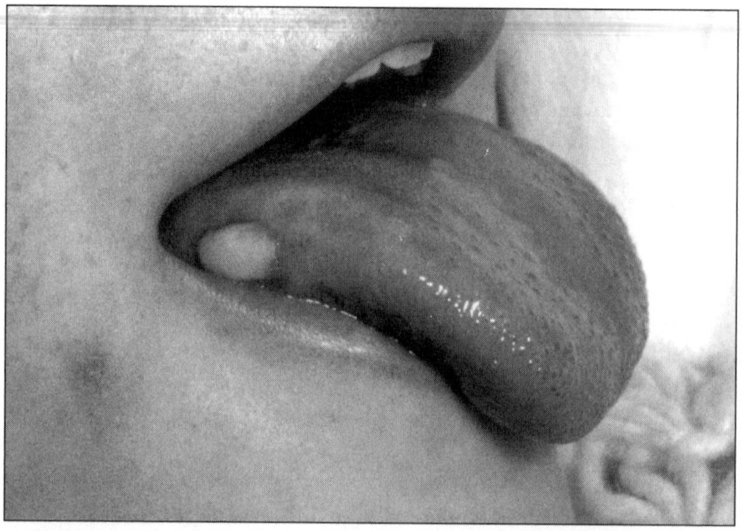

A malignant tumor of the edge of a tongue. (John Radcliffe Hospital/Photo Researchers, Inc.)

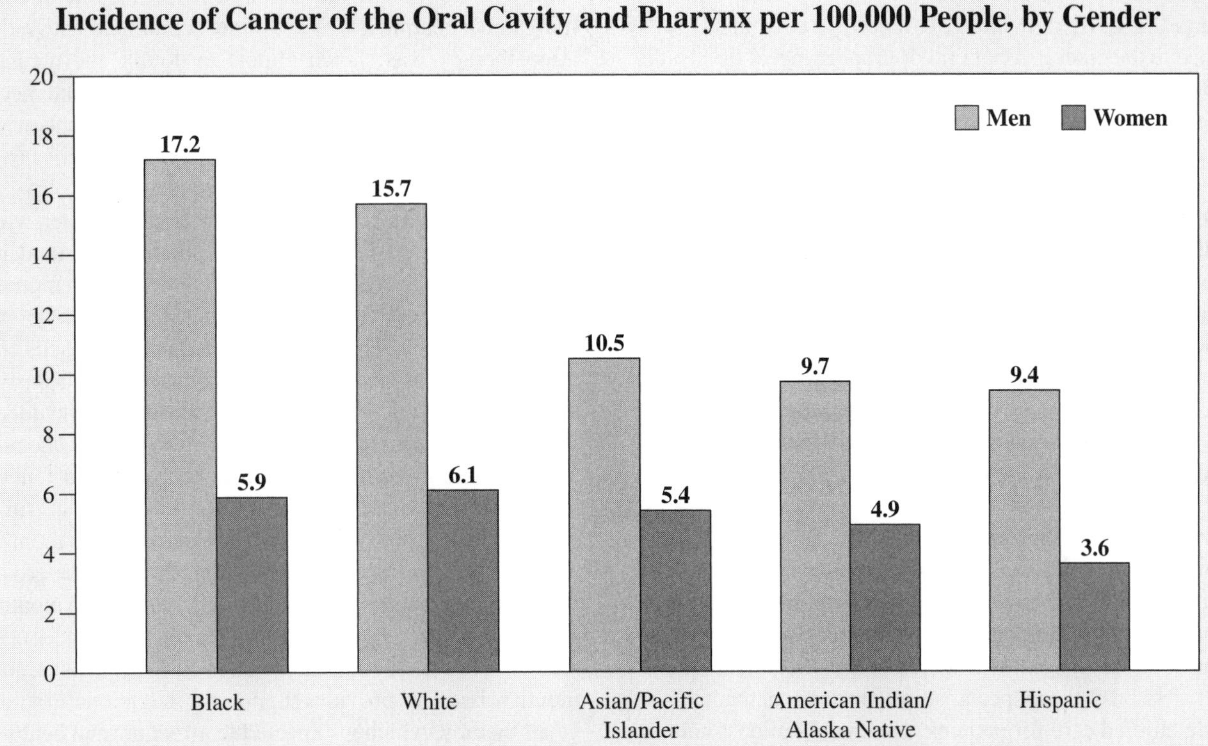

Source: Data from National Cancer Institute, Surveillance Epidemiology and End Results, Cancer Stat Fact Sheets, 2008
Note: Based on cases diagnosed in 2000-2004

and oropharyngeal cancers are carcinomas of the squamous cells, the flat cells that make up the mucosal epithelium, the layer of cells lining the inside of the mouth, nose, larynx, and throat. Less common are lymphomas, lymphoepitheliomas, and minor salivary gland carcinomas. A rare type of oral cancer is verrucous carcinoma, which usually does not metastasize but can penetrate deeply into nearby tissue.

Incidence: According to the American Cancer Society, there are approximately 30,990 new cases of oral and oropharyngeal cancer annually in the United States, with an estimated 7,430 deaths from oral and oropharyngeal cancer each year. The incidence is higher in men than in women. Oropharyngeal cancer is still a relatively rare type of cancer, and both oral and oropharyngeal cancer rates have been decreasing since 1975 in the United States.

Symptoms: Symptoms of oral and oropharyngeal cancer include lumps of white, red, or dark patches inside the mouth that do not recede with time, mouth sores that do not heal or that enlarge over time, lumps in the neck, persistent pain in the mouth, thickening of the cheek, swelling or pain in the jaw, soreness in the throat or a feeling that something is caught in the throat, difficulty chewing or moving the tongue (late-stage symptom), difficulty moving the jaw (late-stage symptom), pain around the teeth, loosening of the teeth, numbness of the tongue or mouth, and changes in the voice.

Screening and diagnosis: Frequent oral examinations are the best way to detect signs of oral and throat cancer. When a tumor is detected, it is graded or staged to determine how benign or aggressive it is. The TNM (tumor/lymph node/metastasis) staging system is a standard way of classifying tumors. T stands for the size of the primary tumor and which tissues of the oral cavity or oropharynx the tumor has spread to, if any. N refers to the extent of spread to regional lymph nodes. M is used to denote whether the tumor has metastasized to other organs. The most common metastatic site is the lungs, followed by the liver and the bones. Within each of these designations, there are several subcategories.

Following TNM staging, the tumor is classified as Stage 0, I, II, III, or IV. Stage 0 refers to a tumor that is confined to the outer layer of oral or oropharyngeal tissue and has not penetrated deeper or metastasized. Stage I tumors are 2 centimeters (cm) or smaller in diameter and have not metastasized. Stage II tumors are between 2 cm and 4 cm in diameter and have not metastasized. Stage III tumors are larger than 4 cm in diameter and have not metastasized, although they may have invaded one of the nearby lymph nodes. Stage IV is further divided into three substages: Stage IVA, in which tumors have spread to nearby sites and may or may not have invaded one or more nearby lymph nodes, Stage IVB, in which tumors may or may not have spread to nearby sites but have spread to one or more lymph nodes, and Stage IVC, in which tumors have metastasized to distant organs.

Treatment and therapy: Primary care physicians will often refer patients to specialists, including oral and maxillofacial surgeons, otolaryngologists (ear, nose, and throat doctors), medical oncologists, radiation oncologists, and plastic surgeons. At specialized cancer treatment facilities, several of these specialists often work together to provide tailored care for patients. Treatment options include radiation therapy, oral chemotherapy, and surgery, as well as combinations of these treatments. The most commonly used treatment is a combination of radiation therapy and chemotherapy with the drug cisplatin. In some cases, surgery may be necessary to remove the cancer cells from a localized region. The surgery is often followed by radiation therapy to destroy any remaining cancer cells. Chemotherapy is sometimes given before other treatments to potentially enhance effectiveness of the follow-up treatment. In addition, treatments for symptoms and the side effects of therapies are often administered concomitantly.

Radiation therapy can take the form of external radiation from specialized equipment or internal radiation, when radioactive substances are placed in seeds, needles, or plastic tubes and inserted in the tissue. A newer form of radiation therapy, intensity-modulated radiotherapy, focuses radiation to more selectively kill the tumor instead of the surrounding healthy tissue. Surgery can be performed to remove tumors in the mouth or throat, or lymph nodes in the neck.

In addition to radiation, chemotherapy, and surgery, targeted therapies are also available. These include cetuximab (Erbitux), docetaxel (Taxotere), and angiogenesis inhibitors. Cetuximab is a monoclonal antibody directed at a protein that is abundant on cancer cells in this region. In a phase III clinical trial conducted at multiple locations in the United States and Europe (lead author James A. Bonner, of the University of Alabama at Birmingham), treatment with cetuximab combined with radiation therapy was shown almost to double the median survival of patients with nonmetastatic head and neck cancer. Another phase III study showed that patients with inoperable head and neck cancer who were administered multidrug chemotherapy that included docetaxel, followed by radiation therapy, survived four months longer with fewer side effects compared with patients on standard therapy. Another study involved 358 patients with inoperable head and neck cancer that had metastasized to lymph nodes in the neck. These patients were randomly selected to receive either standard chemotherapy with cisplastin and 5-fluorouracil, or cisplastin, 5-fluorouracil, and docetaxel. Both groups received radiation therapy after chemotherapy. The group treated with docetaxel had a longer median survival time and progression-free survival (time during which the cancer does not progress)—18.6 months and 12.7 months, respectively—compared with the group that was treated with standard chemotherapy—14.5 months and 8.4 months, respectively. Docetaxel was also associated with fewer side effects such as vomiting, nausea, and mouth sores. This provides support for the rationale of targeted therapy, which is expected to affect normal healthy tissues less than more nonspecific chemotherapy drugs.

Before starting any treatment, it is important for patients to ask their physicians about the treatment length and procedure, risks, side effects, and the results that may be expected.

Prognosis, prevention, and outcomes: The prognosis is good if detected and treated early. However, oral and throat cancers are often not diagnosed until they are late stage, often because they may be painless at early stages or cause minor pains similar to a toothache. The stage of cancer will also determine the type of treatment to use. After treatment, the cancer may reappear (recur or relapse). The recurrence can occur in the mouth or throat (local recurrence), in the lymph nodes (regional relapse), or in a distant site in the body, often the lungs (distant recurrence). A relapse is associated with a poorer prognosis. The five-year relative survival rate is a statistic that calculates the survival of cancer patients relative to the expected survival for people without cancer. This statistic can be used as a guide, but other factors, such as age, health, and tumor properties, must be considered before arriving at a complete prognosis. By studying patients treated between 1985 and 1991, the five-year relative survival rate for oral cavity cancer was calculated to range from 83 percent for Stage I cancer to 47 percent for Stage IV tumors. The one-year survival rate for all stages was 84 percent. The five-year relative survival rate for oropharyngeal cancer ranges from 57 percent for Stage I cancer to 30 percent for Stage IV cancer.

Ing-Wei Khor, Ph.D.

▶ For Further Information

Bonner, J. A., et al. "Radiotherapy plus Cetuximab for Squamous-Cell Carcinoma of the Head and Neck." *New England Journal of Medicine* 354 (2006): 567-578.

D'Souza, G., et al. "Case-Control Study of Human Papillomavirus and Oropharyngeal Cancer." *New Enland Journal of Medicine* 357 (2007): 1944-1956.

Genden, Eric M., and Mark A. Varvares, eds. *Head and Neck Cancer: An Evidence-Based Team Approach.* New York: Thieme, 2008.

Lydiatt, William M., and Perry J. Johnson. *Cancers of the Mouth and Throat: A Patient's Guide to Treatment.* Omaha, Neb.: Addicus Books, 2001.

Nikolakakos, Alexios P., ed. *Oral Cancer Research Advances.* New York: Nova Biomedical Books, 2007.

Vermorken, J. B., et al. "Cisplatin, Fluorouracil, and Docetaxel in Unresectable Head and Neck Cancer." *New England Journal of Medicine* 357 (2007): 1695-1704.

▶ Other Resources

American Cancer Society
Detailed Guide: Oral Cavity and Oropharyngeal Cancer
Http://www.cancer.org/docroot/CRI/CRI_2_3x.asp?rnav=cridg&dt=60.

Cancer Research UK
Types of Mouth and Oropharyngeal Cancer.
Http://www.cancerhelp.org.uk/help/default.asp?page=13033

MayoClinic.com
Oral and Throat Cancer
Http://www.mayoclinic.com/health/oral-and-throat-cancer/DS00349

National Cancer Institute
Oral Cancer
http://www.cancer.gov/cancertopics/types/oral

See also Candidiasis; Chewing tobacco; Cigarettes and cigars; Coal tars and coal tar pitches; Cordectomy; Electrolarynx; Endoscopy; Epidemiology of cancer; Epidermoid cancers of mucous membranes; Epstein-Barr virus; Erythroplakia; Esophageal speech; Glossectomy; Head and neck cancers; Hypopharyngeal cancer; Laryngeal cancer; Laryngeal nerve palsy; Laryngectomy; Laryngoscopy; Leukoplakia; Lip cancers; Oral and maxillofacial surgery; Salivary gland cancer; Throat cancer; Tobacco-related cancers.

▶ Orbit tumors

Category: Diseases, symptoms, and conditions
Also known as: Eye socket tumors, rhabdomyosarcomas, dermoid cysts, capillary hemangiomas, lymphoid tumors, cavernous hemangiomas, neurofibromas, schwannomas, optic gliomas, skin cancers of the eyelids, osteomas

Related conditions: Arteriovenous malformations, gene mutations, trauma, systemic diseases, congenital anatomic defects, chronic inflammation or infection, metastasis from adjacent or distant primary tumors

Definition: Orbit tumors are tumors found in the orbit, also known as the eye socket, which encases the eyeball, optic nerve, extraocular muscles, blood vessels, and soft tissue. Orbit tumors can be primary, in which the tumor originates from the orbit, or metastatic, in which the tumor develops from adjacent or distant tissue and invades the orbit. Most orbit tumors are benign but, because of their space-occupying nature, are readily conspicuous.

Risk factors: The presence of an invasive tumor in adjacent tissue may increase the risk of developing an orbit tumor. There are no other clearly identifiable risk factors for developing orbit tumors.

Etiology and the disease process: The etiology of orbit tumors varies and encompasses the etiologies of arteriovenous malformations, gene mutations, trauma, systemic diseases (such as amyloidosis or lymphoma), congenital anatomic defects, chronic inflammation or infection, and metastasis from adjacent or distant primary tumors.

Incidence: Orbit tumors can develop in children and adults, with different incidence rates depending on tumor type. In children, rhabdomyosarcoma is the most common malignant orbit tumor and accounts for 3 percent of orbit tumors; capillary hemangioma, which occurs in 1 to 4 percent of infants, is the most common benign pediatric tumor. The most common orbit tumors in adults are lymphoid tumors, cavernous hemangioma, and metastatic tumors, which respectively make up 4 to 13 percent, 4 percent, and 8 percent of all orbital neoplasms. Other orbit tumors include dermoid cysts, neurofibromas, schwannomas, optic gliomas, skin cancer of the eyelid, and osteomas.

Symptoms: The most common symptom is proptosis (forward displacement of the eye). Eye pain, visual abnormalities such as double vision or even visual loss, orbital edema, and eye redness are other symptoms of orbit tumors.

Screening and diagnosis: The diagnosis of orbit tumors relies on a meticulous patient history, thorough physical exam, and magnetic resonance imaging (MRI) or computed tomography (CT) scans. The diagnosis is confirmed by performing a tissue biopsy, either by fine-needle aspiration biopsy (FNAB) or by open biopsy of the orbit (orbitotomy). Histological analysis will determine the type of orbit tumor and lay the groundwork for a treatment plan.

Treatment and therapy: Treatment depends on the tumor type. Surgical removal is usually the best option, especially with disfiguring, massive lesions. Some tumors require external beam radiotherapy or adjuvant chemotherapy. In pediatric patients, dermoid tumors are best treated by surgical excision, while capillary hemangiomas spontaneously regress, therefore not requiring any intervention. In adults, radiotherapy is the treatment of choice for lymphoid tumors, while surgery effectively treats cavernous hemangioma.

Prognosis, prevention, and outcomes: The prognosis and outcomes depend on the type of tumor. Most primary orbit tumors are benign and therefore have a good prognosis. Metastatic orbit tumors (with a primary source of cancer elsewhere in the body) usually signify a poor prognosis.

Ophelia Panganiban, B.S.

See also Eyelid cancer; Gonioscopy; Lacrimal gland tumors; Neurofibromatosis type 1 (NF1); Ophthalmic oncology; Retinoblastomas; Rhabdomyosarcomas; Rothmund-Thomson syndrome; Sjögren syndrome.

▶ Orchiectomy

Category: Procedures

Also known as: Radical orchiectomy, inguinal orchiectomy, bilateral orchiectomy, unilateral orchiectomy, orchidectomy

Definition: Orchiectomy is a surgical procedure to remove one or both of the testicles in men with testicular or prostate cancer.

Cancers treated: Testicular cancer, prostate cancer

Why performed: Orchiectomy is used to remove one or both testicles as a treatment for testicular cancer. The testicles are the male sex organs that produce sperm and the hormone testosterone. The testicles are located in the scrotum. Nearby lymph nodes may also be removed at the time of orchiectomy. Artificial testicles may be placed at the time of surgery or in a later reconstructive procedure. Radiation therapy and chemotherapy for treatment of testicular cancer may follow orchiectomy. Orchiectomy may be the only treatment needed to cure early-stage testicular cancer.

A radical or inguinal orchiectomy includes removing one or both testicles and the spermatic cord. The spermatic cord is removed to prevent the cancer from spreading to the lymph nodes and the kidneys. An inguinal orchiectomy involves removing the testicles through an incision in the groin area, rather than directly through the scrotum.

Orchiectomy may be used to remove both testicles in men with prostate cancer. The growth of prostate cancer cells requires testosterone, and removing the testicles eliminates the source of this hormone. Without testosterone, the prostate tumor decreases in size, and symptoms are relieved. Orchiectomy does not cure prostate cancer, but it can help prolong the lives of men with advanced prostate cancer.

Patient preparation: Patients having both testicles removed will not be able to father children after orchiectomy. Patients with one testicle should be able to do so. Patients can choose to bank their sperm in case they wish to father children in the future. It is recommended that men with one testicle consider sperm banking as a precaution in case the second testicle needs to be removed in the future.

Orchiectomy can be an outpatient or inpatient procedure. It can be performed at an outpatient surgical center, urology clinic, or hospital surgery department. General anesthesia is most frequently used, in which the patient is not awake. Epidural anesthesia may be used, in which the patient is awake but does not feel anything from the waist down.

Prior to surgery, the patient receives standard blood and urine tests. The patient is advised not to take blood-thinning medications in the two days before the surgery and should not eat or drink for eight hours before the procedure. The patient uses a special antibacterial soap to wash his genitals and groin before surgery. Orchiectomy takes about forty-five minutes to an hour.

Steps of the procedure: The patient lies on his back on the surgical table. The patient is anesthetized, and vital signs are monitored throughout the surgery. The surgeon makes a 3- to 4-inch incision in the lower abdomen. The surgeon moves the testicles up through the inguinal canal and out through the incision. After removal of the testicles and spermatic cord is complete, the area is closed with sutures and bandaged.

After the procedure: The patient is observed in a recovery area until he is alert. He may stay overnight in the hospital or have another person drive him home. The patient receives medication for mild to moderate pain. Bed rest is recommended for a day.

The patient should wear a jock support or support briefs for two to three days and should not participate in strenuous activities for two to four weeks. Pain may be experienced in the abdomen or scrotum for several weeks. The patient should contact his doctor if he experiences increased pain, bleeding, or signs of infection.

Risks: Orchiectomy is considered a low-risk procedure. The risks include infection, bleeding, abscess formation, nerve injury, bladder damage, and the general risks associated with anesthesia. Removing both testicles causes changes in testosterone levels that increase the risk of hot flashes, erectile dysfunction, loss of sexual interest, loss of muscle mass, gynecomastia (enlarged breasts), and osteoporosis.

Results: Removing a cancerous testicle cures the cancer in the testicle. In the case of prostate cancer, removing the testicles prevents the cancer cells from using testosterone and slows the growth of the cancer while reducing symptoms.

Mary Car-Blanchard, O.T.D., B.S.O.T.

▶ For Further Information

Bohle, A. "Long-Term Followup of a Randomized Study of Locally Advanced Prostate Cancer Treated with Combined Orchiectomy and External Radiotherapy Versus Radiotherapy Alone." *International Brazillian Journal of Urology* 32, no. 6 (November/December, 2006): 739.

Cheung, W. Y., et al. "Appropriateness of Testicular Cancer Management: A Population-Based Cohort Study." *Canadian Journal of Urology* 14, no. 3 (June, 2007): 3542-3550.

Mikkola, A., et al. "Ten-Year Survival and Cardiovascular Mortality in Patients with Advanced Prostate Cancer Primarily Treated by Intramuscular Polyestradiol Phosphate or Orchiectomy." *Prostate* 67, no. 4 (March 1, 2007): 447-455.

Ondrus, D., et al. "Nonseminomatous Germ Cell Testicular Tumors Clinical Stage I: Differentiated Therapeutic Approach in Comparison with Therapeutic Approach Using Surveillance Strategy Only." *Neoplasma* 54, no. 5 (2007): 437-442.

Pectasides, D., D. Farmakis, and M. Pectasides. "The Management of Stage I Nonseminomatous Testicular Germ Cell Tumors." *Oncology* 71, nos. 3/4 (July 17, 2007): 151-158.

Sheinfeld, Joel. *Testicular Cancer: An Issue of Urologic Clinics*. Philadelphia: Saunders, 2007.

Sokoloff, M. H., G. F. Joyce, and M. Wise. "Urologic Diseases in America Project: Testis Cancer." *Journal of Urology* 177, no. (June, 2007): 2030-2041.

▶ Other Resources

American Cancer Society
http://www.cancer.org

See also Cryptorchidism; Prostate cancer; Sertoli cell tumors; Testicular cancer.

▶ Organ transplantation and cancer

Category: Diseases, symptoms, and conditions

Related conditions: Immune suppression, Kaposi sarcoma, nonmelanoma skin cancer, lymphoma

Definition: When organs are transplanted, there is a potential to mechanically transmit diseases from the donor to the patient. Infections, malignant conditions, and autoimmune diseases are examples of easily transmittable conditions. Patients who receive transplanted organs must use long-term immunosuppressive therapy, drugs used to prevent organ rejection by suppressing the immune function of the body. If the immune system is weakened, the chance of developing cancer increases. Cancer risk is high for patients on dialysis for end-stage renal disease, often a precursor to kidney transplant.

Risk factors: Those having undergone organ transplantation are at risk for developing cancers.

Etiology and the disease process: An organ such as a liver, lung, or kidney can contain malignant cells or a tumor at the time of transplantation into a patient. Coupled with immunosuppressive therapy, which weakens the immune system, a cancer transplanted with an organ is generally aggressive and difficult to manage. As organs are more difficult to locate for transplant, older donors and donors with health issues may be used, increasing the risk for cancer transmission from a transplanted organ to the patient.

Although the immune system is most effective at fighting infection, it does protect against cancer to a lesser degree by recognizing cells that are abnormal and attempting to control them. When the immune system is suppressed by drugs to prevent organ rejection, the body loses its ability to fight infection and abnormal cells. Cancers with a viral etiology are most encouraged by immunosuppressive therapy. Kaposi sarcoma, tumors just under the skin, may be transmitted by organ donation from donors infected with human herpesvirus 8 (HHV-8) but also may develop in patients with a preexisting infection when the immune system cannot help the body fight the infection. Lymphoma is most likely to occur in the first year after transplant or when treatment for organ rejection is started. The most common cancer in transplant patients is skin cancer. Cancer usually occurs in the first few years following a transplant.

Incidence: The incidence of developing cancer after transplant is 1 to 2 percent higher than it is in the normal population, and there is a fifteen- to twentyfold higher incidence of some cancers. Patients on immunosuppressive therapy have a much greater risk of developing cancer than the normal population. The cumulative probability for cancer after transplant is approximately 15 percent. Nonmelanoma skin cancers account for 90 percent of skin cancers in transplant patients, and skin cancer in the transplant group has a rate 100 times higher than that of the normal population. In a study by the United Network for Organ Sharing, malignancies caused 26 percent of deaths in kidney patients surviving at least ten years. Liver recipients had a 24 percent death rate from cancer at one year after transplant, and 21 percent of deaths in cardiac recipients in the first two years were from cancer. Kaposi sarcoma develops in organ recipients at a rate 500 times that of the normal population. Breast, colorectal, and cervical cancer risks are also increased after transplant.

Symptoms: Symptoms depend on the cancer type that develops after transplantation. Skin cancers may be visible on the surface of the skin.

Screening and diagnosis: Transplant patients need to receive routine screenings for cancer according to recommended cancer screening guidelines and have routine physician visits as part of follow-up care. Patients should inspect their skin monthly for any changes that could indicate skin cancer. An annual examination by a dermatologist is recommended. There is discussion that better screening of donors before organ donation should be a priority to prevent cancer transmission from affected organs. When symptoms present, diagnosis may include radiology tests, laboratory tests, and physical examination. Staging depends on the cancer diagnosed and the status of the tumor, lymph nodes, and presence or absence of metastasis at diagnosis.

Treatment and therapy: Careful dosing of immunosuppressive therapy to prevent organ rejection without totally depressing the immune system is critical. Some cancers may respond to changing the drugs and doses used in immunosuppressive therapy. If cancer is diagnosed, the treatments depend on the disease but generally include chemotherapy, radiation, and surgery.

Prognosis, prevention, and outcomes: The prognosis for patients developing cancer after transplant varies by the type of cancer. Patients should avoid sun exposure because of the high risk of skin cancer. Screening patients and donors carefully before transplant may prevent some cancers. Lower doses of immunosuppressive therapy may contribute to preventing cancer. There are newer types of immunosuppressive drugs that may decrease the incidence of cancer, including one that reverses the presence of skin cancers. Approximately one-third of all organ transplant patients die from cancer.

Patricia Stanfill Edens, R.N., Ph.D., FACHE

▶ For Further Information

Kauffman, H. M., et al. "Deceased Donors with a Past History of Malignancy: An Organ Procurement and Transplantation Network/United Network for Organ Sharing Update." *Transplantation* 84, no. 2 (July 27, 2007): 272-274.

Niederwieser, D., et al. "Transmission of Donor Illness by Stem Cell Transplantation: Should Screening Be Different in Older Donors?" *Bone Marrow Transplant* 34, no. 8 (October, 2004): 657-665.

Serraino, D., et al. "Risk of Cancer Following Immunosuppression in Organ Transplant Recipients and in HIV-Positive Individuals in Southern Europe." *European Journal of Cancer* 43, no. 14 (September, 2007): 2117-2123.

▶ Other Resources

National Cancer Institute
http://www.cancer.gov

National Marrow Donor Program
http://www.marrow.org

United Network for Organ Sharing
http://www.unos.org/qa.asp

See also Azathioprine; Blood cancers; Bone marrow transplantation (BMT); Childhood cancers; Colony-stimulating factors (CSFs); Cyclosporin A; Denys-Drash syndrome and cancer; Graft-versus-host disease (GVHD); Stem cell transplantation; Umbilical cord blood transplantation.

▶ Organochlorines (OCs)

Category: Carcinogens and suspected carcinogens
Also known as: Environmental, occupational, developmental, neuro-, and reproductive toxicants

Definition: Chlorination of hydrocarbons produces organochlorines, which are chemically stable, fatty, and toxic. OCs accumulate in fat and thus are transported via the food chain to top carnivores, including fish, birds, mammals, and humans. OCs are common contaminants of food, air, water, soil, and breast milk. They comprise diverse subgroups, members of which cause various types of health effects ranging from acutely fatal to chronically toxic over generations. Many OCs cause liver hypertrophy and cancer; neurotoxic, embryotoxic, reproductive, developmental, and immunotoxic effects; and various types of cancers in the pubescent children of exposed mothers.

OCs are produced by the chlorination of some of the petroleum hydrocarbons and can remain in the environment decades after being introduced. They are used in insecticides, fungicides, herbicides, miticides, polychlorinated biphenyls (PCBs), flame retardants, metal cleaners, dry-cleaning solvents, polyvinyl chloride (PVC) and other plastics, paints, dyes, synthetic intermediates, refrigerants, rayon and cellulose manufacturing, detergents, degreasers, disinfectants, halothanes, soft PVC surgical equipment, medicines—some eleven thousand common products contain them or use them in the manufacturing process.

The manufacture, use, and disposal of OCs create environmental and health problems. For example, for only one polymer, PVC, the downstream export of products from its synthesis amounts to 1,229 million metric tons. In another example, pulp and paper industries in North America produce 100 million tons of OCs. The waste by-products that pose the most serious health and ecosystem risks of the manufacturing process include PCBs, polychlorinated dibenzodioxins (PCDDs), polychlorinated dibenzofurans (PCDFs), and polychlorinated diphenyl ethers (PCDEs). Other notorious OCs include the pesticides dichlorodiphenyltrichloroethane (DDT) and dichlorodiphenyldichloroethylene (DDE), cyclodiene insecticides, Mirex, hexachlorobenzene, hexachlorocyclohexanes, and various solvents.

PCBs are mixtures of various congeners and isomers, which are chemically stable and viscous, with low volatility. From agriculture to office buildings, automobiles, and homes, PCBs have caused widespread contamination. Major environmental sources of PCBs include manufacturing wastes, careless waste disposal, and dumping.

Related cancers: Liver and testicular cancer

Exposure routes: Food, air, water, mother's milk

Where found: Air, water, food, breast milk

At risk: Those at highest risk for cancers associated with organochlorines (OCs) include embryos, fetuses, suckling newborns, and adults who are occupationally exposed to or living in the vicinity of the sources of release.

Etiology and symptoms of associated cancers: Organochlorines constitute one of the most diverse groups of cancer-causing chemicals considering their volume, categories of use, and persistence. OCs exert both specific and broad-spectrum effects. Out of all known effects, dioxin-like effects are the most serious cause of public concern: estrogenic effect leading to breast cancer; testosterone degradation leading to male infertility; nervous system damage leading to neurobehavioral deficits in offspring of mothers exposed to OCs; immunosuppression issues; development problems (lower birth weights, shorter gestation, birth defects); and occurrence of other types of cancers.

Both U.S. and European farmworkers exposed to OC pesticides have a six-times higher risk of getting testicular cancer. Many workers involved in the manufacture of 2,6-di-tert-butyl-p-cresol (DBPC; commonly used as a food preservative) have high OC concentrations in their bodies, low sperm count, and no children. Twenty-two OCs are endocrine disruptors, mimic estrogens (xenoestrogens), and induce an enzyme that degrades testosterone. An estimated 220 million pounds of farm pesticides per year in the United States act as xenoestrogens, which can also lead to breast cancer and other hormonal effects.

In the United States, DDE residues in women's fat can be transferred to the fetus or to a baby through breast milk and cause testicular cancer in their sons. OC effects are elevated in the womb and just after birth due to fat mobilization. Nursing infants get 4 to 12 percent of their lifetime's dioxin exposure via the intake of breast milk.

The stunning rise in breast cancer since the 1950's has been suspected to be related to only a few OCs. DDE, PCBs, and DDT are suspected of being involved in human breast cancer and are found in the fat and serum of women with breast cancer. In Copenhagen the risk of breast cancer appeared to be twice as high and aggressive in women with the highest serum concentration as compared with those with the lowest concentration of dieldrin. DDT is regarded as a possible human carcinogen, while PCBs are labeled as probable human carcinogens. PCB-180 and DDE may also be linked to non-Hodgkin lymphoma.

History: Organochlorines do occur, although very rarely, in nature, and are usually associated the high-temperature events such as forest fires and volcanoes. The use and manufacture of OCs by people started in the late 1800's. They were heavily introduced into the environment with the beginning of widespread use of pesticides, particularly DDT, in 1939.

Several billion tons of OCs have been used since World War II, and their residues are present in both humans and the environment. Rachel Carson's 1962 best seller *Silent Spring* sounded the alarm for the general public about the dangers of pesticides in the environment. Production and usage of OC pesticides started declining in the 1970's, and those suspected to be carcinogens were banned in the United States and later throughout much of the world, although some countries continued to use them. Millions of tons of OCs per year were still being produced in the early twenty-first century.

Organochlorine residues remain in the environment (air, water, land) and thus in human food and breast milk for decades. Residues of pesticides banned in the 1970's were still present in the food supply in the early twenty-first century. More OCs were targeted to be banned globally in the May, 2001, Stockholm Convention on Persistent Organic Pollutants; however, the George W. Bush administration did not ratify the treaty for the United States. Although many OCs have been banned over the years, others are still registered for use.

M. A. Q. Khan, M.D., Ph.D., and
Samreen F. Khan, M.S.

▶ For Further Information

Colborn, T., D. Dumanoski, and J. P. Myers. *Our Stolen Future*. New York: Dutton Press, 1995.

Khan, M. A. Q., S. F. Khan, and F. Shutari. "Ecotoxicology of Halogenated Hydrocarbons." In *Encyclopedia of Ecology*. Washington, D.C.: National Council of Science and Environment, 2007.

Khan, M. A. Q., and R. H. Stanton. *Toxicology of Halogenated Hydrocarbons*. New York: Pergamon Press, 1980.

Tenenbaum, D. J. "POPS in Polar Bears: Organochlorines Affect Bone Density." *Environmenal Health Perspectives* 112, no. 17 (2004): A1011.

Thornton, J. *Environmental Impacts of Polyvinyl Chloride (PVC) Building Materials*. Washington, D.C.: Healthy Building Network, 2002.

U.S. Environmental Protection Agency. *The Effects of Great Lakes Contaminants on Human Health*. Report to U.S. Congress. EPA 95-R-95-107. Chicago: Author, 1995.

▶ Other Resources

Department of Health and Human Services
Agency for Toxic Substances and Disease Registry
http://www.atsdr.cdc.gov

International Agency for Research on Cancer
http://www.iarc.fr/index.html

U.S. Department of Labor
Occupational Safety and Health Administration (OSHA)
Hazardous and Toxic Substances
http://www.osha.gov/SLTC/hazardoustoxicsubstances/index.html

See also Dioxins; Pesticides and the food chain.

▶ Orthopedic surgery

Category: Medical specialties

Definition: Orthopedic surgery is the branch of medicine concerned with restoring and preserving the normal function of the musculoskeletal system. It focuses on bones, joints, tendons, ligaments, and muscles. Over the last half century, surgeons and investigators in the field of orthopedics have increasingly recognized the importance that engineering principles play both in understanding the normal behavior of musculoskeletal tissues and in designing implant systems to model the function of these tissues.

Orthopedic surgery encompasses the entire process of caring for the surgical patient, from diagnosis to the preoperative evaluation and through the postoperative and rehabilitation period. Although the surgical procedure may be the key step in helping the patient, the preliminary and follow-up care regimens can determine whether the surgery is successful.

Subspecialties: Hand surgery, shoulder and elbow surgery, total joint reconstruction (arthroplasty), pediatric orthopedics, foot and ankle surgery, spine surgery, musculoskeletal oncology, surgical sports medicine, orthopedic trauma

Cancers treated: Tumors of the musculoskeletal system, soft-tissue and bone sarcomas, osteosarcoma, synovial cell sarcoma

Training and certification: Orthopedic surgeons must first graduate from medical school, then complete a general surgery internship and a five-year orthopedic residency program. After residency training, a certification process is initiated. The initial process is a two-step evaluation. Successful completion of a written examination qualifies the candidate to undergo an oral examination based on surgical case studies. Certification is based on the successful completion of both exams. Since 1986, the American Board of Orthopedic Surgery has issued time-limited certificates, requiring recertification every ten years. The ten-year Maintenance of Certification (MOC) process requires:

- 120 orthopedic-related continuing medical education (CME) credits in each of two consecutive three-year cycles, totaling 240 credits over six years
- A minimum of 20 credits of scored and recorded self-assessment examinations within the total 120 CME credits required for each three-year cycle
- Completion of a cognitive examination

Services and procedures performed: Orthopedics is a broad-based medical and surgical specialty. Services and procedures are based on the following:

- Medical history
- Physical examination: investigation of symptoms and complaints
- Use of laboratory studies: biopsy, blood, and urine
- Imaging diagnostics: X ray, computed tomography (CT), magnetic resonance imaging (MRI), ultrasound, and nuclear medicine
- Staging and classification: of injury, fracture, metabolic condition, or tumor

Treatment protocols are based on selective data. Often treatment of sarcomas requires surgical excision, limb salvage or amputation, joint reconstruction, and the concomitant use of adjuvant therapies (drugs, chemotherapy, and radiation). Rehabilitation (physical and occupational therapies) is also part of orthopedic treatment.

Related specialties and subspecialties: Orthopedics, which is dedicated to the prevention, evaluation, and treatment of diseases and injuries of the musculoskeletal system, has become subdivided into several subspecialties: trauma, sports medicine, spine, oncology (specialized treatment of benign and malignant tumors of bones, joints, and muscles), adult reconstructive surgery, foot and ankle, hand and microsurgery, pediatrics, and musculoskeletal rehabilitation (gait, amputation, prosthetics, and orthotics).

John L. Zeller, M.D., Ph.D.

▶ For Further Information

Bernstein, J., ed. *Musculoskeletal Medicine*. Rosemont, Ill.: American Academy of Orthopedic Surgeons, 2003.

Canale, S. Terry, ed. *Campbell's Operative Orthopaedics*. 9th ed. St. Louis, Mo.: Mosby, 1998.

Green, W. B., ed. *Netter's Orthopedics*. Philadelphia: Saunders/Elsevier, 2006.

Menendez, L., ed. *Orthopaedic Knowledge Update: Musculoskeletal Tumors*. Rosemont, Ill.: American Academy of Orthopedic Surgeons, 2002.

Miller, M., and M. Brinker, eds. *Review of Orthopedics*. 4th ed. Philadelphia: W. B. Saunders, 2004.

Skinner, H. B., ed. *Current Orthopedics: Diagnosis and Treatment*. 4th ed. New York: Lange Medical Books/McGraw-Hill, 2006.

Weinstein, S. L., and J. A. Buckwalter, eds. *Turek's Orthopaedics: Principles and Their Application*. Philadelphia: Lippincott Williams & Wilkins, 2005.

Wold, L. E., C. Adler, F. Sim, and K. Unni, eds. *Atlas of Orthopedic Pathology*. 2d ed. Philadelphia: Saunders, 2003.

▶ Organizations and Professional Societies

American Academy of Orthopedic Surgeons (AAOS)
http://www.aaos.org
6300 North River Road
Rosemont, IL 60018

American Board of Orthopedic Surgery (ABOS)
http://www.abos.org
400 Silver Cedar Court
Chapel Hill, NC 27514

See also Amputation; Giant cell tumors (GCTs); Hematologic oncology; Limb salvage; Liposarcomas; Medical oncology; Pediatric oncology and hematology.

▶ Otolaryngology

Category: Medical specialties
Also known as: Otolaryngology-head and neck surgery; otorhinolaryngology; ear, nose, and throat medicine

Definition: Otolaryngology is the study, diagnosis, and treatment of disorders of the ear, nose, throat, and other structures of the head and neck. To emphasize the discipline's focus on surgery, the American Academy of Otolaryngology voted to change the specialty's name to otolaryngology-head and neck surgery in 1980.

Subspecialties: Head and neck diseases, including treatment of tumors; facial plastic and reconstructive surgery; otology/neurotology (ear); rhinology (nose); laryngology (throat); allergy; pediatrics; sleep

Cancers treated: Any cancer occurring in the head or region of the neck above the collarbone (but not the brain or eye), including the thyroid, voice box, throat, mouth, tongue, lymph nodes, bones, nerves, and base of the skull

Training and certification: Otolaryngologists must complete at least five years of specialty training beyond medical school in an accredited residency program. Residency training involves one to two years of general surgery followed by four years of otolaryngology. After completing five years of residency training, doctors are eligible to become board certified in otolaryngology-head and neck surgery by passing examinations administered by the American Board of Medical Specialties or the Royal College of Physicians and Surgeons of Canada. Many otolaryngologists go on to complete one- or two-year fellowships after their residencies to become certified in an otolaryngology subspecialty. For example, some otolaryngologists may focus on head and neck surgery and treat patients with a variety of different kinds of cancers; others may focus entirely on diseases of the larynx.

During their training, otolaryngologists learn general surgical techniques and gain experience performing surgery, specifically on the head and neck. They also learn diagnostic techniques for the throat and airway such as laryngoscopy, bronchoscopy, and esophagoscopy, as well as how to interpret results of magnetic resonance imaging (MRI), computed tomography (CT), and other scanning methods. Otolaryngologists must also be knowledgeable about radiotherapy and chemotherapy because these treatments may be used to treat cancer either in conjunction with or instead of surgery.

Depending on their subspecialties, otolaryngologists must renew their certifications every few years. Otolaryngologists may obtain additional certification in other specialties that may be relevant to their particular area of expertise. For example, an otolaryngologist who focuses on treating cancer may also be board certified in pathology or radiation oncology.

Services and procedures performed: Otolaryngologists often receive referrals from other physicians if a patient is having ear, nose, throat, or airway symptoms. Therefore, otolaryngologists are often the ones who make the initial diagnosis of cancer. They will perform and interpret tests that stage the tumor and extent of its spread. Because otolaryngologists are trained in both medicine and surgery, patients with head or neck cancer do not need to be referred to another physician for treatment, as is often the case for other cancers.

The overall goal for the otolaryngologist in treating cancer is to remove or control the cancer while also preserving to the extent possible a patient's ability to swallow, breathe, eat, taste, smell, and hear. Because cancers of the head and neck may also involve the respiratory or digestive system, major nerves, the brain, or the eyes, otolaryngologists will often work with other specialists such as gastroenterologists, pulmonologists, ophthalmologists, radiation oncologists, and neurosurgeons in developing the best treatment plan for the patient.

Otolaryngologists can often treat early-stage cancers with radiotherapy or chemotherapy alone. Late-stage cancers typically require surgery, sometimes extensive, in addition to radiotherapy or chemotherapy. Because disfigurement due to tissue loss can occur with head and neck cancer treatments, many head and neck surgeons are also skilled in performing reconstructive or cosmetic plastic surgery. Otolaryngologists are also increasingly employing minimally invasive surgical techniques such as laser endoscopy to excise tumors. Minimally invasive methods not only preserve healthy tissue but also lead to shorter hospital stays and less risk of postsurgery complications.

Related specialties and subspecialties: Otolaryngologists may employ advanced practice nurses in the care of their patients. These are registered nurses who have obtained a master's degree in nursing. Some nurses obtain board certification in otolaryngolic nursing by passing an examination administered by the Society of Otolaryngology-Head and Neck Nurses.

Because the treatment of head and neck cancers can significantly impair a patient's ability to breathe, speak, or swallow, a speech pathologist may also be involved in a patient's care. In particular, speech pathologists work with patients who have lost their vocal cords to cancer and must learn alternative methods of voicing.

The major effects head and neck cancer can have on a patient's physical appearance and lifestyle can often cause anxiety and depression. A patient's care team may therefore also include a social worker or psychologist who can help the patient cope emotionally with the cancer and the effects of treatment.

Pamela S. Cooper, Ph.D.

▶ For Further Information

Corbridge, Roger, and Nicholas Steventon. *Oxford Handbook of ENT and Head and Neck Surgery*. New York: Oxford University Press, 2006.

Spiegel, Jeffrey H., and Scharukh Jalisi, eds. "Contemporary Diagnosis and Management of Head and Neck Cancer." *Otolaryngolic Clinics of North America* 30, no. 1 (2005).

Ward, Elizabeth C., and Corina J. van As-Brooks. *Head and Neck Cancer: Treatment, Rehabilitation, and Outcomes*. San Diego: Plural, 2007.

▶ Organizations and Professional Societies

American Academy of Otolaryngology-Head and Neck Surgery
http://www.entnet.org
One Prince Street
Alexandria, VA 22314

American Board of Otolaryngology
http://www.aboto.org
5615 Kirby Drive, Suite 600
Houston, TX 77005

American Head and Neck Society
http://www.headandneckcancer.org
11300 West Olympic Boulevard, Suite 600
Los Angeles, CA 90064

American Society of Head and Neck Radiology
http://www.ashnr.org
2210 Midwest Road, Suite 207
Oak Brook, IL 60523

▶ Other Resources

National Cancer Institute
Head and Neck Cancers
http://www.cancer.gov/cancertopics/types/head-and-neck

Support for People with Oral and Head and Neck Cancer
http://www.spohnc.org

See also Acoustic neuromas; Laryngeal nerve palsy; Oral and maxillofacial surgery; Oral and oropharyngeal cancers; Throat cancer.

▶ Ovarian cancers

Category: Diseases, symptoms, and conditions
Also known as: Cancer of the ovaries

Related conditions: Abdominal cancer, colon cancer, cancer of the diaphragm, lymphatic cancer, peritoneal cancer, stomach cancer

Definition: Ovarian cancers result from the development of a malignant tumor in the ovaries and can be divided into three main types. The most common is epithelial ovarian cancer, which originates in the surface cells of an ovary. The second type, germ-cell ovarian cancer, starts in the interior cells of an ovary, where eggs are produced. A third main type, stomal ovarian cancer, begins in the connective tissue cells that hold an ovary together and generate the female hormones estrogen and progesterone.

Risk factors: One of the most important risk factors involved in the development of ovarian cancers is inherited gene mutations. Inheritance of mutated breast cancer genes, *BRCA1* and *BRCA2*, is responsible for up to 10 percent of all ovarian cancers. Other factors include having had breast or colon cancer, having a family history of ovarian cancer, not having given birth, taking fertility drugs, and using hormone replacement therapy after menopause. Age is an important risk factor. More than half of the deaths caused by ovarian cancer occur in women between the ages of fifty-five and seventy-four.

Etiology and the disease process: The exact cause of ovarian cancers is still unknown. Some specialists have suggested that ovarian cancer in younger women is related to the tissue-repair process subsequent to ovulation. The formation and division of new cells at the site where an egg is released through a small tear in the ovarian follicle may produce genetic errors. Other specialists believe that the origin of ovarian cancers in younger women is related to the production of abnormal cells associated with the increased hormone levels that occur before and after ovulation.

Ovarian cancers are classified according to the histology of the tumor. Between 85 and 90 percent of ovarian cancers are epithelial ovarian cancers, which are classified by cell type and graded from 1 to 3. About 5 percent of ovarian cancers are germ-cell tumors, which develop in the egg-producing cells of the ovary and generally occur in younger women. Another type of ovarian cancer develops in the stomal cells, the tissue that holds the ovary together.

Ovarian cancer cells metastasize by spreading into the naturally occurring fluids in the abdominal cavity. These cells frequently become implanted in other peritoneal structures, particularly the uterus, the intestines, the omentum, and the urinary bladder. New tumor growths often occur in these areas. In rare instances, ovarian cancer cells spread through the bloodstream or lymphatic system to other parts of the body.

Incidence: Ovarian cancer is the fifth leading cause of cancer-related death in women. Each year, more than

20,000 women in the United States are diagnosed with ovarian cancers and about 15,000 succumb to the disease. Ovarian cancers are most common in industrialized nations. In the United States, a woman has a 1.4 to 2.5 percent chance of developing ovarian cancer in her lifetime.

Symptoms: In the majority of cases, ovarian cancer produces no symptoms or only mild symptoms until it progresses to an advanced stage. Symptoms include general abdominal discomfort, such as bloating, cramps, pressure, and swelling; nausea, diarrhea, or constipation; frequent urination; loss of appetite or feeling bloated after a light meal; and the loss or gain of weight for no apparent reason. Other symptoms can include fatigue, back pain, pain during sexual intercourse, abnormal bleeding from the vagina, menstrual irregularities, shortness of breath, and fluid around the lungs.

Screening and diagnosis: A medical doctor first evaluates a patient's medical and family history, then performs, a thorough physical examination of the pelvic region. The presence of any abnormal growths should be further investigated using ultrasound imaging and computed tomography (CT) scans. Ultrasound can detect the difference between healthy tissues, fluid-filled cysts, and tumors. CT scans produce detailed cross-sectional images of regions within the body. In some cases, X rays of the colon and rectum following a barium enema help identify the presence of ovarian cancers. The level of cancer antigen 125 (CA 125) should be assessed with a blood test; however, this marker identifies only about 10 percent of early ovarian cancers. The amount of four other cancer-related proteins in the blood shows some promise for diagnosing ovarian cancers.

A biopsy must be performed for a definitive diagnosis of ovarian cancer. Biopsies are usually done on tumors removed during surgery, although sometimes they are done during a laparoscopy or using a needle guided by ultrasound or CT scans. If ovarian cancer is present, the stage of the disease is assessed. Staging for ovarian cancer is as follows:

- Stage I: The cancer is limited to one or both ovaries.

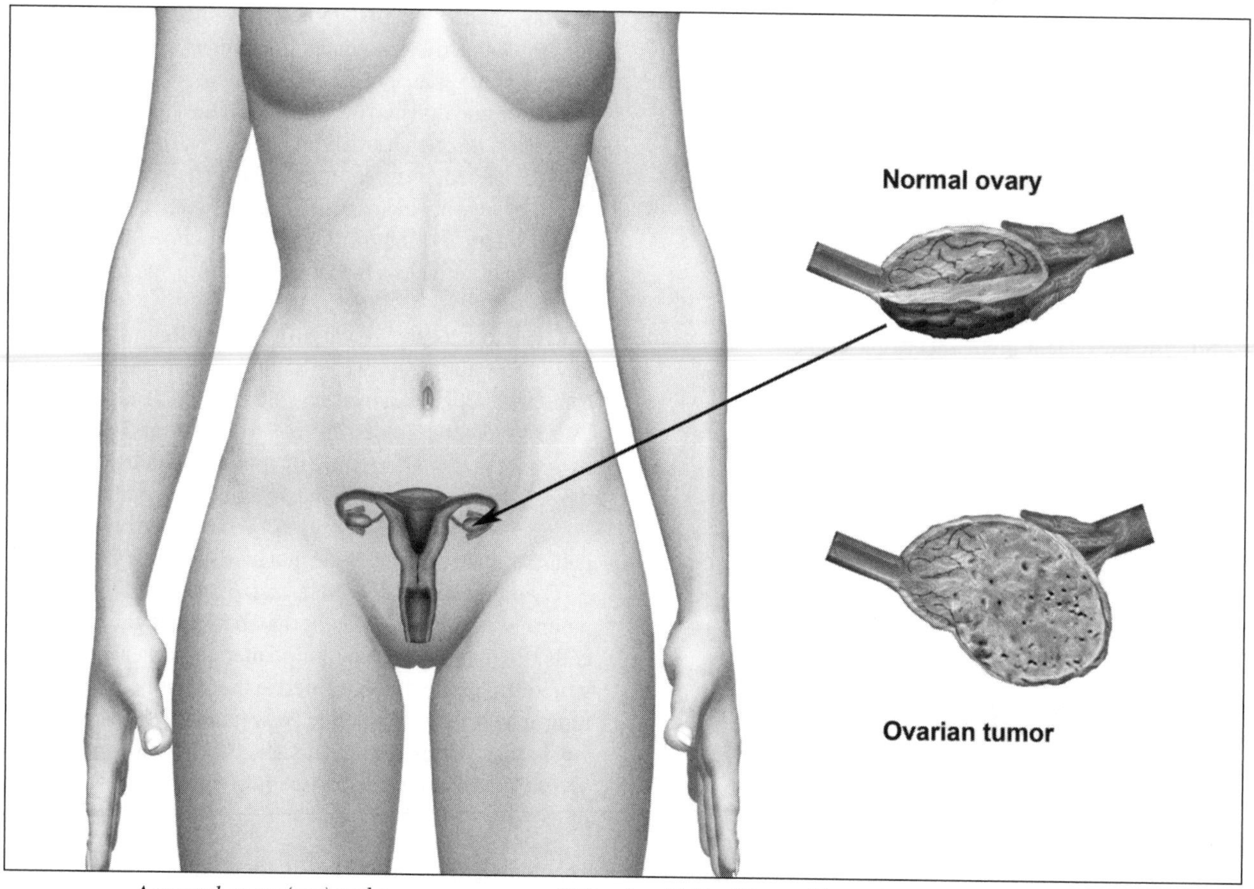

A normal ovary (top) and a cancerous ovary. (©Carol and Mike Werner/Phototake—All rights reserved)

Stage at Diagnosis and Five-Year Relative Survival Rates for Ovarian Cancer, 1996-2004

Stage	*Cases Diagnosed (%)*	*Survival Rate (%)*
Localized[a]	19	92.4
Regional[b]	7	71.4
Distant[c]	68	29.8
Unstaged	7	24.8

Source: Data from National Cancer Institute, Surveillance Epidemiology and End Results, Cancer Stat Fact Sheets, 2008

[a]Cancer still confined to primary site

[b]Cancer has spread to regional lymph nodes or directly beyond the primary site

[c]Cancer has metastasized

- Stage II: The cancer has extended into the pelvic region, such as the uterus or Fallopian tubes.
- Stage III: The cancer has spread outside the pelvis or is limited to the pelvic region but is present in the small intestine, lymph nodes, or omentum.
- Stage IV: The cancer has metastasized to the liver or tissues outside of the peritoneal cavity.

These stages are further broken down into levels of seriousness from A to C.

Treatment and therapy: Depending on the stage of ovarian cancer, surgery is often performed to remove the ovaries, uterine tubes, uterus, omentum, and associated lymph nodes. This process is referred to as surgical debulking. The stage of the disease determines whether additional therapy is needed. Typically, chemotherapy is employed, and if the cancer is localized, radiation therapy is sometimes used. The most effective chemotherapy drugs used in treating ovarian cancers are carboplatin and paclitaxel (Taxol), administered intravenously. The combination reduces cell division in ovarian tumors.

Intraperitoneal therapy, or pumping chemotherapy drugs directly into a patient's abdomen, extends the lives of ovarian cancer victims by an additional year or more; however, it can cause side effects such as stomach pain, numbness in the extremities, and possible infection. In January, 2006, the National Cancer Institute recommended an individualized combination of intravenous and intraperitoneal therapy for ovarian cancer patients. New chemotherapy drugs, vaccines, gene therapy, and immunotherapy treatments are being explored as options for treating ovarian cancers.

Prognosis, prevention, and outcomes: More than 60 percent of ovarian cancer patients are in Stage III or IV at the time of diagnosis, so the prognosis is not promising. The five-year survival rate for all stages of epithelial ovarian cancer is only 35 to 38 percent. With early diagnosis, aggressive surgery, and chemotherapy, the five-year survival rate is above 90 percent and the long-term survival rate approaches 70 percent. For germ-cell ovarian cancer, the prognosis is better than for epithelial ovarian cancer.

Eating well, exercising, and properly managing stress help produce good overall health and reduce the risk of developing ovarian cancers. Measures that help prevent ovarian cancer include having children and breast-feeding them, using oral contraceptives (30 percent reduction), and having a tubal ligation. For women who have a high risk of developing ovarian cancers, removal of the ovaries may be the best prevention.

Alvin K. Benson, Ph.D.

▶ For Further Information

Bardos, A. P., ed. *Trends in Ovarian Cancer Research.* Hauppauge, N.Y.: Nova Science, 2004.

Bartlett, John M. S. *Ovarian Cancer: Methods and Protocols.* Totowa, N.J.: Humana Press, 2000.

Conner, Kristine, and Lauren Langford. *Ovarian Cancer: Your Guide to Taking Control.* Sebastopol, Calif.: O'Reilly, 2003.

Dizon, Don S. *One Hundred Questions and Answers About Ovarian Cancer.* 2d ed. Sudbury, Mass.: Jones and Bartlett, 2006.

Icon Health. *Ovarian Cancer: A Medical Dictionary, Bibliography, and Annotated Research Guide to Internet References.* San Diego, Calif.: Author, 2004.

Nathan, David G. *The Cancer Treatment Revolution: How Smart Drugs and Other New Therapies Are Renewing Our Hope and Changing the Face of Medicine.* New York: Wiley, 2007.

▶ Other Resources

American Cancer Society

Detailed Guide: Ovarian Cancer

http://www.cancer.org/docroot/CRI/CRI_2_3x.asp?dt=33

MayoClinic.com

Ovarian Cancer

http://www.mayoclinic.com/health/ovarian-cancer/DS00293

National Institutes of Health

http://www.cancer.gov/cancertopics/types/ovarian/

Ovarian Cancer National Alliance
http://www.ovariancancer.org/

See also Cervical cancer; Endometrial cancer; Fallopian tube cancer; Fertility drugs and cancer; Gynecologic cancers; Ovarian cysts; Ovarian epithelial cancer; Uterine cancer; Vaginal cancer; Vulvar cancer.

▶ Ovarian cysts

Category: Diseases, symptoms, and conditions
Also known as: Functional ovarian cysts, physiologic ovarian cysts

Related conditions: Ovarian cancer, uterine cancer, lymphatic cancer, peritoneal cancer

Definition: Ovarian cysts are growths that develop within or on the surface of an ovary. They may consist of fluid-filled sacs, semisolid material, or solid material. Fluid-filled cysts are not likely to be cancerous. Most cysts that develop during a woman's childbearing years are not cancerous.

Risk factors: No specific risk factors have been identified. Most ovarian cysts develop as part of the ovulation process. The likelihood of an ovarian cyst causing cancer increases with the size of the growth and the age of the woman. Women over the age of fifty with ovarian cysts have a higher risk of developing ovarian cancer.

Etiology and the disease process: Functional ovarian cysts, which are not disease related, commonly occur during a woman's normal menstrual cycle. Tiny cysts develop to hold the eggs. When an egg matures, the cyst breaks open to allow the egg to move through the Fallopian tube. Typically, the cyst then dissolves. When the cyst continues to grow and does not break open to release the egg, it is termed a follicular cyst. Follicular cysts usually disappear within sixty days. If follicular cysts continue to grow inside an ovary during repeated menstrual cycles, the patient is said to have polycystic ovaries. If a cyst continues to grow after the egg is released, it is called a corpus luteum cyst. This type of cyst can grow as large as four inches in diameter and will sometimes twist the ovary, causing pelvic or abdominal pain. These cysts can also fill with blood and rupture, causing internal bleeding and intense pain. Corpus luteum cysts typically disappear within a few weeks.

Other types of ovarian cysts include endometriomas, cystadenomas, and dermoid cysts. If tissue from the uterine lining grows outside the uterus, a condition known as endometriosis, it sometimes attaches to an ovary and forms a cystic growth known as an endometrioma. These growths can be very painful during menstruation or sexual intercourse. Growths that develop from the outer epithelial cells of an ovary, known as cystadenomas, typically fill with a fluid, can become twelve inches in diameter or larger, and generate much pain by twisting the ovary. Dermoid cysts form from the germ cells that produce human eggs. They can grow rather large and produce painful twisting of an ovary. They are seldom cancerous.

Incidence: Virtually all women who have menstrual periods will develop ovarian cysts of one type or another. About 20 percent of women have polycystic ovaries. Up to 60 percent of women with endometriosis have endometriomas. The vast majority of ovarian cysts are not cancerous.

Symptoms: Although many women experience no symptoms associated with ovarian cysts, some signs may include abdominal pressure or pain, backache, incomplete urination, unexplained weight gain, painful menstrual periods and abnormal bleeding, pelvic pain during sexual intercourse, tender breasts, and nausea and vomiting. If sudden, severe abdominal or pelvic pain occurs, or pain accompanied by fever and vomiting develops, medical attention should be sought immediately.

Dermoid Cysts

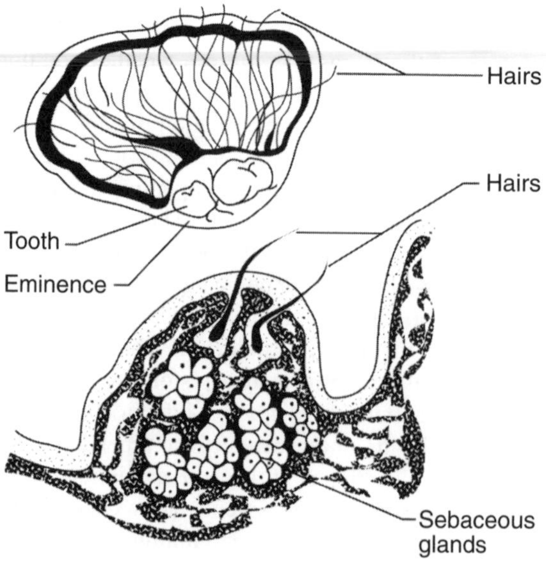

Screening and diagnosis: Ovarian cysts are usually found during routine pelvic exams. If a cyst is found, ultrasonic imaging is used to determine its shape, size, location, and content. To determine whether the cyst is malignant, a cancer antigen 125 (CA 125) blood test is sometimes done. For some women with ovarian cancer, this protein occurs in increased levels. Functional uterine fibroids and endometriosis can also increase the CA 125 level. CA 125 tests are recommended for patients over the age of thirty-five who have a high risk for ovarian cancer.

Treatment and therapy: For women still in their childbearing years who have fluid-filled cysts, the most common approach is to wait and watch. If a cyst persists, gets larger, looks unusual, causes too much pain, or the patient goes through menopause, surgical removal may be the best option. For smaller cysts that do not look abnormal in ultrasound images, a laparoscopy may be performed. Using a small incision near the navel, a scope is used to further investigate the cyst. If nothing unusual is found, the cyst is removed. For larger, suspicious-looking cysts, a laparotomy is done. Through larger openings in the stomach, the cyst is removed and tested for cancer by the pathologist. If the cyst is malignant, the doctor will proceed to remove the affected ovary and associated uterine tissues and lymph nodes.

Prognosis, prevention, and outcomes: Although ovarian cysts cannot be prevented, regular pelvic examinations are important to diagnose any problems as early as possible. Any mentrual cycle changes that are abnormal or persist should be discussed with a medical doctor. For women who frequently develop ovarian cysts, a doctor may prescribe birth control pills to reduce the risk of their formation by preventing follicle formation. In most cases, fluid-filled cysts are benign.

Alvin K. Benson, Ph.D.

▶ For Further Information

Bartlett, John M. S. *Ovarian Cancer: Methods and Protocols*. Totowa, N.J.: Humana Press, 2000.

Conner, Kristine, and Lauren Langford. *Ovarian Cancer: Your Guide to Taking Control*. Sebastopol, Calif.: O'Reilly, 2003.

Hammerly, Milton, and Cheryl Kimball. *When the Doctor Says It's PCOS (Polycystic Ovarian Syndrome)*. Beverly, Mass.: Fair Winds Press, 2003.

Icon Health. *Ovarian Cysts: A Medical Dictionary, Bibliography, and Annotated Research Guide to Internet References*. San Diego, Calif.: Author, 2004.

Reznek, Rodney, ed. *Cancer of the Ovary*. Cambridge, England: Cambridge University Press, 2007.

Vliet, Elizabeth Lee. *It's My Ovaries, Stupid!* 2d ed. Tucson, Ariz.: Her Place Press, 2007.

▶ Other Resources

American Cancer Society
Detailed Guide: Ovarian Cancer
http://www.cancer.org/docroot/CRI/CRI_2_3x.asp?dt=33

MayoClinic.com
Ovarian Cancer
http://www.mayoclinic.com/health/ovarian-cancer/DS00293

National Institutes of Health
http://www.cancer.gov/cancertopics/types/ovarian/

Ovarian Cancer National Alliance
http://www.ovariancancer.org/

See also Amenorrhea; Antiestrogens; CA 27-29 test; CA 125 test; Cervical cancer; Endometrial cancer; Fallopian tube cancer; Fertility drugs and cancer; Gynecologic cancers; Hysterectomy; Ovarian epithelial cancer; Peutz-Jeghers syndrome (PJS); Uterine cancer; Vaginal cancer; Vulvar cancer.

▶ Ovarian epithelial cancer

Category: Diseases, symptoms, and conditions
Also known as: Epithelial carcinoma

Related conditions: Abdominal cancer, colon cancer, lymphatic cancer, peritoneal cancer

Definition: Epithelial ovarian cancer results from the development of a malignant tumor that originates in the cells on the outer surface of an ovary. Between 85 and 90 percent of all ovarian cancers are epithelial ovarian cancers.

Risk factors: A history of ovarian cancer within a family—particularly in a woman's mother, sister, or daughter—increases the risk that a woman will develop epithelial ovarian cancer. Inherited gene mutations, specifically the mutated breast cancer genes *BRCA1* and *BRCA2*, are responsible for 5 to 10 percent of all epithelial ovarian cancer. The risk of developing epithelial ovarian cancer is higher in women who have had breast or colon cancer and is highest among women aged fifty and older.

Etiology and the disease process: The exact cause of ovarian epithelial cancer is unknown but it originates in the cells of tissue that cover an ovary. Epithelial ovarian cancer cells can be readily distinguished under a microscope. These cells are differentiated and classified as serous, mucinous, endometrioid, or clear cell types. Serous epithelial cancer cells are the most common. Undifferentiated epithelial ovarian cancer cells tend to grow and spread more rapidly than the four differentiated types. Epithelial ovarian cancers are classified by cell type and graded from 1 to 3. Grade 1 cells look similar to normal tissue and are less dangerous to the patient. Grade 3 cells look quite different from normal tissue and have the worst prognosis.

Epithelial ovarian cancer cells often metastasize by spreading into the abdominal cavity, where they can become implanted in the uterus, the intestines, the omentum, or the bladder. Sometimes they will metastasize to the lungs. On rare occasions, epithelial ovarian cancer cells spread into the bloodstream or lymphatic system and move to many other parts of the body.

Incidence: Epithelial ovarian cancer is one of the leading causes of cancer-related deaths in women. Each year, more than 18,000 women in the United States are diagnosed with ovarian epithelial cancer and about 14,000 succumb to the disease.

Symptoms: Epithelial ovarian cancer is often not detected until it has progressed to an advanced stage. Symptoms include bloating, swelling, or pain in the abdominal area and gastrointestinal problems involving nausea, diarrhea, or constipation.

Screening and diagnosis: If epithelial ovarian cancer is suspected, a doctor will conduct a thorough physical examination of the pelvic region. The shape, size, and position of the uterus and ovaries are assessed. If any growths or abnormal areas are found, they will be further investigated with ultrasonic imaging and computed tomography (CT) scans. The level of cancer antigen 125 (CA 125), which is raised with ovarian cancer, is measured with a blood test. Levels of other cancer-related proteins in the blood are being evaluated for diagnosing ovarian epithelial cancer.

Definitive diagnosis of epithelial ovarian cancer is made through biopsy. Usually when the tumor is removed, a sample of the tissue is analyzed and the stage of the disease is assessed. The staging of epithelial ovarian cancer is as follows:

- Stage I: The cancer is limited to one or both ovaries.
- Stage II: The cancer has metastasized into other parts of the pelvic region.
- Stage III: The cancer has spread to areas outside of the pelvis or has extended into the small intestine or omentum.
- Stage IV: The cancer has metastasized outside the peritoneal cavity.

Depending on the degree of seriousness, these stagings are further broken down into categories ranging from A to C.

Treatment and therapy: Depending on the stage of epithelial ovarian cancer, surgery is often performed to remove the ovaries, uterus, omentum, and associated lymph nodes. After recovery, the patient typically undergoes a regimen of chemotherapy. The most effective chemotherapy drugs used in treating ovarian epithelial cancers are carboplatin and paclitaxel (Taxol), adminstered intravenously. A combination of intravenous chemotherapy and intraperitoneal therapy, the pumping of chemotherapy drugs directly into a patient's abdomen, is recommended by the National Cancer Institute in the treatment of epithelial ovarian cancer patients.

Prognosis, prevention, and outcomes: Because epithelial ovarian cancer is not usually detected until it is in an advanced stage, the prognosis is not promising. The five-year survival rate for all stages of epithelial ovarian cancer is 35 to 38 percent. With early diagnosis, aggressive surgery, and chemotherapy, the five-year survival rate is above 90 percent, and the long-term survival rate approaches 70 percent.

The risk of developing ovarian epithelial cancer can be reduced with a good diet, exercise, and proper management of stress. Other factors that reduce the risk are bearing children and breast-feeding them if possible. Women with a high risk of developing ovarian epithelial cancer may consider removal of the ovaries as a preventive measure.

Alvin K. Benson, Ph.D.

▶ For Further Information

Parker, James N., and Philip M. Parker, eds. *The Official Patient's Sourcebook on Ovarian Epithelial Cancer*. San Diego, Calif.: Icon Health, 2002.
Pfragner, Roswitha, and R. Ian Freshney, eds. *Culture of Human Cancer Cells*. Hoboken, N.J.: Wiley-Liss, 2004.
Reznek, Rodney, ed. *Cancer of the Ovary*. New York: Cambridge University Press, 2007.

▶ Other Resources

American Cancer Society
Detailed Guide: Ovarian Cancer
Http://www.cancer.org/docroot/CRI/CRI_2_3x.asp?dt=33

MayoClinic.com
Ovarian Cancer
http://www.mayoclinic.com/health/ovarian-cancer/DS00293

National Institutes of Health
http://www.cancer.gov/cancertopics/types/ovarian/

Ovarian Cancer National Alliance
http://www.ovariancancer.org/

See also Cervical cancer; Endometrial cancer; Fallopian tube cancer; Fertility drugs and cancer; Gynecologic cancers; Ovarian cancers; Ovarian cysts; Uterine cancer; Vaginal cancer; Vulvar cancer.

▶ Overtreatment

Category: Social and personal issues

Definition: Overtreatment of cancer patients generally refers to the aggressive treatment of cancer in a patient whose cancer is considered extremely unlikely to spread. It can also refer to the use of an unnecessarily aggressive treatment strategy.

Causes: Standard procedure is to treat anyone who has cancer in the way that is believed best to destroy the cancer. Some people, however, believe that not every person who has cancer is best served by an aggressive cancer treatment plan and that in some cases it may be in the patient's best interest not to treat the cancer at all.

A growing body of evidence suggests that it is not in the best interest of every patient to aggressively treat every cancer. Treatment of prostate and breast cancers especially has come under scrutiny. Researchers have found that there are a surprising number of cases in which an autopsy has revealed a case of prostate cancer but the man had no symptoms of the cancer while alive. This type of evidence is often the basis for arguments against aggressively treating every case of cancer.

Some types of cancer are very slow to grow or may never grow at all and are considered extremely unlikely to spread. Therefore, an approach of watchful waiting may be more appropriate for some individuals than an aggressive treatment plan involving surgery, chemotherapy, radiation therapy, or a combination of treatments.

Side effects: Cancer treatments have many side effects that can significantly decrease people's quality of life. These can include pain, fatigue, nausea, hair loss, appetite loss, and depression. Cancer patients should discuss with their health care team all the benefits of prompt, aggressive treatment as well as the likely side effects and the possible risks of a watchful waiting approach.

The elderly: The elderly may be the group most likely to be affected by the overtreatment of cancer. If a person is of a very advanced age when a slow-growing cancer is diagnosed, it may be unrealistic to assume that the person is going to have enough benefit from treating the cancer to outweigh the negative impact on daily life from the cancer treatment being considered. Instead, it may be more beneficial for the patient to make regular appointments with a doctor to check and ensure the cancer has not grown or spread.

Helen Davidson, B.A.

See also Advance directives; Counseling for cancer patients and survivors; Do-not-resuscitate (DNR) order; End-of-life care; Financial issues; Home health services; Hospice care; Insurance; Living with cancer; Palliative treatment; Psychosocial aspects of cancer; Watchful waiting.

▶ Paget disease of bone

Category: Diseases, symptoms, and conditions
Also known as: Osteitis deformans, Paget's disease

Related conditions: Metabolic and endocrine bone diseases

Definition: Paget disease of bone (osteitis deformans) is a bone disorder in which excessive bone resorption is followed by excessive bone formation. The primary disturbance is an exaggeration of activity by a cell called the osteoclast, which is responsible for removing bone in the remodeling process. Frenzied osteoclastic activity results in localized bone loss followed by a period of hectic bone formation. The osteoblast cell responds by regenerating new bone that is primitive (woven), disorganized, and weaker. The resultant effect of this cycle is a net gain in bone mass; however, the newly formed bone is structurally unsound. The disease process also results in extensive vascularity (increased number of blood vessels and blood flow) and increased fibrous connective tissue within the adjacent bone marrow space. Paget disease can produce a variety of skeletal, neuromuscular, and cardiovascular complications.

Risk factors: Although the exact cause of Paget disease remains unknown, being older than forty-five years and having a family history of the disease are the only known risk factors. Of patients with Paget disease, 15 to 30 percent have a family history. Family studies suggest that a person with a first-degree relative has a seven times higher risk of developing this condition. In families with early-onset or severe Paget disease, the risk is even greater.

Etiology and the disease process: Named after the nineteenth century English surgeon Sir James Paget, Paget disease was first described in 1876 as an inflammatory condition that affects the normal biological processes of bone. The exact cause or mechanism of this disease process remains unknown. Scientists have discovered several genes that appear linked to this disorder. Other investigators believe Paget is related to a viral infection in the bone cells that may be present for many years before problems appear.

As living tissue, bone is engaged in a continual process of renewal; old bone is removed and replaced by new bone. This process of remodeling is disrupted in Paget disease. In the initial, or lytic, phase, old bone starts breaking down faster because of the erratic and accelerated activity of osteoclast cells. The body responds by generating new bone at a faster than normal rate. This mixed phase is devoted to osteoblastic cell activity. In the final osteosclerotic phase, the exhausted cells become quiescent. A mosaic pattern of bone is identifiable. The new bone is coarsely thickened but soft, porous, and lacking structural stability. These microscopic aspects make the bone vulnerable to deformation and to fracture under stress.

A variety of tumors and tumor-like conditions develop in the chaotic activity associated with pagetic bone. The most dreaded complication is the development of sarcomas (bone cancers), which occurs in 5 to 10 percent of patients with severe disease. The prognosis of patients who develop secondary sarcomas is exceedingly poor, but in the absence of malignant transformation, Paget disease usually follows a relatively benign course.

Incidence: Paget disease usually begins in the fifth decade of life, becomes progressively more common thereafter, and has a slight male predominance. There is a striking variation in prevalence both within certain countries and throughout the world. Paget disease is relatively common in England, France, Austria, regions of Germany, Australia, and New Zealand, affecting 5 to 11 percent of the populations in these countries. In the United States, Paget disease is estimated to occur in 1 to 3 percent of people over

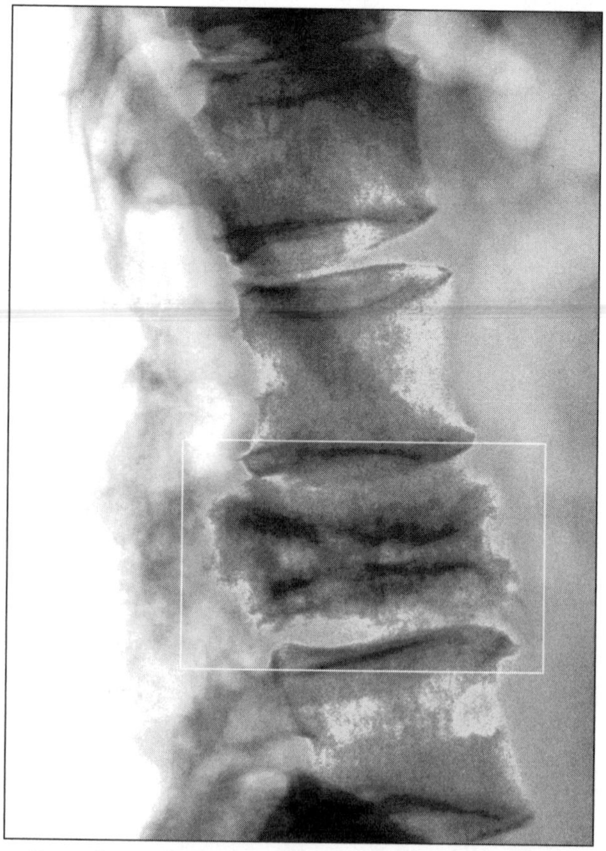

Paget disease in the spine. (Custom Medical Stock Photo)

the age of forty-five. Paget disease is rare before the age of twenty; the estimated incidence among individuals older than eighty is 10 percent. In contrast, Paget disease is rare in the native populations of Scandinavia, China, Japan, and Africa.

Medications Used in Treatment of Paget Disease

Pain Medications
- aspirin, other nonsteroidal anti-inflammatory drugs
- acetaminophen

Medications That Slow the Rate of Bone Turnover
- calcitonin
- etidronate
- alendronate
- pamindronate
- risedronate

Bisphosphonates (help body produce normal bone)
- etidronate disodium
- pamidronate disodium
- alendronate sodium
- tiludronate disodium
- risedronate sodium

Antibiotic
- plicamycin

Sources: The Arthritis Society and National Institutes of Health

Symptoms: Paget disease affects each person differently. Most people with Paget disease have no symptoms. Initial discovery may be the result of a screening X ray for other purposes. When symptoms do occur, they may be widespread but typically arise in the areas affected by the disease, which include bones, joints, and nerves.

The most common bone sites include the spine, pelvis, skull, femur (involved in up to 80 percent of cases), and tibia. Patients will complain of bone pain characterized as constant, aching, deep, and most severe at night. Skull involvement may produce enlargement of the head (frontal bossing). Deafness may result from disease of the temporal bone or ossicles (bones of the middle ear). Involvement at the base of the skull can lead to compression of the brain stem, resulting in symptoms of ataxia (difficulty walking), weakness, or respiratory compromise. Compression fractures of the spine can result in spinal cord injury and spinal deformity.

Hip and knee joints are commonly affected. The cartilage lining the joints near affected bones is damaged. This additional factor coupled with normal wear and tear leads to accelerated osteoarthritis, which may cause joint pain, swelling, and stiffness.

Enlarged bones can compress the spinal cord or the nerves exiting from the brain or spinal cord. Pain resulting from nerve compression is often more severe than bone pain. The location of the pain caused by nerve compression depends on the nerve that is affected. If lumbar nerves from the spine are compromised, this leads to radiating pain from the lower back and into the legs (sciatica). Nerve compression can result in limb weakness, pain, or paralysis. Nerve compression has been implicated in hearing and vision loss along with facial weakness and numbness.

Screening and diagnosis: Diagnosis depends on the following tests:

- Blood test: Alkaline phosphatase is a chemical substance produced by bone cells that are responsible for forming new bone, and its serum level is elevated in Paget disease.
- X ray: The first indication of Paget disease usually is an abnormality found on an X ray. X-ray images delineate areas of bone reabsorption, enlargement of bones, and bone deformities.
- Bone scan: In some cases, bone scans can pick up Paget disease before it is seen on an X ray. In a bone scan, radioactive tracers are injected into the body. The tracers are preferentially taken up by areas of the bone that are metabolically active. Areas of pagetoid bone are seen as darker than areas of normal bone.
- Bone biopsy: Biopsy of the bone provides definitive evidence of the disease. Slides of the sectioned tissue show the classic mosaic pattern of bone. Biopsy can also be useful in staging the disease process.

Treatment and therapy: Asymptomatic patients may not need treatment. Treatment is recommended when the disease is active (indicated by elevated serum levels of alkaline phosphatase). Treatment can help alleviate pain and may halt the damage done to the bones. In many cases, treatment can cause a remission of the disease although not a cure. Medications, surgery, and self-care remain the essential elements in most treatment regimens.

Drug therapy incorporates the use of nonsteroidal anti-inflammatory medications, analgesics, and muscle relaxants that lessen pain and discomfort but do not alter the natural course of the disease. The two major pharmaceuticals employed are calcitonin (a hormone that inhibits osteoclast activity and affects extent of bone resorption, provides relief of acute symptom, and lowers alkaline phosphatase levels) and the bisphosphonates, which are the most effective agents in reducing bone resorption.

Surgery, in rare cases, may be required to stabilize a fracture or to replace a damaged joint. If Paget disease affects the spine or skull, decompressive surgery (removal of excess bone) is needed to reduce the pressure on the nerves, thereby restoring normal neurologic function.

Prognosis, prevention, and outcomes: In most cases, Paget disease progresses slowly. The condition can be managed effectively in nearly all people and is rarely fatal. A nutritional diet, regular exercise, and maintaining a healthy weight are important aspects of any treatment protocol. Certain individuals may require a corset or brace to relieve back pain and provide support. If symptoms become severe, the use of analgesics and muscle relaxants is recommended. Medical supervision and examination are necessary since major complications of this disease can include fractures, osteoarthritis, heart failure, and cancer.

John L. Zeller, M.D., Ph.D.

▶ For Further Information

Kumar, V., A. Abbas, N. Fausto, and R. Mitchels, eds. *Robbins Basic Pathology*. 8th ed. Philadelphia: Saunders/Elsevier, 2007.

Schwamm, H. A., and C. L. Millward. *Histologic Differential Diagnosis of Skeletal Lesions*. New York: Igaku-Shoin, 1996.

Singer, F. "Paget's Disease of the Bone." In *Endocrinology*, edited by L. J. DeGroot. Philadelphia: W. B. Saunders, 1995.

▶ Other Resources

American College of Rheumatology
http://www.rheumatology.org

Paget Foundation
http://www.paget.org

See also Bone cancers; Bone pain; Bone scan; Genetics of cancer; Nuclear medicine scan.

▶ Pain management medications

Category: Chemotherapy and other drugs

Definition: Cancer pain management is a crucial aspect of supportive care of the cancer patient and may involve medication therapy, behavioral modifications, and other lifestyle adjustments. Because pain associated with cancer results from numerous sources and manifests through multiple mechanisms, treatment options are widespread. Although pain cannot always be completely relieved, oral analgesic therapy can be successful in up to 85 percent of patients.

Cancers diagnosed or treated: Medications and other therapies that control pain symptoms are used in patients with any type of cancer; types of treatment depend on the type of pain experienced, which can be determined by the type of cancer or type of treatment (chemotherapy, radiation, surgery) used.

Subclasses of this group: Numerous classes of drugs are useful in the treatment of cancer pain, including nonopioid analgesics, opioid analgesics, tricyclic antidepressants, and anticonvulsants.

Delivery routes: These drugs may be administered orally in tablets, capsules, or solutions; topically as patches, creams, or intranasal sprays; rectally as suppositories; submucosally as lozenges; or intravenously, intramuscularly, or subcutaneously as injectable solutions and suspensions. The drugs may be administered in outpatient, inpatient, or drop-in clinic settings.

How these drugs work: Cancer pain has historically been a cause for concern in patients and caregivers alike. The treatment of pain as a whole and in cancer patients is often poorly or inadequately managed, despite numerous available treatment options. Implementation of pain management guidelines and increased awareness of health professionals about the role of pain and the importance of pain assessment in cancer therapy, however, have improved the control of many types of cancer pain.

Different types of pain require different forms of treatment. Two main types of pain include nociceptive pain—resulting from actual damage to or inflammation of a tissue or organ (visceral pain) or to bone (somatic pain)—and neuropathic pain, which results from nerve damage or compression. Any source of pain may cause acute, chronic, or breakthrough pain.

Nociceptive or neuropathic pain occurring in the cancer patient may result from various sources, all with differing mechanisms. Approximately 70 percent of cancer-related pain results from the tumor itself because of invasion or compression of soft tissue, bone, or nerves. Another 20 percent results from treatments such as radiation, chemotherapy, and surgical biopsy, all of which can be associated with mucositis, neuropathy, infection, and other complications.

Although many options are available to control cancer pain, pharmacologic therapy is the primary, most successful method. Other options include removal of cancer in patients whose tumor compression is the pain source; neurosurgical treatments such as epidural blocks in patients whose pain is not adequately controlled with other options; complementary therapies such as relaxation tech-

Common Medications for Cancer Pain

Drug Class	*Individual Drug Examples*	*Brands*	*Delivery Mode*	*Primary Pain Type Treated*
Anticonvulsants	phenytoin, valproate, carbamazepine, clonazepam	Dilantin, Depakote, Tegretol, Klonopin	Oral, injectable	Neuropathic pain
Benzodiazepines	midazolam, diazepam, alprazolam	Versed, Valium, Xanax	Oral, injectable	Neuropathic pain; muscle spasm or anxiety
Corticosteroids	dexamethasone, prednisone	Decadron, Sterapred	Oral, injectable	Somatic pain from swelling; neuropathic pain
Nonopioids	acetaminophen, aspirin, NSAIDs (e.g., ibuprofen, naproxen)	Tylenol, Motrin, Anaprox	Primarily oral	Mild-to-moderate chronic pain
Opioids	oxycodone, propoxyphene, hydrocodone, morphine, hydromorphone, meperidine, fentanyl	Percocet, Darvocet, Lorcet, Duragesic, Dilaudid, MS Contin, Vicodin	Oral, injectable, transdermal, submucosal, intrarectal	Moderate-to-severe or severe chronic pain; short-acting for breakthrough pain
Tricyclic antidepressants	amitriptyline, desipramine, nortriptyline	Elavil, Norpramin, Pamelor	Oral, injectable	Neuropathic pain; depression

niques, massage, and transcutaneous electrical nerve stimulation (TENS); and psychological treatments that include behavioral or lifestyle changes and support groups.

Analgesic pharmacotherapy and adjuvant medications are primarily used to control cancer pain, and 75 percent of patients experience pain severe enough to require opioid analgesia. Pain falls into many categories, which then dictate treatment options. These categories include mild-to-moderate pain, moderate-to-severe pain, breakthrough pain, and neuropathic pain. Most types of pain in cancer patients are considered chronic, with only breakthrough pain being an acute situation that requires quick-acting relief.

Mild-to-moderate pain may be relieved with nonopioid medications; aspirin, acetaminophen, and ibuprofen or other nonsteroidal anti-inflammatory drugs (NSAIDs) are the primary options. Nonopioid analgesics act primarily on the peripheral nervous system to reduce pain or inflammation at the tissue, organ, bone, or incision site. The anti-inflammatory activity of NSAIDs is useful in particular for bone pain, muscle compression, and some tissue pains from swelling.

Moderate-to-severe pain often requires opioid analgesic therapy. Drugs in the opioid class include oxycodone, propoxyphene, hydrocodone, morphine, hydromorphone, meperidine, and fentanyl. Opioids work in the central nervous system by binding to pain receptors, namely mu, kappa, and/or delta, to induce analgesia. Opioids fall into three categories of activity: pure agonists (such as morphine, codeine, fentanyl, hydromorphine, oxycodone, methadone), pure antagonists (such as naloxone) used to reverse opioid toxicity but without their own analgesia, and mixed or partial agonists/antagonists (such as pentazocine, butorphanol, buprenorphine) that are used in more acute settings because of limited analgesic activity. Pure receptor agonists are primarily used for the control of chronic pain. Most opioid agonists are mu or kappa receptor-selective, although individual agents may have varying amounts of activity at the two receptor subtypes and can be synergistic with each other. Because each opioid agonist interacts uniquely and to differing degrees with mu and kappa receptors, and because patient response to each drug varies, substitutions within the class should be considered before giving up on opioid therapy when pain control is incomplete.

Cancer patients often require high doses of opioids for long periods of time. Important considerations in the long-term management of pain using analgesic therapy are tolerance, withdrawal, addiction, inadequate control, and breakthrough pain. Psychological dependence, or addiction, is uncommon with the appropriate use of opiates, even when doses are increased in response to tolerance. Although the mechanisms driving opiate tolerance are unclear, dosage increases usually improve tolerance of a single agent and are limited only by side effects. Although withdrawal symptoms are possible as a result of physical dependence, tapering doses in reverse often ameliorates these concerns. Adequate control is difficult because of the highly subjective nature of pain. Patients respond differently to pain and to pain medications, and they often fail to report inadequate relief because of personal concerns about dependence or addiction. Communication between health care professionals and patients, however, often resolves this concern, and patients become comfortable with around-the-clock pain control.

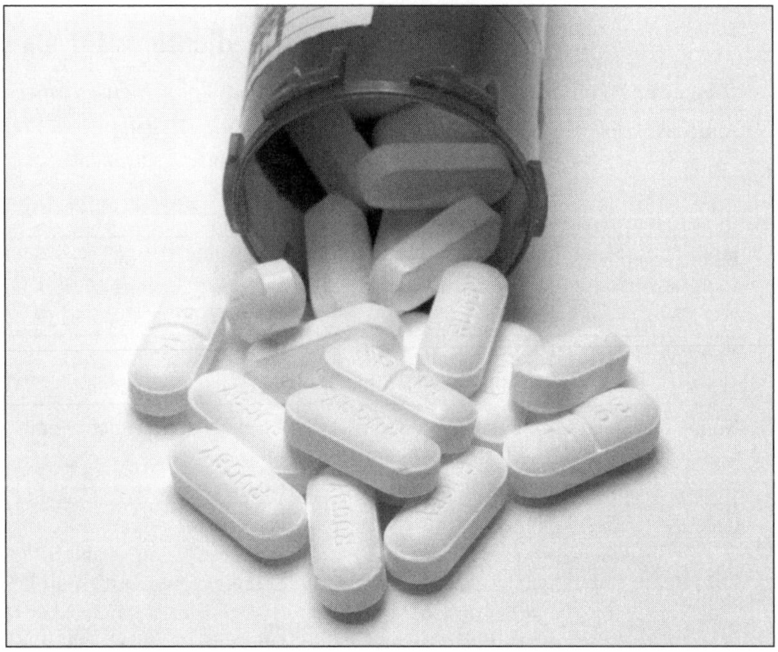

Hydrocodone (Vicodin) tablets. (Custom Medical Stock Photo)

Breakthrough pain, or pain that occurs despite existing pain medications, usually requires a quick-acting, short-acting secondary medication (such as immediate-release morphine tablets or submucosal fentanyl) to provide relief.

For reasons not clearly studied or understood, opioids do provide confirmed relief of peripherally mediated neuropathic pain as well. Adjuvant therapies also play a large role in the treatment of specific pain situations, including neuropathic pain. Common adjuvant drug classes used for neuropathic pain control include tricyclic antidepressants, anticonvulsants, benzodiazepines, and corticosteroids. Tricyclic antidepressants (such as amitriptyline, nortriptyline, and desimpramine) provide established analgesic effects for chronic neuropathic pain through monoamine-related pain-modulating systems in addition to and often prior to the separate relief of depressive symptoms by neurotransmitter alterations. Anticonvulsants (such as phenytoin, valproate, carbamazepine, and clonazepam) usually provide analgesia through the reduction of neuronal excitation or abnormal discharge. Benzodiazepines (such as diazepam and midazolam) have established benefits, through psychotropic and muscle-relaxant activity, in the treatment of neuropathic pain, and they reduce anxiety and associated muscle spasm. Finally, corticosteroids (such as dexamethasone) provide nonselective analgesic effects that are useful for malignant, advanced pain at long-term, low doses and for severe, unresponsive neuropathic pain at short-term, very high doses. Steroids also have nonanalgesic anti-inflammatory benefits that reduce tumor-associated swelling.

Side effects: Because of the varied treatments used to control cancer pain, side effects also differ. General concerns include breakthrough pain, medication tolerance, and withdrawal symptoms. Withdrawal symptoms vary with medication choice and length of use but include rapid breathing, yawning, perspiration, agitation, increased heart rate, muscle twitching, and loss of appetite.

Nonopioid analgesics are not associated with dependence, tolerance, or addiction, although all have a maximum analgesic dose. Select concerns with these agents include liver function damage with acetaminophen and gastrointestinal disturbances or damage with aspirin and NSAIDs.

Opioid side effects include constipation (which can be prophylactically treated with stool softeners), nausea, vomiting, pruritis, and sedation. Respiratory depression is possible in patients with decreased pulmonary function. Many side effects can limit the potential use of a particular opiate but do not rule out the entire class, because the side effects (like the analgesic effects) are linked to specific mu and kappa receptors. For example, constipation and respiratory depression are linked to mu receptor activity.

Adjuvant side effects vary drastically; overlapping toxicities are a primary concern, because adjuvant medications are often combined with each other or with opioids to provide pain relief.

Nicole M. Van Hoey, Pharm.D.

▶ For Further Information

Ballantyne, J. C. "Opioid Analgesia: Perspectives on Right Use and Utility." *Pain Physician* 10, no. 3 (May, 2007): 479-491.

Brennan, F., D. B. Carr, and M. Cousins. "Pain Management: A Fundamental Human Right." *Anesthesia & Analgesia* 105, no. 1 (July, 2007): 205-221.

Burton, A. W., et al. "Chronic Pain in the Cancer Survivor: A New Frontier." *Pain Medicine* 8, no. 2 (March, 2007): 189-198.

Fisch, Michael J., and Allen W. Burton, eds. *Cancer Pain Management*. New York: McGraw-Hill, 2007.

▶ Other Resources

Cancer.Net

http://www.cancer.net/portal/site/patient

See also Acupuncture and acupressure for cancer patients; Adjuvant therapy; Antinausea medications; Bone pain; Breakthrough pain; Brief Pain Inventory (BPI); Brompton cocktail; Cordotomy; Do-not-resuscitate (DNR) order; End-of-life care; Hospice care; Medical marijuana; Nonsteroidal anti-inflammatory drugs (NSAIDs); Opioids; Palliative treatment.

▶ Palliative treatment

Category: Chemotherapy and other drugs

Definition: Palliative treatment is defined as active and compassionate care primarily directed toward symptom management and improving quality of life. It is targeted toward patients who are not candidates for curative cancer therapies. Because of the proliferation of supportive treatments that can extend life, palliative care can be lengthy, lasting for months to many years.

Symptom management and control: For the cancer patient, physical symptoms and discomfort may change in nature, quality, and intensity within short, unpredictable time periods, often requiring close monitoring and therapeutic modifications at regular but nonspecific time intervals. Further, possible or actual changes in mentation, functioning, and personal control may precipitate intense emotions that are unfamiliar, unwanted, and anxiety provoking. Chronicity, remissions, and exacerbations of a variety of uncomfortable symptoms; family separation; financial strain; functional limitations; and role disruptions are but a few of the issues that characterize the lives of individuals with advanced, progressive, or incurable cancer. Even for those who experience lengthy disease-free intervals, the challenge of reducing cancer's presence in their lives can be difficult, and assistance from multiple specialists is often needed. Common symptoms that are treated and controlled or relieved by palliative care interventions can include the following:

- Pain
- Difficulty breathing
- Loss of appetite and weight loss
- Fatigue
- Weakness
- Sleep problems
- Depression and anxiety
- Confusion

Palliative treatment in context: The palliative treatment experience must be examined within the context of the health care delivery system for its potential and its pitfalls to be fully understood. Treatment advances, societal attitudes, and changes in health care structure and financing have all had a dramatic impact on the delivery of palliative care and the creation of gaps between the philosophy and delivery of palliative care services. The secrecy that prevailed in the 1960's and prohibited disclosure of a cancer diagnosis by most physicians has given way to the practice of routinely imparting the particulars of diagnosis, treatment options, and prognosis. Despite this change, it has been observed that persistent cancer-related fears and negative attitudes among health care providers have led to a discrepancy between words and actions, resulting in communication of emotionally laden information in a fashion ranging from overprotective and paternalistic to blunt and matter of fact. Further, patients who are not candidates for curative treatment often find themselves without adequate information and resources to manage their abundant physical and psychosocial problems.

Discrepancies between attitude and practice have been demonstrated by clinicians who have been found to avoid clear, open discussions of topics such as prognosis and death despite consistently expressed beliefs regarding the importance of openness and honesty with all mentally competent patients. Therefore, while the prevailing attitude in health care supports disclosure of medical information and active involvement by patients in decisions that affect them, the actual behavior of health care providers reflects a more limited improvement in patient care. Clinician concerns and personal issues can affect communication with patients at key decision-making and transition points along the continuum of palliative care. The need for clinician support and access to resources is recognized as key in helping members of the palliative care team to assist patients fully, but there is much need for improvement and more resources in this area.

Psychiatric and medical comorbidity: The time during which palliative treatment is necessary has lengthened, causing an increase in the number of cases in which patients need psychiatric care alongside medical care. This phenomenon, although largely ignored, is putting inordinate stress on patients, families, professional caregivers, and the health care system at large. Psychiatric problems tend to be treated based on whether reimbursement is provided, and reimbursement occurs only when psychiatric symptoms emerge as disease states. Insurance rarely covers psychiatric interventions targeted toward symptom management and quality-of-life enhancement, although comprehensive, low-cost interventions supported by scientific evidence of their efficacy are available. Multisystem problems are generally not addressed well by the medical system, which is fragmented and oriented toward specialty care.

Because recipients of palliative cancer treatment are not candidates for curative therapies, they are faced with their own mortality and are vulnerable to intense fear and psychological distress. However, the health care system is oriented toward cure and survival, and it typically places a lower priority on treating and addressing psychosocial issues. Patients receiving palliative care are often concerned about issues such as impending death, pain or other physical discomfort that cannot be relieved, disfigurement, functional decline and increasing dependency on others, loss of mental acuity and bodily functions, and the effects of their illness on their families and friends. These patients need to be closely monitored to manage changes in symptoms and functional status and to evaluate the level of relief achieved through targeted interventions.

Ethical aspects: Care providers must be mindful that the psychological vulnerability of patients receiving palliative care may put some individuals at risk for unnecessary suffering, exploitation, and victimization based on the cure-oriented values inherent in modern health care. For example, an issue that repeatedly surfaces among patients, family members, and professional care providers pertains to the use of aggressive treatment protocols in the presence of progressive, incurable disease. Patients may seek or be recruited for participation in experimental protocols even when treatment is not expected to extend their lives. Questions of ethics and the meaning of informed consent arise in regard to the participation of terminally ill subjects in experimental protocols. Some experts question whether having a particular medical conditions or status (such as being terminally ill) diminishes full participation in the process of informed consent.

The need for health care professionals to establish structured dialogue with patients, family members, and care providers regarding treatment goals and expectations is essential. Treatment planning should take into account the fact that certain individuals with a terminal illness may respond to participation in an investigational treatment with increased hope of survival, regardless of their real chances of survival. These issues, however, become even more complex as changes in health care financing prohibit reimbursement for experimental therapies. Some people will be unable to undergo experimental therapies, and others may assume the cost of aggressive yet often medically futile treatments, creating compelling ethical issues and tensions. These are weighty issues that require active dialogue and debate. The combination of rapid medical and technological advances, diminishing ability to finance rising health care costs, growing numbers of chronically ill patients living longer periods of time, and an ever widening gap between the affluent and poor is adding to the problem.

Patients, their families, and health care providers need to separate and clarify personal values, thoughts, and emotional reactions to these delicate issues if individualized, quality palliative care is to be provided. Psychiatric consultation-liaison nurses, psychiatrists, social workers, and chaplains can be invaluable in assisting patients, family members, and staff to grapple with these issues in a meaningful and productive manner.

Dying and terminal care: Once the terminal care period has begun, it is usually not the fact of dying, but the quality of dying, that is primary for patients and families. Palliative care that continues into the terminal stage of cancer should continue to relieve physical and psychological symptoms and promote comfort and well-being until the patient dies. Often patients and families who have received palliative services in earlier stages of the illness will be more open and accepting of palliative efforts in the final stage of life. In addition, it is important that professional and family caregivers recognize that their work is emotionally draining, and they should seek guidance and support whenever possible.

Professional caregivers should target therapeutic interventions toward increasing the dying patients' sense of personal control and self-efficacy within the context of their functional decline and increased dependency. It is also therapeutic in most cases to inform patients of available resources aimed at discussing and addressing any concerns regarding death and dying. From a practical standpoint, professional caregivers may help patients by inquiring about any unfinished business, including wills and conversations with family and friends, and to provide them with the necessary support and encouragement to accomplish these final goals.

Factors including personal values, socioeconomic status, cultural background, and religious beliefs can influence patients' expectations and experiences as they approach death. For example, a stoic attitude that minimizes or negates discomfort may be related to a cultural value learned and reinforced through years of family experiences. Similarly, an extremely emotional response to routine events during the terminal phase of illness does not necessarily signal mental maladjustment but rather the person's cultural norm. Awareness of the person's cultural, religious, ethnic, and socioeconomic background is important in the process of understanding individual behaviors and limiting value judgments.

Psychiatric complications and terminal care: Delirium, depression, suicidal ideation, and severe anxiety are among the most commonly occurring psychiatric complications encountered in terminally ill cancer patients. When severe, these problems require urgent and aggressive assessment and treatment by psychiatric personnel who can initiate pharmacologic and psychotherapeutic treatment strategies. It should be stressed that psychiatric emergencies require the same rapid intervention as medical crises. In spite of the seemingly overwhelming nature of psychosocial responses in cancer patients, most of them do indeed cope effectively, and it is important to recognize that intense emotions are not one and the same as maladaptive coping.

Hospice care: Hospice care involves structured programs that offer supportive and palliative care at the end of life. The patient, family, and health care team decide when hospice care should begin, but typically patients are eligible for a hospice program when they have about six months to live. Hospice care can be home or institution based. Hospice care aims to manage physical and emotional symptoms with the overriding goal of allowing patients to live their last days with dignity and as high a quality of life as possible. Most hospice programs offer family-centered care, meaning that they involve the patient and family in decision making, which reduces distress and enhances control. A hospice team usually consists of a physician, an advanced practice nurse, a bedside nurse, nursing assistants, social workers, and chaplains. Goals of hospice treatment may include increased time of survival, symptom control, and enhanced quality of life.

Jeannie V. Pasacreta, Ph.D., A.P.R.N.

▶ For Further Information

Barnett, Laura, ed. *When Death Enters the Therapeutic Space: Existential Perspectives in Psychotherapy and Counseling*. New York: Routledge, 2008.

Boog, Kathryn M., and Claire Tester. *A Practical Guide to Palliative Care: Finding Meaning and Purpose in Life and Death*. New York: Elsevier, 2008.

Jacobs, Léa K., ed. *Coping with Cancer*. New York: Nova Science, 2008.

Kuebler, Kim, Debra E. Heidrich, and Peg Esper. *Palliative and End of Life Care: Clinical Practice Guidelines*. 2d ed. St. Louis: Saunders/Elsevier, 2007.

Lewis, Milton J. *Medicine and Care of the Dying: A Modern History*. New York: Oxford University Press, 2007.

Lynn, Joanne, et al. *Improving Care for the End of Life: A Sourcebook for Health Care Managers and Clinicians*. 2d ed. New York: Oxford University Press, 2008.

Werth, James L., and Dean Blevins, eds. *Decision Making Near the End of Life: Issues, Development, and Future Directions*. New York: Brunner-Routledge, 2008.

▶ Other Resources

American Academy of Hospice and Palliative Medicine
http://www.aahpm.org

American Hospice Foundation
http://www.americanhospice.org

American Pain Society
http://www.ampainsoc.org

American Psychosocial Oncology Society
http://www.apos-society.org

Americans for Better Care of the Dying
http://www.abcd-caring.org

National Palliative Care Research Center
http://www.npcrc.org

See also Acupuncture and acupressure for cancer patients; Bone pain; Breakthrough pain; Brief Pain Inventory (BPI); Brompton cocktail; Cordotomy; Do-not-resuscitate (DNR) order; End-of-life care; Hospice care; Medical marijuana; Nonsteroidal anti-inflammatory drugs (NSAIDs); Opioids; Pain management medications.

▶ Palpation

Category: Procedures
Also known as: Manual examination, feeling, probing, touching, manipulation

Definition: Palpation is the careful manual examination of the size, shape, firmness, consistency, texture, tenderness, or location of some body part or organ. Health care professionals use palpation during a physical examination for screening and diagnostic purposes.

Cancers diagnosed: Cancers of the breast, prostate, uterus, ovaries, liver, abdomen, pancreas, skin, bladder, lower colon and rectum, or lymph nodes

Why performed: Despite the technological advances in health care diagnostics, health care providers still acquire valuable information through direct interaction with the patient. By providing a physical examination, providers can screen patients for possible abnormalities. Sometimes cancer can be discovered through palpation of various body parts or organs. For example, a provider can use palpation to screen for cancers of the breast, prostate, uterus, ovaries, liver, abdomen, pancreas, skin, bladder, lower colon and rectum, or lymph nodes. A woman can use palpation in her monthly breast examination to detect lumps or thickening tissue that could indicate cancer.

Palpation is a noninvasive procedure that is less costly than procedures involving technology and can be a highly reliable initial step. When an abnormality is discovered, further diagnostics are performed to diagnose the cancer and determine treatment alternatives.

Patient preparation: Patient preparation depends on the type of palpation procedure. The patient should receive a thorough explanation of what is involved in the examination. Any anticipated discomfort should be disclosed to the patient, and any patient questions should be answered prior to the examination. Successful physical palpation depends of the skill of the provider and a thorough preparation of the patient.

Steps of procedure: The steps of the procedure depend on the area palpated during the physical examination.

After the procedure: The patient should be informed of any possible discomfort, tenderness, or soreness that may occur after the examination, which is generally minimal with palpation. Though palpation does not provide a definitive diagnosis, the practitioner can provide immediate feedback to the patient about cancer possibilities and make plans for further tests.

Risks: One advantage of palpation as a means of screening for cancer and other health care problems is that there is little risk of an adverse event to the patient. Palpation usually results in minimal and/or short-term discomfort for the patient.

Results: A skillful practitioner can use palpation as an effective way to screen a patient for cancer. Immediate follow-up plans can be made for further diagnostics without waiting for the return of other test results.

Marylane Wade Koch, M.S.N., R.N.

See also Breast self-examination (BSE); Clinical breast exam (CBE); Digital rectal exam (DRE); Fibroadenomas; Gynecologic cancers; Pelvic examination; Screening for cancer; Testicular self-examination (TSE).

▶ Pancolitis

Category: Diseases, symptoms, and conditions
Also known as: Universal colitis

Related conditions: Inflammatory bowel diseases, various types of colitis

Definition: Pancolitis is inflammation of the entire large intestine.

Risk factors: People with inflammatory bowel disease, with specific gastrointestinal infections, or who have had abdominal or pelvic radiation therapy or cancer, are at risk for developing pancolitis.

Etiology and the disease process: For unknown reasons, the immune system sometimes attacks the digestive tract, resulting in inflammatory bowel disease (IBD). The two main types of inflammatory bowel disease are ulcerative colitis (UC) and Crohn disease (CD). In these diseases, large quantities of white blood cells migrate into the colon and repeatedly damage it. This can result in inflammation of the entire colon, or pancolitis.

Other causes of pancolitis include the following:

- Infections of the colon with certain microorganisms that cause community-acquired colitis
- Antibiotic-related pseudomembranous colitis, which is brought on by treatments with antibiotics such as clindamycin, ampicillin, or cephalsporins that kill off the common microbial occupants of the colon and allow the growth of another microorganism (*Clostridium difficile*) that damages the colon
- Ischemic colitis, which is caused by blockage of the blood vessels that feed the colon

- Radiation colitis, whereby radiation damage blocks blood flow to the colon
- Cancers that spread to the colon

Incidence: The incidenc of ulcerative colitis is between 35 and 100 cases per 100,000 people, and of Crohn disease, 7 cases per 100,000 people. Between 2 and 5 percent of those who receive abdominal or pelvic radiation therapy suffer from radiation colitis.

Symptoms: The hallmarks of pancolitis are blood discharge after each bowel movement, urgency to defecate, spasm of the anal sphincter (tenesmus), abdominal pain, and rapid weight loss.

Screening and diagnosis: The standard means to diagnose pancolitis is a colonoscopy, which should show continuous, inflamed, bleeding ulcers on the wall of the colon. Colon biopsies are also necessary to determine the exact cause of pancolitis. X rays or computed tomography (CT) scans in which contrast is provided by a barium enema are also used to diagnose pancolitis or its complications.

Treatment and therapy: Colonic inflammation is inhibited by 5-aminosalicylic acid (5-ASA) agents such as mesalamine, sulfasalazine, and balsalazide. Other immune system inhibitors, including infliximab, azathioprine, cyclosporine, methotrexate, and 6-mercaptopurine, are used if 5-ASAs are ineffective. Steroids such as prednisone, methylprednisolone, and budesonide quell active episodes. Surgical removal of the colon (colectomy) is recommended in recalcitrant cases.

Prognosis, prevention, and outcomes: Untreated pancolitis is usually fatal. Inflammatory bowel diseases are usually controlled with therapy, but patients are at increased risk for colon cancer. Colectomy cures many pancolitis cases. For Crohn disease, therapy becomes less effective with time, and surgery is required in two-thirds of patients.

Michael A. Buratovich, Ph.D.

See also Azathioprine; Coloanal anastomosis; Colon polyps; Colonoscopy and virtual colonoscopy; Colorectal cancer; Crohn disease; Enterostomal therapy; Fecal occult blood test (FOBT); Ileostomy; Immunoelectrophoresis (IEP); Inflammatory bowel disease; Premalignancies; Risks for cancer.

▶ Pancreatectomy

Category: Procedures
Also known as: Pancreatoduodenectomy, Whipple procedure, distal pancreatectomy, total pancreatectomy

Definition: Pancreatectomy is a surgical procedure done to remove all or part of the pancreas.

Cancers treated: Pancreatic cancer

Why performed: Pancreatectomy is done to remove all or part of the pancreas. This procedure may be performed when trying to cure the cancer by removing all of it, or it can be done as palliative care to reduce or prevent symptoms from cancer that has already spread to other areas.

Patient preparation: The first step of patient preparation is a thorough evaluation by the cancer care team to ensure that the patient is a good candidate for a pancreatectomy. It is a very difficult procedure that usually has a long recovery time, and it is not appropriate for many individuals. The procedure is appropriate only for individuals who have cancer that is expected to be fully removable by the procedure. As few as 10 percent of individuals diagnosed with pancreatic cancer are good candidates for this surgery. In some cases, pancreatectomy may also be appropriate as a palliative treatment.

Some patients receive radiation or chemotherapy before pancreatectomy. This may be done in an attempt to shrink the tumor to make complete removal more likely. It may also be done before the procedure, because the high risk of complications and long recovery time often mean that necessary additional treatments cannot begin until many weeks after the surgery. In the days before the procedure, patient preparation is generally similar to that for other major surgical operations. Patients may be instructed to avoid food or liquids for a certain amount of time before the procedure or be given antibiotics or other medications to help minimize the risk of complications.

Steps of the procedure: Three main types of pancreatectomy are performed. Which one is performed depends on where the cancer is located and the extent of the cancer's spread. If the goal is palliative, then the procedure performed will depend on the symptoms being treated or prevented. The three types of procedures differ in the amount and section of the pancreas that is removed.

The most common type of procedure is known as a pancreatoduodenectomy, also called the Whipple procedure. During this procedure, the surgeon removes the head of the pancreas (the part closest to the small intestine). The

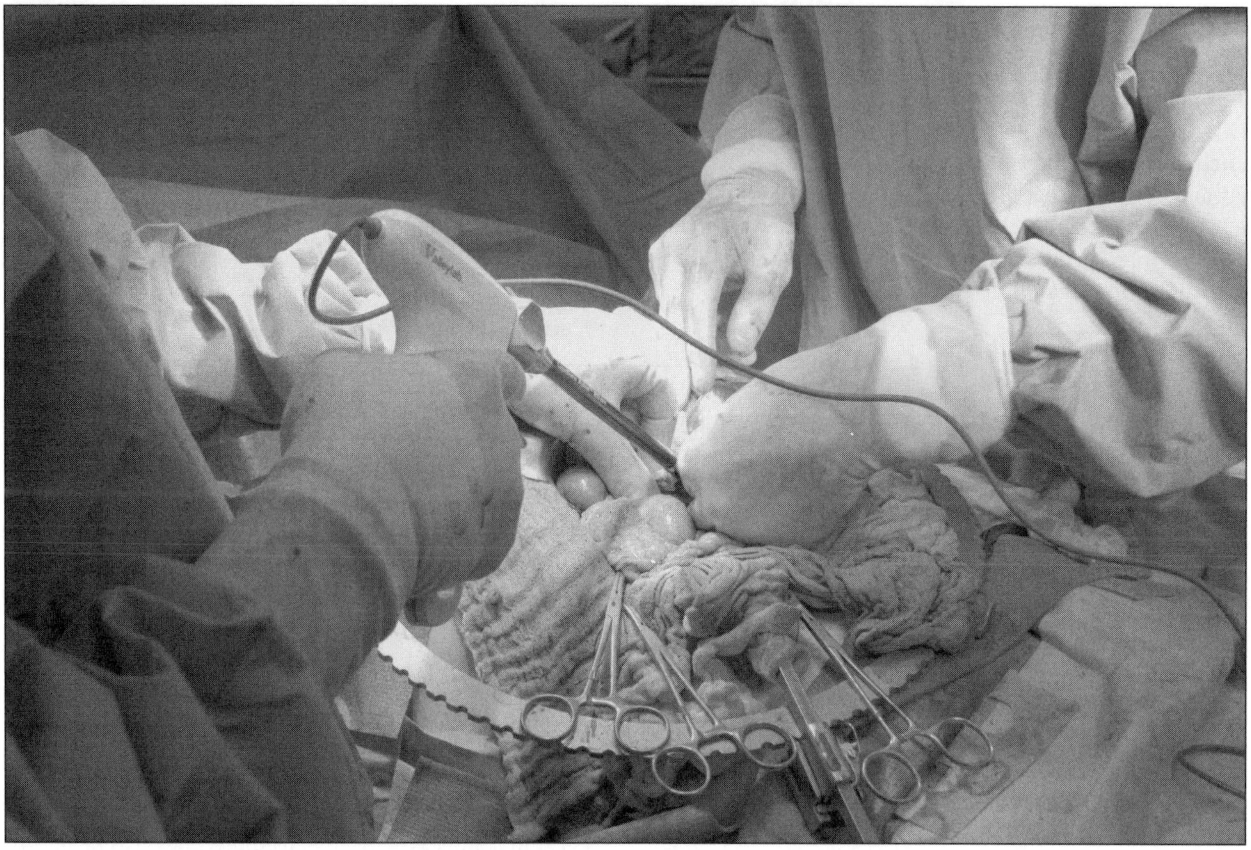

Surgeons remove the pancreatic head, part of the duodenum, and surrounding tissue in a Whipple procedure used to treat pancreatic cancer. (©Barry Slaven, MD, PhD/Phototake—All rights reserved)

surgeon also usually removes the duodenum, the gallbladder, and part of the bile duct. In some cases, the surgeon removes part of the stomach as well. The part of the pancreas that remains is then surgically connected to the patient's small intestine.

Another procedure in which only part of the pancreas is removed is known as a distal pancreatectomy. When performing this procedure, the surgeon removes only the tail end (the thinner end) of the pancreas. In some cases, the spleen is also surgically removed at the same time. This procedure is appropriate only when the tumor is relatively small and localized in the distal end of the pancreas.

When the entire pancreas is removed, the procedure is known as a total pancreatectomy. When this is done, the surgeon takes out all of the pancreas and usually the spleen. This procedure is used when the cancer is located within the body of the pancreas.

After the procedure: Pancreatectomy is a major surgical procedure and usually requires a prolonged hospital stay. Most patients remain in the hospital for two or more weeks after the procedure. During this time, the patient is carefully monitored to check for complications such as infection and bleeding. If the surgery was done using an open technique, then the wound requires care and monitoring. Patients who did not receive chemotherapy or radiation therapy before the pancreatectomy generally receive it as soon as it is feasible after the surgery. If the entire pancreas, or a very large portion of the pancreas, was removed, then the patient may be given a regimen of medications to take to correct insulin and other imbalances if the pancreas no longer produces sufficient quantities for good health.

Risks: There are many significant risks associated with pancreatectomy. According to the American Cancer Society, when a pancreatoduodenectomy is performed by an extremely skilled and experienced surgeon at a hospital or center where the health care team is very experienced in the procedure, 2 to 5 percent of patients die as a direct result of complications of the surgery. When the procedure is performed by a less experienced surgeon at a small hospital that may not be prepared for possible complications, up to 15 percent of patients may die. Nonfatal complications from the procedure are very common. They can include infection, bleeding, and leakage at one of the points a surgical connection was made.

Results: The results from pancreatectomy vary depending on the type of procedure performed and the extent to which the cancer has spread to other areas of the body. For patients who had cancer that is considered completely removable through the pancreatectomy, the five-year rate of survival is about 20 percent.

Robert Bockstiegel, B.S.

▶ For Further Information

DeVita, Vincent T., Jr., Samuel Hellman, and Steven A. Rosenberg, eds. *Cancer: Principles and Practice of Oncology—Pancreatic Cancer.* Philadelphia: Lippincott Williams & Wilkins, 2006.

Lowy, Andrew M., Steven D. Leach, and Philip Philip, eds. *Pancreatic Cancer.* New York: Springer, 2008.

Riess, H., A. Goerke, and H. Oettle, eds. *Pancreatic Cancer.* New York: Springer, 2008.

Suda, Koichi, ed. *Pancreas: Pathological Practice and Research.* New York: Karger, 2007.

▶ Other Resources

American Cancer Society
http://www.cancer.org

Pancreatica
http://www.pancreatica.org

See also Alcohol, alcoholism, and cancer; Bile duct cancer; Cholecystectomy; Endocrine cancers; Endocrinology oncology; Endoscopic retrograde cholangiopancreatography (ERCP); Gallbladder cancer; Islet cell tumors; Multiple endocrine neoplasia type 1 (MEN 1); Pancreatic cancers; Pancreatitis; Percutaneous transhepatic cholangiography (PTHC).

▶ Pancreatic cancers

Category: Diseases, symptoms, and conditions
Also known as: Adenocarcinoma of the pancreas, cystadenocarcinoma

Related conditions: Acinar cell carcinoma, insulinoma, gastrinoma, glucoganoma

Definition: Pancreatic cancers are malignant tumors occurring anywhere in the pancreas. The pancreas is an organ behind the stomach containing exocrine and endocrine glands. The exocrine glands, where most pancreatic cancer occurs, release digestive juices, which break down fats, proteins, and carbohydrates, and neutralize stomach acids. The endocrine glands produce insulin and glycogen, hormones used by the body to metabolize, or break down, sugar to use as energy.

Risk factors: Factors implicated in the development of pancreatic cancer include advanced age, diabetes, cigarette smoking, chronic pancreatitis, and a family history of the disease. Some 90 percent of those who develop pancreatic cancer are older than age fifty-five, and the average age at time of diagnosis is seventy-two.

Diabetes and pancreatic cancer have been linked, but it is not clear whether diabetes is a cause or a symptom of pancreatic cancer. Research indicates that 1 percent of people diagnosed after the age of fifty with type II diabetes (in which the body does not produce adequate amounts of insulin, a hormone manufactured in the pancreas) will be diagnosed with pancreatic cancer within three years of diagnosis. This suggests that initial onset of diabetes at age fifty and older may be an early symptom of pancreatic cancer. A study in the *British Journal of Cancer* found that people with type I, or juvenile-onset, diabetes have twice the normal risk of developing pancreatic cancer as those without the condition. According to a study of more than four hundred women who developed gestational diabetes and were followed for a mean of thirty-eight years, those who develop gestational diabetes are at increased risk of developing pancreatic cancer years later.

An estimated 25 to 30 percent of pancreatic cancer cases can be attributed to cigarette smoking. The cancer-causing chemicals in cigarette smoke are thought to enter the bloodstream and damage the pancreas, creating a two to three times greater risk among smokers.

The role of diet in developing pancreatic cancer is inconclusive, although diets high in fat and processed meats appear to present some increased risk, and diets high in fruit, vegetables, and fiber appear to protect against cancer. Obesity and lack of physical activity are also risk factors, as is occupational exposure to chemicals and pesticides.

Long-term inflammation of the pancreas, or chronic pancreatitis, is a risk factor, but the majority of people with this condition do not develop cancer of the pancreas without the presence of other risk factors. However, having a family history of pancreatitis at a young age has been implicated in the development of pancreatic cancer years later. Individuals who have had peptic ulcer surgery with a partial gastrectomy (partial removal of the stomach) may be at increased risk of developing pancreatic cancer.

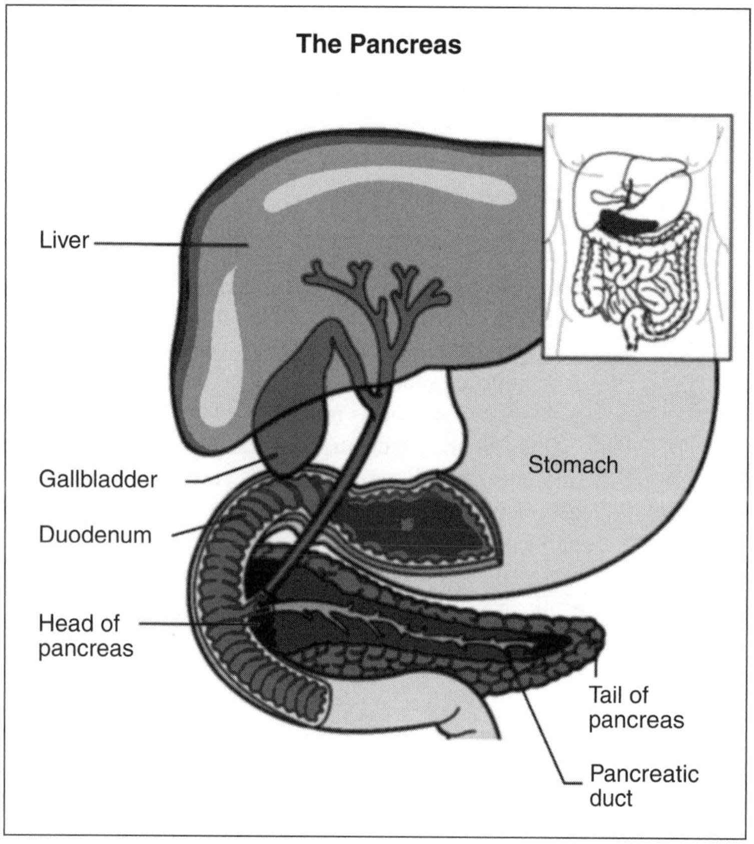

Helicobacter pylori infection also has been linked to pancreatic cancer.

According to the National Familial Pancreas Tumor Registry (NFPTR) at Johns Hopkins University, 5 to 10 percent of cases of pancreatic cancer are due to familial factors. Particularly among those with two or more relatives who have had pancreatic cancer, inherited deoxyribonucleic acid (DNA) mutations are believed to play a part. People of Ashkenazi Jewish descent may be at greater risk because of the presence of an inherited mutation in the breast cancer gene *BRCA2* (each individual inherits two such genes, one from the mother and one from the father). However, the presence of one defective *BRCA2* does not increase an individual's risk of developing pancreatic cancer in the absence of other genetic and environmental factors.

Further, individuals with a rare hereditary disease, Peutz-Jeghers syndrome, in which affected family members develop polyps from the surface of the intestine, may be at increased risk of developing pancreatic cancer. Individuals with hereditary nonpolyposis colorectal cancer (HNPCC) also may be at increased risk of developing cancer of the pancreas.

Etiology and the disease process: Pancreatic cancer occurs when abnormal cells grow in pancreatic tissue. The vast majority of abnormal cells occur in the ducts carrying pancreatic juices from the exocrine glands. Although the exact cause of pancreatic cancer is not known, inherited or acquired changes in DNA are believed to be behind most cases. Many pancreatic cancers are not detected until they are locally advanced and have invaded the vascular system or have spread to lymph nodes. If the tumor blocks the common bile duct and bile cannot be released into the digestive system, the patient's skin and whites of the eyes become jaundiced and the urine may become darker. The cancer may spread and cause pain in the upper abdomen and sometimes the back.

Incidence: Pancreatic cancer is the fourth-leading cause of cancer death in the United States because it grows aggressively and causes few symptoms in the initial stages. However, it is relatively rare compared with other forms of cancer. About 30,000 new cases are diagnosed each year, as compared with 200,000 new cases of breast cancer and 170,000 of lung cancer. According to the American Cancer Society, rates of pancreatic cancer have dropped since the 1980's. The incidence rate of pancreatic cancer is 11.4 per 100,000 men and women, although this type of cancer is more prevalent among men than women. The incidence of pancreatic cancer is 50 to 90 percent higher in the African American population than in other racial or ethnic groups in the United States, probably because of the higher rates of obesity, poverty, cigarette smoking, and type II diabetes in this group.

Symptoms: Many people do not experience symptoms of pancreatic cancer until the tumor has spread to the lungs, liver, or lymph nodes. The majority (80 percent) of pancreatic cancers occur in the head of the organ, creating symptoms associated with blockage of this area closest to the bile duct. One common symptom is jaundice, a yellowing of the skin and the whites of the eyes resulting from an accumulation of bilirubin in the blood. At least half of those with pancreatic cancer will experience jaundice. Other symptoms include nausea and diarrhea, a swollen gallbladder or liver, pain in the midback, fatigue, a slow metabolism, light-colored stools, and itchy skin.

The 20 percent of pancreatic cancers occurring in the tail of the pancreas often obstruct the vein draining the spleen, resulting in an enlarged spleen and pressure in varicose veins around the stomach and esophagus. An individual may experience this as pain in the midback, pain in the stomach several hours after a meal, blood clots in the legs, and loss of appetite. Tumors or cystadenocarcinoma affecting the hormone-secreting functions of the pancreas, though rare, can produce symptoms of fatigue, dizziness, chills, diarrhea, or muscle spasms.

If the pancreatic cancer occurs in the islet cells, which produce insulin and other hormones, the cells may produce too much insulin, causing the affected individual to feel dizzy and weak and to experience chills, muscle spasms, and diarrhea. This type of endocrine pancreatic cancer is considered highly treatable.

Screening and diagnosis: A high blood level of cancer antigen 19-9 (CA 19-9), a product released into the blood by pancreatic cancer cells, serves as a marker indicating the presence of a pancreatic tumor. However, this marker is used only to assess response to therapy and not as a screening test.

Because there is no screening test for pancreatic cancer, people should report any sudden onset of abdominal pain, loss of appetite, or unexplained weight change to their physician. If pancreatic cancer is suspected, the physician will palpate for presence of an abdominal tumor and order blood tests that will indicate changes in blood sugar or the presence of anemia. However, the pancreas is hidden behind other organs and cannot be felt during a routine physical exam. A differential diagnosis should rule out any liver-related causes of jaundice.

If a pancreatic tumor is present, diagnostic tests such as ultrasound, computed tomography (CT) scans, and endoscopic retrograde cholangiopancreatography (ERCP), a type of X ray, will be ordered to stage the progression of the disease. An ultrasound has been shown to be more useful than a CT scan in detecting the presence of small tumors. A CT scan can be used to guide a needle in obtaining a biopsy. During a positron emission tomography (PET) scan, a form of sugar that is readily absorbed by cancer cells is injected into the patient's blood to assess the location and spread of cancer cells. A combination PET/CT scan has been found useful in detecting the spread of cancer that surgery cannot remove, for staging, and even for detecting early-stage cancer. ERCP can be used to examine the pancreatic duct while a tissue biopsy is taken to study the cancer cells. An angiogram can be used to show any blockage or impediment of blood flow in vessels caused by the tumor or abnormality of blood vessels to assess the likelihood of removing the cancer surgically.

If surgery such as a laparoscopy is performed, a biopsy may be taken to determine the location and spread of the disease. Laparoscopy is a diagnostic procedure in which an incision is made in the abdomen and a laparoscope, or lighted tube, is inserted to view the pancreas. Alternatively, the physician may choose to perform a laparotomy, a diagnostic surgical procedure in which a large incision is made to examine organs in the abdomen for extent of disease.

Staging for pancreatic cancer is as follows:

- Stage IA: Tumor is confined to pancreas and is no larger than 2 centimeters (cm).
- Stage IB: Tumor is confined to pancreas and is larger than 2 cm.
- Stage IIA: Cancer has metastasized to nearby organs and tissues but not into large blood vessels or to lymph nodes.
- Stage IIB: Cancer has metastasized to nearby lymph nodes and may have spread to nearby tissues and organs but not distant sites.
- Stage III: Cancer has reached blood vessels near the pancreas and may have spread to lymph nodes but not distant sites.
- Stage IV: Cancer, regardless of tumor size, has metastasized to distant organs, and may also be in tissues near the pancreas or in lymph nodes.

Alternatively, some physicians stage the pancreatic cancer on the basis of the likelihood that the tumor can be

Relative Survival Rates for Pancreatic Cancer by Stage at Diagnosis, 1988-2003

	Survival Rates (%)					
Stage	*1-Year*	*2-Year*	*3-Year*	*5-Year*	*8-Year*	*10-Year*
Localized[a]	40.5	24.5	19.5	17.4	16.8	16.6
Regional[b]	38.0	16.7	10.5	7.2	5.7	5.3
Distant[c]	10.5	4.1	2.6	1.6	0.9	0.7
Unstaged	20.8	9.3	6.2	4.7	4.1	3.6

Source: Data from National Cancer Institute, Surveillance Epidemiology and End Results, Cancer Stat Fact Sheets, 2008

[a]Cancer still confined to primary site

[b]Cancer has spread to regional lymph nodes or directly beyond the primary site

[c]Cancer has metastasized

removed surgically according to the following stages: resectable (can remove entire tumor); locally advanced, unresectable (wherein complete removal of the tumor is not possible); and metastatic (where the cancer has spread and surgery would be undertaken only to relieve symptoms or complications).

Treatment and therapy: The Whipple procedure, or pancreatectomy, a major surgery with a high risk of complications, is used when it is likely that surgery will cure the individual of the entire pancreatic tumor. The head of the pancreas and parts of the stomach and small intestine, bile duct, and gallbladder are removed. After this surgery, the pancreas is still able to produce insulin and digestive juices. A total pancreatectomy involves removal of the entire pancreas, part of the stomach and small intestine, the common bile duct, and the gallbladder, spleen, and nearby lymph nodes.

Palliative surgery may relieve pain and complications associated with the impact of the cancer on digestion, particularly blockage of the bile duct. When surgery cannot remove the entire tumor, during the course of an ERCP, a biliary stent is placed to relieve biliary obstruction and allow vessels to move bile. Inserting an endoscopic or percutaneous biliary stent can relieve jaundice, particularly for those with cancer in the head of the pancreas.

Radiation therapy may be administered five times a week for several weeks or months before surgery, after surgery, or as a primary treatment in conjunction with chemotherapy when the cancer is isolated in the pancreas but cannot be removed surgically.

Chemotherapy alone, particularly gemcitabine, is often used for palliative care of metastatic pancreatic cancer that has spread distally to other organs or body parts. Gemcitabine (Gemzar) has resulted in clinical improvement in 25 percent of these patients. The use of erlotinib (Tarceva), which stops signals that instruct cancer cells to multiply, in combination with gemcitabine has proved to be more effective than using gemcitabine alone. However, patients must be healthy and functioning well enough to be able to tolerate the side effects of chemotherapy. Common side effects of chemotherapy treatment with gemcitabine include fatigue, lowered production of blood cells, increased incidence of infection, tiredness, breathlessness, and bruising.

Ongoing clinical trials involve a vaccine for pancreatic cancer that is used to treat existing disease by causing an immune response to the pancreatic cancer.

Prognosis, prevention, and outcomes: The mortality rate for pancreatic cancer based on National Cancer Institute data collected between 2000 and 2004 is 10.6 deaths per 100,000 men and women. Overall five-year survival rates for this cancer are 5 percent. The majority of pancreatic cancers (52 percent) are diagnosed when they have already metastasized.

The five-year survival rate following diagnosis for those with cancers of the exocrine pancreas, the most common type, is 20.3 percent when the cancer is localized. However, when it has spread to nearby organs and tissues, the survival rate falls to 8.0 percent, and 1.7 percent when the cancer has spread to distant organs.

Recommendations for preventing pancreatic cancer include health education to reduce tobacco consumption and referring those at increased risk for familial reasons to genetic counseling and possibly genetic testing.

Susan H. Peterman, M.P.H.

▶ For Further Information

Hassan, M. N., et al. "Risk Factors for Pancreatic Cancer: Case-Control Study." *American Journal of Gastroenterology* 102, no. 12 (August, 2007): 2696-2707.

Reber, Howard, ed. *Pancreatic Cancer: Pathogenesis, Diagnosis, and Treatment*. Totowa, N.J.: Humana Press, 1998.

Risch, H. A. "Etiology of Pancreatic Cancer, with a Hypothesis Concerning the Role of N-Nitroso Compounds and Excess Gastric Acidity." *Journal of the National Cancer Institute* 95, no. 12 (July 2, 2003): 948-960.

Wiederpass, E., et al. "Occurrence, Trends and Environment Etiology of Pancreatic Cancer." *Scandinavian Journal of Environmental Health* 24, no. 3 (June, 1998): 165-174.

▶ Other Resources

American Cancer Society
Detailed Guide: Pancreatic Cancer
http://www.cancer.org/docroot/CRI/content/CRI_2_4_1X_What_is_pancreatic_cancer_34.asp

Medical University of South Carolina Digestive Disease Center
http://www.ddc.musc.edu

Pancreatic Cancer Action Network
http://www.pancan.org/

Pancreatica.org
http://www.pancreatica.org

Sol Goldman Pancreatic Cancer Research Center
http://www.pathology.jhu.edu/pancreas

See also Alcohol, alcoholism, and cancer; Bile duct cancer; *BRCA1* and *BRCA2* genes; CA 19-9 test; Cholecystectomy; Endocrine cancers; Endocrinology oncology; Endoscopic retrograde cholangiopancreatography (ERCP); Gallbladder cancer; Islet cell tumors; Multiple endocrine neoplasia type 1 (MEN 1); Pancreatectomy; Pancreatitis; Percutaneous transhepatic cholangiography (PTHC); Peutz-Jeghers syndrome.

▶ Pancreatitis

Category: Diseases, symptoms, and conditions
Also known as: Inflammation of the pancreas

Related conditions: Diabetes mellitus, alcoholism, pancreatic cancer, gallstones

Definition: Pancreatitis, inflammation of the pancreas, appears in acute and chronic forms. Acute pancreatitis comes on suddenly and typically resolves quickly, but it may be severe and life-threatening. Chronic pancreatitis slowly destroys the pancreas.

Risk factors: Alcohol abuse, trauma, high lipid or calcium levels are all associatted with pancreatitis.

Etiology and the disease process: The pancreas is a glandular organ that lies behind the stomach. It produces hormones and digestive enzymes. Specialized pancreatic cells produce the hormones glucagon and insulin. Glucagon stimulates the liver to convert stored glycogen into glucose, raising blood glucose (sugar) levels. As blood glucose levels rise, the pancreas responds by secreting insulin. Insulin helps transport glucose into the body's cells, where it is used for energy. Other cells located throughout the pancreas secrete digestive enzymes. These enzymes are secreted in fluid that travels from the pancreas through the pancreatic duct to the duodenum (portion of the small intestine), where they become activated and aid digestion.

In pancreatitis, the flow of pancreatic enzymes becomes obstructed by gallstones or spasm and edema at the ampulla of Vater, the area where the pancreatic and liver ducts enter the duodenum, and the enzymes begin digesting the pancreas.

Incidence: More than 300,000 people are hospitalized with acute pancreatitis annually; additionally, 85,000 are hospitalized with chronic pancreatitis.

Symptoms: Mild pancreatitis may manifest with upper abdominal pain centered near the umbilicus. As pancreatitis progresses, abdominal pain becomes severe and persistent and may radiate to the back. It commonly occurs after eating a large meal or drinking alcohol. Other symptoms may include abdominal distension and tenderness, bruising in the flank or around the umbilicus, fever, nausea, rapid pulse, and low blood pressure.

Screening and diagnosis: Physical examination, blood tests to detect elevated pancreatic enzyme (amylase and lipase) levels, and abdominal computed tomography scan confirm the diagnosis. Abdominal ultrasonography may detect gallstones.

Treatment and therapy: Treatment depends on the severity of symptoms. Mild pancreatitis may abate without treatment. Severe pancreatitis requires withholding food and fluids, administering replacement fluids and electro-

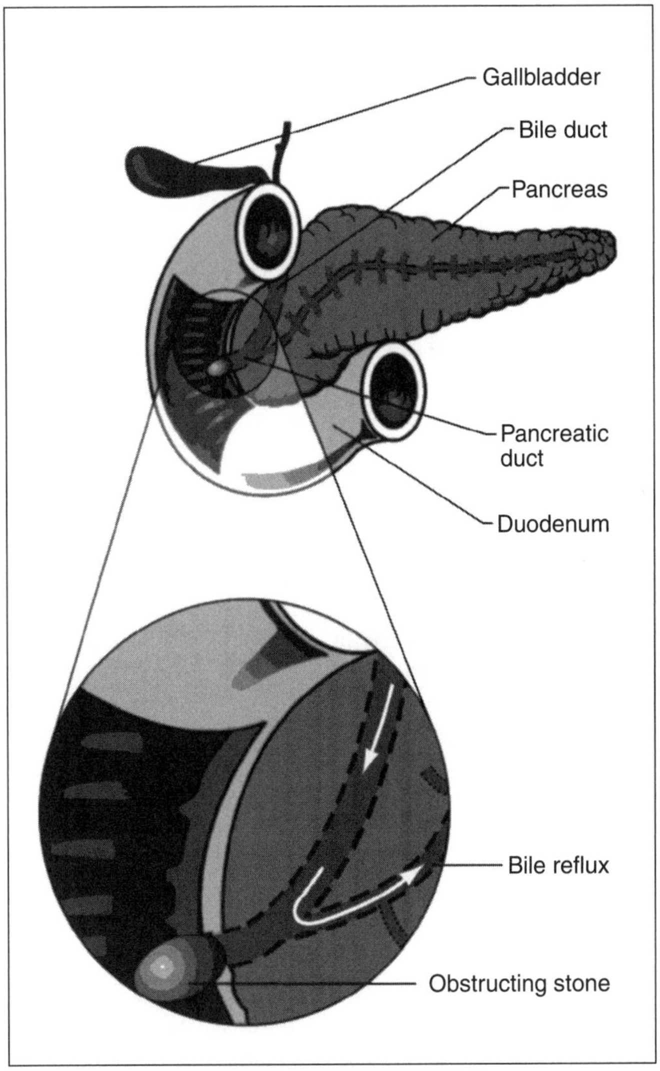

The pancreas, showing the pancreatic duct.

lytes intravenously, and inserting a nasogastric tube to decrease abdominal distension. Medications such as hydromorphone or morphine are commonly prescribed to control pain. Surgical drainage of a pancreatic abscess or pseudocyst may be necessary.

Prognosis, prevention, and outcomes: Pancreatitis causes approximately 3,500 deaths annually. The prognosis is good when pancreatitis results from biliary tract disease but poor when it is a complication of alcoholism. Pancreatitis increases the risk for pancreatic cancer.

Collette Bishop Hendler, R.N., M.S.

See also Alcohol, alcoholism, and cancer; Bile duct cancer; Cholecystectomy; Endocrine cancers; Endocrinology oncology; Endoscopic retrograde cholangiopancreatography (ERCP); Gallbladder cancer; Islet cell tumors; Multiple endocrine neoplasia type 1 (MEN 1); Pancreatectomy; Pancreatic cancers; Percutaneous transhepatic cholangiography (PTHC).

▶ Pap test

Category: Procedures
Also known as: Pap smear, Papanicolaou test, gynecological exam

Definition: A Pap test is the removal of microscopic cells from the cervix, the opening between the vagina and uterus in females, for laboratory evaluation.

Cancers diagnosed: Cervical cancer

Why performed: The Pap test is a diagnostic procedure performed for early detection of cervical cancer. The test can also detect abnormal, noncancerous cells and certain vaginal infections. Cervical cancer has been linked to certain strains of the human papillomavirus (HPV), which is sexually transmitted. These viruses can be detected with current Pap test technology. According to guidelines from the American College of Obstetricians and Gynecologists, a female patient should have the first Pap test within three years of having sexual intercourse or at age twenty-one, whichever comes first. Until age thirty, women should have annual testing. After age thirty, if the woman is in a monogamous sexual relationship and has had three consecutive normal Pap tests, testing can be done every three years. For women over the age of sixty-five with three normal tests and no abnormal tests for the prior ten years, testing may be discontinued. Women who have had a hysterectomy may stop having Pap tests, unless the hysterectomy was performed because of cancer. These are general

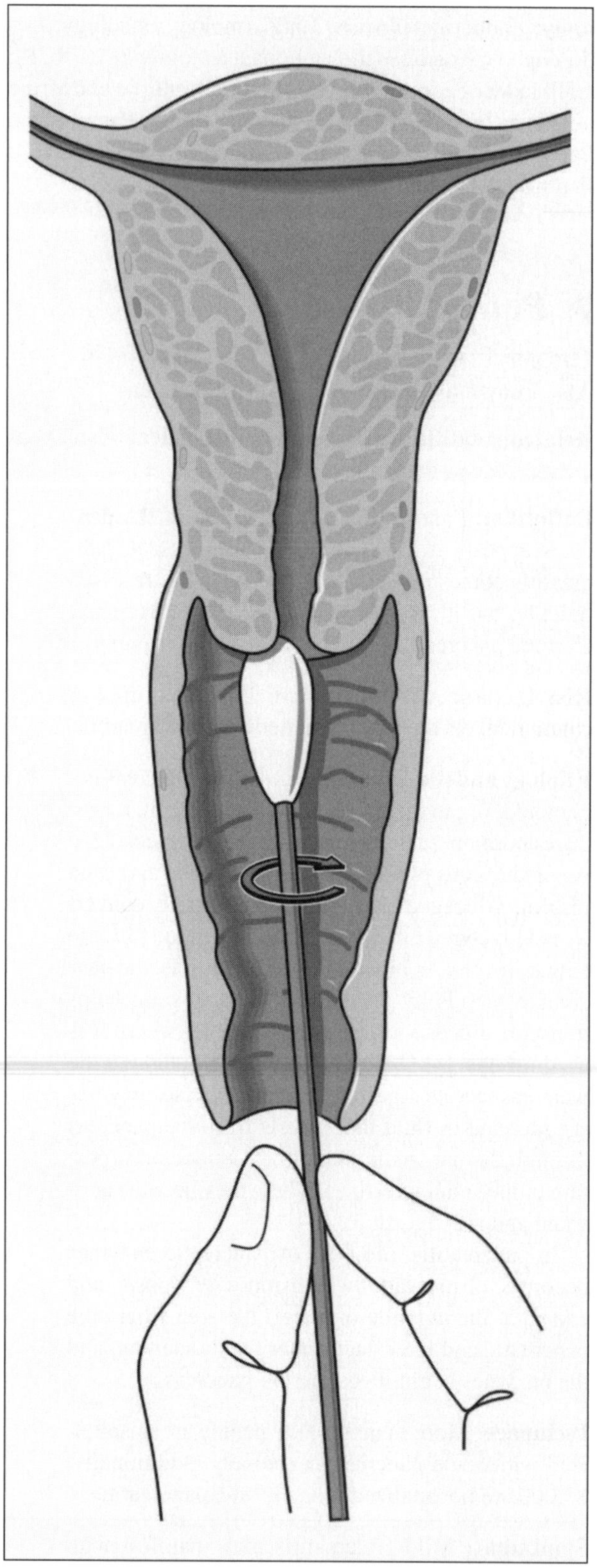

Obtaining a Pap smear. (LifeART© 2008 Wolters Kluwer Health, Inc.-Lippincott Williams &Wilkins. All rights reserved.)

guidelines for testing; individual situations must be considered by the health care provider.

Patient preparation: The patient must not be menstruating at the time of testing. It is recommended that the patient avoid sexual intercourse, tampons, douching, and vaginal medications, creams, or sprays for two days before the test. The patient should empty her bladder immediately before the procedure and then undress from the waist down. A patient gown or drape will be provided.

Steps of the procedure: The test is usually done in a health care provider's office during a gynecological examination, which includes a breast and pelvic examination. The patient is placed in lithotomy position on the examination table. In this position, the patient is lying on her back with feet in stirrups at the end of the table and is draped with a sheet.

The examiner will push the patient's knees apart to inspect the external genital area. A plastic or metal speculum is lubricated with water or a water-based gel and is inserted into the vagina. The curved blades of the speculum are opened and the cervix is located. A thin plastic brush with an end that looks like a broom is inserted into the opening of the cervix and is rotated 360 degrees to collect endocervical cells. The patient may feel a slight pinching sensation. The collection device and the speculum are removed. The broom end is placed into a small container with preservative chemicals and is sent to the laboratory for evaluation of the cervical cells. In the past, samples of cells were obtained with a small wire brush and smeared on a glass slide and sent to the laboratory. Newer technology with the broom is more accurate than the older methods.

After the Pap test, the provider will then place lubricant on two fingers and insert them into the vagina while feeling with the other hand on top of the abdomen. This is done to feel the uterus, cervix, and ovaries for any abnormalities, tenderness, or masses. Then, a rectal examination may be done in some patients. The rectal wall lies against the back of the vaginal wall. A tilted uterus may be examined during a rectal examination.

After the procedure: The patient may need to remove lubricant if it is used during the test. The patient is allowed to go home immediately after the examination and resume previous levels of activity.

Risks: Brief mild discomfort may occur in some patients during a Pap test. Some may experience a small amount of vaginal bleeding or spotting during or after the test. Some women may experience embarrassment during the examination. These risks are minor given the benefits of early detection of cervical cancer with the likelihood of successful treatment.

Results: The results are generally available within one week. A normal or negative Pap test will have no abnormal cells or infectious agents present. An abnormal Pap test may show abnormal noncancerous cells, abnormal cancer cells, or infection. If a patient has an abnormal Pap test, then further evaluation is needed. A repeat Pap test may be performed in approximately three months. This time lapse is to allow possible infections to be resolved that may be the cause of the abnormal test. Other patients may have a more detailed test or a biopsy. If cancer is detected, then surgery is generally performed. Rarely, the test may give a false negative result when the test is actually abnormal. This may occur from a poor sample or from laboratory error.

Amy Bull, D.S.N., A.P.N.

▶ For Further Information

Carlson, Karen J., Stephanie A. Eisenstat, and Terra Ziporyn. *The New Harvard Guide to Women's Health.* Cambridge, Mass.: Harvard University Press, 2004.

Minkin, Mary Jane, and Carol V. Wright. *A Woman's Guide to Sexual Health.* New Haven, Conn.: Yale University Press, 2004.

Rosenthal, M. Sara. *The Gynecological Sourcebook.* 4th ed. New York: McGraw-Hill, 2003.

▶ Other Resources

National Cervical Cancer Coalition
http://www.nccc-online.org

National Women's Health Information Center
http://www.4women.gov/faq/pap.htm

See also Antiviral therapies; Cervical cancer; Colposcopy; Conization; Diethylstilbestrol (DES); Endometrial cancer; Fertility drugs and cancer; Gynecologic cancers; Human papillomavirus (HPV); Hysterectomy; Hystero-oophorectomy; Loop electrosurgical excisional procedure (LEEP); Pelvic examination; Pregnancy and cancer; Vaccines, preventive; Virus-related cancers.

▶ Paracentesis

Category: Procedures
Also known as: Abdominal tap, abdominal paracentesis, peritoneal tap

Definition: Paracentesis is the insertion of a needle or catheter through the peritoneum, the membrane that lines the abdominal cavity, to sample or drain excess fluid.

Cancers diagnosed or treated: Most metastatic cancers, especially liver cancer, mesothelioma, and ovarian cancer

Why performed: Primarily a diagnostic but sometimes a therapeutic procedure, paracentesis is performed to identify new cancer cells that have metastasized to the abdomen, or to analyze the extent of an existing cancer that is causing fluid buildup (ascites) in the peritoneal space. In the latter case, physicians may perform paracentesis to remove a large amount of fluid and relieve the patient of pain in the lungs, kidneys, and bowels.

Patient preparation: The physician will discuss risks, benefits, and alternatives with the patient and ask him or her to sign an informed consent form. A few days before the procedure, the patient undergoes blood tests to confirm that there are no clotting or bleeding problems in the abdomen. On the day of the procedure, a radiologist will perform an ultrasound scan of the peritoneal space to assess the size and area of the ascites. Immediately before the test, the patient must urinate to leave an empty bladder.

Steps of the procedure: Non-emergency paracentesis is scheduled in an outpatient setting. The abdominal area is cleaned with an antiseptic soap, and a local anesthetic such as lidocaine is injected into the patient's abdomen. Based on the ultrasound and percussion of the abdomen, the physician chooses the insertion site for paracentesis. Typically, the patient sits in a semi-recumbent position, so a site just below the navel is optimal for insertion and fluid aspiration. A nurse will shave this area of the abdomen if needed. When enough fluid has been removed (10 to 50 milliliters in diagnostic paracentesis and up to 10 liters in therapeutic paracentesis), the physician withdraws the needle from the abdomen and applies direct pressure to the puncture site with a sterile dressing. Large accumulations of fluid require the insertion of a vacuum-pressurized catheter through which the fluid can drain into a container. Results are sent to the laboratory for analysis right away. The entire procedure takes ten to thirty minutes.

After the procedure: The patient rests for one to four hours while vital signs, incision site, and fluid drainage are monitored. If large amounts of fluid are drained, then nurses will actively monitor the patient's blood pressure for hypotension and shock. An intravenous (IV) line may be inserted to avoid fluid shifts in the body and prevent kidney failure. Slight fluid drainage from the puncture site may continue for one to two days. Normally, the patient does not require an overnight stay.

Risks: Paracentesis is a relatively safe procedure. Although the incidence of any particular complication is rare, a range of intraprocedure complications may occur. The paracentesis needle may perforate the bladder, bowels, or blood vessels in the abdomen, causing internal bleeding or hemorrhage. Infection of the peritoneal fluid or the spread of cancer inside the abdomen are also risks associated with the paracentesis needle. The risk of external infection around the puncture site is increased if there is persistent leakage from the puncture site.

Results: Patients undergo paracentesis only if they have ascites, an abnormal condition, in the abdomen. Several laboratory tests are performed on the peritoneal fluid to assess the abnormality. A high white blood cell count may indicate inflammation, bacterial perotinitis, infection, or cancer in the abdomen. High albumin protein content in the fluid, as compared to the content in the patient's blood serum, may indicate tuberculosis, kidney disorder, pancreatitis, or cancer. Lower protein content may indicate liver cirrhosis or portal hypertension. A high level of the enzyme lactate dehydrogenase in the fluid may indicate infection or cancer. A high level of the enzyme amylase may indicate pancreatitis. A low level of glucose may indicate infection. To confirm the type of infection or cancer, cells from the fluid will undergo culture and pathology in the laboratory. A biopsy may also be performed.

Bharat Burman, B.A.

▶ For Further Information

Aziz, K., and G. Y. Wu. *Cancer Screening: A Practical Guide for Physicians*. Totowa, N.J.: Humana Press, 2002.

Foley, K. M., et al. *When the Focus Is on Care: Palliative Care and Cancer*. Atlanta: American Cancer Society, 2005.

Waller, A., and N. L. Caroline. *Handbook of Palliative Care in Cancer*. Boston: Butterworth-Heinemann, 2000.

▶ Other Resources

American Cancer Society
Treatment of Mesothelioma by Stage
http://www.cancer.org/docroot/CRI/content/CRI_2_4_4X_Treatment_Options_by_stage_29.asp?sitearea=

National Cancer Institute
Screening and Testing to Detect Cancer
http://www.cancer.gov/cancertopics/screening

See also Ascites; Mesothelioma.

▶ Paraneoplastic syndromes

Category: Diseases, symptoms, and conditions
Also known as: Paraneoplastic disorders

Related conditions: Cushing syndrome, Lambert-Eaton myasthenic syndrome, dermatomyositis-polymyositis, malignant carcinoid syndrome, leukemoid reaction, disseminated intravascular coagulation (DIC), syndrome of inappropriate antidiuretic hormone (SIADH)

Definition: Paraneoplastic syndromes are a large group of clinical symptoms that may arise from the presence of a malignancy. These symptoms, while they can be considered distinct clinical entities in themselves, are an indirect result of the biochemical by-products of the primary neoplastic entity.

Risk factors: The risk factors for developing one or more paraneoplastic syndromes depend on a family history of malignant cancer and the type of primary tumor. For instance, specific tumors such as small-cell lung carcinoma are associated with a higher predilection for Cushing syndrome from adrenocorticaltropic hormone (ACTH) secretion.

Etiology and the disease process: The origin of most paraneoplastic syndromes is generally attributed to the unabated production of different types of chemical messengers by tumor cells. These chemicals include cytokines, hormones and their precursors, autoantibodies, enzymes, and fetal proteins. The corresponding effect of these substances on metabolic, biochemical, and physiologic pathways can be observed clinically. Because these substances circulate through the body, the primary site of the tumor may be distant from the organ systems involved. In a similar manner, a paraneoplastic syndrome alone may herald the presence of malignancy bearing a poor prognosis.

Incidence: The incidence of paraneoplastic syndromes is estimated at 10 to 15 percent in patients with malignant cancer. The exact figure may be within the range of 2 to 20 percent, as these syndromes can masquerade as nonmalignant diseases on manifestation and thus are poorly accounted for.

Symptoms: Symptoms of paraneoplastic syndromes are very broad and may initially occur as nonspecific complaints such as an unexplained, persisting fever; noninduced loss of appetite; and involuntary weight loss. More specific symptoms point to an affected organ system, although the primary tumor may remain unknown. Vague joint and muscle pain may be associated with bone joint thickening or connective tissue proliferation (scleroderma or amyloidosis). Weakness, diarrhea, and mental status changes can be attributed to electrolyte imbalances of sodium, potassium, and phosphorus; acid-base disorders caused by adrenocorticotropic hormone, antidiuretic hormone, or intestinal hormone secretion; kidney damage; or malabsorption of nutrients. Bleeding from underproduction or overactivation and depletion of coagulation components (disseminated intravascular coagulation, cryoglobulinemia), migratory sites of spontaneous intravascular clotting, or abnormal excesses of or deficits in red blood cells or white blood cell subtypes (anemia, erythrocytosis, thrombocytosis) may also be present. Itching is the most common skin complaint of cancer patients. Other skin lesions may appear and include loss or excess of hair (alopecia, hypertrichosis), stress-induced flushing, scalelike changes (icthyosis), shingles (herpes zoster), and black pigmentation of skin (acanthosis nigricans, dermic melanosis). Cushingoid symptoms (fatigue, lethargy, psychosis, buffalo hump, hypertension, purple striae, central obesity) is suggestive of excess ACTH-like molecule secretion. Muscular weakness around the pelvic girdle and scapular areas that improves throughout the day and decreased tendon reflexes are characteristic of Lambert-Eaton syndrome (LEMS).

Screening and diagnosis: There is currently no screening available for paraneoplastic syndromes, as they depend on the underlying cause. Establishing the etiology of a paraneoplastic syndrome depends on clinical and confirmatory investigation of a suspected neoplasm through a combination of laboratory, imaging, and pathology studies of biopsy specimens. Bleeding disorders can often be assessed with blood tests such as complete blood counts, as well as assessments of platelet function, platelet factors, and clotting mechanisms. Multistep diagnostics such as the dexamethasone suppression test can be used to rule out a pituitary cause of Cushingoid symptoms by measuring ACTH and cortisol levels in response to low and high doses of dexamethasone if a twenty-four-hour screening for urine cortisol before testing is positive. In spite of all these investigations, a definitive "diagnosis" is truly established only once the primary tumor is located and biopsied, if not excised. Decrease in antidiuretic hormone secretion by the tumor is often resistant to changes in serum levels by withholding water intake.

Autoantibodies such as anti-Hu, anti-Ri, and antibodies against amphyphysin are present in some patients exhibiting neurologic symptoms and syndromes such as neuronopathy, encephalitis, opsoclonus/myoclonus syndrome, and stiff man syndrome. Cancer-associated autoantibodies

Cancers Commonly Associated with Paraneoplastic Syndromes

- Breast cancer
- Gastric cancers
- Hepatocellular carcinoma
- Leukemias
- Lung cancer
- Lymphomas
- Neural cancers
- Ovarian cancer
- Pancreatic cancers
- Renal carcinoma

such as the antineuronal antibody Ma2 are seen in testicular cancer.

Treatment and therapy: Treatment and therapy are directed toward tumor detection and elimination. This may involve a combination of surgical, chemotherapeutic, and radiologic interventions depending on the type of tumor found. Treatment of the paraneoplastic disease itself will often fail if the location of the primary tumor is not established.

In cases in which an immune-mediated etiology is present, immunosuppression may be of help. Agents used include cyclosporine, antithymocyte globulin, and prednisone.

Prognosis, prevention, and outcomes: Prognosis is widely variable and depends on the clinical presentation of the paraneoplastic disease. For example, disseminated intravascular coagulation may indicate a poor prognosis while less life-threatening diseases fare better. Generally, treatment of the tumor results in resolution of the paraneoplastic disease. However, severity of the specific disease may prolong recovery. There are no preventive measures.

Aldo C. Dumlao, M.D.

▶ For Further Information

Kelloff, Gary, Ernest T. Hawk, and Caroline C. Sigman, eds. *Cancer Chemoprevention*. 2 vols. Totowa, N.J.: Humana Press, 2004-2005.

Montgomery, Hugh, Neil Goldsack, and Richard Marshall. *My First MRCP Book*. London: Remedica, 2003.

Rose, Noel R., and Ian R. Mackay. *The Autoimmune Diseases*. Amsterdam: Elsevier/Academic Press, 2006.

▶ Other Resources

National Institute of Neurological Disorders and Stroke
Paraneoplastic Syndromes Information Page
http://www.ninds.nih.gov/disorders/paraneoplastic/paraneoplastic.htm

MayoClinic.com
Paraneoplastic Syndromes of the Nervous System
http://www.mayoclinic.com/health/paraneoplastic-syndromes/DS00840

See also Carcinoid tumors and carcinoid syndrome; Cushing syndrome and cancer; Disseminated intravascular coagulation (DIC); Endocrine cancers; Hormonal therapies; Lambert-Eaton myasthenic syndrome (LEMS); Syndrome of inappropriate antidiuretic hormone production (SIADH).

▶ Parathyroid cancer

Category: Diseases, symptoms, and conditions
Also known as: Parathyroid carcinoma

Related conditions: Primary hyperparathyroidism, hypercalcemia

Definition: Parathyroid cancer is an uncommon endocrine malignancy of the parathyroid glands. The parathyroid glands, which are at the upper and lower poles of the thyroid gland, are usually distinguishable as four distinct glands; however, more or less than four have been found during surgeries.

The parathyroid glands help normalize the body's metabolism by regulating calcium concentrations in the blood. The hormone that is released by the parathyroid gland acts on bones, kidney structures, and tissues of the intestines. Parathyroid cancer has been known to cause increased production and activity of the glands, or hyperparathyroidism. Because of the infrequency of this form of cancer, limited studies have been made of its natural history and underlying biologic basis.

Risk factors: Increased risk of parathyroid cancer is associated with hereditary hyperparathyroidism and a related condition called hyperparathyroidism-jaw tumor syndrome (HPT-JT). Previous radiation to the neck is known to be a slight risk factor for head and neck cancer. No association between gender and parathyroid cancer has been reported.

Etiology and the disease process: What causes parathyroid cancer is unknown. However, a related cancer-producing gene (oncogene) has been located on chromosome 11. Also, some cases of parathyroid cancer in patients under twenty years of age indicate a genetic factor as a potential causative factor in this form of cancer. As the disease progresses, parathyroid hormone levels become elevated and as high as 10.2 times the upper limit of normal.

Even a very small metastatic deposit may produce significant release of parathyroid hormone and cause severe increases of calcium levels. Parathyroid cancer grows slowly and metastasizes late, with the lungs being a common (20 to 40 percent) area of involvement. Other sites that may be affected include bones, the pleura, pericardial tissue surrounding the heart, and the pancreas. Because the disease is usually slow growing, most patients die of metabolic complications rather than the cancer itself.

Incidence: Parathyroid cancer is one of the rarest of all human cancers, with an estimated incidence of 0.015 per 100,000 population and an estimated prevalence of 0.005 percent in the United States. The incidence of hyperparathyroidism has increased since 1974, yet studies show that the incidence of parathyroid cancer among patients with primary hyperparathyroidism is around 1 percent.

Symptoms: Parathyroid cancer usually manifests with symptoms consistent with severe hyperparathyroidism. Because most of the parathyroid cancer tumors preserve the ability to produce active parathyroid hormone, hypercalcemia is a common feature. There is a greater incidence of renal and bone disease compared with patients with benign hyperparathyroidism. Hoarseness with recurrent laryngeal nerve involvement is rare. However, its presence in a patient with primary hyperparathyroidism who has not had prior neck surgery is very suggestive of parathyroid cancer.

Screening and diagnosis: Diagnosis of parathyroid cancer is considered with a palpable neck mass, significant elevated calcium and parathyroid hormone (PTH) levels, and combined renal and bone disease. Hypercalcemia, the hallmark of hyperparathyroidism, is usually severe in patients with parathyroid cancer. For patients suspected to have this form of cancer, computed tomography (CT) scanning is thought to be the most useful for detecting the primary tumor, its local extent, and metastases. Ultrasonography in conjunction with CT scans and magnetic resonance imaging (MRI) may be useful in the evaluation of the disease in the neck and better detects distant metastases in the chest or abdomen. If any of these noninvasive tests is unsuccessful in localizing the tumor, specific venous sampling or arteriography is a useful option.

Researchers Ashok R. Shaha and Jatia P. Shah have proposed a staging system, with subgroups based on tumor size and metastases, for these relatively rare tumors.

Tumor size:

- T1 = Primary tumor less than 3 centimeters (cm) in size
- T2 = Primary tumor greater than 3 cm
- T3 = Primary tumor of any size with invasion of the surrounding soft tissues
- T4 = Massive central compartment disease invading the trachea and esophagus or recurrent parathyroid cancer

Metastases:

- N0 = No regional lymph node metastases
- N1 = Regional lymph node metastases
- M0 = No evidence of distant metastases
- M1 = Evidence of distant metastases

Stage grouping:

- Stage I: T1N0M0

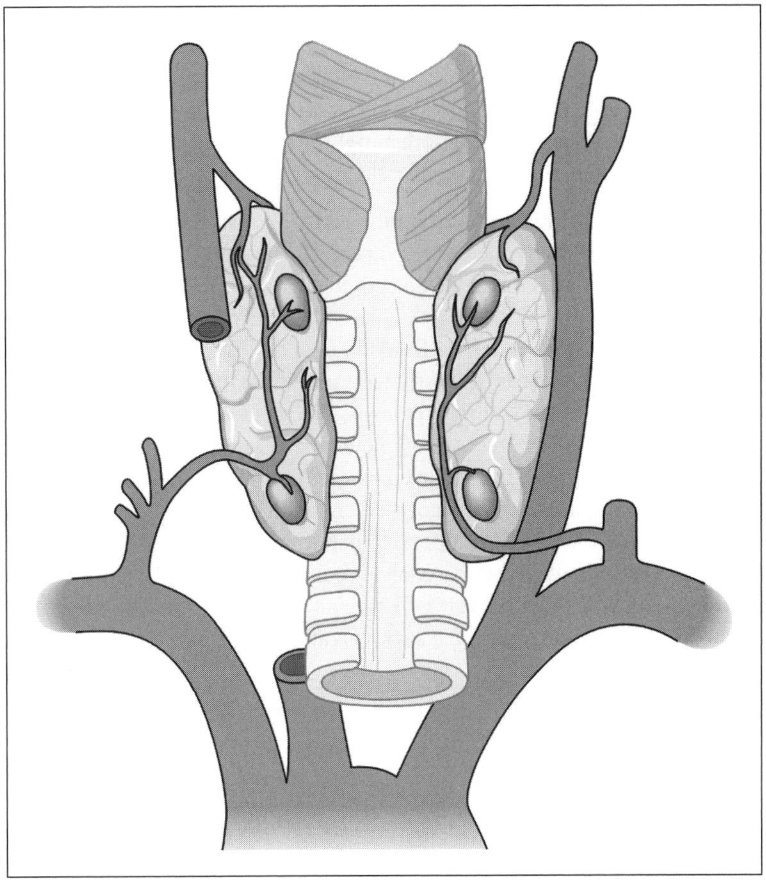

In this posterior view of the trachea, two small paired parathyroid glands can be seen embedded in each lobe of the thyroid gland. (LifeART© 2008 Wolters Kluwer Health, Inc.-Lippincott Williams &Wilkins. All rights reserved.)

Relative Survival Rates for Parathyroid Cancer by Gender, 1988-2001

Gender	*Survival Rate (%)* 1-Year	3-Year	5-Year	10-Year
Men	93.8	93.8	89.6	71.7
Women	94.0	93.1	93.1	88.4
Total	94.1	94.1	93.1	81.6

Source: Data from L. A. G. Ries et al., eds., *Cancer Survival Among Adults: U.S. SEER Program, 1988-2001—Patient and Tumor Characteristics*, NIH Pub. No. 07-6215 (Bethesda, Md.: National Cancer Institute, 2007)

- Stage II: T2N0M0
- Stage IIIA: T3N0M0
- Stage IIIB: T4N0M0
- Stage IIIC: Any T, N1, M0
- Stage IV: Any T, any N, M1

Treatment and therapy: Initial therapeutic treatment for parathyroid cancer involves surgical resection of the entire tumor. Patients who are not surgical candidates, such as those in whom the tumor has invaded neck structures, undergo radiation therapy or chemotherapy; however, these therapies have met with limited success.

Prognosis, prevention, and outcomes: The prognosis for individuals with parathyroid cancer varies. The best prognosis results from early detection and complete removal of the tumor during the initial surgery. The average time between the initial surgery and the first potential recurrence is around two to three years. Recurrence earlier than this is an unfavorable factor regarding prognosis. The recurrence-free survival rate is 30 percent. Complete cure is reported unlikely once the tumor has recurred, yet lengthened survival can be possible with surgery or chemotherapy or both. Radiation therapy for inoperable parathyroid carcinoma is usually ineffective. In cases of recurrence of the tumor, the five-year overall survival rate is reported to be about 50 percent and the ten-year survival rate varies from 13 to 49 percent.

Jeffrey P. Larson, P.T., B.S., A.T.C.

▶ For Further Information

Copstead, Lee-Ellen C., and Jacquelyn Banasik. *Pathophysiology: Biological and Behavioral Perspectives*. 3d ed. Philadelphia: Saunders, 2005.

Kulkarni, P. S., and Purvish M. Parikh. "The Carcinoma of Parathyroid Gland." *Indian Journal of Cancer* 41 (April 1, 2004): 51-59.

Wiseman, Sam M., et al. "Parathyroid Carcinoma: A Multicenter Review of Clinicopathologic Features and Treatment Outcomes." *Ear, Nose and Throat Journal* 83, no. 7 (July 1, 2004): 491-494.

▶ Other Resources

MedlinePlus

Parathyroid Cancer

http://www.nlm.nih.gov/medlineplus/ency/article/007264.htm

National Cancer Institute

Parathyroid Cancer

http://www.cancer.gov/cancertopics/types/parathyroid/

See also Endocrine cancers; Endocrinology oncology; Family history and risk assessment; Giant cell tumors (GCTs); Hypercalcemia; Multiple endocrine neoplasia type 1 (MEN 1); Multiple endocrine neoplasia type 2 (MEN 2); Neuroendocrine tumors; Nuclear medicine scan; Pheochromocytomas; Pituitary tumors; Ultrasound tests; Zollinger-Ellison syndrome.

▶ Pathology

Category: Medical specialties

Also known as: Pathobiology, anatomical pathology, clinical pathology

Definition: Pathology is a science that seeks to understand the changes in function and structure of organs, tissues, cells, and body fluids that lead to disease and death. The word "pathology" comes from the Greek word *pathos*, meaning feeling, pain, or suffering, and the suffix *ology*, which signifies "the study of."

Pathologists, in concert with the scientists and technicians who assist them, investigate the nature and causes of disease in anatomical and metabolic systems at molecular and genetic levels. These molecular-level processes must be fully understood in order to diagnosis a disease. An accurate differential diagnosis is the basis for the choice of therapy and potential return to health.

Anatomical pathology, the study of structural and cellular changes in disease processes, includes surgical pathology; autopsy services that identify clues for the coroner or medical examiner, who determines causes of death; and forensic pathology, which provides the scientific link between medicine and the law

Clinical pathology focuses on the cellular and chemical changes in body cells and fluids that differentiate health from disease and includes the disciplines of microbiology, immunology, hematology, immunohematology/blood banking/transfusion services, and chemistry.

Subspecialties: Pathology is a unique specialty in the sense that pathologists do not typically see a patient but instead consult with the patient's physician. Pathology includes ten certifiable clinical and anatomical subspecialties at the physician level. Clinical pathology specialties are blood banking/transfusion medicine/immunohematology, chemical pathology, hematology, medical microbiology, and molecular genetics and are supported by clinical laboratory scientists and technicians. Anatomical pathology specialties are cytopathology, dermatophathology, neuropathology, pediatric pathology, and forensic pathology and are supported by pathology assistants, histologists, cytologists, and cytogeneticists.

Anatomical pathology. When a patient undergoes surgery for tumor evaluation and removal, it is the surgical pathologist who advises the surgeon if the mass is cancer or not. While the patient remains under anesthesia, the surgeon passes the tissue to the surgical pathologist, who examines the specimen both by gross examination with the naked eye in its entirety and by frozen section at the time of the operation.

In the case of tumor removal, it is the surgical pathologist who is looking at the margins of the excision and telling the surgeon if they are clean (free of cancer) or not. It is the surgical pathologist who informs the surgeon if the entire tumor has been removed, whether the lymph nodes are involved, and whether the tissue is metastatic, a manifestation of malignancy as a secondary growth arising from the primary tumor. In this way, the surgical pathologist plays a pivotal role in determining what the surgeon will ultimately choose as the next step.

When tissue is removed, it is passed to the histology department, where histologists stabilize the tissue by fixation. The tissue is then immersed in multiple baths to dehydrate and clear it, and finally impregnate it with wax. After embedding, sectioning, and staining, the tissue is once again reviewed by the pathologist, who is often determining whether cancer or particular receptors for cancer such as HER2/neu are present.

In cytopathology the anatomical pathologists work closely with cytologists who process, stain, and review all cell preparations. These specialists study cell structures, cell composition, the interaction of cells with other cells, and the larger environment in which cells exist. Cytologists look for too many of one kind of cell or note when a particular cell type is missing. Suspicious smears are referred to the pathologist.

One common cytological procedure is the PAP test, the medical screening method to detect premalignant and malignant changes in the ectocervix. The Pap smear has become a routine procedure during a woman's annual gynecological examination. The cytologist looks at the cell structures to detect the early formation of cancer cells. Early detection leads to greater survival rates.

Clinical pathology. In the clinical laboratory, thousands of medical tests are available, including those designed to diagnose and track cancer. Examples include tests for cancer antigens (CA), alpha-fetoprotein (AFP), carcinoembryonic antigen (CEA), lipid-associated sialic acid (LASA), prostate-specific antigen (PSA), and the T-lymphocyte cluster of differentiation (CD) markers.

General chemistry and hematology tests identify cancers or may function to demonstrate the degree to which the body is tolerating therapies and provide guidance to the patient's physician in making adjustments to treatment. As genomics and proteomics become more commercially available, the clinical laboratory will provide personalized profiles that will permit the treating physician to tailor therapies specific to the particular cancer and to the individual for more effective protocols leading to a cure.

New and potentially useful markers for cancer diagnoses are continuously being discovered. Time and tedious research are required to determine which ones will result in earlier diagnoses, increasingly targeted and cost-effective treatment, and ultimately prevention.

Training and certification: Although pathology departments are in the background, away from the public eye, they are complex, multifaceted operations supporting the practitioners who care for patients. Directors of full-service laboratories must be licensed physicians or individuals who have earned a doctor of philosophy degree in chemical, physical, biological, or clinical laboratory science.

Certified pathologists are licensed physicians who have first graduated from an approved medical school or college of osteopathic medicine and who select specialty training in a pathology residency program that is accredited by the Accreditation Council for Graduate Medical Education or the Royal College of Physicians and Surgeons of Canada. After three or four years of graduate medical education, candidates pass an objective written and practical examination.

There are three pathology certifications: anatomic pathology (AP), clinical pathology (CP), and combined anatomic pathology and clinical pathology (AP/CP). After January, 2006, new diplomates were required to renew certificates after ten years.

Within the pathology department are cadres of scientists and specialists in chemistry, microbiology, hematology, transfusion service, immunology, cytology, and histology with certifications that require baccalaureate and associate degrees.

Services and procedures performed: In addition to performing surgical diagnostic procedures, anatomical pathologists examine tissue that is acquired through biopsy from all parts of the body. After providing a gross examination of the specimen, histologists prepare tissue slides that are then stained and reviewed for a final diagnosis by the pathologist.

The clinical pathologist is responsible for the quality assurance of all the biological tests performed in the chemistry, hematology, immunology, immunohematology, and microbiology laboratories. These responsibilities include method selection, quality control, and interpretation of test results.

Forensic pathologists are trained to assist law enforcement in homicide cases. They establish the cause of death, estimate the time of death, infer the type of weapon used, distinguish homicide from suicide, establish the identity of the deceased, and determine the effect of trauma or preexisting conditions to the consequential death.

Related specialties and subspecialties: Pathologists, clinical laboratory scientists, cytologists, cytogeneticists, histologists, pathology assistants, and phlebotomists work together as a team to deliver diagnostic and monitoring laboratory test results to the primary care physicians who actually interact with patients and their families. Each of these professional groups has academic, certification, and continuing education requirements to support changing and emerging practice in the specialty.

Clinical laboratory scientists have bachelor's degrees, and clinical laboratory technicians have associate degrees. Both are certified to perform testing procedures in chemistry, microbiology, hematology, transfusion services, and immunology. Phlebotomists collect blood and other body fluids for analysis in the clinical laboratories and may be certified.

Histologists are technologists with associate or bachelor's degrees who are certified to process, embed, stain, and cut tissue to the thickness of a single layer for the purpose of demonstrating cellular morphology, chemical composition, and function of normal and abnormal tissue.

Cytologists, cytogenecists, and pathology assistants all have obtained a bachelor's degree and certification. Cytologists are trained to process and prepare cells for review. Suspicious cells are passed to pathologists for final identification. Cytogeneticists are trained to process cells and thus reveal information coded in the chromosomes to describe the heredity of the individual as this information relates to particular diseases. Pathology assistants are specifically trained to provide anatomical services under the direction of a pathologist, including the gross examination of surgical pathology specimens and autopsies.

Jane Adrian, M.P.H., Ed.M., M.T. (ASCP)

▶ For Further Information

Benson, Ellis S., Barbara F. Atkinson, and Martin Alax. *Career Guide in Pathology*. Chicago: American Society for Clinical Pathology, 1998.

McClatchey, Kenneth D., ed. *Clinical Laboratory Medicine*. 2d ed. Philadelphia: Lippincott Williams & Wilkins, 2002.

Pagana, Kathleen Deska, and Timothy J. Pagana. *Mosby's Diagnostic and Laboratory Test Reference*. Philadelphia: Elsevier-Mosby, 2006.

Sloan, Sheila B., and John L. Dusseau. *Word Book in Pathology and Laboratory Medicine*. 2d ed. Philadelphia: Elsevier/Saunders, 1995.

Thomas, Lewis. *The Fragile Species*. New York: Collier Books, 1992.

_______. *The Lives of a Cell: Notes of a Biology Watcher*. New York: Viking Press, 1974.

▶ Organizations and Professional Societies

American Association of Bioanalysts
http://www.aab.org
906 Olive Street, Suite 1200
St. Louis, MO 63101-1434

American Association of Clinical Chemistry
http://www.aacc.org
1850 K Street NW, Suite 625
Washington, D.C. 20006-2213

American Association of Pathologists' Assistants
http://www.pathologistsassistants.org
Rosewood Office Plaza, Suite 300N
1711 West County Road B
Roseville, MN 55113

American Board of Pathology
http://www.abpath.org
P.O. Box 25915
Tampa, FL 33622-5915

American Osteopathic College of Pathologists
http://www.doaocp.org
142 East Ontario Street
Chicago, IL 60611-8224

American Society for Clinical Pathology
http://www.ascp.org
33 West Monroe, Suite 1600
Chicago, IL 60603

American Society of Cytopathology
http://www.cytopathology.org
400 West 9th Street, Suite 201
Wilmington, DE 19801

Clinical Laboratory Management Association
http://www.clma.org
989 Old Eagle School Road, Suite 815
Wayne, PA 19087

College of American Pathologists
http://www.cap.org/apps/cap.portal
325 Waukegan Road
Northfield, IL 60093-2750

Intersociety Council for Pathology Information
http://www.pathologytraining.org
9650 Rockville Pike
Bethesda, MD 20814-3993

National Accrediting Agency for Clinical Laboratory Sciences
http://www.naacls.org
8410 West Bryn Mawr Avenue, Suite 670
Chicago, IL 60631

National Credentialing Agency for Laboratory Personnel
http://www.nca-info.org
18000 West 105th Street
Olathe, KS 66061-7543

▶ Other Resources

Lab Tests Online
http://www.labtestsonline.org

MyBiopsy.org
http://www.mybiopsy.org

U.S. Food and Drug Administration
CLIA—Clinical Laboratory Improvement Amendments
http://www.fda.gov/cdrh/clia

See also Breslow's staging; Cancer biology; Carcinomatosis; Cytology; Gleason grading system; Grading of tumors; Hematologic oncology; Immunocytochemistry and immunohistochemistry; Malignant tumors; Medical oncology; Metastasis; Molecular oncology; Needle biopsies; Staging of cancer; Stereotactic needle biopsy; TNM staging; Tumor markers; Urinalysis.

▶ PC-SPES

Category: Complementary and alternative therapies
Also known as: PC-CARE, Ponicidin

Definition: PC-SPES is a mixture of eight herbs marketed as a dietary supplement for prostate health and as a complementary and alternative medicine (CAM) for prostate cancer. It should not be confused with SPES, a different product.

Cancers treated or prevented: Prostate cancer

Delivery routes: Oral by capsule

How this substance works: PC-SPES (a name derived from the initials for "prostate cancer" and the Latin word for "hope," *spes*) is a dietary supplement alleged to support prostate health and limit the growth of prostate cancer. The ingredients include eight herbs used in traditional Chinese medicine: Baikal skullcap (*Scutellaria baicalensis*), licorice (*Glycyrrhiza glabra L.* or *Glycyrrhiza uralensis*), reishi mushroom (*Ganoderma lucidum*), isatis (*Isatis indigotica*), ginseng (*Panax ginseng* or *Panax pseudoginseng var. notoginseng*), chrysanthemum flowers (*Dendranthema morifolium*), *Rabdosia rubescens* (*Isodon rubescens*), and saw palmetto (*Serenoa repens*). In the 1990's, PC-SPES showed promise both in preventing cell damage and in limiting tumor growth in cases of prostate cancer.

Between 1997 and 2002, PC-SPES was marketed in the United States as a dietary supplement; it therefore did not need to meet the U.S. Food and Drug Administration (FDA) standards for drug safety and efficacy and did not require a prescription. In early studies in which cancer cells from rats were mixed with PC-SPES, the mixture limited the growth of the tumor cells. When testing revealed, however, that some forms of PC-SPES illegally contained warfarin (a blood thinner), diethylstilbestrol (DES, a hormonal therapy for prostate cancer), and indomethacin (an anti-inflammatory), PC-SPES was taken off the market. Forms of PC-SPES without these drugs remain on the market but are unstandardized.

How PC-SPES may work without the prescription drugs is unknown but is being studied. The herbs contain plant estrogens (phytoestrogens) that may be effective in limiting the action of testosterone, the male hormone that contributes to tumor growth. Patients respond to PC-SPES similarly to those responding to estrogen therapy using DES. The National Center for Complementary and Alternative Medicine (NCCAM) is conducting studies on drug-free forms of PC-SPES to determine its efficacy, and clinical trials may be planned once a standard formula is established.

Side effects: Users of PC-SPES have noted side effects including breast swelling and tenderness, loss of libido, impotence (erectile dysfunction), and, less frequently, blood clots in the legs and diarrhea. PC-SPES may also have interactions with drugs, including anticancer drugs.

Christina J. Moose, M.A.

See also Cartilage supplements; Chemoprevention; Complementary and alternative therapies; Dietary supplements; Diethylstilbestrol (DES); Gerson therapy; Herbs as antioxidants; Lutein; Lycopene; Nutrition and cancer prevention; Nutrition and cancer treatment; Prostate cancer; Saw palmetto; Sun's soup.

▶ Pediatric oncology and hematology

Category: Medical specialties
Also known as: Pediatric cancer treatment

Definition: Pediatric oncology and hematology is the medical specialty for the diagnosis and treatment of childhood and adolescent cancerous diseases and blood disorders. Most pediatric oncology and hematology programs treat children and young adults from birth through age twenty.

Pediatric oncology and hematology practices can be found in university medical centers, large community hospitals, specialized children's hospitals, comprehensive cancer centers, and specialty pediatric cancer centers.

Certain medical centers are designated as comprehensive cancer centers by the National Cancer Institute because they meet certain research and patient treatment criteria, including having a multidisciplinary team of professionals with expertise and training in pediatric and adolescent hematologic and malignant disorders, clinical services connected to research, clinical trials and basic laboratory research, cancer information services, and psychosocial support services. Research has shown that children and adolescents who are treated in a center with specialized cancer services and specialists have better outcomes.

A child's pediatrician or family doctor can provide a referral to a pediatric cancer program.

Subspecialties: Pediatric hematology, pediatric radiation oncology, neuro-oncology, ortho-oncology

Cancers treated: Many childhood and adolescent cancers, particularly leukemia, lymphoma, osteogenic sarcoma, rhabdomosarcoma, Ewing sarcoma, neuroblastoma, non-Hodgkin lymphoma, brain tumors, bone tumors, musculoskeletal and soft-tissue tumors, solid tumors of the kidney and liver, tumors of the eye, Langerhans cell histiocytosis, and Wilms' tumor (nephroblastoma)

Training and certification: In addition to having a four-year medical degree from an accredited program and board certification from the American Board of Pediatrics, pediatric hematologists-oncologists have completed three years of postgraduate residency training in general pediatrics and at least three years of fellowship training in pediatric hematology and oncology.

After completing a minimum of three years of successful training, pediatric hematologist-oncologist fellows are eligible to take a certification examination offered by the Subboard of Hematology/Oncology of the American Board of Pediatrics. Once certified, pediatric hematologists-oncologists may further their training by participating in one or more years of clinical or laboratory research.

Pediatric hematologists-oncologists are trained in the basic science and clinical expression of cancer and blood diseases in children and adolescents. They are involved in patient care, medical teaching, and research. They study the etiology of cancer and its evaluation, diagnosis, and management in ambulatory and hospitalized patients. Specific areas of study include chemotherapy, oncology, hemostatis-thrombosis, hematology, sickle cell treatment, neuro-oncology, stem cell transplantation, hematopathology, clinical pathology, blood banking, and radiation oncology. Hematologist-oncologists often focus on treating patients with either cancer or blood disorders, although they receive training in diagnosing and treating both conditions.

Pediatric hematology and oncology clinical practice guidelines, quality standards, and quality assurance measures have been established by these organizations:

- Children's Oncology Group (COG): A network of research groups, sponsored by the National Cancer Institute, with more than two hundred international member institutions that conduct pediatric and adolescent clinical trials to identify cancer causes and introduce new treatments that address long-term childhood cancer survival.
- American Society of Pediatric Hematology/Oncology (ASPHO): A professional association for pediatric hematologist-oncologists. ASPHO established standard requirements for pediatric hematology and oncology programs.
- American Academy of Pediatrics (AAP): A professional organization of more than sixty thousand pediatricians and pediatric subspecialists that creates clinical practice guidelines.

Services and procedures performed: A pediatric hematologist-oncologist plans and coordinates the diagnosis and treatment of newly diagnosed or recurring malignancies and blood disorders in children and adolescents. The pediatric hematologist-oncologist is part of a multidisciplinary team of pediatric cancer providers whose goals are to provide early detection; accurately diagnose the condition; offer prompt, appropriate treatment to reduce morbidity and improve quality of life and survival; reduce long-term effects of chemotherapy and radiation therapy; and provide long-term follow-up. Pediatric hematologist-oncologists are trained and skilled in chemotherapy drug indications and toxicities so they can safely administer these therapies while minimizing side effects.

Related specialties and subspecialties: Pediatric hematologist-oncologists work with a multidisciplinary team that includes the primary care pediatrician and also may include pediatric surgical specialists such as urologic surgeons, orthopedic surgeons, and neurosurgeons; diagnostic radiologists; radiation oncologists; infectious disease specialists; pediatric pathologists; pediatric oncology nurses; consulting pediatric specialists; physical therapists; pediatric oncology social workers and other allied health care professionals, such as child-life specialists, educational specialists, registered dietitians, and pharmacologists. Communication between the pediatric hematologist-oncologist and the patient's primary care pediatrician is essential to ensure the continuum of care.

Laparoscopy and thoracoscopy are among the surgical techniques used by pediatric surgeons to diagnose and treat cancers in children and adolescents. Pediatric surgeons first obtain a four-year medical degree from an accredited program and board certification from the American Board of Surgery, then complete five years of residency training in an accredited general surgery program and at least two years of fellowship training in pediatric surgery. Pediatric oncology surgeons receive additional training in the surgical diagnosis and treatment of pediatric cancers.

Diagnostic radiologists capture and interpret medical images for the purpose of diagnosis. They must have a four-year medical degree from an accredited program, must have board certification from the American Board of Radiology or the American Osteopathic Board of Radiology, and must have passed a licensing examination and completed at least four years of residency training in an accredited radiology program.

Radiation oncologists use radiation to treat cancers. In the United States, most of them have completed residency training in their field in a program approved by the American Council of Graduate Medical Education or the American Board of Radiology.

Infectious disease specialists are pediatricians who are experts in the diagnosis and treatment of infectious diseases. In addition to having a four-year medical degree from an accredited program and board certification from the American Board of Pediatrics, infectious disease specialists have completed three or more years of residency training and two to three years of additional training in infectious diseases.

Pediatric pathologists are physicians who are experts in the pathology of hematologic malignancies and solid tumors in children and adolescents. They use immunochemistry and molecular techniques to assess malignancies. Pediatric pathologists obtain a four-year medical degree from an accredited program and board certification from the American Board of Pediatrics, then complete three or more years of residency training and one to two years of additional training in pathology.

The Association of Pediatric Oncology Nurses provides a certification program for pediatric oncology nurses. The organization also facilitates the professional development of pediatric oncology nurses. Pediatric oncology nurses provide medical care, educate patients and their families, and administer medications. Pediatric oncology clinical nurse specialists are registered nurses with a master's degree in oncology nursing. They have experience in managing complications of cancer treatment, understand pediatric protocols, and prepare and administer medications, including chemotherapy. Pediatric oncology nurse practitioners are registered nurses with a master's or doctoral degree.

▶ For Further Information

Altman, Arnold J., ed. *Supportive Care of Children with Cancer: Current Therapy and Guidelines from the Children's Oncology Group*. Baltimore: Johns Hopkins University Press, 2004.

American Academy of Pediatrics. "Guidelines for the Pediatric Cancer Center and Role of Such Centers in Diagnosis and Treatment." *Pediatrics* 113, no. 6 (June, 2004): 1833-1835.

Lanzkowsky, Philip. *Manual of Pediatric Hematology and Oncology*. 3d ed. San Diego, Calif.: Academic Press, 2000.

Pizzo, P. A., and D. G. Poplack. *Principles and Practice of Pediatric Oncology*. 5th ed. Philadelphia: Lippincott Williams & Wilkins, 2005.

Stocker, J. T., and L. P. Dehner, eds. *Pediatric Pathology*. 2d ed. Philadelphia: Lippincott Williams & Wilkins, 2001.

▶ **Organizations and Professional Societies**

American Society of Pediatric Hematology/Oncology
http://www.aspho.org
4700 West Lake Avenue
Glenview, IL 60025

Association of Pediatric Oncology Nurses
http://www.apon.org
4700 W. Lake Avenue
Glenview, IL 60025-1485

Children's Oncology Group
http://www.curesearch.org
Research Operations Center
440 East Huntington Drive, Suite 400
Arcadia, CA 91006-3776

National Childhood Cancer Foundation/CureSearch
http://www.curesearch.org
4600 East West Highway, Suite 600
Bethesda, MD 20814-3457

▶ **Other Resources**

Candlelighters Childhood Cancer Foundation
http://www.candlelighters.org

Children's Cancer Association
http://www.childrenscancerassociation.org

National Children's Cancer Society
http://www.nationalchildrenscancersociety.org

Ronald McDonald House Charities
http://www.rmhc.com

Angela M. Costello, B.S.

See also Childbirth and cancer; Childhood cancers; Endocrinology oncology; Ewing sarcoma; Family history and risk assessment; Hematologic oncology; Histiocytosis X; Juvenile polyposis syndrome; Medical oncology; Molecular oncology; Nephroblastomas; Neurologic oncology; Pregnancy and cancer; Wilms' tumor; Wilms' tumor aniridia-genitourinary anomalies-mental retardation (WAGR) syndrome and cancer; Young adult cancers.

▶ Pelvic examination

Category: Procedures
Also known as: Female gynecologic examination, reproductive health examination

Definition: A pelvic examination is a visual inspection of external female genitalia, followed by insertion of a speculum into the vagina to visualize the cervix and a bimanual examination of the uterus and adnexa (ovaries, Fallopian tubes, and uterine ligaments) for masses, tenderness, and overall impression.

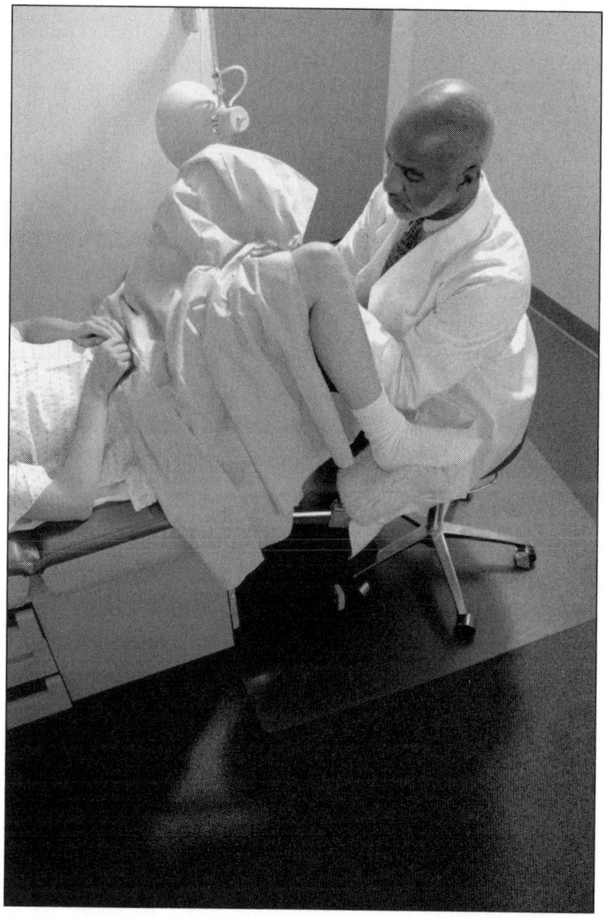

Pelvic examinations allow doctors to check for several types of cancer. (PhotoDisc)

Cancers diagnosed: If a collection of cells for a Pap (Papanicolaou) test is done as part of the pelvic examination, then screening for cervical cancer and precursor cellular changes (precancerous conditions) is included; visual inspection of the external genitalia may reveal abnormal tissue to be biopsied for the detection of vulvar or vaginal cancer.

Why performed: A pelvic examination allows for examination of internal and external genitalia as well as the collection of specimens. Some pelvic examinations include laboratory specimen collection for Pap testing (with the collection of cervical and endocervical samples either by fixed slides or the newer liquid cytologic methodology); examination of vaginal discharge for bacterial vaginosis, trichomonas, or yeast vaginitis; and testing for common infections such as gonorrhea and chlamydia. Any particular pelvic examination, however, may include only some or none of these tests. It is important for patients to be aware that not all pelvic examinations include Pap testing. Exams may be performed for routine screening, including a Pap smear, or for symptomatic gynecologic problems.

Patient preparation: The patient should empty her bladder prior to the exam and should have a chance to express any concerns or apprehensions. She should not douche prior to the exam. It is preferable for patients not to be menstruating when examined, although this may not be possible depending on the reason for the visit. Having the patient move down to the far end of the table relieves some pressure from the speculum.

Steps of the procedure: A pelvic exam involves the external examination and palpation of the genitalia, followed by insertion of a vaginal speculum, collection of specimens, and a bimanual examination with palpation of uterine and adnexal size, mobility, position, contours, presence of masses, and tenderness with palpation.

After the procedure: The physician will help the patient sit up slowly when the exam is completed. Bleeding is possible following a pelvic examination but is not a cause for alarm unless excessive or prolonged.

Risks: Pelvic examinations may be embarrassing and emotionally and physically uncomfortable for some patients, but they carry no known risks.

Results: The results of a pelvic examination depend on visual examination and any clinical or laboratory findings.

Clair Kaplan, R.N., M.S.N., A.P.R.N. (WHNP), M.H.S., M.T. (ASCP)

See also Antiviral therapies; Cervical cancer; Colposcopy; Conization; Diethylstilbestrol (DES); Endometrial cancer; Fertility drugs and cancer; Gynecologic cancers; Human papillomavirus (HPV); Hysterectomy; Hysterooophorectomy; Loop electrosurgical excisional procedure (LEEP); Pap test; Pregnancy and cancer; Transvaginal ultrasound; Uterine cancer; Vaccines, preventive; Vaginal cancer; Virus-related cancers; Vulvar cancer.

▶ Penile cancer

Category: Diseases, symptoms, and conditions
Also known as: Cancer of the penis, penile carcinoma, penile malignancies, penile carcinoma in situ (CIS), erythroplasia of Queyrat, Bowen disease

Related conditions: Male reproductive cancers, urethral cancer, dermatologic malignancies, squamous cell carcinomas, human papillomavirus infections, testicular cancer, prostate cancer, recurrent balanitis, phimosis

Definition: Penile cancer is cancer on the skin and deeper tissues of the penis.

Risk factors: Poor hygiene, exposure to human papillomavirus (especially subtypes 16 and 18), and lack of circumcision are major risk factors for development of penile cancer. Age is also a risk, as most cases appear in men aged fifty and older. Smoking is an additional risk

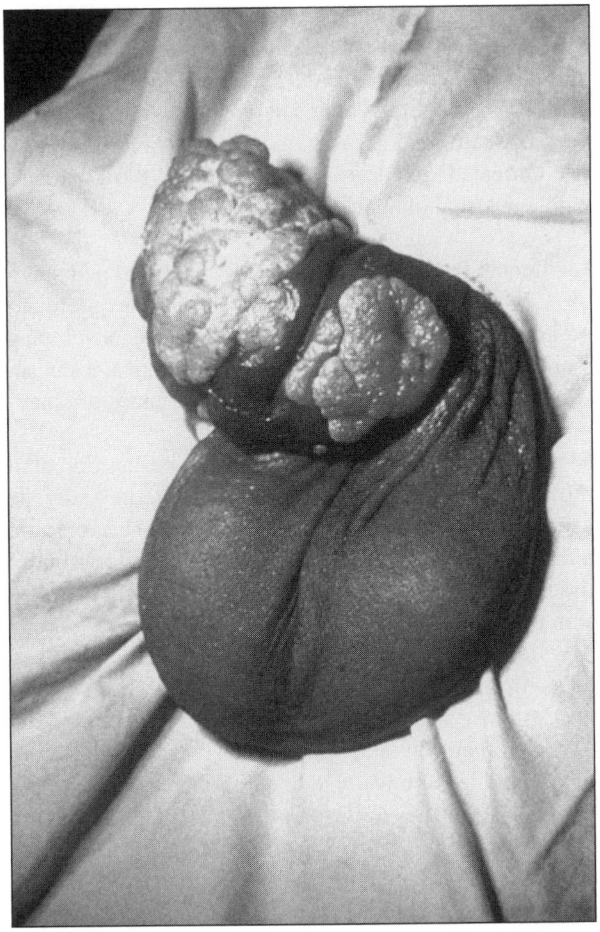

This penile cancer is a giant condyloma of Buschke and Löwenstein. (Centers for Disease Control and Prevention)

factor. The most important risk is phimosis, a narrowing of the opening of the prepuce that results in a foreskin that cannot be retracted. This is a painful condition in which the foreskin of uncircumcised men becomes inflamed with a chronic buildup of smegma under the foreskin, often due to lack of hygiene. Circumcision is an operation, usually done on newborns, that removes the foreskin from the penis. In the United States about two-thirds to three-quarters of newborns are circumcised, although this varies around the world, with circumcision being rare in many parts of the developing world.

Etiology and the disease process: Penile cancer most commonly begins as small lesions (sores) on the skin of the glans of the penis or prepuce, the opening of the foreskin. Lesions are usually squamous cell carcinomas, which may remain on the skin, then invade deeper into the tissues and spread (metastasize) into the bloodstream and lymph nodes. Delays in seeking treatment, due to misinformation, embarrassment, and fear, result in many cases being diagnosed at an advanced stage. Penile cancer that has metastasized into the adjacent lymph nodes can cause death from sepsis or hemorrhage. Metastasis into the blood, liver, bone, and brain are rare unless the cancer has been untreated and has reached a very advanced stage. If left untreated, penile cancer is fatal for most patients within a period of about two years.

Incidence: Penile cancer is quite rare in developed countries. In the United States, around 1,300 cases are diagnosed each year; however, in parts of the developing world, such as Asia, Africa, and South America, it can account for anywhere from 6 to 30 percent of cancers in men.

Symptoms: Symptoms include sores, rashes, or skin growths on the penis and foul-smelling material under the foreskin of uncircumcised men. The foreskin can obscure a lesion that is not healing and may not be detected until tissue death (necrosis) produces material under the foreskin that has a foul odor.

Screening and diagnosis: Screening for penile cancer is not customary, but men should have a genital examination as part of their routine physicals. Diagnosis is made from biopsy and is more likely to be performed early on a suspected lesion if patients seek care from a urologist. Staging of the cancer determines how much it has spread (invasiveness) and if lymph nodes have been affected. Biopsy of sentinel lymph nodes may also be done to determine the degree of spread to the lymphatics. Staging is generally done using the TNM (tumor/lymph node/metastasis) system, which classifies the tumor based on the presence or absence of spread, involvement of lymph nodes, and existence of more distant metastases.

Relative Survival Rates for Penile Cancer, 1988-2001

Years	*Survival Rates (%)*
1	87.4
3	76.7
5	71.4
10	62.6

Source: Data from L. A. G. Ries et al., eds., *Cancer Survival Among Adults: U.S. SEER Program, 1988-2001—Patient and Tumor Characteristics*, NIH Pub. No. 07-6215 (Bethesda, Md.: National Cancer Institute, 2007)

Treatment and therapy: Treatment for penile cancer is usually surgery to remove the cancerous area. Radiation therapy and chemotherapy may also be used to kill cancer cells. Although laser therapy can sometimes be used, most often more radical forms of surgery are necessary, although penis-sparing surgery is used whenever possible. Penectomy is surgery that removes all or part of the penis. A partial penectomy may preserve sexual function and the ability to urinate from the penis. A total penectomy completely removes the penis and creates a new outlet for urination, usually located behind the testicles. Plastic surgery to create a new penis is possible, but function may be limited. Mohs micrographic surgery is an advanced technique that uses microscopy to remove cancerous tissue and allows for maximal sparing of penile tissue. Radiation is less likely to be used than surgical treatment but may involve external beams or implantation of a radioactive source near the tumor. Chemotherapy may be locally applied or, in cases of metastatic cancer, given systemically.

Prognosis, prevention, and outcomes: Prognosis depends on the time between first appearance of penile cancer and initiation of treatment, and the status of lymph nodes is the most important clinical indicator of prognosis. Occurrence of penile cancer is rare in men who have been circumcised as newborns; however, circumcision itself carries risks, and medical authorities have not agreed that there is enough evidence to support recommendations for routine neonatal circumcision. Adult circumcision does not prevent development of the disease. It is not yet known if the development of a vaccine against the human papillomavirus can reduce incidence of penile cancer.

Outcomes depend on state of progression (especially lymph node involvement) when the cancer is detected, treatments used, and response to treatment. Cure rates in men without lymph node involvement who have had surgical treatment may average 80 to 100 percent, whereas cure rates are 32 to 50 percent in men with lymph node involvement. In cases where penis-sparing therapies have been used, surveillance for recurrence is important. Any consideration of outcomes should address the emotional toll of the disease and necessary treatments.

Clair Kaplan, R.N., M.S.N., A.P.R.N. (WHNP), M.H.S., M.T. (ASCP)

▶ For Further Information

Busby, J. E., and C. A. Pettaway. "What's New in the Management of Penile Cancer?" *Current Opinion in Urology* 15, no. 5 (September, 2005): 350-357.

Jemal, A., et al. "Cancer Statistics." *CA: A Cancer Journal for Clinicians* 57 (2007): 43-66.

McDougal, W. S. "Advances in the Treatment of Carcinoma of the Penis." *Urology* 66, suppl. 5 (November, 2005): 114-117.

Micali, G., M. R. Nasca, D. Innocenzi, and R. A. Schwartz. "Penile Cancer." *Journal of the American Academy of Dermatology* 54, no. 3 (March, 2006): 369-391.

▶ Other Resources

American Family Physician
Penile Cancer
http://www.aafp.org/afp/20040201/617ph.html

M. D. Anderson Cancer Center
Penile Cancer Facts
http://www.mdanderson.org/diseases/penile-cancer/?gclid=CMzR0b2Axo4CFQp7PAodSwLixw

National Cancer Institute
Penile Cancer
http://www.cancer.gov/cancertopics/types/penile/

See also Bowen disease; Infectious cancers; Oncogenic viruses; Prostate cancer; Prostatectomy; Sexuality and cancer; Skin cancers; Testicular cancer; Testicular self-examination (TSE); Urethral cancer; Urinary system cancers; Urologic oncology.

▶ Percutaneous transhepatic cholangiography (PTHC)

Category: Procedures
Also known as: Operative cholangiography, T-tube cholangiography, cystic duct cholangiography

Definition: Percutaneous transhepatic cholangiography (PTHC) is a diagnostic test used to visualize the the liver or bile ducts. Although this procedure is frequently performed in the operating room at the time of exploration of the biliary tract for nonpalpable stones or tumors, it can also be performed postoperatively in the radiology suite to assess catheter patency and drainage and to evaluate for the presence of residual stones or residual narrowing or obstruction of the biliary tract.

Cancers diagnosed: Bile duct carcinoma, pancreatic cancer

Why performed: The main application of PTHC is to avoid common bile duct surgical exploration and to identify calculi that have escaped palpation, as well as to evaluate for the presence of biliary tract tumors or pancreatic tumors. The intrapancreatic segment of the common bile duct is often altered by pancreatic cancer, and PTHC can be used for its evaluation. Postoperative cholangiography is usually performed in the X-ray suite prior to removal of the T tube placed at the time of surgery to demonstrate the patency of the common duct, the absence of retained stones, and the free passage of bile into the duodenum.

Patient preparation: This procedure is frequently performed in the operating room at the time of exploration of the biliary tract for nonpalpable stones or tumor. Therefore, patient preparation is determined by the surgeon prior to the procedure and commonly involves the usual preadmission testing performed before any surgical procedure, as well as instructions such as nothing by mouth after midnight the night before the procedure.

Steps of the procedure: Radiopaque material is injected by the surgeon into the cystic duct while the patient is still in the operating room. Alternatively, after surgery, radiopaque material may be injected into the T tube by a radiologist in the radiology suite. This tube was placed in the common duct intraoperatively using sterile technique under fluoroscopic guidance. In both situations, X-ray films are then taken. In some cases, a trained interventional radiologist, under fluoroscopic control and using sterile technique, can insert a fine needle directly into the biliary tree and outline the intrahepatic ducts, the common hepatic ducts, and the common bile duct using a contrast medium.

After the procedure: If a T tube was placed in the common duct intraoperatively, then the procedure is performed as an inpatient procedure (during the patient's hospital stay). Patients should consult their health care providers if they have any questions or concerns regarding the use of a T-tube cholangiogram or PTHC.

Risks: Patients will consult with their health care providers regarding the need for the study, its risks, how it will be done, and what the results indicate.

Results: The X-ray films taken during the procedure are read by the radiologist the same day. The patient will need to contact the doctor or health care provider for the radiology report and for follow-up therapy. Results are dependent on the reason for the study, such as exploration of the biliary tract for nonpalpable stones or tumors.

Debra B. Kessler, M.D., Ph.D.

See also Bile duct cancer; Gallbladder cancer.

▶ Pericardial effusion

Category: Diseases, symptoms, and conditions
Also known as: Dropsy of pericardium, malignant pericardial effusion, pericarditis, swollen heart, fluid around the heart

Related conditions: Any number of cancers that have spread throughout the body

Definition: Pericardial effusion is an increase in the amount of fluid between the pericardium and the heart. The pericardium is a thin layer of tissue that forms the pericardial sac, a pouch that holds the heart and the ends of the major blood vessels. The pericardium keeps the heart confined to the chest cavity and prevents it from enlarging if blood flow to the heart increases. The sac normally contains a small amount of fluid. Too much fluid puts pressure on the heart and affects its normal functioning.

When the buildup of excess fluid is caused by infection of the pericardium, the condition is known as pericarditis. When the buildup is a result of inflammation or cancer it is called pericardial effusion. When the amount of fluid reaches a dangerous level, it is called malignant pericardial effusion. Effusions in cancer patients are malignant about half of the time.

Risk factors: For cancer patients, the disease itself poses the greatest risk. A less serious but still common risk is earlier radiation treatments to the chest, especially for lung cancer.

Some Causes of Malignant and Nonmalignant Pericardial Effusion

Causes of Malignant Pericardial Effusion
- Cancer of pericardium or heart muscle
- Cancers that have metastasized from the lung, breast, esophagus, thymus, and lymph system

Causes of Nonmalignant Pericardial Effusion
- Acquired immunodeficiency syndrome (AIDS)
- Heart attack
- Infection of pericardium; can be a side effect of radiation therapy or chemotherapy
- Injury
- Lupus
- Surgery
- Underactive thyroid gland

Source: National Cancer Institute

Etiology and the disease process: The causes of effusions in patients who do not have cancer are many. The cause of malignant pericardial effusion in cancer patients is cancer that develops in the pericardium or the heart muscle, or cancer that has metastasized from almost anywhere else in the body, including the lungs, breasts, esophagus, colon, prostate, and even bone marrow (leukemia) and skin (melanoma).

Cancerous cells rub against the pericardium. This irritant causes fluid to build up, much the way a blister forms under the skin. Some cancers produce little fluid but cause the pericardium to thicken and become rigid. Both conditions are serious.

An effusion can be chronic (present over time) or acute (occurring suddenly). If the fluid collects slowly over time, the pericardium may stretch enough to hold it. The patient usually feels no symptoms until a large amount of fluid accumulates. When the volume of fluid reaches a critical amount or when fluid accumulates rapidly—even a relatively small amount of fluid—a condition known as cardiac tamponade occurs. At this stage, the effusion surrounds and squeezes at the heart. This interferes with the heart's ability to effectively pump blood. Cardiac tamponade is a medical emergency that can be fatal if not promptly treated.

Incidence: Because effusions develop from a number of different diseases or conditions, any patient with any of the many conditions that can produce an effusion may be stricken with one. Effusions affect both sexes, all age groups, and all racial and ethnic groups.

Malignant pericardial effusion is more common in cancer patients than in patients who do not have cancer. Studies have revealed that 33 percent of patients with lung cancer have an effusion caused by the spread of their cancer at the time of their death. Further, 33 percent of pericardial effusions are a result of the spread of lung cancer. Lung cancer is the most common cancer found in malignant pericardial effusions in men.

Breast cancer causes 25 percent of pericardial effusions, and about 25 percent of patients with breast cancer have pericardial effusion. Breast cancer is the most common cancer found in malignant pericardial effusions in women.

Cancers that affect the blood (such as leukemia and Hodgkin disease) account for 15 percent of malignant pericardial effusions.

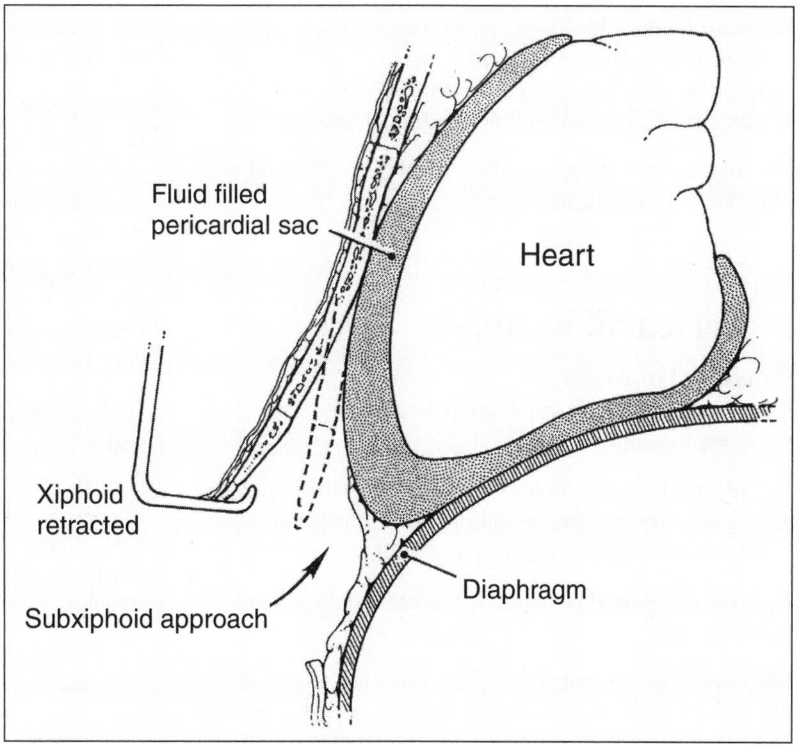

A surgical approach to treating cardiac tamponade. (LifeART© 2008 Wolters Kluwer Health, Inc.-Lippincott Williams &Wilkins. All rights reserved.)

Symptoms: Symptoms of an effusion are similar to symptoms associated with heart problems and include chest pain, rapid heartbeat, shortness of breath, dizziness or fainting, difficulty in swallowing, cough, and low blood pressure.

Screening and diagnosis: Spotting an effusion is relatively easy for doctors. X rays and other imaging techniques reveal the characteristic "water-bottle" shape of the swollen pericardial sac. Sometimes doctors perform a pericardiocentesis, a procedure that uses a needle to withdraw some of the fluid. Doctors then analyze the fluid to determine the cause of the effusion.

Treatment and therapy: For cancer patients, treatment generally involves relief of symptoms, because pericardial effusions usually arise in the later stages of cancer, often in the last few week of life. Doctors use various noninvasive and surgical procedures to drain the fluid, thus offering the patient some relief. In addition, doctors prescribe aspirin and anti-inflammatory drugs.

Prognosis, prevention, and outcomes: There is no way to prevent an effusion in cancer patients. The prognosis for cancer patients with malignant pericardial effusion is poor. One study showed that of patients diagnosed with malignant pericardial effusions, 86 percent died within a year of diagnosis. About one-third died within the first month. In 43 percent of the cases studied, pericardial effusion was the first sign of cancer.

Wendell Anderson, B.A.

▶ For Further Information

Gornik, H., M. Gerhard-Herman, and J. Beckman. "Abnormal Cytology Predicts Poor Prognosis in Cancer Patients with Pericardial Effusion." *Journal of Clinical Oncology* 23, no. 22 (August 1, 2005): 5211-5216.

Laham, R., et al. "Pericardial Effusion in Patients with Cancer: Outcome with Contemporary Management Strategies." *Heart* 75, no. 1 (January, 1996): 67-71.

Moore, K., and L. Schmais. *Living Well with Cancer: A Nurse Tells You Everything You Need to Know About Managing the Side Effects of Your Treatment.* New York: Putnam Publishing Group, 2001.

▶ Other Resources

MayoClinic.com

Pericardial Effusion: What Are the Symptoms?
http://www.mayoclinic.com/health/pericardial-effusion/HQ01198

National Cancer Institute
Malignant Pericardial Effusions
http://www.nci.nih.gov/cancertopics/pdq/supportivecare/cardiopulmonary/Patient/page4

See also Lactate dehydrogenase (LDH) test; Mesothelioma; Pericardiocentesis.

▶ Pericardiocentesis

Category: Procedures
Also known as: Pericardial tap, percutaneous pericardiocentesis

Definition: Pericardiocentesis is the insertion of a needle or catheter through the pericardium, the membrane that surrounds the heart, to drain excess fluid.

Cancers diagnosed or treated: Mesothelioma, advanced breast cancer

Why performed: Primarily a therapeutic but sometimes a diagnostic procedure, pericardiocentesis is performed to remove from the pericardium excess fluid that is inhibiting the heart's pumping action. If this pericardial effusion has accumulated rapidly, causing a life-threatening condition known as cardiac tamponade, then the procedure is performed on an emergency basis to avoid sudden death. In cases of suspected metastatic cancer, fluid buildup requires both relief and pathology.

Patient preparation: A few days before the procedure, an electrocardiogram (EKG), an echocardiogram, and blood tests confirm that it is safe to perform the operation. Patients must not eat or drink for several hours beforehand.

Steps of the procedure: Nonemergency pericardiocentesis is scheduled in a hospital. An intravenous (IV) line is inserted in the patient's arm or hand for medications. The puncture site is sterilized and a local anesthetic given. With the patient's head elevated 30 to 60 degrees, the physician, guided by an image on a video monitor, inserts a needle beneath the breastbone and into the pericardium. When enough fluid has been removed, the needle is withdrawn and direct pressure is applied. Large accumulations of fluid require the insertion of a catheter through which the fluid can drain into a bag. Extreme cases require general anesthesia and open surgery.

After the procedure: The patient stays in an intensive care unit while vital signs, the incision site, and fluid drainage are monitored. Nurses especially watch for bulging of the jugular vein in the neck, which suggests problems with blood flow. The length of the hospital stay may be as short as overnight or as long as a few days.

Risks: With guided imaging, pericardiocentesis is relatively safe, with a 5 percent risk of these side effects: air embolism (air in a blood vessel, blocking blood flow); infection of the pericardial membranes (pericarditis) or at the incision site; irregular heartbeat (arrhythmia); heart attack (myocardial infarction); pneumopericardium (introduction of air into the pericardial sac); and puncture of the heart muscle (myocardium), stomach, lungs, liver, or a coronary artery.

Results: Normal pericardial fluid is clear, straw-colored, and low in viscosity. High viscosity, low clarity, and the presence of blood, bacteria, abnormal cells, high levels of protein, or an excessive number of white blood cells indicate an abnormal result. The latter three conditions particularly suggest the spread of cancer to the pericardium, which is confirmed with biopsy and pathology.

Christina J. Moose, M.A.

See also Acupuncture and acupressure for cancer patients; Bronchoalveolar lung cancer; Mediastinoscopy; Mesothelioma; Pericardial effusion; Thoracoscopy; Thymomas.

▶ Peritoneovenous shunts

Category: Procedures
Also known as: Peritoneovenous ascites shunts

Definition: Peritoneovenous shunts are surgically implanted devices used to relieve intractable cases of ascites. This condition, characterized by excess buildup of fluids in the peritoneal (abdominal) cavity, generally results from chronic liver disease but also from malignancy in one out of ten cases. The shunt—a plastic or silicone rubber tube—serves to drain fluid from the abdominal cavity into the jugular vein in the neck.

Cancers treated: Ovarian, endometrial, colon, gastric, breast, and pancreatic cancers

Why performed: Tumor-induced ascites is difficult to manage and is usually a manifestation of late-stage cancer. It causes abdominal swelling, nausea, loss of appetite, and shortness of breath as a result of fluid accumulation in the chest cavity. Peritoneovenous shunting carries potential risks but may be recommended to ease discomfort when medical therapy consisting of salt restriction, diuretics, repeated fluid aspirations, chemotherapy, or immunotherapy fails to reduce ascites.

Patient preparation: Before surgery, the patient undergoes routine laboratory tests, including a coagulation profile and liver panel, and imaging tests, such as computed tomography (CT) scan and ultrasonography, to assess the extent of ascites and the condition of the veins selected for shunting. The operation is contraindicated if an additional test shows that the ascitic fluid is infected.

Steps of the procedure: The patient is given a sedative and undergoes either local or general anesthesia at the hospital. The surgeon makes a small incision and inserts a shunting tube under the skin of the chest that will run from the abdominal cavity to the jugular vein. The tube is then passed down to the superior vena cava, a large vein that returns blood to the heart. With a pump chamber and a one-way valve that prevents backflow, the shunt drains ascitic fluid into the systemic circulation.

After the procedure: After surgery, the patient's vital signs are monitored by a nursing staff, and for up to forty-eight hours the shunt is checked to make sure that it functions properly. Antibiotics and pain medication are prescribed as needed. Patients are instructed to pump the shunt daily to remove fluid from the abdomen, to take their prescribed medication, and to restrict sodium intake.

Risks: Complications are common and include shunt malfunction, infection, blood clots, edema, leakage of ascitic fluid, and heart failure.

Results: The procedure is deemed successful when fluid in the abdomen gradually ceases to accumulate after surgery, but frequently a blood clot or scar tissue will form around the shunt and block the valve or tube.

Anna Binda, Ph.D.

See also Ascites; Cytology; Gallbladder cancer; Gastrointestinal cancers; Krukenberg tumors; Mesothelioma; Pancreatic cancers; Paracentesis.

▶ Personality and cancer

Category: Social and personal issues

Definition: The question of whether certain personality traits make some people more prone to develop or die from diseases such as cancer dates back to the time of Hippocrates, the ancient Greek physician.

Research: The ancient Greeks classified personality types based on humours: sanguine (blood—arrogant, impulsive), choleric (yellow bile—a leader, ambitious), melancholic (black bile—depressive, creative), and phlegmatic (phlegm—unemotional, rational). Twentieth century psychologist Hans Eysenck categorized personality by examining four factors based on character traits: extraversion (social and lively), neuroticism (anxious and emotionally unstable), psychoticism (aggressive, cold, egocentric, and tough-minded), and "lie" (conforming, socially naïve, and dissimulating). Many other classification schemes exist. Multiple studies have looked at whether certain personality types or traits increase a person's risk of developing or dying from cancer. Some studies reported an association between personality traits and risk of developing cancer or dying from cancer, while others found no association.

Researcher Naoki Nakaya and his colleagues, from Tohoku University in Japan, reviewed these studies and found limitations that make it impossible to come to any conclusions about their findings. For example, one study did not assess personality traits before the cancer diagnosis, making before-and-after comparisons impossible. Further studies by Nakaya and other scientists continued to yield mixed results. Studies of Japanese men and women and Swedish twins did not find an increased risk of developing or surviving cancer among people based on personality traits. However, Nakaya's study in a large group of Danish cancer patients did find a strong association between neuroticism and rate of survival. In 2008, Eveline M. A. Bleiker of the Netherlands Cancer Institute and her colleagues published the results of a follow-up study of about 9,700 women with breast cancer. Although the original study, in 1996, had found a weak link between antiemotionality, or a lack of emotional behavior, and a higher risk of developing breast cancer, their study thir-

Eysenck Personality Questionnaire

The Eysenck Personality Questionnaire (1975) was the product of Hans Eysenck (1916-1997), a German-born English psychologist. He based his theory of personality on physiology and genetics and focused on temperament, or the part of the personality that is from nature, not nurture. He was one of the first psychologists to use factor analysis, a statistical method, in the study of personality. His first personality test, the Maudsley Medical Questionnaire (1959), focused on neuroticism/stability. With the Maudsley Personality Inventory (1959), he added extraversion/introversion. With the Eysenck Personality Inventory (1964), he added a lie scale, which measured a person's tendency to dissimulate. The 1975 version added psychoticism/socialization, which looked at aggressiveness and impulsivity. Eysenck's personality tests have been widely used.

teen years later found no connection between personality traits and an increased risk for breast cancer.

Linking personality traits to cancer risk is difficult because there are so many things that may be more closely related to a person's cancer risk, such as stress, depression, or a person's behaviors and decisions. For example, neuroticism can lead to distress and stress, which in turn can weaken the immune system and leave people vulnerable to illness. In addition, neuroticism has been linked to depression, and studies have found an association between depression and survival from certain types of cancers. Researchers from the National Institute on Aging studied a group of men and women over seventy-one years of age and found an 88 percent higher risk of developing cancer in those who were chronically depressed (depressed for at least six years).

Risky behavior: The American Cancer Society takes the position that lifestyle and behavior are better predictors than personality in assessing people's risk for developing or dying from cancer. About 75 to 80 percent of cancer cases and deaths result from things people do, such as smoking or chewing tobacco, not exercising or not eating right, and not visiting the doctor regularly. In 2000 almost 5 million people worldwide died prematurely from a smoking-related disease. At least 30 percent of cancer deaths and 87 percent of lung cancer deaths are related to smoking. In addition, 33 percent of cancer deaths are linked to poor diet and exercise habits and being overweight or obese. Neglecting personal health ranks high on the list of risky behaviors that can and often will lead to poorer outcomes after a cancer diagnosis. Early detection and treatment of cancer can save a person's life. Screenings and guidelines are available for breast, cervix, colon, rectum, prostate, mouth, and skin cancers through the American Cancer Society.

Perspective and prospects: Research has not definitively established personality as a risk factor for cancer. The main risk factors remain behaviors and lifestyle issues (tobacco use, poor diet, physical inactivity, and obesity) along with environmental factors (carcinogens, infectious agents). Rather than an individual's personality, that person's mental state (chronic depression or stress) may be a better predictor of an individual's risk of developing or surviving cancer.

Christine G. Holzmueller, B.L.A.

▶ For Further Information

Bleiker, E. M., et al. "Personality Factors and Breast Cancer Risk: A Thirteen Year Follow-Up." *Journal of the National Cancer Institute* 100, no. 3 (February 6, 2008): 213-218.

Dalton, Susanne Oksbjerg, et al. "Depression and Cancer Risk: A Register Based Study of Patients Hospitalized with Affective Disorders, Denmark, 1969-1993." *American Journal of Epidemiology* 115, no. 12 (2002): 1088-1095.

Nakaya, Naoki, Pernille E. Hanson, et al. "Personality Traits and Cancer Survival: A Danish Cohort Study." *British Journal of Cancer* 95 (2006): 146-152.

Nakaya, Naoki, Yoshitaka Tsubono, et al. "Personality and Risk of Cancer." *Journal of the National Cancer Institute* 95 (2003): 799-805.

▶ Other Resources

American Cancer Society
http://www.cancer.org

National Cancer Institute
Psychological Stress and Cancer: Questions and Answers
http://www.cancer.gov/cancertopics/factsheet/Risk/stress

See also Anxiety; Complementary and alternative therapies; Depression; Ependymomas; Non-Hodgkin lymphoma; Oligodendrogliomas; Pineoblastomas; Psychosocial aspects of cancer; Self-image and body image; Singlehood and cancer; Stress management; Symptoms and cancer.

▶ Pesticides and the food chain

Category: Carcinogens and suspected carcinogens
RoC status: Dichlorodiphenyltrichloroethane (DDT), reasonably anticipated human carcinogen since 1985
Also known as: Insecticides—chlorinated hydrocarbons, organophosphates, carbamates, dinitrophenols, thiocyanates, growth regulators, inorganics (arsenicals and fluorides), microbials; herbicides—amides, acetamides, carbamates, thiocarbamates, phenoxy compounds, dinitrophenols, dinitroanilines; fungicides—dicarboximides, chlorinated aromatics, dithiocarbamates, mercurials; algicides—organotins; molluscicides—chlorinated hydrocarbons; nematocides—halogenated alkanes; rodenticides—anticoagulants, botanicals, fluorides, inorganics, thioureas

Related cancers: Lymphoma, brain tumors, leukemia, cancers of the breast, skin, stomach, prostate, ovaries

Definition: Pesticides refer to any substance or mixture of substances intended for preventing, destroying, repelling, or lessening the damage of any pest. A pest is any living organism that could harm crops and people or other animals, or is in an undesirable location. Pesticides may be chemical, biological, or antimicrobial. They are released into the environment primarily through the spraying of insecticides on fruits and vegetables and other crops, such as corn, wheat, rice, and cotton, and by the use of herbicides on grass. Pesticides are believed to be responsible for a number of cancers.

Exposure routes: Ingestion, inhalation, absorption

Where found: Pesticides are found in the environment, in streams, rivers, lakes, groundwater, and the soil, including fields (where chlorophenols, particularly in the form of weed killers, build up over the years) and chemically treated lawns. DDT, banned in the United States in 1972, still exists in the soil and is stored in the fatty tissues of individuals; it may also be on products imported into the United States from countries where it is allowed.

Pesticides have entered the food chain: Chemicals from pesticides get into groundwater or streams, then into the grass and other vegetation, then into carnivorous animals and then omnivorous animals such as humans. Those animals at the top of the food chain, such as humans or scavengers, fare worse than those below them, as the buildup of toxins is much greater at the top. In the aquatic food chain, chemicals from pesticides enter agricultural runoff or wastewater, then are taken up by algae and plankton, then smaller organisms, then larger fish, and finally humans. Fish containing mercury or other chemicals can be lethal to people.

At risk: People who produce or distribute pesticides, agricultural workers and people living in close proximity to fields, people who use pesticides in and around their homes, and people who eat fish or pesticide-treated fruits and vegetables

Etiology and symptoms of associated cancers: Studies have shown that human bodies contain hundreds more chemicals—including those contained in pesticides—than they did fifty years ago. Pesticides are linked to lymphoma, a cancer of the white blood cells. Of the two kinds of lymphoma, Hodgkin disease and non-Hodgkin lymphoma (NHL), the latter is most associated with pesticide carcinogens. Non-Hodgkin lymphoma begins when a blood cell (lymphocyte) becomes malignant and subsequently produces descendants of the single cell in which mutations (errors) have occurred. Although lymphoma can occur in any part of the body, tumors typically form in the lymphatic system, meaning bone marrow, lymph nodes, the spleen, and blood. The initial symptoms are usually perceived as swelling around the lymph nodes at the base of the neck, fever, fatigue, and unexplained weight loss.

Breast cancer is linked to organochlorine pesticides, which affect the endocrine system. Absorbed through ingested foods, the pesticides mimic, alter, or modulate hormonal activity and are therefore known as endocrine disruptors. Raising the activity and quality of estrogens the human body produces causes tumors to form. Pesticides are also linked to ovarian cancer, in that malignant ovarian tumors are endocrine related and hormone dependent.

Atrazine, used on 96 percent of the United States corn crop, exists in most drinking water supplies in the Midwest and has been linked to birth defects in farmers' children. Long-term exposure to atrazine has been linked to weight loss, cardiovascular damage, retina and muscle degeneration, and cancer.

Organophosphate pesticides, which have largely replaced organochlorine pesticides, are connected with skin and eye problems, headaches, dizziness, nausea, vomiting, and abdominal pain. The thirty-seven compounds that make up this group destabilize a key enzyme in the brain known as cholinesterase, causing trauma to the brain and nervous system. Studies have related pesticide risk with respiratory problems, memory disorders, dermatologic conditions, cancer, depression, neurologic deficiencies, miscarriages, and birth defects. Primarily, these pesticides affect the nervous system by disrupting the enzyme that regulates acetylcholine, a neurotransmitter.

Definitive proof that DDT is a human carcinogen is still lacking, but it has been associated with liver, lung, and thyroid tumors.

History: More than four thousand years ago, Sumerians dusted sulfur on their crops to kill insects, and more than two thousand years ago, ancient Greeks used pesticides to protect their crops. By the fifteenth century, arsenic, mercury, and lead—highly toxic chemicals—were used on crops to eliminate insects. During the seventeenth century, farmers used nicotine sulfate, derived from tobacco leaves, as an insecticide, and in the nineteenth century, pyrethrum, extracted from chrysanthemums, and rotenone, removed from roots of tropical vegetables, were used as pesticides.

In 1939 Swiss scientist Paul Müller discovered the potency of a compound made of carbon and hydrogen called dichlorodiphenyltrichloroethane (DDT), first used in World War II against typhus, plague, malaria, and dengue and yellow fevers. After the war, DDT use in the United States soared. Farmers killed pests such as boll weevils that were devastating cotton crops, and the government used low-flying crop-dusting planes to rid the forests of gypsy moths. Other parts of the world began using DDT to combat malaria; after homes and huts were sprayed in North Africa, Asia, India, and Zanzibar, the number of malaria cases declined drastically.

In 1962 Rachel Carson published *Silent Spring*, the product of more than four years of research, in which she maintained that pesticides were harming wildlife and the environment. Using meticulous documentation, Carson claimed that the government knew little about the dangers of pesticides. Although the book was criticized as well as praised, it spurred concerns about pesticides and other pollutants, leading to the beginning of the environmental movement and President Richard M. Nixon's creation of the Environmental Protection Agency (EPA) in 1970. Soon the EPA targeted DDT, eventually banning it in 1972. Although time has proven Carson's position on the harm from pesticides to wildlife correct, the idea that DDT is a human carcinogen is still being contested.

In the years since its ban, DDT has been replaced by a huge array of insecticides, herbicides, and pesticides that have been tentatively linked with tumors and cancers of the lymphatic, endocrine, neurological, respiratory, and reproductive systems but have not been proven to to be carcinogens. Although studies have shown an increase in the rates of tumors or cancers in agricultural areas where large amounts of pesticides are used, scientific proof of the connection is inconclusive. Because of the gap in time between exposure and the first symptoms of illness (frequently decades) and the inability to pinpoint a particular pesticide as the carcinogen, definite scientific proof is hard to provide.

Nevertheless, strict regulations are in effect: The EPA must approve any pesticide for sale or use in the United States, and the Food Quality Protection Act (1996) requires the oversight of the manufacture, distribution, and use of pesticides. Although the causal relationship between pesticides and cancer is hard to establish, pesticides have other proven health risks, and many people in the United States are trying to minimize or avoid their use. The EPA provides many suggestions on how to use pesticides more safely, and some people have turned to organically grown products as a way to avoid most pesticides.

Because of the carcinogenic potential of pesticides, the organic foods industry has grown. The Organic Foods Production Act (1990) authorized national standards for the production, handling, and processing of organically grown agricultural products. Essentially, organic farming is an ecological system that avoids chemical pesticides, promotes soil conservation, and integrates the parts of the farming system into an ecological whole. Although organic farming cannot guarantee that the soil does not contain pesticide residue, the practice follows methods designed to minimize contamination from air, soil, and water. Organic meat, poultry, eggs, and dairy products come from animals that are not given any antibiotics or growth hormones. Organic food is produced without using conventional pesticides or fertilizer made from synthetic ingredients or sewage sludge. Organic farms use cover crops, green manures, animal manures, and crop rotation to manage weeds, insects, and diseases and promote biological activity and long-term soil health.

Mary Hurd, M.A.

▶ For Further Information

Beres, Samantha. *Pesticides: Critcal Thinking About Environmental Issues*. Farmington Hills, Mich.: Greenhaven Press, 2002.

Carson, Rachel. *Silent Spring*. 1962. Reprint. Boston: Mariner Books, 2007.

Dunn, Jancie. "Toxic Overload: Teflon, Pesticides on Golf Courses, Plastic Bottles—An Explosion of Research Is Investigating Environmental Links and Breast Cancer." *Vogue*, October, 2006, 326ff.

Hemingway, Jean. "An Overview of Pesticide Resistance." *Science* 5, no. 298 (October 4, 2003): 96-97.

Izakson, Orna. "Farming Infertility: Country Living May Be Hazardous to Your Potency." *E/The Environmental Magazine* 15, no. 1 (January/February, 2004): 40-41.

Levine, Marvin J. *The Toxic Time Bomb in Our Midst*. Westport, Conn.: Praeger, 2007.

National Research Council. *Carcinogens and Anticarcinogens in the Human Diet*. Washington, D.C.: National Academy Press, 1996.

_______. *Pesticides in the Diets of Infants and Children*. Washington, D.C.: National Academy Press, 1993.

Rosenberg, Tina. "What the World Needs Now Is DDT." *The New York Times*, May 23, 2004, p. 8.

U.S. Department of Health and Human Services, Public Health Service, National Toxicology Program. *Eleventh Report on Carcinogens*. Research Triangle Park, N.C.: Author, 2005.

Wright, Karen. "Testing Pesticides on Humans." *Discover* 3, no. 12 (December, 2003): 66-69.

▶ Other Resources

National Cancer Institute

Cancer Trends Progress Report—2007 Update: Pesticides
http://progressreport.cancer.gov/doc_detail.asp?pid=1&did=2007&chid=71&coid=713&mid=

U.S. Environmental Protection Agency
Pesticides
http://www.epa.gov/pesticides/index.htm

See also Acrylamides; Agent Orange; Aplastic anemia; Arsenic compounds; Astrocytomas; Bisphenol A (BPA); Coal tars and coal tar pitches; Coke oven emissions; Curcumin; Dietary supplements; Diethanolamine (DEA); Dioxins; Epstein-Barr virus; Erionite; Herbs as antioxidants; Macrobiotic diet; Neuroectodermal tumors; Non-Hodgkin lymphoma; Occupational exposures and cancer; Organochlorines (OCs); Pancreatic cancers; Premalignancies; Prevention; Richter syndrome; Risks for cancer; Vinyl chloride.

▶ Peutz-Jeghers syndrome (PJS)

Category: Diseases, symptoms, and conditions
Also known as: PJS, polyps and spots syndrome

Related conditions: Unexplained hamartomatous mixed polyposis

Definition: Peutz-Jeghers syndrome (PJS) is a rare disorder that causes the growth of multiple benign polyps in the stomach and small intestines. Most people with PJS have a family history of this inherited disorder, but it can also affect those without such a history. Polyps characteristic of the syndrome usually begin to develop during childhood or adolescence and have even been found in newborns. They often cause such medical problems as recurrent bowel obstructions, chronic bleeding, and abdominal pain, and they tend to become cancerous over time. PJS has also been found to increase an affected person's risk of developing other cancers throughout the body, including breast, ovarian, uterine, pancreatic, testicular, and lung cancer.

Risk factors: Peutz-Jeghers syndrome is genetically linked, meaning that it is associated with a defect, or mutation, in one or more genes. A person at increased risk of developing this disorder usually has family members with the disease. The risk factors for people who develop PJS without a familial link are unknown. In these cases, the disease appears to result from new mutations in the gene responsible for the disorder, so exposure to chemicals in the environment may also be a risk factor.

Etiology and the disease process: Peutz-Jeghers syndrome is caused by a mutation in a gene that aids in the control of cell growth and division. Normally, during conception, two copies of each gene are passed on to the child, one from the mother and one from the father. In PJS, one inherited copy of a gene called serine/threonine-protein kinase 11, or *STK11*, is defective and is present in all cells, disrupting the cells' ability to control division. Research has shown that an additional gene mutation is necessary for PJS to cause cancer, either in the second copy of the *STK11* gene or in another gene. Whether the person develops cancer and which organs will be affected depends on which cells are affected by the second mutation. It is believed that the defective *STK11* gene is only one requirement in a process that involves mutations in other genes. Some people with defective *STK11* genes do not develop cancer because the other mutations do not occur.

Incidence: Peutz-Jeghers syndrome is considered a rare disorder; however, with estimates of its incidence ranging from 1 in 25,000 to 1 in 280,000 births, it is uncertain how many cases go undiagnosed.

Symptoms: Individuals with Peutz-Jeghers syndrome commonly develop small, dark blue or brown spots that resemble freckles around the eyes, lips, and nostrils; inside the mouth; around the anus; and, frequently, on the hands and feet. They typically appear during infancy or early childhood and gradually fade as the person ages. Many symptoms depend on the location and extent of the polyps or cancer and can include abdominal cramps and pain,

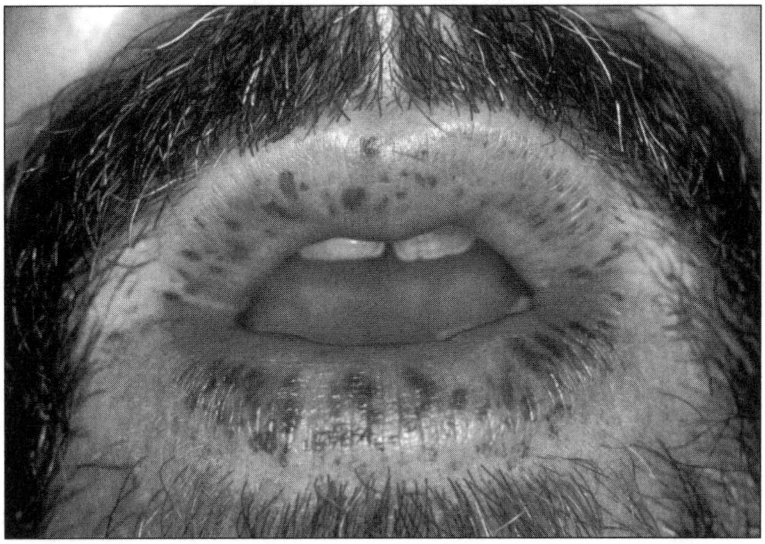

Pigmentation on the lips of a male patient with Peutz-Jeghers syndrome. (©Watney Collection/Phototake–All rights reserved)

bloody urine and stools, anemia, and vomiting (possibly with blood). Gynecomastia, an abnormal enlargement of the breasts, typically precedes the development of testicular, ovarian, and uterine cancer. Other findings in a patient with PJS include ovarian cysts, benign ear tumors, rectal prolapse, intussusception (part of the bowel folds into itself), and bladder, ureteral, intestinal, bronchial, and nasal polyps.

Screening and diagnosis: Screening for Peutz-Jeghers syndrome includes a blood test to look for a mutation in the *STK11* gene. It is not routinely performed unless PJS is suspected or other family members have been diagnosed with the disorder.

An accurate family history and extensive physical examination, including testing, are essential for the diagnosis of PJS. The syndrome is suspected when someone has a family history of PJS and the characteristic spots that accompany the disorder. Diagnostic tests should include an X ray of the abdomen, upper and lower gastrointestinal studies, stools for occult blood, mammography, testicular ultrasound, and colonoscopy or sigmoidoscopy.

Staging of PJS is based on the cancers that develop.

Treatment and therapy: Treatment of Peutz-Jeghers syndrome may include surgery to remove polyps that are causing chronic problems and to decrease bowel loss caused by intussusception. Repeated surgery to remove part of the intestine is common in PJS and often results in short-bowel syndrome, a condition that develops after bowel surgery, when there is not enough surface area in the bowel to absorb sufficient nutrients from food. If this occurs, special nutritional interventions are required.

The primary goal in treating PJS, however, is the early identification of malignancies. Physical examinations and screening tests should be scheduled at recommended intervals to monitor polyps and detect cancers. Surveillance programs typically recommend that colon and testicular cancer screenings start between ages eight and ten and that screening for most other cancers starts by age twenty.

Other treatments are specific to any cancers that may be identified.

Prognosis, prevention, and outcomes: The incidence of cancer in people with Peutz-Jeghers syndrome is high; it is estimated that 93 percent will develop cancer by age sixty-four. Breast (50 percent), colorectal (40 percent), pancreatic (35 percent), and stomach (30 percent) cancers are among the most common. Deaths result from complications of polyps, repeated surgeries, or cancer. There is no known method of preventing PJS.

Dorothy P. Terry, R.N.

▶ For Further Information

Bourke, B., et al. "Peutz-Jeghers Syndrome and Management Recommendations." *Clinical Gastroenterology and Hepatology* 4, no. 12 (December, 2006): 1550.

Gunabushanam, G., et al. "Peutz-Jeghers Syndrome." *Pediatric Radiology* 36, no. 8 (August, 2006): 888-889.

Hearle, N., et al. "Frequency and Spectrum of Cancers in the Peutz-Jeghers Syndrome." *Clinical Cancer Research* 12, no. 10 (May 15, 2006): 3209-3215.

▶ Other Resources

Genetics Home Reference

Peutz-Jeghers Syndrome
http://ghr.nlm.nih.gov/condition=peutzjegherssyndrome

Peutz-Jegher's Syndrome

http://www.peutz-jeghers.com/

See also Colon polyps; Colonoscopy and virtual colonoscopy; Colorectal cancer screening; Family history and risk assessment; Gastric polyps; Hereditary mixed polyposis syndrome; Hereditary polyposis syndromes; Juvenile polyposis syndrome; Pancreatic cancers; Polyps; Sertoli cell tumors; Small intestine cancer.

▶ Pharmacy oncology

Category: Medical specialties

Also known as: Oncology pharmacy, hematology/oncology pharmacy

Definition: Pharmacy oncology is the specialized practice of pharmacy with the specific goals of reducing the cancer care burden and of promoting optimal, cost-effective, safe cancer care. According to the Board of Pharmacy Specialties, which certifies oncology pharmacists, pharmacy oncology specialists "recommend, design, implement, monitor, and modify pharmacotherapeutic plans to optimize outcomes in patients with malignant diseases." The practice of oncology pharmacy, when incorporated into multidisciplinary care, provides cancer patients with the best access and control of treatment options. It also provides educational and research support to other members of the interdisciplinary cancer care team.

Subspecialties: Community oncology pharmacy, chemotherapeutics

Cancers treated: All

Training and certification: Clinical, registered pharmacists with a bachelor of science in pharmacy (BSP) or doctor of pharmacy (Pharm.D.) may be found working in hospital or clinical settings and in nontraditional community oncology settings, such as individual oncologist offices or retail pharmacies that specialize in chemotherapeutic treatments. In addition to practical experience in drug information, intravenous (IV) admixture, and patient interaction, pharmacists have structured educational opportunities to become pharmacy oncology specialists. On-site training with an existing oncology pharmacist and the oncology team is often provided to individual pharmacists in institutional or community pharmacies, and residencies and fellowships in oncology are available to newly graduated or practicing pharmacists with a doctor of pharmacy. Residency programs entail one full year of practical study in general clinical pharmacy; thereafter, students apply for a specialty residency in oncology. The specialty oncology residency requires another full year of practical study in a purely cancer-based setting. For this residency, the pharmacist is mentored by an existing specialty oncology pharmacist and participates in patient care as part of the health professional team. Examples of educational instruction topics for oncology residencies include adult medical oncology, bone marrow transplantation, pediatric oncology, palliative and pain care, surgical oncology, immunotherapy, radiation oncology, and pharmaceutical management. Residency programs typically require a doctor of pharmacy for application and, after successful completion, provide the pharmacist the necessary requirement for more intense training.

For pharmacists interested in training beyond residency programs, fellowship positions in oncology are available. Such postdoctoral fellowships are generally two-year positions that provide pharmacists an opportunity to focus their knowledge in oncology topics. Fellowship programs are often highly specific and include instruction on topics such as the clinical pharmacology of chemotherapeutic and related medications, study design and analysis techniques, presentation and publication of scientific data, pharmacokinetic and pharmacodynamic modeling, therapeutic drug monitoring of individual agents, and drug information management and analysis. Deeper involvement with the oncology care team and with oncology research is provided in fellowship positions.

An oncology specialty certification may be awarded by the Board of Pharmacy Specialties to pharmacists who meet the following minimum criteria: The registered pharmacist must have completed at least three years of practice, with a substantial amount of that time spent in oncology settings, or must have completed a specialty residency in oncology pharmacy plus one year of practice, with a substantial portion of that year spent in oncology settings. In addition, the pharmacist must pass a stringent written test, the Oncology Pharmacy Specialty Certification Examination. After meeting these criteria and applying to the Board of Pharmacy Specialties for certification, the pharmacist may be designated a board-certified oncology pharmacist (BCOP). The pharmacist may retain this title as long as recertification requirements are met every seven years, by either retaking and passing the examination or completing one hundred hours of continuing education; both the exam and education are provided by the Board of Pharmacy Specialties.

Services and procedures performed: Oncology pharmacists provide numerous services to the health care team and to patients. Oncology pharmacists may be found in hospital-based or office-based oncology clinics or in standalone community pharmacies that service nearby cancer providers. Although they vary between settings, all services provided by oncology pharmacists fall into a handful of categories: educational and counseling services, drug administration and monitoring services, supportive care services, research and guidelines development services, medication safety services, and economic benefits.

Oncology pharmacists regularly provide educational services to other members of the health care team and counseling services to patients. Pharmacists provide safe-handling instructions to nurses who handle and administer cytotoxic drugs. They provide intravenous (IV) admixture instruction to pharmacists and technicians to prevent chemotherapy incompatibilities and provide IV administration instruction to nurses to prevent medication errors. Oncology pharmacists educate all members of the health care team about medication-error prevention, including instruction about confusing, similar-sounding or similarly written medication names. They often contribute to the development and enforcement of the institution's best practices in cancer care.

In direct interactions with patients, pharmacists provide safe handling and administration instructions of cytotoxic drugs, and they provide dosing suggestions and methods to manage medication side effects. In addition, pharmacists who counsel cancer patients have the opportunity to reinforce the treatment goals and address adherence issues or other patient concerns. In community settings especially, oncology pharmacists contribute to the continuity of care by supporting and managing even complex outpatient treatments, thus keeping patients out of the hospital for longer durations and by providing another source of communication between the patient and primary cancer care provider.

Drug information services are a primary responsibility

of pharmacists on the oncology care team. In addition to providing specific drug suggestions and knowledge about drug interactions and incompatibilities, side effects, and handling risks associated with chemotherapy, pharmacists are able to evaluate pharmacokinetic and pharmacodynamic effects of drugs and regimens. They interpret laboratory changes and other treatment-related problems and adjust chemotherapy regimens accordingly. By performing therapeutic drug monitoring for specific agents, pharmacists anticipate and prevent drug toxicities or subtherapeutic risks as well. In addition to providing information about chemotherapy regimens, oncology pharmacists are trained to safely perform chemotherapy admixture and can provide this service even to outpatients in a community oncologist office setting.

Supportive care services offered by the oncology pharmacist include antiemetic and pain-control care. By developing and implementing antiemetic regimens according to the emetic potential of chemotherapy regimens, oncology pharmacists help minimize or even eliminate this common side effect of chemotherapy. Pharmacists often oversee the provision of pain management and palliative care with medications. Because of their extensive medication knowledge, oncology pharmacists are able to manage these cancer-related concerns and also anticipate and prevent the associated side effects or drug interactions that may occur with the drug therapy of pain or emesis.

Pharmacists often contribute to the interdisciplinary team by providing access to drug-related databases and by presenting new research findings on drug therapy or updated regimens, within an institution in a brown-bag or continuing-education setting or to the larger medical field through publications in journals. In addition, oncology pharmacists play a role in developing institutional treatment guidelines for specific cancers or cancer-related health issues along with other team members and in evaluating medication use practices and offering improvements. Related to these contributions, oncology pharmacists provide medication safety services, such as reporting medication errors to MedWatch or other oversight and reporting organizations. They also ensure that cytotoxic medications are properly stored and prepared by professionals and ensure that professionals use appropriate protective measures during preparation.

Lastly, oncology pharmacists reduce cancer-care costs to patients and to providers by ensuring the smooth delivery of cancer care. In particular, oncology pharmacists are able to recommend affordable treatment options, to decrease waste from incorrect medication handling, and to streamline treatment plans by removing unnecessary or replacing overly toxic medications.

Related specialties and subspecialties: Related specialties in the cancer field include medical oncology, nursing oncology, and radiation oncology. Together with oncology pharmacists, members of these fields make up a typical interdisciplinary cancer care team.

Related specialties in the pharmacy field include IV admixture pharmacy, nutrition pharmacy, pain-management pharmacy, and clinical pharmacology and pharmaceutics. Pharmacists may also complete certification programs in nutrition pharmacy and in clinical pharmacology.

Nicole M. Van Hoey, Pharm.D.

▶ For Further Information

Holdsworth, M. T. "State of Oncology Pharmacotherapy." *The Annals of Pharmacotherapy* 40, no. 12 (December, 2006): 2238-2239.

Liekweg, A., M. Westfeld, and U. Jaehde. "From Oncology Pharmacy to Pharmaceutical Care: New Contributions to Multidisciplinary Cancer Care." *Support Care Cancer* 12, no. 2 (February, 2004): 73-79.

Nygren, P. "The Pharmacist and Quality of Cancer Chemotherapy." *Acta Oncologica* 46, no. 6 (2007): 715-716.

Semaan, N. "Integration of Complementary Disciplines into the Oncology Clinic. Part III, Herbal Medicine-Drug Interactions: The Role of the Pharmacist." *Current Problems in Cancer* 24, no. 4 (July/August, 2000): 213-222.

▶ Organizations and Professional Societies

American Society of Health-System Pharmacists (ASHP)
http://www.ashp.org/s_ashp/index.asp
7272 Wisconsin Avenue
Bethesda, MD 20814

Hematology/Oncology Pharmacy Association (HOPA)
http://www.hoparx.org
175 Wall Street
Princeton, NJ 08540

▶ Other Resources

Board of Pharmacy Specialties
http://www.bpsweb.org

Canadian Association of Pharmacy in Oncology
http://www.capho.org/about.htm

International Society of Oncology Pharmacy Practitioners
http://www.isopp.org

See also Case management; Overtreatment; Palliative treatment.

▶ Phenacetin

Category: Chemotherapy and other drugs; carcinogens and suspected carcinogens
RoC status: Reasonably anticipated human carcinogen since 1980
Also known as: Saridon, Acetophenetidin

Related cancers: Urothelial neoplasms, especially transitional cell carcinoma of the renal pelvis and bladder

Definition: Phenacetin is an analgesic and antipyretic introduced in 1887. It was linked to urothelial neoplasms, especially transitional cell carcinoma of the renal pelvis and bladder, as well as interstitial nephritis in combination with renal papillary necrosis and was removed from the market in 1983.

Exposure routes: Oral ingestion

Where found: Sold as an analgesic and antipyretic (fever-reducing) medication

At risk: All who have taken medications containing phenacetin

Etiology and symptoms of associated cancers: The cause and mechanism of the nephropathic change due to phenacetin in humans is unknown, but the renal lesion sometimes seen was interstitial nephritis in combination with renal papillary necrosis.

When administered in the diet, phenacetin caused benign and malignant tumors of the urinary tract in mice and rats of both sexes and of the nasal cavity in rats of both sexes, according to studies by the International Agency for Research on Cancer (IARC). There is limited evidence for the carcinogenicity of phenacetin in humans because this medication was usually taken mixed with other drugs.

History: Phenacetin, first introduced in 1887, was used principally as an analgesic and fever reducer. Its analgesic effects are reportedly because of its actions on the sensory tracts of the spinal cord. In addition, phenacetin acts as a negative inotrope on the heart, weakening the heart's muscular action. Phenacetin also was once used as a stabilizer for hydrogen peroxide in hair-bleaching preparations. Many case reports provided evidence that abuse of analgesic mixtures containing phenacetin resulted in kidney cancer (cancer of the renal pelvis). It was implicated in kidney disease (nephropathy) and renal papillary necrosis due to abuse of analgesics and was withdrawn from the U.S. market in 1983.

Phenacetin was first listed in the *First Annual Report on Carcinogens* (RoC; 1980), and analgesic mixtures containing phenacetin were first listed in the *Fourth Annual Report on Carcinogens* (1985).

Debra B. Kessler, M.D., Ph.D.

See also Adenocarcinomas; Bladder cancer; Gallbladder cancer; Gastrointestinal oncology; Kidney cancer; Renal pelvis tumors; Transitional cell carcinomas; Urethral cancer; Urinary system cancers.

▶ Phenolics

Category: Complementary and alternative therapies
ATC code: D08AE
Also known as: Phenols

Definition: Phenolics are a class of compounds grouped together because of their chemical structure; they are aromatic compounds (containing benzene rings), usually with hydroxyl groups. Their function varies, however, and they may have a protective role against many cancers. Subclasses of this group are benzenediols, capsaicinoids, monolignols, and phenol ethers.

Cancers treated or prevented: Primarily breast cancer

Delivery routes: Oral in diet, pills, or capsules

How these compounds work: Phenolic acids have become the topic of much study for their protective role against many cancers. Examples of phenolics include gallic acids, curcumin, and ferulic acids. Found in abundance in many plants, phenolics in even low concentrations decrease cell proliferation, which makes them critically important in the shrinkage of cancer cells and concurrent reduction in size of tumors. Though the exact mechanisms by which phenolics work as antiproliferative substances in the treatment of cancer is unclear, a diet consisting of many fruits and vegetables seems to play an important role in cancer prevention and aids in cancer treatment by reducing tumor size and spread.

Proposed mechanisms by which these phenolic acids function include antioxidant effects, steroid receptor binding, direct interaction with intracellular elements and signaling systems, and aryl hydrocarbon receptor (AhR) binding and modification of subsequent pathways. Polyphenols and phenolic acids are rich in antioxidants, which reduce the concentration of harmful free radicals in the human body. Binding to receptor sites and inhibiting particular enzymes inhibits cell growth and prevents the inflammatory response of surrounding healthy tissues. As a result of their oxidation-reduction properties, they efficiently inactivate oxyl radicals and repair amino acid and deoxyribonucleic acid (DNA) base radicals. Phenols also induce apoptosis (scheduled cell death) and restrict the formation of new blood vessels. This active mechanism of phenolics is an important feature, since both growth and metastasis of a tumor depends heavily on angiogenesis (blood vessel formation) to provide oxygen and nutrients to the growing tumor cells.

Numerous laboratory studies have shown that phenolic acids inhibit the growth of cancerous cell in vitro. Unfortunately, studies performed in vivo do not show such clear benefits. Much of this may be attributable to differences in lifestyle or genetics. One promising study, however, showed that individuals who were prescribed low doses of aspirin had a decreased risk of developing colon cancer. The main metabolite of aspirin is a phenolic acid called salicylic acid. Salicylic acid is also found in plants, where it exists as a protective hormone. Its presence in fruits and vegetables may explain their oncoprotective role when made a staple in the human diet. Many more studies are currently being conducted on this matter.

Side effects: There are no known side effects of phenolics in the diet, but phenolics can be toxic at excessive levels for those who have phenol sulfotransferase (PST) deficiency, a disease that results from a difficulty in processing phenols into useful or at least nonharmful substances. In this case, phenols in the diet should be reduced or an agent used to facilitate processing.

Dwight G. Smith, Ph.D.

See also Angiogenesis; Antioxidants; Beta-carotene; Bioflavonoids; Breast cancer in children and adolescents; Breast cancer in men; Breast cancer in pregnant women; Breast cancers; Calcium; Carotenoids; Chemoprevention; Clinical breast exam (CBE); Coenzyme Q10; Complementary and alternative therapies; Cruciferous vegetables; Curcumin; Dietary supplements; Essiac; Free radicals; Fruits; Garlic and allicin; Glutamine; Green tea; Herbs as antioxidants; Isoflavones; Lutein; Lycopene; Nutrition and cancer prevention; Phytoestrogens; Resveratrol; Wine and cancer.

▶ Pheochromocytomas

Category: Diseases, symptoms, and conditions
Also known as: Chromaffin cell tumors, PCC

Related conditions: Early-onset hypertension, medullary thyroid cancer, multiple endocrine neoplasia type 2 (MEN 2), von Hippel-Lindau (VHL) disease, neurofibromatosis type 1, and abnormalities in succinate dehydrogenase subunit B (SDHB) and succinate dehydrogenase subunit D (SDHD)

Definition: Pheochromocytomas are tumors of chromaffin cells, neuroendocrine cells of the sympathetic nervous system (SNS). Their primary locations are in the adrenal medulla and sympathetic nervous system ganglia. These cells produce and secrete norepinephrine and epinephrine, vital agents in human survival that contribute to the fight-or-flight stress response. Pheochromocytomas are predominantly adrenal medulla tumors but may be found in other chromaffin cell locations, including the abdomen, thorax, and neck. Extra-adrenal tumors are called paragangliomas. Pheochromocytomas and paragangliomas may be benign or malignant.

Risk factors: The risk factors for the majority of the cases of pheochromocytomas are unknown. However, in cases where there is a family history of the disease, the primary risk factor is having a parent with the disease. Inheritance is by the autosomal dominant mechanism, so a person with the disease has a 50 percent chance of passing the abnormal gene and therefore the disease to his or her child.

Etiology and the disease process: The majority of pheochromocytomas have no known genetic basis and are termed sporadic. However, approximately 25 percent have a genetic etiology and are associated with specific syndromes such as multiple endocrine neoplasia type 2 (MEN 2), von Hippel-Lindau disease, neurofibromatosis type 1 (NF1), succinate dehydrogenase subunit B (SDHB), and succinate dehydrogenase subunit D (SDHD) abnormalities.

The MEN syndromes, caused by abnormalities on chromosome 10, make certain endocrine glands become overactive. MEN 2a causes pheochromocytomas, medullary thyroid cancer in early adulthood, and hyperparathyroidism, while MEN 2b manifests as pheochromocytomas, medullary thyroid cancer in early childhood, and neuromas, especially of the lips and tongue.

Von Hippel-Lindau disease is characterized by angiomas in the eye, hemangioblastomas of the brain and spinal cord, renal cell cancer, and pheochromocytomas. The *VHL* gene located on chromosome 3 normally functions as a tumor suppressor and inhibits uncontrolled cell proliferation. Mutations result in tumor growth.

Neurofibromatosis type 1 is a neurocutaneous disorder characterized by multiple café-au-lait spots and neurofibromas of the skin and nerves. Malignant connective or other soft-tissue neoplasms are common. The *NF1* gene is also a tumor suppressor. Located on chromosome 17, this gene can undergo mutations that result in abnormal cell growth and tumor formation.

Succinate dehydrogenase (SDH) is a component of the Krebs cycle and the mitochondrial respiratory chain. Four subunits have been identified: SDHA, SDHB, SDHC, and SDHD. SDHB and SDHD mutations correlate with extra-adrenal malignant paragangliomas, SDHB more so than SDHD mutations. Metastasis is common and precludes a cure.

Incidence: The rate of occurrence of pheochromocytoma is between 1 in 2,000 and 1 in 6,000 people. The annual occurrence rate is between 500 and 1,000 cases per year. Additional occurrences have been detected on autopsy.

Symptoms: Symptoms are related to elevated levels of catecholamines and metanephrines. Since pheochromocytomas release these agents intermittently, symptoms are paroxysmal. The most common symptoms include autonomic disturbances such as hypertension, tachycardia, palpitations, tachypnea, and sweating. In addition headache, flushing of the face, nausea and vomiting, chest pain, anxiety, nervousness, panic, and a sense of impending doom are often noted.

Screening and diagnosis: Detection of a pheochromocytoma can involve multiple and repeated testing, which can be time-consuming and expensive. The failure to detect the presence of a pheochromocytoma can be life-threatening to the individual.

Laboratory evaluation includes urine and blood sampling. Urinary tests are done for the presence of metanephrines and vanillyl mandelic acid (VMA). Plasma measurements are done for metanephrines and catecholamines. Urine testing is less sensitive and specific.

Metanephrines (normetanephrine and metanephrine) are metabolites of norepinephrine and epinephrine, the catecholamines normally secreted by the adrenal medulla but with increased levels in pheochromocytoma. A negative test reliably excludes the presence of a pheochromocytoma and avoids the sometimes false negative results obtained when plasma catecholamine values are obtained. Generally, a negative metanephrine plasma test precludes further testing. Accurate evaluation requires the avoidance of caffeine and acetaminophen before testing.

When a pheochromocytoma is diagnosed by laboratory methods, radiological evaluation helps identify the location and extent of any tumors. Magnetic resonance imaging (MRI), metaiodobenzylguanidine (MIBG) scintigraphy, and dopa positron emission tomography (PET) scanning are the most reliable methods of choice.

Treatment and therapy: Treatment of pheochromocytomas is by surgical removal, either through a traditional open incision or by newer laparoscopic techniques using several small incisions, a small camera, and long instruments. If only one adrenal gland is affected, typically the entire gland is removed. When bilateral involvement is present, attempts may be made to salvage the adrenal cortex. If this is not possible, lifelong adrenal medication supplementation will be required. It is possible that in the future, drugs will be developed to prevent endocrine gland overactivity and inhibition of angiogenic factors.

In patients with metastatic pheochromocytomas, a regimen of chemotherapy, radiation, somatostatin analogs, and 131I-MIBG is utilized. The survival rate is poor.

Prognosis, prevention, and outcomes: Since about 15 percent of patients with pheochromocytomas have a genetic basis for associated syndromes, they are candidates for genetic counseling and chromosomal analysis. Surgical removal of the pheochromocytoma alleviates symptoms associated with sympathetic nervous system involvement. Early and consistent screening for medullary thyroid cancer development leads to diagnosis and treatment in earlier stages of the disease, making a cure more possible. Total thyroidectomy prevents thyroid cancer but requires the patient to undergo lifelong thyroid medication supplementation. Malignant pheochromocytomas and paragangliomas have a mean survival rate of three years.

Wanda Todd Bradshaw, R.N.C., M.S.N.

Relative Survival Rates for Malignant Pheochromocytoma, 1988-2001

	Survival Rates (%)			
Gender	*1-Year*	*3-Year*	*5-Year*	*10-Year*
Men	83.9	73.4	67.3	29.7
Women	85.1	72.6	62.4	58.9
Total	84.5	73.0	64.8	44.0

Source: Data from L. A. G. Ries et al., eds., *Cancer Survival Among Adults: U.S. SEER Program, 1988-2001—Patient and Tumor Characteristics*, NIH Pub. No. 07-6215 (Bethesda, Md.: National Cancer Institute, 2007)

▶ **For Further Information**

Benn, Diana E., et al. "Clinical Presentation and Penetrance of Pheochromocytoma/Paraganglioma Syndromes." *Journal of Clinical Endocrinology and Metabolism* 91, no. 3 (2005): 827-836.

Neumann, Hartmut P., B. Bausch, et al. "Germ-Line Mutations in Nonsyndromic Pheochromocytoma." *New England Journal of Medicine* 346 (2002): 1459-1466.

Neumann, Hartmut P., A. Vortmeyer, et al. "Evidence of MEN-2 in the Original Description of Classic Pheochromocytoma." *New England Journal of Medicine* 357 (2007): 1311-1315.

Scholz, Tim, et al. "Current Treatment of Malignant Pheochromocytoma." *Journal of Clinical Endocrinology and Metabolism* 92, no. 4 (2006): 1217-1225.

▶ **Other Resources**

National Cancer Institute

Pheochromocytoma

http://www.cancer.gov/cancertopics/types/pheochromocytoma

Pheochromocytoma Organization

http://www.pheochromocytoma.org/sys-tmpl/door/

See also Adrenal gland cancers; Antidiarrheal agents; Endocrine cancers; Endocrinology oncology; Hemangioblastomas; Medulloblastomas; Multiple endocrine neoplasia type 1 (MEN 1); Multiple endocrine neoplasia type 2 (MEN 2); Neuroendocrine tumors; Neurofibromatosis type 1 (NF1); Nuclear medicine scan; Parathyroid cancer; Thyroid cancer; Von Hippel-Lindau (VHL) disease.

▶ Pheresis

Category: Procedures

Also known as: Apheresis, automated blood collection

Definition: Pheresis is a process in which the patient's blood is withdrawn from the body, the white blood cells or platelets are removed from the blood, and then the blood is returned back to the patient. Therapeutic pheresis is used to treat patients who have an elevated white blood count or

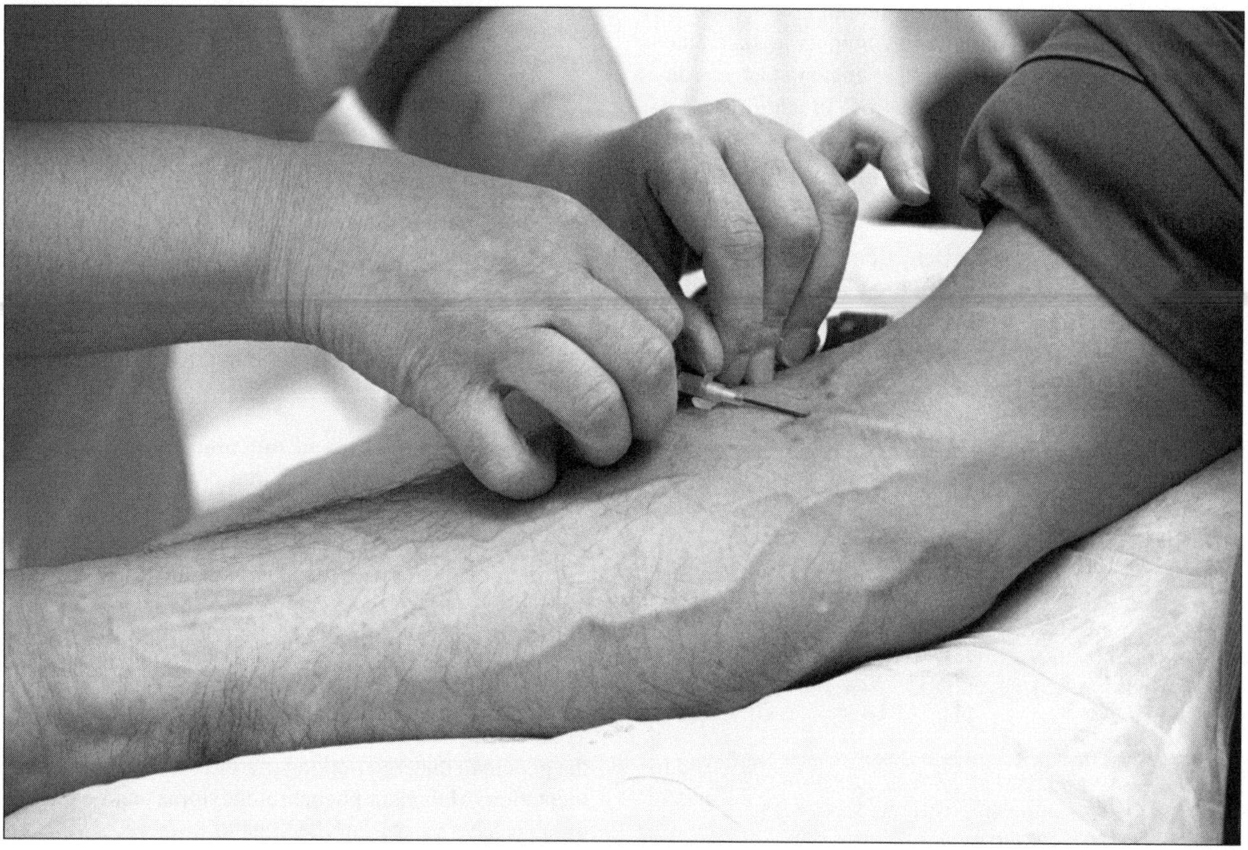

Here pheresis is being used to treat a patient with chronic lymphoblastic leukemia. (Antonia Reeve/Photo Researchers, Inc.)

platelet count related to a cancer disease process. Pheresis is also used to collect donor platelets from healthy people to be given to cancer patients who have no platelets.

Cancers treated: Hematological (blood) cancers

Why performed: Blood cancers can cause the bone marrow to malfunction and produce too many platelets or white blood cells, creating a life-threatening situation if the levels of these cells are not decreased. Oral medications can be given if levels are only slightly elevated, but for more acute cases, pheresis may be used. Specialized pheresis treatments are also performed. Photopheresis is used to treat graft-versus-host disease as well as lymphoma. Pheresis is also used to harvest stem cells for bone marrow transplantation. Therapeutic plasma exchange is used to treat the side effects of lung cancer, breast cancer, colon cancer, thymomas, and Hodgkin disease.

Patient preparation: Patients who have low levels of calcium may need to take a calcium supplement prior to having pheresis done. Patients may also receive calcium tablets during the procedure to help with the side effects associated with low calcium counts.

Steps of the procedure: The patient is positioned for comfort, usually in a recliner or a bed. An intravenous (IV) line is placed in the arm, usually the inner elbow, to allow for the blood to be withdrawn. The blood travels from the IV through a tube and then circulates through the pheresis machine to pull out the cells. The blood is then returned into the other arm through another IV that is placed there. This procedure can take two to three hours to perform and is done in a variety of settings. Pheresis can be done at the bedside, in a clinic, or even in a mobile pheresis lab.

After the procedure: After pheresis, the patient will be monitored for bleeding from the IV site. Pressure may need to be applied for five to ten minutes directly to the insertion site. Patients will also be monitored for tingling of the face and arms, which indicates low calcium levels, as well as dizziness. Cancer patients with an elevated platelet count or white blood cell count have their counts lowered to a safe level and then are placed on an oral agent or receive chemotherapy to maintain the safe levels.

Risks: Bleeding and infection may occur. Rare episodes of an air embolus have occurred with the removal of access lines.

Results: The patient will have the blood count lowered to a safe level in order to receive chemotherapy for the underlying cancer diagnosis. If a patient is given pheresis because the count is too high and does not follow up with additional medications, then the count will again rise to an unsafe level and the patient will need to receive pheresis therapy again.

Katrina Green, R.N., B.S.N., O.C.N.

▶ For Further Information

Tabuchi, T., et al. "Granulocyte Apheresis as a Possible New Approach in Cancer Therapy: A Pilot Study Involving Two Cases." *Cancer Detection & Prevention* 23, no. 5 (1999): 417-421.

▶ Other Resources

American Cancer Society
http://www.cancer.org

American Red Cross
http://www.redcross.org

National Cancer Institute
http://www.cancer.gov

See also Blood cancers; Bone marrow transplantation (BMT); Breast cancers; Chronic myeloid leukemia (CML); Infection and sepsis; Lambert-Eaton myasthenic syndrome (LEMS); Leukapharesis; Lymphomas; Myasthenia gravis; Mycosis fungoides; Myeloproliferative disorders; Side effects; Waldenström macroglobulinemia (WM).

▶ Photodynamic therapy (PDT)

Category: Chemotherapy and other drugs
ATC code: 101XD

Definition: Photodynamic therapy (PDT) is an emerging modality for treating local precancerous and cancerous lesions of epithelial origin. The technology relies on a class of anticancer drugs called photosensitizers that become active when exposed to specific light wavelengths, usually from a laser beam. Minimally invasive, PDT is also used to treat nonmalignant diseases, particularly the ocular condition known as wet age-related macular degeneration.

Cancers treated: Esophageal cancer, lung cancer, bladder carcinoma, nonmelanoma skin cancer

Subclasses of this group: Currently, most of the clinically approved photosensitizers are porphyrins, but other drugs under clinical investigation belong to the chlorin or purpurin family.

Delivery routes: Intravenous or topical, depending on the drug's chemical structure and the type of cancer and its location

Common Photosensitizers

Drug (Other Names)	Brands	Subclass	Delivery Mode	Conditions Treated
Aminolevulinic acid (5-aminolevulinic acid, ALA)	Levulan	Porphyrin	Topical	Actinic keratosis (precancerous skin lesion)
Methyl aminolevulinate (m-ALA)	Metvix	Porphyrin	Topical	Actinic keratosis, skin cancer
Porfimer sodium	Photofrin	Porphyrin	IV	Barrett esophagus (precancerous lesion), esophageal cancer, cervical cancer, lung cancer, stomach cancer, superficial bladder cancer
Temoporfin (meta-tetrahydroxyphenylchlorin, mTHPC)	Foscan	Chlorin	IV	Head and neck cancer

How these drugs work: The first clinical application of PDT was reported in 1903 by two German researchers, who used a topical coal tar dye called eosin in combination with visible light to treat skin cancer. The isolation of safer and more effective photosensitive dyes, called porphyrins, has propelled the field forward. Photosensitizers preferentially accumulate in abnormal tissues and cause little damage to surrounding healthy cells.

PDT is a two-part process. First, a nontoxic photosensitizer is administered to the patient. The lesion site is then exposed to light that is of a suitable wavelength to excite the photosensitive drug. Activated drug molecules initiate cytotoxic reactions that destroy tumor cells. They transfer energy to molecular oxygen, which, in turn, generates reactive oxygen species (ROS), such as singlet oxygen. These active molecular species damage deoxyribonucleic acid (DNA) and cause the oxidation of proteins and lipids. As a result, cancer cells undergo necrosis or apoptosis, the natural process of cell death. Because light needed to activate most photosensitizers cannot penetrate deeply into tissue, the therapeutic potential of PDT is limited to the treatment of local superficial tumors rather than large tumors or metastases.

Side effects: One side effect of PDT is increased sensitivity to light (sunburn-like reactions), which may last for several weeks after administration. Other side effects include constipation, irritation at the injection site, back pain, chest pain, fever, flulike syndrome, and general weakness.

Anna Binda, Ph.D.

See also Basal cell carcinomas; Bile duct cancer; Bladder cancer; Bone cancers; Bowen disease; Cutaneous breast cancer; Esophageal cancer; Keratosis; Laser therapies; Lung cancers; Skin cancers; Squamous cell carcinomas.

▶ Phyllodes tumors

Category: Diseases, symptoms, and conditions
Also known as: Phylloides tumors, cystosarcoma phyllodes

Related conditions: Fibroadenomas

Definition: Phyllodes tumors are masses that originate in the connective tissue of the breast. The term "phyllodes" comes from a Greek word meaning leaf. The tumor is so-named because it has leaflike projections seen on cross section. Most are benign, or noncancerous, and the rate of malignancy is estimated to be from 23 to 50 percent. A small percentage of phyllodes tumors occur in men, usually in the breast and occasionally in the stromal tissue of the prostate gland.

Risk factors: Women with a history of fibroadenoma, a benign breast tumor, may be at higher risk.

Etiology and the disease process: The cause of phyllodes tumors is not known. They develop in the connective, or stromal, tissue of the breast and can penetrate into ductal tissue or cystic spaces. They usually have a glandular component as well. These tumors may grow slowly for years, then enlarge rapidly over a period of weeks or months. Because of their rapid growth, most phyllodes tumors are discovered on self-examination. If left untreated, they can encompass the entire breast.

Incidence: Phyllodes tumors are rare, making up less than 1 percent of breast masses, or about 1 in 100,000. The overall risk of malignancy is low, about 2 per 1 million women. Phyllodes tumors usually occur in adult women, the average age at diagnosis being forty to fifty years, though they sometimes occur in adolescents or the elderly.

Symptoms: The most common symptom of phyllodes tumors is a firm, moveable, rapidly enlarging breast mass. Pressure from the tumor mass can compress the skin of the breast and cause it to appear translucent or bluish with dilated blood vessels. Tumors sometimes break through the skin and cause ulceration. Some tumors are painful; others are not. Metastasis, or spread to other parts of the body, from cancerous tumors can cause pain at the site of metastasis.

Screening and diagnosis: Mammograms reveal phyllodes tumors to be smooth or lobular masses with well-defined borders. Ultrasound examination or other imaging techniques, including computed tomography (CT) and magnetic resonance imaging (MRI), may be used to locate and size phyllodes tumors, but, because of similarities between benign and malignant phyllodes tumors and between phyllodes tumors and fibroadenomas, diagnosis is based on histology, or microscopic examination, of a tumor sample. Fibroadenomas can be diagnosed by needle biopsy and imaging studies, but these methods are not adequate for diagnosis of phyllodes tumors. Excisional or core biopsy is essential to their diagnosis. Histologic factors that help differentiate benign from malignant phyllodes tumors, and both from other tumors, include degree of cellularity, cellular atypia, and growth pattern. Immunostaining of tumor cells is useful in differentiating phyllodes tumors from fibroadenomas because of markedly increased stromal cellularity in phyllodes tumors.

Phyllodes tumors are classified as benign, borderline, or malignant. Benign tumors have largely normal cell growth and differentiation. Malignant tumors have a high number of mitotic figures, or rapidly dividing cells (10 or more per 10 high power fields), infiltrating margins, and marked atypia of cells (2-3+). Borderline tumors have some features of both benign and malignant growths, with 5 to 9 mitotic figures per 10 high power fields, pushing or infiltrating margins, and 2+ cellular atypia. Even within these guidelines, phyllodes tumors are difficult to evaluate, and their growth is unpredictable. For this reason, more than one review of tumor cells is warranted in every case.

Treatment and therapy: The most common treatment for phyllodes tumors is surgical excision, or removal, of the lesion. A wide margin of normal cells (1 to 2 centimeters, or cm) is removed with the tumor to reduce the chance of recurrence. Tumor size varies from about 5 to 30 cm. Mastectomy, or removal of the entire breast, may be the treatment of choice for large tumors or for any tumor that recurs. The treatment is the same for benign and malignant tumors, as chemotherapy, radiation, and hormone therapy have not, in most cases, been effective against cancerous phyllodes tumors.

Prognosis, prevention, and outcomes: The prognosis, or most likely outcome, for phyllodes tumors varies because growth and chance of recurrence are unpredictable. Benign tumors can recur, sometimes with more aggressive or malignant growth. The recurrence rate is reported to be from 1 to 35 percent for benign tumors and 27 to 35 percent for malignant tumors. About one-fourth of malignant tumors metastasize. The lungs, bones, chest wall, and abdominal organs are the most common sites of metastasis. Metastasis is usually fatal within three years of diagnosis. Because treatment options are limited, close follow-up, even for benign tumors, is essential for the best long-term results.

Cathy Anderson, R.N., B.A.

▶ For Further Information

Beers, M. H., and R. Berkow, eds. "Cystosarcoma Phyllodes." In *The Merck Manual of Diagnosis and Therapy*. Whitehouse Station, N.J.: Merck Research Laboratories, 2004.

Esposito, N. N., et al. "Phyllodes Tumor: A Clinicopathologic and Immunohistochemical Study of Thirty Cases." *Archives of Pathology and Laboratory Medicine* 130, no. 10 (2006): 1516-1521.

Jacobs, T. W., et al. "Fibroepithelial Lesions with Cellular Stroma on Breast Core Needle Biopsy: Are There Predictors of Outcome on Surgical Excision?" *American Journal of Clinical Pathology* 124, no. 3 (2005): 342-354.

Wang, Z. C., A. Buralmoh, J. D. Iglehart, and A. Richardson. "Genome-Wide Analysis for Loss of Heterozygosity in Primary and Recurrent Phyllodes Tumor and Fibroadenoma of Breast Using Single Nucleotide Polymorphism Arrays." *Breast Cancer Research and Treatment* 97, no. 3 (2006): 301-309.

▶ Other Resources

American Cancer Society
What Is Breast Cancer?
http://www.cancer.org/docroot/CRI/content/CRI_2_4_1X_What_is_breast_cancer_5.asp

American Society of Breast Disease
http://www.asbd.org

See also Benign tumors; Breast cancer in children and adolescents; Breast cancer in men; Breast cancer in pregnant women; Breast cancers; Computed tomography (CT) scan; Fibroadenomas; Imaging tests; Magnetic resonance imaging (MRI).

▶ Phytoestrogens

Category: Lifestyle and prevention
Also known as: Soy isoflavones (genistein, daidzein, glycitein, formononetin), lignans (secoisolariciresinol, matairesinol, pinoresinol, lariciresinol), coumestans (coumestrol)

Definition: Phytoestrogens are naturally occurring, estrogen-like chemicals found in many plants. There are three basic categories of phytoestrogens: isoflavones, lignans, and coumestans. They come primarily from food sources.

Cancers treated or prevented: May mitigate breast, prostate, uterine, and possibly lung and colon cancers

Delivery routes: Oral through diet, pill, or capsule

How these compounds work: Phytoestrogens have been touted as natural substances that help prevent certain types of cancer, especially hormone-related cancers such as breast, prostate, and uterine cancer. Phytoestrogens can provide hormonal modulation, which naturally regulates hormones. Though not conclusive, some studies demonstrate that phytoestrogens may also provide some protection against lung and colon cancers.

Phytoestrogens can be absorbed into the body chemistry either to act as estrogens at low levels or to block the estrogen effect at high levels. These substances can mimic a weak estrogen to stimulate or to inhibit the growth of cells. Research has shown that increased exposure to certain hormones can increase the risk of cancer. Phytoestrogens appear to protect the body from hormones that can produce cancer.

The best sources of phytoestrogens occur naturally in plants. More than three hundred foods contain phytoestrogens. The most common ones are whole grains such as oats, wheat, and corn; edible seeds such as flax and sesame; legumes such as lentils, soybeans, sprouts, black beans, and chickpeas; vegetables such as leafy greens, fennel, celery, asparagus, carrots, parsley, and seaweed; fruits such as oranges, bananas, and strawberries; olive, safflower, and pumpkin oils; nuts such as pistachios, chestnuts, and walnuts; and other sources such as garlic, onions, and red wine. Soy products such as tofu (bean curd), soy milk, tempeh, and soy yogurt are well-known sources of isoflavone phytoestrogens. Certain herbs also contain phytoestrogens, such as red clover, green tea, hops, alfalfa, licorice, citrus peel, and flax seeds; herbal teas are considered longevity tonic.

Phytoestrogens are also marketed in pill and capsule form as food supplements. The U.S. Food and Drug Administration (FDA) does not regulate food supplements for safety and effectiveness; these supplements are not recommended, as their safety has not been established and could increase the incidence of cancer.

Phytoestrogens consumed in food are generally considered safe when taken in moderate amounts. Though some research studies have shown that phytoestrogens may protect against cancer, others dispute this effect. More studies are needed to fully assess the effect of phytoestrogens on the body chemistry.

Side effects: Patients taking hormone therapies for cancer, such as tamoxifen or other antiestrogenic drugs, should seek the advice of their health care providers before taking supplementation of phytoestrogens, as these phytonutrients may interfere with drug therapy.

Marylane Wade Koch, M.S.N., R.N.

See also Antioxidants; Beta-carotene; Bioflavonoids; Breast cancers; Calcium; Carotenoids; Chemoprevention; Coenzyme Q10; Complementary and alternative therapies; Cruciferous vegetables; Curcumin; Dietary supplements; Essiac; Free radicals; Fruits; Garlic and allicin; Glutamine; Green tea; Herbs as antioxidants; Isoflavones;

Food Sources of Phytoestrogens

Phytoestrogen content of foods, from highest to lowest combined isoflavones (genistein, daidzein, glycitein, formononetin), lignans (secoisolariciresinol, matairesinol, pinoresinol, lariciresinol), and coumestan (coumestrol), in micrograms per 100 grams.

Food	*mcg/100g*	*Food*	*mcg/100g*
Flax seeds	379,380.0	Dried dates	329.5
Soy beans	103,920.0	Sunflower seeds	216.0
Tofu	27,150.1	Chestnuts	210.2
Soy yogurt	10,275.0	Olive oil	180.7
Sesame seeds	8,008.1	Almonds	131.1
Flax bread	7,540.0	Green beans	105.8
Multigrain bread	4,798.7	Peanuts	34.5
Soy milk	2,957.2	Onions	32.0
Hummus	993.0	Blueberries	17.5
Garlic	603.6	Corn	9.0
Mung bean sprouts	495.1	Coffee, regular	6.3
Dried apricots	444.5	Watermelon	2.9
Alfalfa sprouts	441.4	Milk, cow	1.2

Lutein; Lycopene; Macrobiotic diet; Nutrition and cancer prevention; PC-SPES; Phenolics; Prevention; Prostate cancer; Resveratrol; Soy foods; Uterine cancer; Wine and cancer.

▶ Pineoblastomas

Category: Diseases, symptoms, and conditions
Also known as: Pinealoblastomas

Related conditions: Supratentorial primitive neuroectodermal tumors, pineocytomas

Definition: Pineoblastomas, made up of immature cells in the pineal gland (a small organ near the center of the brain), are fast-growing, cancerous tumors that primarily affect young children. The pineal gland is made up of two main cell types: glial cells, which give it its form, and pineocytes, neural cells with photosensory and neuroendocrine functions that produce several hormones, including melatonin, which helps to control the sleep-wake cycle. Pineoblastomas are invasive tumors that spread to nearby areas of the brain and cerebrospinal fluid and can cause bleeding into the brain's ventricles. Pineoblastomas should not be confused with pineocytomas, which are slow-growing, benign tumors that primarily develop in middle-aged and older adults.

Risk factors: The risk factors for pineoblastoma are unknown; however, some researchers believe that gene mutations may be involved.

Etiology and the disease process: The cause of pineoblastomas is unknown. Researchers studying other diseases have noticed an increased incidence of pineoblastoma in patients with hereditary, bilateral retinoblastoma, caused by the retinoblastoma gene (*RB1*). They believe that this gene may play a role in the development of pineoblastoma in addition to affecting its response to treatment. Because of the rarity of pineoblastoma, however, research is limited and this theory has not been investigated sufficiently.

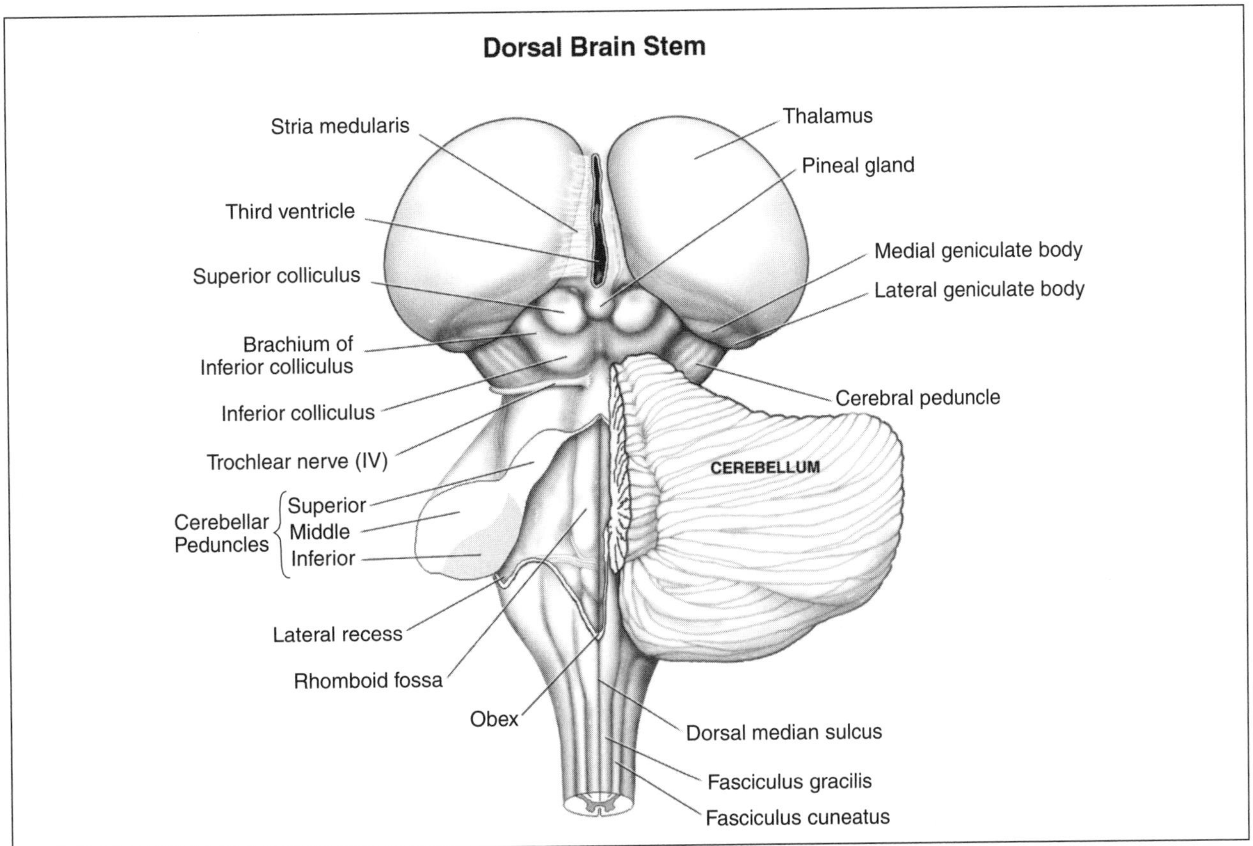

Posterior view of the brain stem, showing the pineal gland (top center) along with other structures. (©F. D. Giddings/Phototake. All rights reserved.)

As pineoblastomas grow, they cause increased pressure in the brain and block the flow of cerebrospinal fluid, causing many neurologic symptoms. Because cells in the pineal gland produce hormones needed for normal body functions, pineoblastomas also cause changes in other body systems. In a process called seeding, they tend to produce multiple, initially small, tumors that are deposited into the cerebrospinal fluid early in the disease process. Pineoblastomas then spread through the brain and spinal cord via the cerebrospinal fluid. When they spread to other body areas, the most common sites are the bones and lungs.

Incidence: After leukemia and lymphoma, brain tumors are the most common type of childhood cancer. However, pineoblastomas are extremely rare among these brain tumors, with only about a 0.4 to 1.0 percent incidence out of all brain tumors. Each year, cancer of the brain and spinal cord occurs in about 2,200 children younger than age fifteen in the United States. Of that number, only between 10 and 40 will be diagnosed with pineoblastoma.

Symptoms: Pineoblastomas cause symptoms related to an increase in pressure inside the brain and blockage of cerebrospinal fluid. They can vary depending on the size of the tumor, its location, and the child's age. Most symptoms of pineoblastomas are similar to those of other brain tumors, including nausea and vomiting, seizures, changes in personality or behavior, unusual sleepiness, headaches, double vision, and developmental delays or failure to thrive. Hydrocephalus, an excessive accumulation of fluid in the brain, and hormonal abnormalities may also occur.

Screening and diagnosis: Screening for abnormal brain function takes place whenever a medical practitioner makes a physical examination of a child and takes a growth and development history. When abnormalities appear, the practitioner will typically order laboratory tests and possibly imaging studies. Laboratory tests usually include a complete blood count, electrolyte levels, and liver, thyroid, and kidney function tests. Imaging studies include a chest X ray, bone scan, magnetic resonance imaging (MRI), and computed tomography (CT) scanning. An examination of the cerebrospinal fluid, called a lumbar puncture, will be performed to look for cancer cells as well as to rule out other diseases. If the child's condition permits, a definitive diagnosis of pineoblastoma is made during surgery, after a pathologist examines the tumor cells.

For pineoblastoma, the extent of the cancer is usually described as risk groups instead of stages. The tumor is called "average risk" when the child is older than age three, most or all of the tumor was removed by surgery, and the cancer has not spread beyond the pineal gland. It is called "poor risk" when the child is younger than age three, the tumor was near the center of the brain, some of the tumor was not removed by surgery, or the cancer has spread to other parts of the brain or body, including the spinal cord.

Treatment and therapy: Treatment for pineoblastoma is based on the child's age and risk group. When the child is younger than age three, surgical removal of most or all of the tumor is performed. If the child is considered a poor risk, chemotherapy is used after surgery. When the child is older than age three, surgery is followed by radiation treatment of the entire brain and spinal cord. Any child considered a poor risk might also be given chemotherapy.

Prognosis, prevention, and outcomes: There is no known prevention for pineoblastoma. The prognosis for pineoblastomas varies with the child's age and risk group but is typically poor, with an estimated survival time of sixteen to twenty-five months. Although some children do survive five years or more, the tumors commonly recur or develop in other parts of the body. When they do, they are almost always fatal.

Dorothy P. Terry, R.N.

▶ For Further Information

Amendola, B. E., et al. "Pineal Tumors: Analysis of Treatment Results in Twenty Patients." *Journal of Neurosurgery* 102 (January, 2005): 175-179.

Bruce, J. N., and A. T. Ogden. "Surgical Strategies for Treating Patients with Pineal Region Tumors." *Journal of Neurooncology* 69, nos. 1-3 (August/September, 2004): 221-236.

Gururangan, S., et al. "High-Dose Chemotherapy with Autologous Stem-Cell Rescue in Children and Adults with Newly Diagnosed Pineoblastomas." *Journal of Clinical Oncology* 21, no. 11 (June 1, 2003): 2187-2191.

▶ Other Resources

American Cancer Society

Treatment of Specific Types of Brain and Spinal Cord Tumors
http://www.cancer.org

National Cancer Institute

Childhood Supratentorial Primitive Neuroectodermal Tumors and Pineoblastoma
http://www.nci.nih.gov/cancertopics/pdq/treatment/childSPNET

See also Brain and central nervous system cancers; Childhood cancers; Cobalt 60 radiation; Computed tomography (CT) scan; Imaging tests; Lumbar puncture; Magnetic resonance imaging (MRI); Neuroendocrine tumors; Retinoblastomas.

▶ Pituitary tumors

Category: Diseases, symptoms, and conditions
Also known as: Pituitary adenomas, pituitary carcinomas, teratomas, germinomas, choriocarcinomas, Rathke cleft cysts, gangliocytomas, prolactinomas

Related conditions: Multiple endocrine neoplasia type 1 (MEN 1), acromegaly, Cushing syndrome, panhypopituitarism, hypogonadism, diabetes insipidus, hyperthyroidism

Definition: Pituitary tumors are found in the pituitary gland, a small organ that sits in the sella turcica (a small bony space) in the center of the brain just above the nose. Almost all pituitary tumors are adenomas, which are benign (not cancerous) glandular tumors. Malignant tumors (for example, pituitary carcinomas) are rare. Among those, teratomas, germinomas, and choriocarcinomas usually occur in children or young adults. Rathke cleft cysts and gangliocytomas of the pituitary are usually found in adults. Cancers that metastasize to the pituitary from other sites are classified by their primary site and not as pituitary tumors.

Risk factors: People with multiple endocrine neoplasia type 1 (MEN 1), a hereditary condition, have a very high risk of developing tumors of the pituitary along with tumors of two other glands, the parathyroid and pancreas. About 50 percent of the children of an affected parent will inherit the defective gene that causes MEN 1.

Etiology and the disease process: The pituitary gland produces hormones that regulate the functions of other glands in the body. Most pituitary tumors start in the anterior pituitary gland. Pituitary adenomas remain confined to the skull but may grow into the walls of the sella turcica and surrounding nerves, vessels, and coverings of the brain. An enlarged pituitary can damage nearby parts of the brain. For example, damage to the optic nerve can lead to vision problems or even vision loss. About 75 percent of pituitary adenomas produce hormones and are therefore termed functional, while the rest do not and are termed nonfunctional. Pituitary tumors can cause overproduction of hormones; however, damage to pituitary tissue can also lead to hormone deficiency.

Adenomas are categorized into two types: microadenomas, tumors that are smaller than 1 centimeter (cm), and macroadenomas, which are larger than 1 cm. Microadenomas generate symptoms because of hormone overproduction and rarely because of damage to surrounding tissue, whereas macroadenomas cause symptoms by both hormone overproduction and tissue damage. Adenomas are further classified by the specific hormones produced: prolactin (prolactinomas, about 43 percent of all pituitary adenomas), growth hormone (GH, about 17 percent), adrenocorticotropin (ACTH, about 7 percent), thyroid-stimulating hormone (TSH, about 3 percent), and gonadotropin (which with null-cell, or nonfunctional, adenomas make up about 30 percent).

About 3 percent of all pituitary tumors are caused by inherited mutations in deoxyribonucleic acid (DNA) in people with MEN 1. Some 40 percent of GH-secreting adenomas have an acquired mutation in a specific protein called Gs alpha. It is not clear yet whether abnormal genes are essential for pituitary tumor formation. However, gene alterations probably result in the loss of regulatory mechanisms for hormone production and growth of glandular cells, thereby promoting tumor growth.

Incidence: In the United States, pituitary tumors represent between 10 and 15 percent of all intracranial tumors. The incidence of acromegaly, a condition produced when the body creates too much growth hormone, is approximately 3 per 1 million people and similar in men and women.

Symptoms: All adenomas can cause headaches and visual problems when they grow large enough to affect nearby tissues. Macroadenomas can lead to neurologic symptoms such as double or blurred vision due to paralysis of eye movement, loss of peripheral vision, sudden blindness, facial numbness or pain, headaches, dizziness, and even loss of consciousness. The destruction of normal pituitary tissue by macroadenomas and pituitary carcinomas leads to a lack of normal body hormones such as cortisone, thyroid hormone, and sex hormones. This can result in nausea, weakness, weight loss or gain, irregular menses, erectile dysfunction, and decreased libido (mainly in men). Macroadenomas and pituitary carcinoma can also cause diabetes insipidus as a result of a lack of production of vasopressin (also called the antidiuretic hormone, ADH). If severe and untreated, this condition can lead to coma and death.

GH-secreting adenomas in children can stimulate excessive bone growth, leading to gigantism. Symptoms are being very tall and experiencing very rapid growth, joint pains, and increased sweating. Adults with GH-secreting adenomas may develop acromegaly, characterized by growth of the skull, hands, feet, and facial bones, leading to changes in the appearance of the face; joint pain; deepening of the voice; increased sweating; diabetes mellitus; kidney stones; heart disease; headaches; unusual hair growth; and thickening of the tongue, palate, and skin.

ACTH-secreting adenomas can stimulate the production of steroid hormones by the adrenal gland and subsequently cause a condition called Cushing syndrome. The symptoms are weight gain, increased body hair, fat deposits in the neck, mood swings, irregular menses, high blood pressure, high blood sugar, osteoporosis, easy bruising, and purple stretch marks on the abdomen.

Prolactin-producing adenomas (prolactinomas) are difficult to spot in children. They are most common in young women, in whom high prolactin levels can cause irregular menses and abnormal breast milk production (galactorrhea), and in older men, in whom they cause impotence or loss of libido.

TSH-secreting adenomas cause hyperthyroidism, with symptoms such as an enlarged thyroid, weight loss, increased appetite, rapid heartbeat, tremor, anxiousness, sleeping problems, frequent bowel movements, and feeling warm or hot.

Gonadotropin-secreting adenomas are not very common. They produce follicle-stimulating hormone (FSH) and luteinizing hormone (LH), which may cause irregular menses.

Nonfunctional adenomas may be the most common pituitary tumors, but they are rarely detected, as they do not cause symptoms and are typically detected by magnetic resonance imaging (MRI) or computed tomography (CT) scans taken for other reasons.

Screening and diagnosis: Knowing what hormone an adenoma produces is critical in choosing the treatment and determining the prognosis. Biochemical testing for GH-secreting adenomas includes a check for excessive production of GH and insulin-like growth factor 1 (IGF-1). If both levels are very high, the patient clearly has a pituitary tumor. If the levels are only slightly increased, a glucose suppression test is done.

Biochemical testing for ACTH-secreting adenomas includes measuring levels of ACTH and cortisol in blood samples and of cortisol and other steroid hormones in urine samples taken at different times during the day. These tests may be repeated after taking dexamethasone, a cortisone-like drug. These tests are also used to distinguish patients with ACTH-secreting adenomas from patients

Hormones Secreted by the Pituitary Gland and Their Functions

Hormone	*Functions*
Adrenocorticotropic hormone (ACTH)	• stimulates adrenal glands to release cortisol, which controls blood pressure and metabolism of fat, protein, and carbohydrates • controls fight-or-flight response through adrenal glands
Antidiuretic hormone (ADH); also known as vasopressin	• increases amount of water reabsorbed into the blood by kidneys
Endorphin	• reduces the sensation of pain • helps control immune system
Follicle-stimulating hormone (FSH)	• stimulates maturation of ovarian follicles • helps support sperm cell maturation
Growth hormone (GH)	• controls growth and metabolism • stimulates muscle development and reduces fat tissue
Luteinizing hormone (LH)	• triggers ovulation • stimulates production of testosterone
Melanocyte-stimulating hormone	• governs production of melanin in the skin
Oxytocin	• contracts uterus in labor • promotes ejection of milk in breast-feeding
Prolactin	• stimulates the production of breast milk after giving birth
Thyroid-stimulating hormone (TSH)	• stimulates thyroid to control basal metabolic rate • stimulates thyroid to guide growth and maturation

with other diseases, such as adrenal gland tumors, which cause similar symptoms.

Tests to measure blood levels of prolactin, TSH, LH, and FSH can identify patients with prolactinomas, TSH-secreting adenomas, or gonadotropin-secreting tumors. If tests for excessive hormone production are negative or the levels are lowered, a pituitary adenoma is considered nonfunctional.

Macroadenomas and pituitary carcinomas—and particularly metastatic cancer—can damage the part of the pituitary gland that produces vasopressin, leading to diabetes insipidus. This can also occur as a side effect of the surgical treatment of pituitary tumors. Diagnosis of diabetes insipidus is made by tests to measure sodium levels and total salt concentration (osmolality) of the blood and urine. In addition, a water deprivation test may be necessary.

Imaging tests (MRI and CT scans) are used to visualize tumors. Venous blood sampling may be necessary to confirm the presence of ACTH-secreting adenomas if they are too small to be detected by MRI scans. Testing of vision and visual fields also helps to detect pituitary tumors. A closer analysis of the type of tumor can be done by taking a biopsy.

No staging system exists for pituitary tumors as they are nearly always benign. Pituitary carcinomas are too rare for development of a staging system. The most useful information in treating an adenoma is whether it is a macroadenoma or a microadenoma, whether it produces hormones, and which hormones it produces.

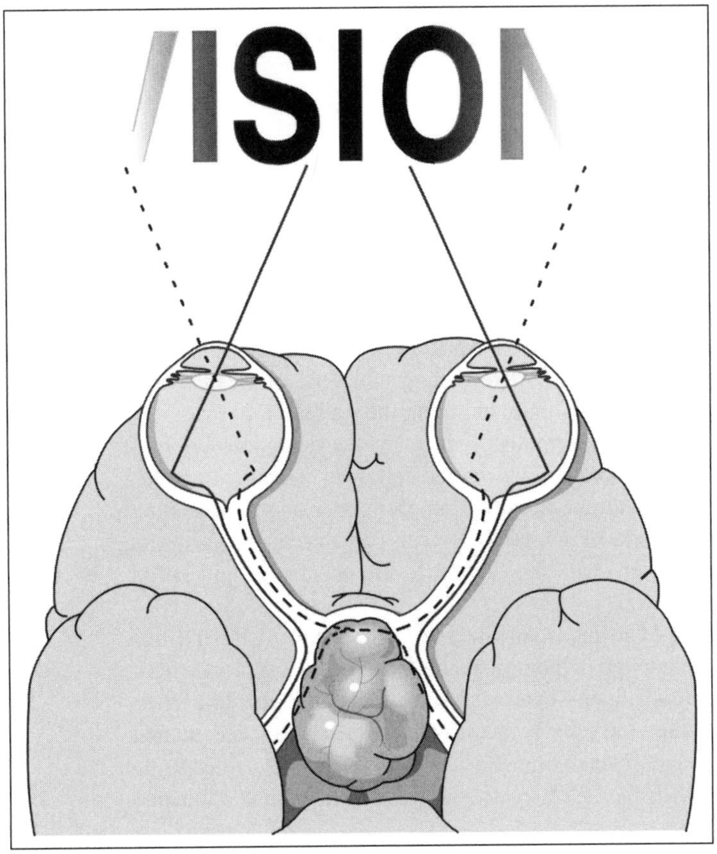

A pituitary tumor in the area of the optic chiasma affects a person's peripheral vision. (LifeART© 2008 Wolters Kluwer Health, Inc.-Lippincott Williams &Wilkins. All rights reserved.)

Treatment and therapy: Pituitary tumors may be treated surgically, medically, radiotherapeutically, or with combinations of these therapies. Which therapy is used depends on the type of tumor.

Prognosis, prevention, and outcomes: Pituitary tumors are usually curable. Prognosis depends on the type of pituitary tumor and on the patient's general health and age.

Nicola E. Wittekindt, Dr.Sc. (ETH Zürich)

▶ For Further Information

Kufe, Donald W., et al., eds. *Holland Frei Cancer Medicine 7*. 7th ed. Hamilton, Ont.: BC Decker, 2006.

Nussey, S. S., and S. A. Whitehead. *Endocrinology: An Integrated Approach*. London: Taylor & Francis, 2001.

Weinberg, Robert A. *The Biology of Cancer*. New York: Garland Science, Taylor & Francis, 2007.

▶ Other Resources

National Cancer Institute

Pituitary Tumors Treatment

http://www.nci.nih.gov/cancertopics/pdq/treatment/pituitary/patient/

National Institute of Neurological Disorders and Stroke

Pituitary Tumors Information Page

http://www.ninds.nih.gov/disorders/pituitary_tumors/pituitary_tumors.htm

Pituitary Network Association

http://www.pituitary.org

See also Acrylamides; Amenorrhea; Cushing syndrome and cancer; Endocrine cancers; Endocrinology oncology; Family history and risk assessment; Multiple endocrine neoplasia type 1 (MEN 1); Neuroendocrine tumors.

▶ Placental alkaline phosphatase (PALP)

Category: Cancer biology

Definition: Placental alkaline phosphatase (PALP) is one of the four isoenzymes of alkaline phosphatase, a group of enzymes that hydrolyze organic phosphate esters. Alkaline phosphatase isoenzymes associated with the liver, bone, and intestine are normally present in serum. When the serum alkaline phosphatase level is above established reference ranges, determining which fraction is elevated may be helpful in pinpointing the source of disease.

PALP is normally produced by the syncytiotrophoblast of the placenta. This unique cell layer is in direct contact with maternal blood during pregnancy and is considered the source of rising PALP levels in maternal plasma during gestation, with the highest levels occurring right before delivery.

PALP-like isoenzymes are similar to PALP but different enough in their biochemical and physical properties to be considered separate proteins. Several PALP-like isoenzymes have been identified, characterized, and named: Regan, Nagao, and Kasahara. Some authors refer to the PALP-like isoenzymes as germ-cell alkaline phosphatases.

Related cancers: When pregnancy is not a condition of consideration, elevated levels of PALP have been associated with cancers of the testis, ovary, colorectal tract, and lung. In the 1970's and 1980's, researchers investigated the relationship between malignant changes in many tissues with the serum concentration of several fetal-type proteins. They pursued PALP along with alpha-fetoprotein (AFP) and carcinoembryonic antigen (CEA) as tumor markers. Of these, PALP and the PALP-like isoenzymes have yet to be demonstrated as useful markers for screening or monitoring cancer and related conditions.

Ongoing research: Cancer researchers continue to explore a role for PALP as a tumor marker. Antibodies to detect and differentiate PALP and the related PALP-like isoenzymes are being designed and tested. Some of the antibodies are used in immunohistochemistry protocols, requiring a biopsy of the organ where the suspicious tumor is located. These tissue biopsy studies can confirm the presence of PALP and PALP-like isoenzymes, which further choracterizing the tumor and leading to a more specific diagnosis and targeted therapy.

Other researchers are designing antibodies that target PALP and PALP-like isoenzymes in an individual's plasma and thus can serve as noninvasive markers for cancer. To date elevated concentrations of PALP and PALP-like enzymes have been found to be no better than cancer antigen 125 (CA 125) and AFP in monitoring ovarian cancer. However, there is some evidence that PALP and PALP-like isoenzymes may become useful indicators of cancer recurrence in survivors.

Jane Adrian, M.P.H., Ed.M., M.T. (ASCP)

See also Alkaline phosphatase test (ALP); Cancer biology; Immunocytochemistry and immunohistochemistry; Paget disease of bone; Pregnancy and cancer; Staging of cancer; Tumor markers.

▶ Plant alkaloids and terpenoids in chemotherapy

Category: Chemotherapy and other drugs
ATC code: 101C

Definition: Alkaloids and terpenoids are compounds derived from plants, some of which are shown to have anticancer activity and have been developed into useful chemotherapeutic agents. Subclasses of this group include vinca alkaloids, taxanes, podophyllotoxins, epipodophyllotoxins, camptothecins, ellipticine, and colchicine.

Cancers treated or prevented: Breast cancer, ovarian cancer, lung cancer, prostate cancer, lymphomas, leukemias

Delivery routes: Intravenous

How these drugs work: Plants are an important source of natural products effective in treating human cancer, with several useful chemotherapeutic agents currently on the market or in clinical trials. Specifically, many plant-derived alkaloids and terpenoids have significant anticancer properties. Synthetic and semi-synthetic derivatives of alkaloid and terpenoid compounds with anticancer activity have also been developed. In plants, these compounds are produced as secondary metabolites that probably function as defense chemicals that inhibit cell division in invading pathogens. These same cytostatic compounds can be useful in cancer treatment by stopping the growth of cancer cells. Some examples of alkaloids and terpenoids used in chemotherapy are vinca alkaloids, podophyllotoxins, and taxanes.

Alkaloids are naturally occurring amines produced by plants and are grouped into several classifications, usually based on the metabolic pathway through which they are generated. These classifications include indole, purine, pyridine, and isoquinoline, with terpenoids one classifica-

Common Plant Alkaloids and Terpenoids

Drug	*Brands*	*Subclass*	*Delivery Mode*	*Cancers Treated*
9-Aminocamptothecin	9-AC	Camptothecin	IV	Ovarian, stomach cancers
Amsacrine	Amsidine	Epipodophyllotoxin derivative	IV	Germ-cell testicular cancer, bone and soft tissue sarcomas, adult and childhood leukemias
Colchicine		Colchicine	IV	Solid tumors, chronic myelocytic leukemia, other leukemias
Docetaxel	Taxotere	Taxane diterpenoid	IV	Breast, prostate, non-small-cell lung, and other cancers
Elliptinium	Celiptium	Ellipticine	IV	Stomach, lung, and breast cancers
Etoposide	Etophos, Vepesid	Epipodophyllotoxin	IV, oral	Lung, ovarian, and testicular cancers
Irinotecan	CPT-11, Camptostart, Campto	Camptothecin	IV	Metastatic colorectal cancer, bowel cancer
Paclitaxel	Taxol	Taxane diterpenoid	IV	Metastatic breast cancer, advanced lung cancer, head and neck cancers, melanoma, ovarian cancer, lymphomas, non-small-cell lung cancer
Teniposide	Vumon, VM-26	Epipodophyllotoxin	IV	Adult and childhood leukemias, lymphomas, Hodgkin lymphoma, childhood neuroblastoma
Topetecan	Hycamtin	Camptothecin	IV	Ovarian, small-cell lung cancers
Vinblastine	Velbe	Vinca alkaloid	IV	Hodgkin disease; non-Hodgkin lymphomas; leukemia; renal, testicular, head, neck, breast, and lung cancers
Vincristine	Oncovin, Cytocristin, Onococristin-AQ, Vincristine, Vincristine sulfate	Vinca alkaloid	IV	Kaposi sarcoma, non-Hodgkin lymphoma, Hodgkin disease, acute lymphocytic leukemia, small-cell lung cancer, cervical and breast cancer
Vindesine	Eldisine	Vinca alkaloid	IV	Leukemia, lymphoma, melanoma, breast and lung cancers
Vinflunine	Javlor	Vinca alkaloid	IV	Bladder, lung, gastric cancers
Vinorelbine	Navelbine	Vinca alkaloid	IV	Breast cancer, small-cell lung cancer

tion of alkaloids. Terpenoids are sometimes also referred to as isoprenoids and are classified according to the number of isoprene units that they contain. For example, monoterpenoids are made up of two isoprene units, whereas diterpenoids are composed of four isoprene units.

Four structural classes of plant-derived anticancer agents of alkaloid or terpenoid origin are available in the United States: vinca alkaloids, taxanes, epipodophyllotoxins, and camptothecins. These compounds work by affecting cell division and deoxyribonucleic acid (DNA) synthesis or function.

The search for anticancer agents from plants was initiated in 1947 when podophyllotoxins from the American mayapple (*Podophyllum peltatum*) inhibited the growth of tumor cells in laboratory experiments. The subsequent discovery of antileukemic properties of vinblastine and vincristine, bis-indole alkaloids derived from the Madagascar periwinkle (*Catharanthus roseus*), spurred broad investigations of plant-derived compounds for possible anticancer activity. *C. roseus* was found to be a storehouse of more than seventy-five alkaloids, several of which possess anticancer activity. Among other plant species that have provided clinically useful drugs are *Taxus brevifolis*, the source of diterpene taxol; *Ochrosia elliptica*, one of the sources of the pyridocarbazole alkaloid ellipticine; and *Camptotheca acuminata*, which contains camptothecin.

While being used to treat other conditions, the leaves of *C. roseus*, formerly *Vinca roseus*, were found to contain cytotoxic compounds. Among these compounds were two terpenoid indole alkaloids, vinblastine and vincristine, which subsequently became the first natural anticancer agents used clinically. Vinblastine and vincristine, together with a number of semi-synthetic derivatives, are collectively termed the vinca alkaloids. Although they have been in clinical usage since the 1970's, the vinca alkaloids are still extremely useful chemotherapeutic agents with well-known antimitotic activity. Vinca alkaloids work by binding specific sites on tubulin and preventing assembly of tubulin into microtubules, which are essential for cell division.

Soon after the introduction of vinblastine and vincristine, intensive chemical research was undertaken to try to develop semi-synthetic derivatives that had higher activity, lower toxicity, and broader anticancer effects. Several successful semi-synthetic derivatives were developed, including vindesine, vinorelbine, and vinflunine. Vindesine has a vincristine-like spectrum of activity and is used mainly to treat melanoma, acute lymhoblastic leukemia, and advanced non-small-cell lung cancer. Vinorelbine has reduced side effects and is now widely used in treatment of non-small-cell lung cancer and breast cancer, with utility toward other cancers, including lymphoma and esophageal and prostate cancers, under clinical investigation. Vinflunine is a semi-synthetic fluorinated derivative of vindesine and is currently in clinical trials for treatment against various cancers, including bladder, lung, and gastric cancers.

Another class of plant alkaloids used in chemotherapy is the taxanes. Taxanes are derived from either the bark or the needles of some species of yew tree. Taxanes currently used as chemotherapeutic agents include paclitaxel and docetaxel. Paclitaxel is derived from the bark of the European yew tree (*Taxus baccata*), while docetaxel is derived from the pine needle of the Pacific yew tree (*Taxus brevifolia*). Paclitaxel, marketed under the name Taxol, is one of the most effective plant-derived chemotherapeutic agents. Patients with refractory ovarian cancer, metastatic breast cancer, advanced lung cancer, cancers of the head and neck, melanoma, and lymphomas respond positively to treatment with Taxol. The taxanes work by increasing the stability of microtubules, which inhibits cell division by preventing the separation of chromosomes during anaphase.

Other classes of plant alkaloids used in chemotherapy include the podophyllotoxins, camptothecins, ellipticines, and colchicine. Podophyllotoxins, or epipodophyllotoxins, are alkaloids naturally occurring in the root of the American mayapple or mandrake (*Podophyllum emodi*). A rare Himalayan mayapple (*Podophyllum hexandrum*) has also recently been found to contain active compounds, but this plant is endangered and consequently limited in supply. Efforts to obtain these compounds through recombinant technologies are under way. Some epipodophyllotoxin derivatives, etoposide and teniposide, are currently used in cancer treatment. Semi-synthetic derivatives such as amsacrine and etoposide phosphate also exist. Podophyllotoxins and their derivatives work by preventing cell division in tumor cells by keeping cells from entering the cell cycle and undergoing DNA replication.

Camptothecin is a quinoline alkaloid isolated from *C. acuminata*. Examples of camptothecins used in chemotherapy include topotecan and irinotecan. Topotecan is currently used to treat ovarian cancer, and irinotecan is currently marketed for treatment of metastatic cancer of the colon or rectum. Another compound, 9-aminocamptothecin, is also being investigated for treatment of ovarian and stomach cancers. Ellipticine is an alkaloid isolated from an evergreen tree of the Apocyanaceae family. Ellipiticine and its derivatives, including elliptinium, are promising anticancer agents and are highly effective against several types of cancer, with limited side effects. Colchicine is a tricyclic tropane alkaloid from the autumn crocus (*Colchicum autumnale*) and gloriosa lily (*Gloriosa superba*). Cochicine has been used effectively to treat chronic myelocytic leukemia, but toxic or near-toxic doses are required for therapeutic benefit. For this reason, colchicine and its analogs are primarily used as tools to study new mitotic inhibitors rather than in chemotherapy.

Although exact mechanisms of action of podophyllotoxins, camptothecins, and ellipticines still have to be elucidated, these compounds and their derivatives are believed to function as either type I or type II topoisomerase inhibitors, enzymes essential for critical steps in cell division—the transcription and replication of DNA. Colchicines prevent tubulin polymerization during the cell cycle.

Side effects: Side effects of plant alkaloids and terpenoids used in chemotherapy include lowered resistance to infection, bruising or bleeding, anemia, constipation, cramps, diarrhea, nausea, peripheral neuropathy (numbness or tingling in hands or feet), headaches, tiredness, and hair loss. Mouth sores and ulcers, changes in taste, and loss of appetite can also occur. Skin rashes and allergic reactions are seen less commonly.

C. J. Walsh, Ph.D.

▶ **For Further Information**

Cutler, S. J., and H. G. Cutler. *Biologically Active Natural Products: Pharmaceuticals*. Boca Raton, Fla.: CRC Press, 2000.

Kintzios, S. E. "Terrestrial Plant-Derived Anticancer Agents and Plant Species Used in Anticancer Research." *Critical Reviews in Plant Sciences* 25 (2006): 79-113.

Mukherjee, A. K., et al. "Advances in Cancer Therapy with Plant Based Natural Products." *Current Medicinal Chemistry* 8 (2001): 1467-1486.

Noble, R. L. "The Discovery of the Vinca Alkaloids—Chemotherapeutic Agents Against Cancer." *Biochemistry and Cell Biology* 68 (1990): 1344-1351.

Perry, Michael C., ed. *The Chemotherapy Source Book*. 4th ed. Philadelphia: Wolters Kluwer Health/Lippincott Williams & Wilkins, 2008.

▶ **Other Resources**

Cancer Backup
http://www.cancerbackup.org.uk

National Cancer Institute
http://www.cancer.gov

National Center for Complementary and Alternative Medicine
http://nccam.nih.gov

See also Antineoplastics in chemotherapy; Antioxidants; Breast cancers; Caffeine; Complementary and alternative therapies; Dietary supplements; Green tea; Herbs as antioxidants; Indoles; Leukemias; Lung cancers; Lymphomas; Nutrition and cancer prevention; Nutrition and cancer treatment; Opioids; Ovarian cancers; Prostate cancer; Stomach cancers.

▶ Plasticizers

Category: Carcinogens and suspected carcinogens

Definition: Plasticizers are chemical substances that are used as additives during the manufacture of various polymers such as polyvinyl chloride (PVC), food packaging, food storage containers, children's toys, and medical devices to impart flexibility, strength, and durability.

Types of plasticizers: A large variety of chemicals are used as plasticizers. They are classified into various categories based on their chemical structure. The most widely used plasticizers are derived from the family of dicarboxylic esters and are commonly known as phthalates: Examples include di(2-ethylhexyl) phthalate (DEHP), di-n-octyl phthalate (DOP), adipates, and maleates. Chemicals from the family of organophosphates and some glycol esters are also used as plasticizers.

Uses: Phthalates such as DEHP are predominantly used in the manufacture of PVC, which is one of the oldest polymers used to make pipes and various plastic containers. Phthalates are also used as plasticizers in medical devices such as dialysis bags, intravenous bags, and tubing. They are also used in detergents, lubricating oils, flooring materials, food-packaging materials, and storage containers.

Environmental exposure: Plasticizers are not covalently bound to the plastic matrix, and they consequently leach out when in contact with oils, fats, and other greasy substances, especially at higher temperatures. This is especially true of phthalates, which are used in food wraps and containers. Plasticizers in food wraps have been shown to migrate into and contaminate fatty foods such as meat, cheese, and oily snacks. Plasticizers are also released into the environment directly during the manufacture of plastics and from discarded plastic containers, wraps, and pipes. As plastics have myriad uses, the plasticizers in them are ubiquitous contaminants of air, water, food, and medicines. Human exposure to plasticizers is mainly through ingesting water and food contaminated with them. Infants are exposed to plasticizers when they chew or suck on plastic toys or pacifiers or drink liquids out of plastic feeding bottles. Another source of exposure is through air, in which plasticizers such as DEHP adhere to aerosol particles. Animal studies have shown that phthalates can cross the placental barrier, and therefore, this can potentially cause prenatal exposure in humans.

Toxicity and metabolism: Toxicity studies on plasticizers (especially the phthalates DEHP and DOP) have been done on rodents through various exposure routes. It has been found that the rodents metabolize phthalates readily, and the liver and kidneys are common target organs for general toxicity. The major concern about the toxicity of phthalates stems from reports from the U.S. National Toxicology Program showing several of them to be carcinogenic in rodents. The mechanism of carcinogenesis in rodents or other species is as yet unclear, and there are no clear-cut studies extrapolating the animal data to humans. Many industry groups and advocacy panels have analyzed the animal data on the toxicity of plasticizers and have failed to come to a consensus because the toxicity patterns vary greatly by species and routes of exposure. Plasticizers have been detected in breast milk and children's blood samples, but there are no studies that clearly relate childhood exposure to the risk of adult human cancers, and therefore childhood exposure to plasticizers is shrouded in controversy.

There are reports in literature that indicate that plasticizers, especially the phthalates, act as hormone disrupters. Hormones are chemical messengers produced by various glands in animals and humans that travel through the bloodstream and regulate growth, reproduction, and metabolic functions in the body. This system, known as the endocrine system, is a very finely tuned mechanism in the body, and endocrine disrupters can readily throw it off balance, creating major health and cancer risks. Young animals and children are more vulnerable to exposure to such disrupters because their systems are still in the developmental stage, so there is a great concern regarding the exposure of infants and children to phthalates.

Preventive measures: Because plasticizers are widely distributed environmental contaminants, there is a great deal of concern regarding cancer and other health risks to adult human populations as a result of exposure of infants and children to environmental endocrine disrupters. The conflicting conclusions from various animal studies and the lack of data extrapolating the animal exposure studies to human infants and adults underscore the complexity of the science. More studies delineating the toxicokinetics of plasticizers, especially in vulnerable subpopulations such as pregnant and lactating women, premature infants, and children, are needed. There are many ongoing studies to assess the risk of exposure to plasticizers and evaluate the potential of early childhood exposure in increasing the risk of cancer in adults.

The European Union has recommended banning the use of certain phthalates. Toy manufacturers are funding research to develop newer plasticizers with greater biodegradability and lower toxicity, such as alkyl citrates and esters of vegetable oils. These environmentally benign plasticizers are being developed for use in food-packaging materials, medical devices, and children's toys. With all the conflicting health and cancer risk data on plasticizers, it makes perfect sense for individuals and industry and government regulatory agencies to take reasonable steps to limit exposure to plasticizers.

Lalitha Krishnan, Ph.D.

▶ For Further Information

Huber, W. W., B. Grasl-Kraupp, and R. Schulte-Hermann. "Hepatocarcinogenic Potential of Di(2-ethylhexyl) Phthalate in Rodents and Its Implications on Human Risk." *Critical Reviews in Toxicology* 26 (1996): 365-481.

Sissell, Kara. "States, Retailers Push to Eliminate Phthalates from Toys." *Chemical Weekly* 170, no. 12 (April 14-21, 2008): 29.

_______. "Study Links Phthalates and Infant Care Products." *Chemical Weekly* 170, no. 5 (February 11-18, 2008): 29.

Voiland, Adam. "More Problems with Plastics: Like BPA, Chemicals Called Phthalates Raise Some Concern." *U.S. News & World Report*, May 19, 2008, p. 54.

Woodward, Kevin N. *Phthalate Esters: Toxicity and Metabolism*. Boca Raton, Fla.: CRC Press, 1988.

▶ Other Resources

Canadian Cancer Society
Phthalates
http://www.cancer.ca/ccs/internet/standard/0,3182,3172_1706523966__langId-en,00.html

National Toxicology Program
http://cerhr.niehs.nih.gov

U.S. Environmental Protection Agency
Consumer Factsheet on: Di (2-ethylhexyl) Phthalate
http://www.epa.gov/OGWDW/dwh/c-soc/phthalat.html

U.S. Food and Drug Administration
FDA Public Health Notification: PVC Devices Containing the Plasticizer DEHP
http://www.fda.gov/cdrh/safety/dehp.html

See also Bisphenol A (BPA); Carcinogens, known; Carcinogens, reasonably anticipated; Childhood cancers; Di-(2-ethylhexyl) phthalate (DEHP); Organochlorines (OCs); Risks for cancer; Vinyl chloride.

▶ Pleural biopsy

Category: Procedures
Also known as: Needle biopsy of the pleura, open pleural biopsy, closed pleural biopsy

Definition: A pleural biopsy is the removal of a sample of the pleura (the membrane that surrounds the lungs) so that it can be tested by a pathologist for cancer or other diseases.

Cancers diagnosed: Lung cancer, metastatic pleural tumor, malignant pleural mesothelioma

Why performed: This test may be used to diagnose mesothelioma, a tumor in the pleural membrane, or lung cancer.

It is indicated when a pleural fluid sample shows possible cancer or when a chest X ray shows a thickening or mass in the pleura.

Patient preparation: Pleural biopsy may be done in a doctor's office or in the hospital using a local anesthetic. A blood test may be required before the test to ensure that the patient does not have a prolonged bleeding or clotting time.

Steps of the procedure: In a percutaneous biopsy, the doctor uses a large-bore needle. The skin around the site is cleaned and injected with a local anesthetic. The patient sits up and may be asked to hold his or her breath to prevent air from entering the chest during the procedure. The physician makes an incision and inserts the needle through the chest wall and into the pleura. Ultrasound can be used to help view the progress of the needle. When it is in place, a biopsy trocar is inserted through the needle to remove a sample of tissue. The doctor usually removes three samples, places them in fixative, and sends them to the laboratory. The procedure can take less than thirty minutes.

To obtain larger specimens of the pleura, the biopsy can also be performed during a thoracoscopy, using a laparoscope (a tube with a tiny camera on the end) that the doctor inserts through the skin and into the chest, or as an open pleural biopsy, a surgery performed under general anesthesia.

After the procedure: A bandage is placed over the incision. The patient is observed for respiratory distress and bleeding. After returning home, the patient should be aware of any shortness of breath. Light-headedness or an increased pulse rate might indicate internal bleeding.

Risks: Potential complications from this procedure include respiratory distress, pneumothorax (presence of air in the chest outside the lung), injury to the lung, infection, and bleeding.

Results: Preparation of a tissue sample and analysis by a pathologist may take several days. The pathologist can identify the presence or apparent lack of cancer cells in the tissue.

Marcia Pinneau, R.N.

See also Bronchoalveolar lung cancer; Lung cancers; Mesothelioma; Needle biopsies; Pleural effusion; Pleurodesis; Thoracentesis; Thoracoscopy.

▶ Pleural effusion

Category: Diseases, symptoms, and conditions
Also known as: Parapneumatic effusion, water or fluid in the chest, pleural fluid

Related conditions: Lung cancer

Definition: A pleural effusion is the abnormal collection of excess fluid between the layers of the pleura, the membranes lining the lungs and chest cavity. Pleural effusions are either malignant or nonmalignant.

Depending on the cause of the pleural effusion, the excess fluid is either rich in protein (exudative) or protein-poor (transudative or watery). Congestive heart failure and abnormal lung pressure are often associated with transudative pleural effusions. Certain cancers, kidney disease, pneumonia, or other lung infections are usually associated with exudative pleural effusions.

Risk factors: The risk factors for pleural effusions include chemotherapy or radiation therapy of the chest, a collapsed lung, lung cancer, breast cancer, lymphoma, and leukemia. Pleural effusions may occur as a complication of abdominal or thoracic surgery or because of chest trauma.

Etiology and the disease process: A small amount of fluid is normally present in the pleural cavity to lubricate the pleural surfaces. The abnormal collection of fluid in the pleural space may occur as the result of cancer treatment such as chemotherapy or radiation therapy or in the presence of a collapsed lung or certain cancers. Cancer causes about 40 percent of symptomatic pleural effusions, according to the National Cancer Institute. In addition, lung cancer, breast cancer, lymphoma, and leukemia account for approximately 75 percent of all malignancy-related pleural effusions. In some cases, the fluid itself is malignant.

Incidence: In the United States, approximately 100,000 cases of pleural effusions are diagnosed per year, and 43 cases are detected per 100,000 hospital admissions, according to the National Cancer Institute.

Symptoms: Symptoms of a pleural effusion include shortness of breath, rapid or labored breathing, chest pain, and dry cough. Additional symptoms are often related to the underlying condition, such as fluid retention and swelling. In some cases, there are no symptoms, but the effusion may be discovered during a routine chest X ray or other diagnostic test.

Screening and diagnosis: The accurate diagnosis of a pleural effusion is essential so that treatment can be targeted for malignant effusions. The first steps in the diagnosis include a medical history and physical exam, lung-function tests, and chest X ray.

Other diagnostic tests include a computed tomography (CT) scan, chest ultrasound, thoracentesis, and pleural fluid analysis (biopsy). A thoracentesis is the removal of pleural fluid by a needle inserted through the chest wall, between the ribs. The pleural fluid is then analyzed in the laboratory. Thoracoscopy (T-scope) and pleural biopsy are performed in some cases when a thoracentesis cannot be done because of the location of the effusion. A thoracoscopy is a minimally invasive surgical procedure performed with a small videoscope instrument (thoracoscope) and surgical instruments. The scope and instruments are inserted through small incisions to examine the chest cavity and remove a tissue sample or pleural fluid sample (pleural biopsy). The sample is then examined in a laboratory.

Treatment and therapy: In cancer patients, not all pleural effusions are malignant but may be the result of malnutrition or the result of a comorbid condition, such as congestive heart failure, pulmonary embolism, or pneumonia. Treatment is directed at the underlying medical condition or type of cancer causing the pleural effusion. The goals of treatment include draining excess fluid, treating infection, and fully expanding the lung. When the effusion is transudative and asymptomatic, no treatment may be needed.

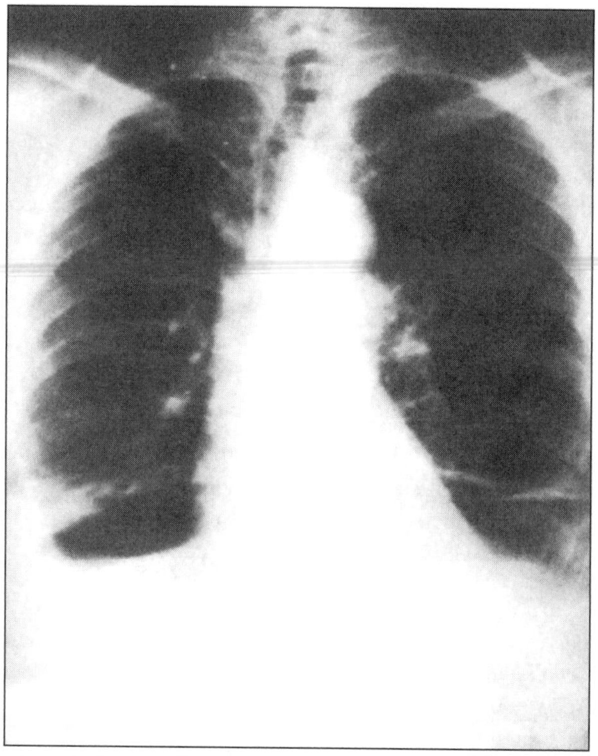

Pleural effusion. (LifeART© 2008 Wolters Kluwer Health, Inc.-Lippincott Williams &Wilkins. All rights reserved.)

Treatment options include thoracentesis, use of sclerosing agents, or surgery. Thoracentesis helps reduce pressure on the lungs by removing excess fluid. It can be used as a palliative treatment to relieve symptoms of advanced cancers. Sclerosing agents such as talc, doxycycline, and bleomycin may be inserted through a chest tube during thoracentesis to prevent a recurring effusion. Sclerosing agents also may be used during pleurodesis, a procedure to close the pleural sac. Pleurodesis is usually performed for cases of recurring malignant effusions in patients with metastatic breast, ovarian, or lung cancer.

Surgical options to drain excess fluid include thoracotomy (open-chest surgery) or minimally invasive video-assisted thoracoscopic surgery. Surgery is recommended for the treatment of infections or when the location of the effusion prohibits the use of thoracentesis for fluid analysis. In some cases, a pleural-peritoneal shunt is implanted to transfer fluid from the pleural cavity to the abdominal cavity, where it can drain more easily. Pleurectomy is another surgery performed under general anesthesia to remove the parietal pleura, the outermost lining around the lungs.

Prognosis, prevention, and outcomes: The outcome of a pleural effusion depends on the underlying condition causing the effusion. Potential complications of a pleural effusion include an empyema (abscess in the pleural space) if the pleural fluid becomes infected and a collapsed lung if the fluid has built up for a long time.

Malignant pleural effusions are often associated with advanced disease and increased morbidity and mortality.

Angela M. Costello, B.S.

▶ For Further Information

Akopov, A. L., et al. "Thoracoscopic Collagen Pleurodesis in the Treatment of Malignant Pleural Effusions." *European Journal of Cardiothoracic Surgery* 28, no. 5 (2005): 750-753.

Colice, G. L., et al. "Medical and Surgical Treatment of Parapneumonic Effusions: An Evidence-Based Guideline." *Chest* 118 (2000): 1158-1171.

Maghfoor, I., D. C. Doll, and J. W. Yarbro. "Effusions." In *Clinical Oncology*, edited by M. D. Abeloff et al. New York: Churchill Livingstone, 2000.

▶ **Other Resources**

American College of Chest Physicians
http://www.chestnet.org

National Cancer Institute
Cardiopulmonary Syndrome Overview
http://www.cancer.gov/cancertopics/pdq/supportivecare/cardiopulmonary

Society of Thoracic Surgeons
Patient Information
http://www.sts.org/sections/patientinformation/

See also Asbestos; Bronchoalveolar lung cancer; Lung cancers; Mesothelioma; Needle biopsies; Pleural biopsy; Pleurodesis; Radiofrequency ablation; Thoracentesis; Thoracoscopy; Ultrasound tests.

▶ Pleurodesis

Category: Procedures

Definition: Pleurodesis is the binding together of the pleural membranes surrounding the lungs to make breathing easier.

Cancers treated: Mesothelioma, lung cancer

Why performed: Pleurodesis is used to help lung cancer patients with malignant pleural effusions breathe more easily. Normally, the membranes of the pleural cavity that surrounds the lungs are coated with fluid that provides surface tension to make them adhere, causing the lungs to inflate when the diaphragm moves during inspiration. Extra fluid in this cavity (pleural effusion) makes it difficult to breathe because pleural surfaces do not stick together and also because the lungs do not have room to expand completely. During pleurodesis, the extra fluid is removed and a sclerosant (chemical irritant) such as sterile talc or an antibiotic is injected into the pleural cavity. The irritation causes inflammation in the membranes, which makes them stick together and also prevents more fluid accumulation. Alternatively, the surfaces can be mechanically irritated (scraped) during a surgical procedure.

Patient preparation: Patients are typically hospitalized, although pleurodesis can also be done on an outpatient basis. Patients should report any allergies to medications or other substances, such as iodine. They may be asked to stop taking medications that can increase the risk of bleeding.

Steps of the procedure: The skin and chest wall are injected with a local anesthetic and a chest tube is inserted into the pleural cavity (a procedure called a thoracotomy). A chest X ray is taken to ensure proper placement. Any fluid in the cavity is drained, in some cases over several days. Before injection of the sclerosant, the patient may receive an analgesic and/or sedative to prevent discomfort. Sometimes the patient is asked to rotate from side to side. Then the excess sclerosant is drained and the doctor removes the chest tube, which may take only a few hours. An occlusive dressing is applied over the opening to prevent air from entering the chest.

After the procedure: Patients are observed for serious complications such as respiratory distress, a collapsed lung, or bleeding. The occlusive dressing is typically left in place for two days; if stitches are used to close the opening, then they may remain in place for a week. Additional pain medication may be needed once the anesthetic has worn off. A low-grade fever is a common response to the inflammation.

Risks: The risks of pleurodesis include respiratory distress, infection, a collapsed lung, and bleeding. Patients may also have a reaction to the irritant.

Results: After a successful pleurodesis, the patient will find breathing is easier. This procedure may be repeated if needed.

Marcia Pinneau, R.N.

See also Bronchoalveolar lung cancer; Lung cancers; Mesothelioma; Pleural biopsy; Pleural effusion.

▶ Pleuropulmonary blastomas

Category: Diseases, symptoms, and conditions
Also known as: Pneumoblastomas, mesenchymal cystic hamartomas, pulmonary rhabdomyosarcomas

Related conditions: Cystic nephromas, renal tumors

Definition: Pleuropulmonary blastomas are rare childhood cancers occurring most commonly in the lungs.

Risk factors: A risk factor for pleuropulmonary blastoma is a familial history of childhood cancers, including lung cysts, kidney cysts, and thyroid tumors, although the specific genetic defect has not been elucidated. Children with pleuropulmonary blastoma may have other types of cancers and neoplastic diseases outside the lung, such as cystic nephroma of the kidney.

Etiology and the disease process: Pleuropulmonary blastoma is almost always intrathoracic or intrapulmonary. Multiloculated or unilocular lung cysts often precede development of pleuropulmonary blastoma. In 40 percent of cases, air-filled cysts were present at diagnosis, and in 25 percent of these cases pneumothorax occurred. Pleuropulmonary blastoma is categorized into three subtypes (I, II, III), and the latter two are aggressive malignancies with metastatic potential. Metastases to contralateral or ipsilateral lung tissue develop relatively frequently. Types II and III pleuropulmonary blastoma may metastasize within or beyond the chest cavity. Metastasis in most pleuropulmonary blastoma cases occurs within twenty-four months after diagnosis but occasionally at thirty-six months and beyond.

Incidence: Pleuropulmonary blastoma is a rare condition that occurs almost exclusively in children under the age of seven to eight years. Type I disease is found more often in younger children, and type III in older children.

Symptoms: Symptoms of pleuropulmonary blastoma include mild to severe respiratory distress, dyspnea (shortness of breath), fever, cough, and chest or abdominal pain due to air-filled cysts or pneumothorax.

Screening and diagnosis: Type I pleuropulmonary blastoma is cystic in appearance with no grossly identifiable nodular disease. Type II is cystic and has identifiable nodular disease. Type III is a nodular disease with no detectable cystic areas. The median age of diagnosing type I pleuropulmonary blastoma is eleven months. The frequency of cerebral metastasis in pleuropulmonary blastoma typically tends to be higher than in other pediatric sarcomas.

Treatment and therapy: Type I pleuropulmonary blastoma patients are treated with surgery with or without adjuvant chemotherapy. Typically children with types II or III pleuropulmonary blastoma are treated with surgery, chemotherapy, or radiation.

Prognosis, prevention, and outcomes: In a study, the overall survival in type I pleuropulmonary blastoma was between 65 and 90 percent. Type I may recur and progress to type II or III, and type II may progress to type III. After recurrence, type II and III pleuropulmonary blastoma has a poor prognosis.

Anita Nagypál, Ph.D.

See also Childhood cancers; Hereditary papillary renal cell carcinomas; Kidney cancer; Lung cancers; Renal pelvis tumors.

▶ *PMS* genes

Category: Cancer biology
Also known as: PMS1 postmeiotic segregation increased 1 (*Saccharomyces cerevisiae*); postmeiotic segregation increased (*S. cerevisiae*) 1; PMS2 postmeiotic segregation increased 2 (*S. cerevisiae*); postmeiotic segregation increased (*S. cerevisiae*) 2

Definition: *PMS* genes, *PMS1* and *PMS2*, encode proteins that are part of the cellular mismatch repair machinery that corrects errors made during deoxyribonucleic acid (DNA) replication. Defects in mismatch repair proteins are seen in hereditary nonpolyposis colorectal cancer, or HNPCC.

Normal cellular function: Each time a cell divides, it must faithfully replicate its genetic material contained within the DNA. Due to the inherent properties of the replication machinery, a number of mutations are made each time the genome is replicated. These mutations are rarely permanent, though, because of the action of a set of proteins that recognize and repair DNA damage. One type of repair mechanism is called the mismatch repair pathway.

Role in cancer: Individuals who inherit a mutation in one of the mismatch repair genes are strongly predisposed to developing certain types of cancer, including colorectal, ovarian, and endometrial. *MLH1* and *MSH2* are the most commonly mutated genes in this pathway, but *PMS1* and *PMS2* are also mutated in some cases of hereditary nonpolyposis colorectal cancer. Cells that have defects in mismatch repair proteins have a mutator phenotype; that is, because the machinery that normally corrects errors is compromised, the frequency of mutations is significantly higher than in normal cells. These cells are more likely to accumulate mutations within genes that are critical for limiting cell growth and proliferation and inducing cell death when damage has been done to the DNA, which are characteristics of cancer cells.

Clinical implications: Because inheriting a mutation in one of the DNA mismatch repair genes greatly predisposes an individual to developing cancer, it is important to identify at-risk individuals so that they can be frequently screened for tumors. People with a strong family history of early-onset colorectal cancer are urged to undergo genetic testing to identify mutations in the mismatch repair genes. Once a tumor has formed, the levels of mismatch repair proteins can provide insight into the patient's prognosis and cancer progression. In addition, knowing the levels of mismatch repair proteins within tumor cells can have implications for the method of treatment that is prescribed. Although the effects vary based on tumor type, there have been data showing that the state of the mismatch repair machinery can affect the efficacy of certain types of chemotherapeutic agents. For example, patients with ovarian cancer resulting from defective mismatch repair show higher levels of cancer recurrence following treatment with cisplatin.

Lindsay Lewellyn, B.S.

See also Endometrial cancer; Family history and risk assessment; Genetic testing; Genetics of cancer; Hereditary cancer syndromes; Ovarian cancers; Turcot syndrome.

▶ Pneumonectomy

Category: Procedures
Also known as: Lung removal, extrapleural pneumonectomy

Definition: Pneumonectomy is the surgical removal of the entire lung. Extrapleural pneumonectomy is the surgical removal of the lung, a portion of the membrane covering the heart, the membrane lining the affected side of the chest cavity, and a portion of the diaphragm.

Cancers treated: Lung cancer, mesothelioma

Why performed: Pneumonectomy is a surgical procedure used to treat lung cancer when the tumor cannot be removed by a less extensive procedure. It may also be performed in the presence of severe chest trauma. Rarely, pneumonectomy is used for treatment of bronchiectasis, lung abscesses, or extensive unilateral tuberculosis. Extrapleural pneumonectomy is sometimes a treatment option for those patients with malignant mesothelioma.

Patient preparation: Before planning surgery, a computed tomography (CT) scan of the head and abdomen and a bone scan are typically performed to confirm that the cancer has not spread to other areas of the body. If the cancer has spread, then pneumonectomy may not be a treatment option.

Before surgery, studies are performed to check for abnormalities and establish a baseline for postoperative comparison. These studies include a chest X ray, electrocardiogram (EKG), bleeding time, and blood tests to check kidney function; electrolyte, hemoglobin, and oxygen levels; and white blood cell count. Pulmonary function tests are performed to evaluate lung function and to determine whether the remaining lung is healthy enough to handle the increased workload. A blood sample is also drawn to check the patient's blood type in case a transfusion is needed during surgery.

A week before surgery, aspirin and anti-inflammatory drugs are stopped. The patient is given special instructions about when to stop taking anticoagulants, if prescribed. The patient must not eat or drink for at least eight hours before surgery, and an intravenous (IV) catheter is inserted for the delivery of fluids and medications. An indwelling urinary catheter is also inserted so that urine output can be monitored closely during and after the procedure.

Steps of the procedure: When the patient arrives in the operating suite, an arterial catheter may be inserted to monitor the patient's blood pressure and oxygenation. An epidural catheter may also be inserted for postoperative pain control. An endotracheal tube is inserted through the nose or mouth to maintain the patient's airway and provide oxygenation during surgery.

After the patient is anesthetized, the surgeon makes an incision into the chest cavity. When the chest cavity is entered, the lung collapses. The surgeon locates and ties off the pulmonary artery supplying the lung and the pulmonary veins. The ribs are spread, and the lung is exposed for removal. In some cases, it is necessary to remove a rib. The mainstem bronchus is divided, and the affected lung is removed. The surgeon staples or sutures the bronchial stump. Chest tubes typically are not inserted into the chest; instead fluid is permitted to accumulate inside the empty chest cavity, preventing mediastinal shift. Finally, after making sure that the bronchial stump is not leaking air, the surgeon closes the chest cavity and applies a sterile dressing.

When an extrapleural pneumonectomy is necessary, the surgeon removes the lung, a portion of the membrane covering the heart, the membrane lining the affected side of the chest cavity, and a portion of the diaphragm and replaces them with synthetic patches.

After the procedure: The patient is transferred to the surgical intensive care unit (SICU) and attached to a monitor that displays the patient's heart rhythm, blood pressure, and oxygen saturation. These devices help the SICU nurses monitor the patient's condition closely. The patient may have an endotracheal tube in place and require mechanical ventilation to assist breathing. If mechanical ventilation is not necessary, then the patient will receive supplemental oxygen through a nasal cannula or facemask. The patient is encouraged to cough, deep-breathe, and use an incentive spirometer to prevent pneumonia. If the patient requires mechanical ventilation immediately after surgery, then early extubation is the goal to prevent ventilator-associated pneumonia. The head of the patient's bed is elevated at least 30 degrees to help prevent pneumonia. The patient is turned every two hours from the back to the nonoperative

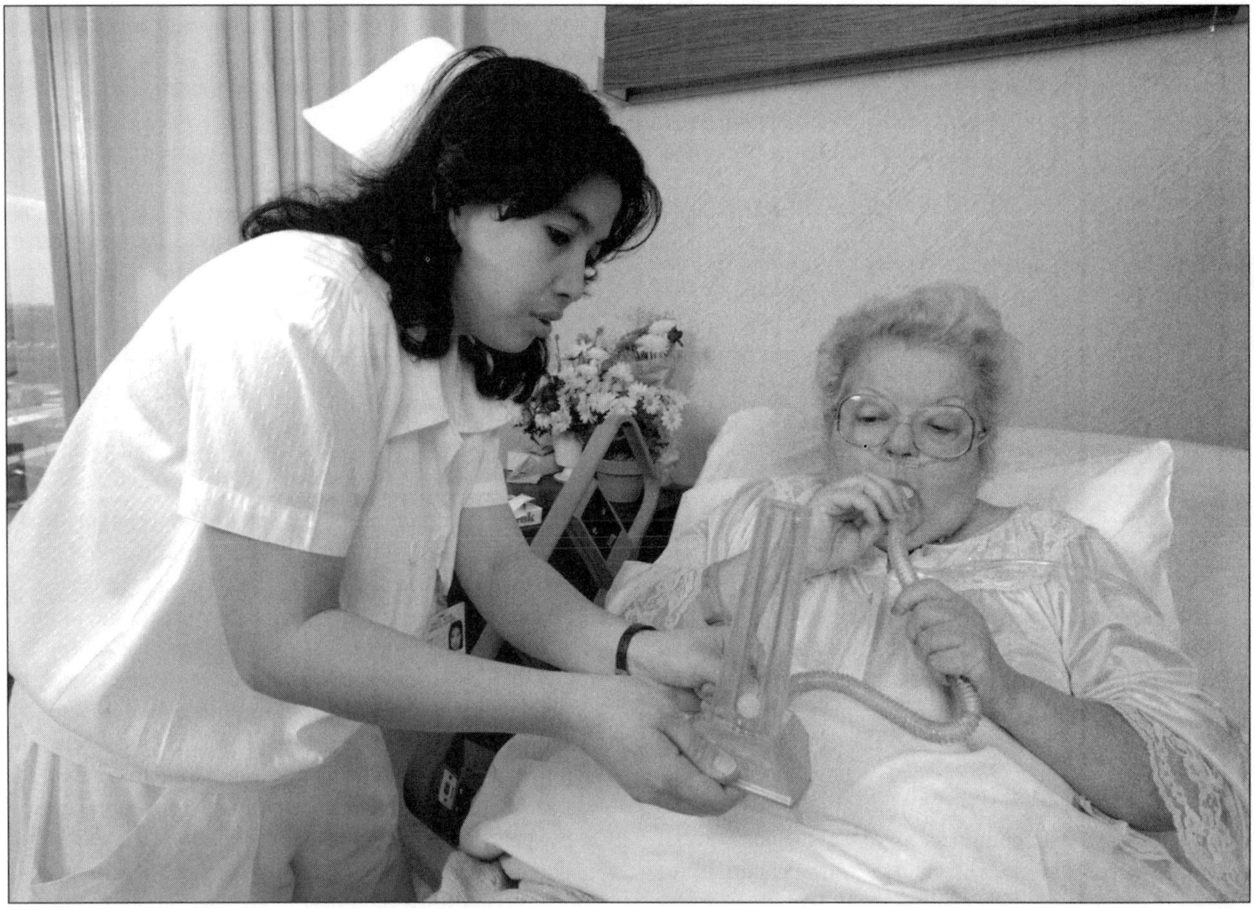

After lung surgery, patients are asked to exercise their lungs by using a spirometer. (Digital Stock)

side to prevent the heart and remaining lung from shifting toward the operative side. Fluids are administered conservatively through an IV infusion pump to prevent fluid overload. Sequential compression devices are attached to the patient's legs to help prevent blood clot formation. Pain medications are administered continuously either through an epidural catheter or through an IV catheter, as needed.

The patient is transferred to a medical surgical floor when considered stable, typically a few days after surgery, and then discharged to home. The patient is instructed to resume activities of daily living slowly in order to allow the remaining lung to compensate for its increased workload. Recovery commonly takes several months because shortness of breath significantly limits the patient's ability to exercise. Some patients require lifelong supplemental oxygen therapy.

Risks: The risks of pneumonectomy include surgical site infection, pneumonia, empyema (pus in the pleural space), hemorrhage, pulmonary edema, myocardial infarction, cardiac arrhythmia, pulmonary embolism, and ventilator-dependent respiratory failure. Rarely, stump failure results in cardiopulmonary arrest.

Results: Pathologic examination of the lung specimen reveals the type of cancer.

Collette Bishop Hendler, R.N., M.S.

▶ For Further Information

Lorigan, Paul. *Lung Cancer*. Dana-Farber Cancer Institute Handbook. Philadelphia: Mosby, 2007.

Smeltzer, Suzanne C., et al., eds. *Brunner and Suddarth's Textbook of Medical-Surgical Nursing*. 11th ed. Philadelphia: Lippincott Williams & Wilkins, 2008.

Surgical Care Made Incredibly Visual! Philadelphia: Lippincott Williams & Wilkins, 2006.

See also Asbestos; Bilobectomy; Bronchoalveolar lung cancer; Lung cancers; Mesothelioma; Pleurodesis; Thoracentesis; Thoracoscopy.

Pneumonia

Category: Diseases, symptoms, and conditions
Also known as: Pneumonitis, bronchopneumonia, community-acquired pneumonia

Related conditions: Aspiration pneumonia, atypical pneumonia, viral pneumonia, walking pneumonia, Legionella pneumonia, pneumocystis carinii pneumonia (PCP), other pneumonia, primary lung cancer, metastatic lung disease

Definition: Pneumonia is a disease of the lungs and respiratory system in which the alveoli (air sacs) become inflamed, infected, or blocked and cannot exchange air (oxygen).

Risk factors: People with respiratory problems tend to be more prone to pneumonia. The elderly, children, and people with complicating health problems are more affected by pneumonia. Pneumonia usually follows a cold or case of the flu. Persons with compromised immune systems such as acquired immunodeficiency syndrome (AIDS) patients, organ transplant patients, and cancer patients are at risk.

Another risk factor is smoking, as this can damage the cilia (microscopic hairs) that naturally sweep impurities out of the lungs. Smoke can paralyze the cilia, allowing secretions to accumulate in the lungs. If these secretions contain bacteria, pneumonia can result.

Exposure to chemicals or other pollutants on the job or in the environment can cause inflammation in the lungs, making it harder to clear the lungs of secretions. People in hospital intensive care units may be exposed to bacteria in the breathing tube of a mechanical ventilator.

Sometimes a tumor will restrict or block a cancer patient's airways, which results in the inability to clear secretions from the lungs. This can predispose the patient to pneumonia. Other risk factors for the cancer patient include radiation therapy, chemotherapy, steroids, malnutrition, surgery, neutropenia (depressed white cell count), limited mobility, antibiotics, and spleenectomy, which results in immune system problems.

Etiology and the disease process: Pneumonia can be caused by bacteria, fungi, viruses, or chemical and physical damage such as inhalation of toxins and cancer. When a person breathes, the air passes through the trachea (windpipe) to the lungs, which branch into tubes called bronchi. The bronchi divide into smaller narrow tubes called brochioles that lead to small saclike alveoli (air sacs). The function of the alveoli is to exchange gases (oxygen and carbon dioxide) with the blood capillaries. In pneumonia, these alveoli become inflamed or blocked so that the exchange of oxygen and carbon dioxide is diminished. How severely this exchange is restricted depends on the underlying cause of the pneumonia and the overall health of the patient.

Incidence: An estimated 4 million Americans develop pneumonia each year. Pneumonia and influenza (together) are the seventh leading cause of death in the United States. In 2003, pneumonia claimed 63,241 lives; every year more than 60,000 American with pneumonia die. About 50 percent of all pneumonia is caused by respiratory viruses. *Streptococcus pneumoniae* (pneumococcus) is the most common pneumonia-causing bacterium.

Symptoms: When people have bacterial pneumonia, they experience difficulty breathing, have shallow rapid breathing, and may have a productive cough. Their cough may produce greenish or yellow sputum (phlegm) or sometimes blood-tinged sputum. Patients with bacterial infections usually experience shaking, chills with fever, and sharp pain in the chest that gets worse when coughing or breathing deeply. Patients with viral pneumonia exhibit more flulike symptoms such as a dry cough, headache, muscle pain, fever, and fatigue. The cough may produce a small amount of clear or white sputum. Viral pneumonia can become bacterial pneumonia (a secondary infection) under the right conditions. Other symptoms include headache, loss of appetite, severe fatigue, sweating and clammy skin, and sometimes mental confusion in older adults.

Screening and diagnosis: Diagnosis is made by physical examination and by listening to the sound of the breath (such as crackles) through a stethoscope. The health care provider usually orders a chest X ray and reviews the scan for consolidations (white or opaque areas) that represent infected or blocked areas. Sometimes the pneumonia is not easy to visualize with an X ray, so computed tomography (CT) may be used.

The health care provider may request a culture of the sputum (Gram-staining procedure) to isolate the causal bacteria and confirm that the bacteria are sensitive to the prescribed antibiotic. A complete blood count test will allow the provider to monitor elevated white cell counts that can indicate bacterial disease. Blood tests for specific organisms may be needed to further define the cause of the pneumonia. In severe cases, arterial blood gases may be used to assess oxygenation of the blood.

The diagnostic health care provider may also use a bronchoscope (flexible tube) to examine the lungs for swelling, inflammation, obstruction, or a tumor if the pneumonia is severe and not responding to treatment.

Treatment and therapy: Pneumonia is treated based on the cause of the disease. Antibiotics are used to treat bacterial pneumonia but are useless for viral pneumonia. Strains of bacteria that are resistant to antibiotics are making the treatment of pneumonia a challenge. Most people can be treated at home unless they have underlying chronic diseases such as cancer or are elderly or very young. In these cases, hospitalization is necessary to stabilize the person with intravenous antibiotics and fluids, and possibly oxygen therapy. Occasionally steroid drugs must be used to decrease inflammation or wheezing.

If a patient is allowed to recuperate at home, the health care provider will encourage increased fluid intake to loosen the lung secretions and allow the patient to expectorate (spit out) phlegm. Key to recovery is rest and symptom control, such as managing fever with acetaminophen or aspirin (no aspirin in children).

Sometimes postural drainage will be ordered for patients who need help removing phlegm. With assistance, the patient will lean over the side of the bed with head down and allow gravity to drain the lungs. Those assisting can gently but firmly pound the patient's upper back to mechanically dislodge mucus. This can be done for about five to fifteen minutes, three times a day, or as tolerated by patients.

Treatment for cancer patients with pneumonia must be aggressive and prompt. Bed rest and taking medications to expel phlegm to clear the airways may be prescribed. The health care provider must choose treatment approaches that complement the therapy that patients are receiving for their cancer so as not to decrease the immune response.

Alternative or complementary treatments offer no cure for pneumonia but may provide some symptom relief. Acupuncture can be used to relieve congestion and may improve generalized fatigue. Some people benefit from a warm bath or room vaporizer using either plain, distilled water or distilled water with essential oils like eucalyptus added. People with asthma should avoid heat inhalations as these can irritate sensitive lung tissue.

Other complementary treatments include massaging the upper back, taking homemade cough syrup of honey and other natural ingredients, and drinking echinacea herbal tea. Supplements such as zinc or vitamins A, C, and E may may support the immune sytem.

Prognosis, prevention, and outcomes: Pneumonia can range in severity from mild to severe to fatal, depending on the cause and the age and health of patients. With adequate treatment of the cause, most pneumonia patients will show improvement within about two weeks. If patients have other compromising diseases, such as cancer, recovery may be slower. If patients fail to respond to treatment, they may die of respiratory failure.

Prevention is especially important for patients with cancer or infected with the human immunodeficiency virus (HIV). Measures to prevent infection include frequent washing of hands after blowing the nose or coughing, going to the bathroom, diapering a baby, and before and after food preparation. Immune-compromised people should avoid contact with anyone who has a cold or flu or has been exposed to these illnesses. They should also use a protective mask when cleaning to decrease exposure to dust and molds. The influenza and pneumonia vaccines may also be options and should be checked out with a health care provider.

Robert W. Koch, D.N.S., R.N.

▶ For Further Information

Baez-Escudero, José L., John N. Greene, Ramon L. Sandin, and Albert L. Vincent. "Pneumocystis Carinii Pneumonia in Cancer Patients." *Abstracts in Hematology and Oncology* 7, no. 1 (2005).

Cunha, Burke A., ed. *Pneumonia Essentials*. Royal Oak, Mich.: Physicians' Press, 2007.

Fein, Alan, et al. *Diagnosis and Management of Pneumonia and Other Respiratory Infections*. Caddo, Okla.: Professional Communications, 1999.

▶ Other Resources

American Lung Association
http://www.lungusa.org

MayoClinic.com
Pneumonia
http://www.mayoclinic.com/health/pneumonia/DS00135

National Lung Cancer Partnership
http://www.nationallungcancerpartnership.org

See also Antiviral therapies; Bacteria as causes of cancer; Bronchial adenomas; Bronchoalveolar lung cancer; Bronchography; Candidiasis; Carcinoid tumors and carcinoid syndrome; Chromium hexavalent compounds; Coughing; Craniotomy; Esophagectomy; Hemoptysis; Infection and sepsis; Insurance; Laryngectomy; Lobectomy; Lung cancers; Mayo Clinic Cancer Center; Mycosis fungoides; Neutropenia; Pleural effusion; Pneumonectomy; Thoracentesis; X-ray tests.

▶ Polycyclic aromatic hydrocarbons

Category: Carcinogens and suspected carcinogens
RoC status: Reasonably anticipated human carcinogen since 1981
Also known as: Polynuclear aromatic hydrocarbons, polyaromatic hydrocarbons, PAHs

Related cancers: Lung, colon, skin, and bladder cancer

Definition: Polycyclic aromatic hydrocarbons (PAHs) refer to a group of chemicals formed from burning wood, coal, oil, gas, and other carbon-containing substances.

Exposure routes: Inhalation, ingestion, skin contact

Where found: In air (from motor vehicle exhaust, burning wood and refuse, tobacco smoke, industrial emissions, smoke from fires), contaminated water and food, meat cooked by certain high-temperature methods (such as grilling), and coal tar products used to treat skin conditions

At risk: Industrial workers in coking plants; coal tar, aluminum, iron, steel, and asphalt production plants; and petroleum refineries; as well as road construction workers, smokers, and those exposed to tobacco smoke

Etiology and symptoms of associated cancers: Polycyclic aromatic hydrocarbons are procarcinogens in that they are converted by the detoxification system in the human body to substances that can cause cancer. Such substances bind to deoxyribonucleic acid (DNA), the molecules that carry a person's genetic blueprint. Studies suggest that this binding causes changes in DNA that lead to cancer.

Some symptoms of associated cancers include shortness of breath, coughing, weight loss (lung cancer); blood in urine (bladder cancer); weight loss, blood in stools, change in bowel habits (colon cancer); change in a wart or mole, or a skin growth that may exhibit redness (skin cancer).

History: Polycyclic aromatic hydrocarbons are naturally present in the environment (such as in coal, peat, and crude oil) and are also formed artificially by various burning processes. The involvement of substances containing polycyclic aromatic hydrocarbons in causing cancer was shown in 1775 when Percival Pott, a British surgeon, described scrotal cancer in chimney sweeps who had been exposed to coal soot. Coal tar was subsequently (1915) found to induce tumors when repeatedly applied to rabbits' ears. In 1933 a specific polycyclic aromatic hydrocarbon isolated from coal tar , benzo(a)pyrene, was shown to cause skin cancer in mice. Animal studies have since shown that repeated administration of this and other polycyclic aromatic hydrocarbons to animals through skin, the air, or diet causes various types of cancer, including breast, skin, stomach, lung, and bladder cancer. Human studies have shown an association between lung, bladder, colon, and skin cancer in industry workers exposed to high levels of polycyclic aromatic hydrocarbons.

Polycyclic aromatic hydrocarbon emissions are regulated by several agencies. The Occupational Safety and Health Administration (OSHA) regulates the exposure of industrial workers to polycyclic aromatic hydrocarbons. The Environmental Protection Agency regulates the amount of polycyclic aromatic hydrocarbons released into surface waters (Clean Water Act) and the air (Clean Air Act) and present in drinking water (Safe Drinking Water Act). The Food and Drug Administration regulates the amount of polycyclic aromatic hydrocarbons in bottled drinking water.

Jason J. Schwartz, Ph.D., J.D.

See also Air pollution; Bronchial adenomas; Carcinogens, known; Carcinogens, reasonably anticipated; Chewing tobacco; Coal tars and coal tar pitches; Coughing; Lung cancers; Mineral oils; Occupational exposures and cancer; Skin cancers; Soots; Tobacco-related cancers.

▶ Polycythemia vera

Category: Diseases, symptoms, and conditions
Also known as: PV

Related conditions: Essential thrombocythemia, idiopathic myelofibrosis

Definition: Polycythemia vera is a rare myeloproliferative disorder that causes chronic overproduction of red blood cells and possibly of white cells and platelets. Although these cells function normally, their overabundance causes increased blood viscosity and decreased blood flow, with possible clot formation and resultant heart attack or stroke, and possible systemic decreases in oxygen supply, resulting in compromised muscle function, lung function, and visual acuity, or in angina, congestive heart failure, or gout.

Risk factors: Polycythemia vera occurs more frequently in men aged sixty and older and in Jews of eastern European descent. Although family history is not a risk factor, polycythemia vera occasionally occurs in more than one family member.

Etiology and the disease process: The cause of polycythemia vera is unknown. Disease progression is slow, as is symptom onset. Polycythemia vera occurs because of a deoxyribonucleic acid (DNA) mutation—in most cases, in the *JAK2* gene—in hemopoietic stem cells (blood-forming cells in bone marrow) that triggers blood cell overproduction.

In rare instances, myelofibrosis—abnormal, fibrous bone marrow tissue—may develop and may lead to acute myelogenous leukemia (AML), an aggressive disease characterized by overabundance in blood and bone marrow of immature white blood cells.

Incidence: The reported incidence ranges from 0.5 to 2.5 per 100,000 people worldwide.

Symptoms: Overabundance of red blood cells and platelets causes the symptoms associated with polycythemia vera. Symptoms may include dizziness, enlarged spleen, fatigue, headache, itchy or flushed skin, kidney stones, profuse sweating, shortness of breath, stomach ulcers, tinnitus, and vision problems.

Screening and diagnosis: Due to its slow progression and delayed expression of nonspecific symptoms, polycythemia vera may be diagnosed via routine blood testing if results indicate a 33 percent or greater increase in hematocrit level, hemoglobin concentration, and red cell count. Other indicators may be elevated platelet count or white cell count, presence of the *JAK2* mutation in blood cells, or low erythopoietin (EPO) level (determined by assay).

Treatment and therapy: Initial options are phlebotomy to reduce blood volume and drug therapy to decrease cell count. The platelet count-lowering drug anagrelide or the myelosuppressive drugs hydroxyurea, interferon alpha, and radioactive phosphorus (^{32}P) may be used. However, side effects are associated with all treatments, including phlebotomy, which can result in anemia.

Prognosis, prevention, and outcomes: There is no cure for polycythemia vera. If untreated, it can lead to death. If treated, life expectancy and quality of life may be unaffected. Response to therapy may be monitored via hematocrit levels and hemoglobin concentrations.

Cynthia L. De Vine, B.A.

See also Bone marrow aspiration and biopsy; Chlorambucil; Chronic myeloid leukemia (CML); Hematologic oncology; Hypercoagulation disorders; Myeloproliferative disorders; Radiopharmaceuticals.

▶ Polypectomy

Category: Procedures
Also known as: Endoscopic polypectomy

Definition: Polypectomy is the removal of a protruding growth (polyp), leaving the underlying tissue.

Cancers diagnosed or treated: Cancers of the colon, rectum, small bowel, stomach, uterus, and nose

Why performed: Most polypectomies are performed to remove polyps that are or are likely to become cancerous, thereby controlling or preventing the disease. Such polyps arise most frequently in the colon and rectum; less frequently in the stomach, small intestine, and uterus; and rarely in the nose. Most polypectomies are performed during a diagnostic endoscopic procedure (such as colonoscopy, gastroscopy, hysteroscopy, or sigmoidoscopy). Polyps that cannot be removed with an endoscope, such as polyps that are too large or too numerous, require local excision or major surgery to remove the polyp and underlying tissue completely with a margin of healthy tissue.

Patient preparation: A few days before the procedure, the patient may need to stop certain medications. For gastrointestinal procedures, the patient may need to cleanse the bowel and may not eat or drink after midnight.

Steps of the procedure: Endoscopic procedures are scheduled in an outpatient setting. For the procedure, sensors are placed to monitor the patient's condition. An intravenous (IV) line is started for fluids and medications. The patient lies on the side, and sedation is given. If the patient has an electronic implant, then special precautions are taken. The appropriate endoscope is inserted through the anus (to examine colonic and rectal polyps), mouth (gastric and small intestinal polyps), or vagina (uterine polyps). The physician slowly withdraws the endoscope, carefully viewing the entire lining. When a polyp is found, its location, size, and appearance are documented. The physician may sample (biopsy), destroy (ablate), or remove (excise and retrieve) the polyp. If the polyp was not totally removed, then its location is marked with a small tattoo. All biopsy samples and excised tissues are taken to the laboratory for histopathologic evaluation.

After the procedure: The patient's condition is monitored until he or she awakens and then the patient may leave, transported by a companion. The next day, the patient resumes normal activities.

Risks: Polypectomy is relatively safe, with a small risk of perforation, bleeding, infection, postpolypectomy coagulation syndrome, or reaction to the sedative.

Results: The completeness of removal varies with the polyp's size and shape (such as broad or stalked) and the removal technique (such as type of excision, with or without ablation). Histopathologic evaluation determines whether each polyp is or is not likely to become cancerous and, if so, whether all diseased tissue was removed. Additional treatment, follow-up examinations, or both may be recommended.

Patricia Boone, Ph.D.

See also Biopsy; Colon polyps; Colonoscopy and virtual colonoscopy; Colorectal cancer; Colorectal cancer screening; *DPC4* gene testing; Hysteroscopy; Infection and sepsis; Juvenile polyposis syndrome; Polyps; Rectal cancer; Sigmoidoscopy; Small intestine cancer; Stomach cancers; Uterine cancer.

▶ Polyps

Category: Diseases, symptoms, and conditions
Also known as: Intestinal polyps, colorectal polyps, gastric polyps, nasal polyps, uterine polyps

Related conditions: Polyps may be related to certain genetic disorders that promote their growth in the colon, stomach, and rectum. Although not cancers themselves, these disorders make the person who inherits the defective gene more susceptible to cancer.

Definition: A polyp is an abnormal mass of tissue that attaches to mucous membranes, tissue linings that protect and keep moist the hollow organs of the body such as the colon, stomach, nose, sinuses, and uterus. Polyps can form on mucous membranes anywhere in the body but most commonly develop in the colon or rectum, both parts of the large intestine. They usually cause no problem, but some turn into colon or rectal cancer, generally called colorectal cancer because the two cancers have so much in common.

Risk factors: Risk factors for colorectal polyps include being past the age of fifty; inheriting a gene that causes polyp growth; previous colorectal, breast, ovarian, or uterine cancer; a personal or family history of polyps; radiation treatments to the stomach or pelvis; eating a diet high in fat and low in calcium and fiber; smoking; excessive alcohol intake; lack of exercise; and obesity.

Etiology and the disease process: Like most cancers, polyps are the result of abnormal cell growth. However, not all polyps are cancerous. Mutations in genes that control cell growth cause polyps to develop. Sometimes they continue to grow and turn cancerous. In general, the larger the polyp, the more likely it is to become cancerous. Doctors consider all polyps, even benign ones, precancerous and remove them whatever their size.

Incidence: Colorectal cancer is the third most common cancer and the second leading cause of death from cancer in the United States. (Lung cancer is the first.) More than 50,000 people die from colorectal cancer each year.

Anyone can get polyps and colorectal cancer, but some people are more susceptible than others. Whites and African Americans are more likely to get polyps and die from colorectal cancer than are Hispanics, Asian Americans, and Native Americans. Women and men under the age of fifty get polyps and die from colorectal cancer at about equal rates. Over the age of fifty, men are more vulnerable than women. Researchers estimate that 30 percent of adults the age of fifty and older have one or more colon or rectal polyps.

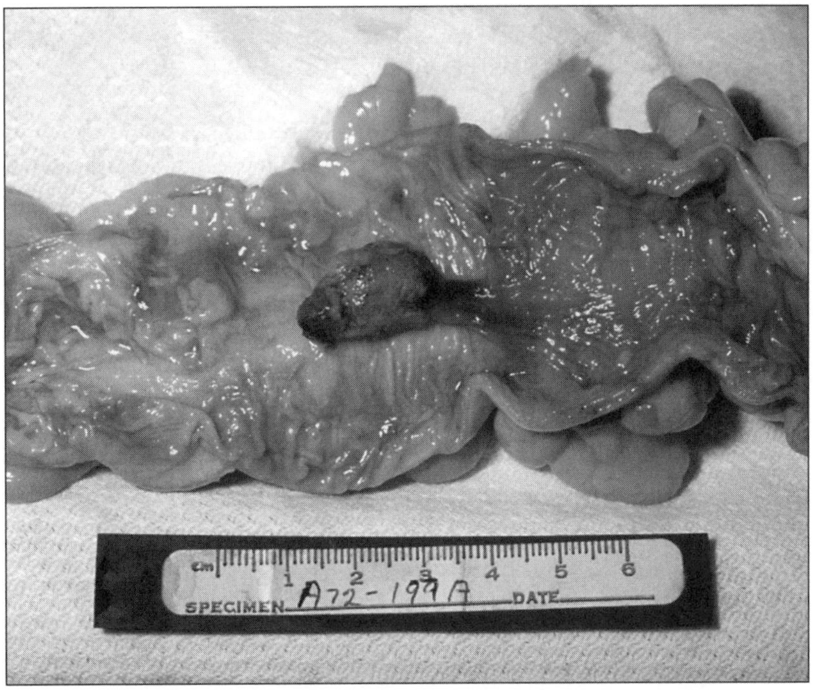

Gross pathology of a colon polyp (center). (Centers for Disease Control/Dr. Edwin P. Ewing, Jr.)

Symptoms: Most polyps generate no symptoms. They are usually found during routine screenings for colon cancer. Very large polyps, however, can cause bleeding from the rectum, bloody stool, and changes in bowel movement patterns.

Screening and diagnosis: The most common screenings for colorectal cancer are as follow:

- Fecal occult blood test: This test checks for blood in the stool.
- Flexible sigmoidoscopy: This test examines the bottom third of the large intestine (the rectum and descending colon). The doctor inserts into the rectum a thin, flexible tube with a small camera on the end that is connected to a video monitor. This enables the doctor to look for polyps in real time.
- Colonoscopy: The procedure for this test is the same as for the sigmoidoscopy, but in this test, the doctor searches the entire large intestine.

Treatment and therapy: When a polyp is discovered during screening, the doctor removes it and tests it for cancer. If the polyp is found to be cancerous, any of four main treatments for colorectal cancer begins.

- Surgery is the main treatment. Surgeons cut out the cancerous tumor and part of the area surrounding it to prevent its spreading.
- Radiation therapy uses high-energy rays to kill or shrink cancer cells. In some cases, radiation is used to shrink the tumor before surgery. Radiation is also used to ease symptoms such as pain and bleeding in late stages of cancer.
- Chemotherapy (cancer-fighting drugs) may be beneficial in the early stages of cancer. The drugs also help relieve symptoms in late stages. Because chemotherapy affects cells other than cancer cells, it sometimes causes serious side effects.
- Targeted therapies use manufactured proteins called monoclonal antibodies that attack only the part of the cancer cells that makes them different from normal cells. This treatment causes fewer side effects than other chemotherapies.

Prognosis, prevention, and outcomes: Outcomes for patients with colorectal cancer are good when the cancer is caught early. Some 90 percent of patients whose cancer is diagnosed and treated before it has spread live at least five years after diagnosis.

Because doctors do not know the exact causes of polyps, prevention measures are inexact. Generally, however, doctors believe that polyps may be prevented by maintaining a diet low in fat and high in fiber and certain cruciferous vegetables such as broccoli and cauliflower, not smoking, avoiding alcohol, exercising and maintaining a healthful weight, and (when prescribed by a doctor) taking aspirin.

Wendell Anderson, B.A.

▶ For Further Information

Adrouny, R. *Understanding Colon Cancer.* Jackson: University of Mississippi Press, 2002.

American Cancer Society. *Quick Facts Colon Cancer: What You Need to Know—Now.* Atlanta: Author, 2007.

Levin, B. *American Cancer Society's Complete Guide to Colorectal Cancer.* Atlanta: American Cancer Society, 2006.

Lipkin, M: "Strategies for Colon Cancer Prevention." *Annals New York Academy of Sciences* 768 (September 30, 1995): 170-179.

▶ Other Resources

American College of Gastroenterology
http://www.acg.gi.org

American Society of Colon and Rectal Surgeons
http://www.fascrs.org

National Cancer Institute
http://www.cancer.gov

National Digestive Disease Information Clearinghouse
What I Need to Know About Colon Polyps
http://digestive.niddk.nih.gov/ddiseases/pubs/colonpolyps_ez/

See also Adenomatous polyps; Benign tumors; Colon polyps; Colonoscopy and virtual colonoscopy; Colorectal cancer; Colorectal cancer screening; Gastric polyps; Gastrointestinal cancers; Hereditary mixed polyposis syndrome; Hereditary polyposis syndromes; Juvenile polyposis syndrome; Sigmoidoscopy.

▶ Positron emission tomography (PET)

Category: Procedures
Also known as: PET scan, ^{18}F-FDG PET, ^{18}F-FET PET

Definition: Positron emission tomography (PET) scanning is a procedure in which a small amount of radioactive glucose or amino acid is injected into a vein and a scanner is used to make detailed, computerized pictures of areas

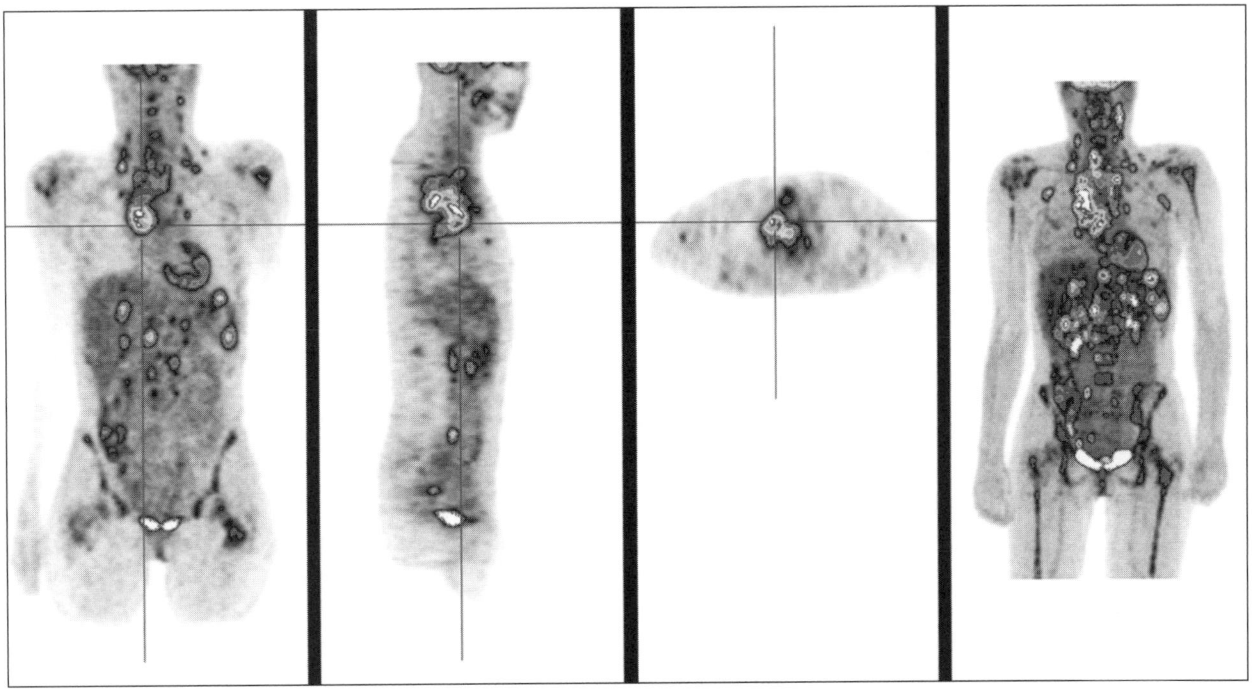

A PET scan shows Hodgkin disease, Stage IV B, with metastases of the bone, lymph nodes, and viscera. (©BSIP/Phototake—All rights reserved)

inside the body. Since cancer cells often utilize more glucose and amino acids than normal cells, the pictures can be used to find cancer cells in the body by looking for areas with higher uptake of these nutrients.

Cancers diagnosed: A wide range of cancers

Why performed: PET scans are used to screen for tumors in cancer diagnosis and to aid in tumor staging, locating metastases, and assessing treatment response, such as tumor recurrence. In addition to cancers, PET scans are effective for determining the presence of infections, heart disease, brain disorders, abnormal blood flow, and bone disorders.

Patient preparation: Patients should restrict the amount of sugar and caffeine consumed on the day before the scan. On the day of the scan, patients should not ingest anything except water for a minimum of six hours before the scan. Prior to the PET scan, blood glucose levels should be less than 120 milligrams per deciliter in nondiabetics and should fall between 150 and 200 milligrams per deciliter in diabetics. Patients are asked to drink 500 milliliters of water after injection of a radioactive compound approximately 1 hour before the PET scan. For renal or pelvic imaging, 20 to 40 milligrams of furosemide may be given ten to fifteen minutes after the injection of radioactive glucose or amino acid. Patients should also refrain from strenuous exercise for twenty-four hours before PET to minimize uptake of the radioactive compound by the muscles during the test. Just before the scan, patients are asked to remove any dentures, jewelry, or metal objects that may interfere with imaging.

Steps of the procedure: Patients are injected with glucose (FDG) or tyrosine (FET) labeled with radioactive fluorine (^{18}F). The compounds are given about an hour to distribute throughout the body. The patient then empties the bladder and lies still on the scanner bed. The PET scan takes approximately forty-five to sixty minutes, depending on the type of scan taken and the model of scanner used. Commonly, an initial whole-body scan is conducted about an hour after injection of the radioactive compound. This scan typically samples from the angle of the jaw to the level of the mid-thigh. A later scan, known as a delayed scan, is then taken approximately two hours after the injection, focusing on the organ or tissue of interest.

A major complication in interpreting PET data is the presence of multiple primary and metastatic lesions throughout the body. The uptake of radioactive glucose or amino acids into these tumors and into the surrounding normal tissues is a dynamic process that peaks at different times, depending on the specific tissues examined, patient preparation, and other factors. Thus if a patient undergoes serial PET scanning, then the time between injection of the radioactive compound and PET imaging should be the same in the baseline study and in subsequent studies. The National Cancer Institute consensus recommendations for FDG-PET scanning in clinical trials states that serial PET scans should be conducted at the same institution, using the same type of camera, the same dose of radioactive compound, the same imaging times, and the same acquisition and reconstruction parameters.

After the procedure: The patient is asked to drink plenty of fluids for a day after the scan in order to flush the radioactive compound from the body. The PET scans are interpreted by a trained radiologist, who sends the results to the referring physician.

Risks: The procedure is completely painless, with no side effects. The amount of radiation exposure is very small and similar to that from a standard X ray. Like any other procedure involving radiation, however, PET is accompanied by a small risk of tissue damage. Some patients may also experience soreness in the arm where the intravenous (IV) line was placed. Pregnant patients should inform the doctor of their condition, as PET scans may be harmful to the fetus.

Results: PET scans can identify regions in the body with abnormal metabolism of nutrients, which may indicate the presence of cancer cells. These areas can then be examined more closely by computed tomography (CT) or magnetic resonance imaging (MRI) to confirm that tumors are present and, if so, where they are located. PET scans may be useful in determining the extent of spread of certain cancers, assessing how the cancer responds to treatment, and determining if the cancer has recurred. Cancers may use more energy than surrounding tissues and therefore appear brighter on the PET scan.

PET scanning can be used in combination with CT scanning to produce anatomical pictures of organs and tissues that show regions of abnormal metabolism. PET/CT scanning machines are now available at many medical centers. This combination method can be more powerful than either technique used alone. R. A. Kuker and colleagues showed that a combination of delayed-phase FDG-PET and CT could identify liver tumors and metastases that could not be detected by CT alone.

Several important factors must be considered when analyzing PET scans. A crucial factor in analyzing PET data is the time of measurement. For example, whole-body images are composites of static images that are obtained at various predetermined times after the injection of the radioactive compound. These scans must be corrected for signal attenuation over time. Other factors that have an impact on data analysis are the volume of distribution, body weight, lean body mass, body surface area, and normal serum glucose or amino acid concentrations. After correcting for these factors, the standardized uptake value (SUV) is the most common assessment used. When suspected lesions are identified on a PET scan, both maximum and mean SUV are determined for regions in the tumor and in normal tissue in the same organ. The tumor-to-normal-tissue SUV (T/N) ratio can be calculated. A value for the maximum SUV T/N ratio, for example, can be set as a threshold above which a suspected lesion is considered positive.

When using PET to determine tumor response to treatment, experts recommend conducting PET studies six to eight weeks after radiation therapy and two weeks after chemotherapy. The SUVs of the target tumors are determined before and after treatment. The SUVs of normal tissue in the organs in which the tumors occur are also obtained as a reference, and T/N ratios are obtained. This ensures that the SUV changes are attributable to either tumor progression or treatment response, and not to normal changes in the cells over time. The shape and size of tumors frequently change during the course of treatment. These changes should be recorded along with the changes in tumor uptake values. The interpretation of PET data is key to obtaining accurate and reliable results. Many types of cancer do not appear on PET scans and may be detected only by imaging techniques with a higher resolution, such as PET/CT or MRI. Some noncancerous tissues can also appear similar to tumors on a PET scan, resulting in false positives.

Ing-Wei Khor, Ph.D.

▶ For Further Information

Christian, Paul E., and Kristen M. Waterstram-Rich, eds. *Nuclear Medicine and PET: Technology and Techniques*. 6th ed. St. Louis: Mosby/Elsevier, 2007.

Kubota, K. "From Tumor Biology to Clinical PET: A Review of Positron Emission Tomography (PET) in Oncology." *Annals of Nuclear Medicine* 15 (2001): 471-486.

Kuker, R. A., G. Mesoloras, and S. A. Gulec. "Optimization of FDG-PET/CT Imaging Protocol for Evaluation of Patients with Primary and Metastatic Liver Disease." *International Seminars in Surgical Oncology* 4 (2007): 17-21. Also available online at http://www.issoonline.com.

Shankar, L. K., J. M. Hoffman, S. Bacharach, et al. "Consensus Recommendations for the Use of ^{18}F-FDG PET as an Indicator of Therapeutic Response in Patients in National Cancer Institute Trials." *Journal of Nuclear Medicine* 47 (2006): 1059-1066.

▶ Other Resources

Cedars-Sinai Health System
http://www.csmc.edu

Mayo Clinic
Positron Emission Tomography (PET) Scan: Detecting Conditions Early
http://www.mayoclinic.com/health/pet-scan/CA00052

National Cancer Institute
http://www.cancer.gov

PETNET solutions
Patient Preparation
http://www.petscaninfo.com/zportal/portals/pat/my_pet_scan/for_patients

See also Angiography; Barium enema; Barium swallow; Bone scan; Bronchography; Computed tomography (CT)-guided biopsy; Computed tomography (CT) scan; Cystography; Ductogram; Endoscopic retrograde cholangiopancreatography (ERCP); Gallium scan; Hysterography; Imaging tests; Lymphangiography; Magnetic resonance imaging (MRI); Mammography; Nuclear medicine scan; Radionuclide scan; Thermal imaging; X-ray tests.

▶ Poverty and cancer

Category: Social and personal issues

Definition: Cancer has higher rates of incidence and mortality among people of lower socioeconomic status. Impoverished people, whether in developed or underdeveloped countries, tend to be poorly educated about cancers and cancer prevention, have little access to screening, and have cancers discovered in later stages. Moreover, they are often unable to access and afford medical treatment.

Description of the population: People living in absolute poverty are defined by the World Bank as earning one or two dollars per day in developing countries such as India and Sierra Leone and about twenty-six dollars per day in the United States. In addition to economic indicators, poverty may be defined as lacking basic human services—such as employment opportunities, safe drinking water, and basic sanitation services—and access to food, health, education, and shelter.

Incidence, death, and survival statistics: According to the World Health Organization, globally the six leading types of cancer in terms of incidence are lung cancer, breast cancer, colorectal cancer, stomach cancer, liver cancer, and cervical cancer. In the United States, the top six types of cancer, according to the American Cancer Society, are prostate cancer, lung and bronchus cancer, breast cancer, colon cancer, urinary bladder cancer, and non-Hodgkin lymphoma. In 2006, approximately three million of the six million deaths from cancer occurred in developing countries. The deaths were mainly attributed to late diagnosis of the disease (in either Stage III or IV), when death is often no longer preventable.

Approximately 23 percent of all malignancies in developing countries are caused by infectious agents such as hepatitis B and hepatitis C viruses (HBV and HCV, which cause liver cancer), human papillomaviruses (HPV, which causes cervical cancer), and *Helicobacter pylori* (*H. pylori*, the bacterial agent that causes stomach cancer) and are preventable with safe health and behavioral practices. In developed countries, only 8 percent of all malignancies are attributable to these infectious agents. The variance in malignancy rates in developing and developed countries suggests that poverty and poor health practices are at least partially responsible.

Breast and cervical cancer rates are steady or decreasing in some developed countries such as the United States, possibly because of early detection, proper and timely treatment, and vaccination; however, the trend is different in many developing countries. For example, Pakistan is continuing to see an increase in cancer prevalence among women. It has the highest prevalence of breast cancer of any Asian country, accounting for about 25 percent of all malignant tumors among Pakistani women. Malaysia also experiences high rates of breast cancer, and 50 to 60 percent of breast cancers were diagnosed late, in Stages III and IV, contributing to low survival rates for breast cancer among Malaysian women.

Cervical cancer, which is preventable through vaccination and safe sex practices, is highly endemic in Central America, Southeast Africa, and India. Approximately 80 percent of all cervical cancer deaths occur in developing countries, where prevention, detection, and treatment strategies are minimal or absent.

Risk statistics: Socioeconomic status, tobacco use, poor nutrition or diet, physical inactivity, and prohibitively expensive health care are major risk factors for cancer globally. Environmental factors also are risk factors. This is particularly true in China, where, according to the Ministry of Health, pollution is the main reason that cancer is the country's leading cause of death.

The main difference between cancer in developing and developed countries is that developing countries are experiencing cancers largely associated with behavior and environment (cervical, liver, and stomach); these cancers are more often detected in early stages and successfully treated in developed countries. In developed countries, cancers that are preventable through diet and nutrition, physical activity, and avoiding tobacco use are endemic. For example, obesity is a leading cause of death in high- to middle-income countries, and obesity is associated with breast and colon cancer. However, developing countries often encounter food shortages, and as a result obesity and its related cancers are less prevelant.

Developing countries often lack a stable health care system to address and treat cancer. If treatment is available, it is often geographically distant or not affordable except by the affluent members of the society. For example, Pakistan has numerous medical facilities that diagnose and treat cancer. However, a majority of Pakistani cancer patients are unable to afford treatment even if the facilities are in their area. Diagnostics are not typically available to socioeconomically disadvantaged groups, while higher-income groups benefit greatly from screening and physical examinations.

Poor health education is a contributing risk factor for cancer. Mexico has high rates of cervical cancer, and the cancer is endemic in groups with low literacy rates and lack of access to proper health care. In 2000, 44 percent of Mexican women who died of cervical cancer lacked formal education. Areas positively correlated with cervical cancer (India, southeastern Africa, and Central America) also have high rates of infection with the human immunodeficiency virus (HIV), suggesting risky sexual practices and poor health education.

Cultural barriers: Financial barriers are not the only reason that people in developing countries do not get cancer screening and treatment. Culture also plays a major role in preventing the early detection and proper treatment of cancer. One large cultural barrier that is often noted among impoverished populations is the role of traditional medicine. Often physicians in developing countries who were trained in and practice Western medicine incorporate traditional beliefs into their practices. In India, Pakistan, and Malaysia, traditional beliefs have been noted to interfere with the timely diagnosis of cancer. Social stigmas—such as the fear that cancer is contagious and that patients will be abandoned by their spouses and communities—also inhibit timely diagnosis and treatment for cancer in developing countries.

Perspective and prospects: Poverty is the greatest barrier to early diagnosis and proper treatment for cancer globally. The poor suffer greater mortality from cancer, particularly in developing countries. Financial and cultural barriers prevent socioeconomically disadvantaged people from seeking early diagnosis and treatment for the disease.

Areas to be addressed in solving this problem include improvement of health education, integration of the socioeconomically disadvantaged into health care systems, and the removal of cultural barriers to prevention and timely diagnosis.

Primarily, health education needs to be emphasized. Safe sex practices may help eliminate cervical and liver cancers by lowering the spread of HPV and hepatitis B and C. Better sanitation may reduce the incidence of *H. pylori* and reduce stomach cancers resulting from this bacterial agent. Additionally, the effects of tobacco use need to be emphasized to reduce global lung cancer rates. Proper health education may also help reduce the social stigmas and cultural barriers attached to cancer and enable more timely diagnosis.

Even if people become educated regarding their health, the medical system needs to be in place and capable of adequately treating cancer. In the United States, Canada, and Western Europe, the health systems are well-equipped to diagnose and treat cancer; however, this is not true of most developing countries. However, because developing countries are often dealing with a high prevalence of infectious diseases, they often give a lower priority to the prevention of chronic diseases. The vaccination of people in developing countries against HPV and hepatitis B could help control the increase in the rates of cervical cancer and liver cancer, respectively.

Samreen F. Khan, M.A.

▶ For Further Information

Ali, Abrar Ashraf, et al. "Carcinoma Breast: A Dilemma for Our Society." *Ann King Edward Medical College* 9, no. 2 (June, 2003): 87-89.

Aziz, Z., et al. "Socioeconomic Status and Breast Cancer Survival in Pakistani Women." *Journal of the Pakistan Medical Association* 54, no. 9 (September, 2004): 448-453.

Bosanquet, Nick, and Karol Sikora. *The Economics of Cancer Care*. Cambridge: Cambridge University Press, 2006.

Hisham, Abdullah, and Cheng-Har Yip. "Overview of Breast Cancer in Malaysian Women: A Problem with Late Diagnosis." *Asian Journal of Surgery* 27, no. 2 (April, 2004): 130-133.

Holtz, Carol, ed. *Global Health Care: Issues and Policies*. Sudbury, Mass.: Jones and Bartlett, 2008.

Jemal, Ahmedin, et al. "Cancer Statistics, 2007." *CA: A Cancer Journal for Clinicians* 57, no. 43 (2007): 43-66.

Pal, S. K., and B. Mittal. "Fight Against Cancer in Countries with Limited Resources: The Post-genomic Era Scenario." *Asian Pacific Journal of Cancer Prevention* 5, no. 3 (July, 2004): 328-333.

Ward, E., et al. "Cancer Disparities by Race/Ethnicity and Socio-economic Status." *CA: A Cancer Journal for Clinicians* 54, no. 2 (2004): 78-93.

▶ Other Resources

American Cancer Society
http://www.cancer.org

Prevent Cancer Foundation
http://www.preventcancer.org/

World Health Organization
Cancer
http://www.who.int/cancer/en/

See also African Americans and cancer; Carcinomatosis; Developing nations and cancer; Epidemiology of cancer; Ethnicity and cancer; Latinos/Hispanics and cancer; Native North Americans and cancer; Obesity-associated cancers; Singlehood and cancer; Statistics of cancer.

▶ Prayer and cancer support

Category: Social and personal issues

Definition: Prayer, the act of communicating with a deity or other "higher force" in which a person has faith, has helped some cancer patients cope with their disease.

History and origin: The idea of healing through faith is not new. Within most formal religions—Hinduism, Buddhism, Judaism, Christianity, and Islam—some form of prayer has evolved as a means of communicating with a deity or spiritual being who the faithful believe has the power to heal and provide physical and mental solace during challenging times. Spirituality, or a strong belief in a higher power, can also exist outside the boundaries of formal religion, and in this case, prayer is often a communication with a higher force or energy that has powers beyond those of humans. An illness such as cancer is a powerful life event that often makes people face mortality and question the purpose and meaning of life. In many instances, this questioning leads them to prayer, spiritual growth, and a positive outlook, which helps them cope. This increased ability to cope as a result of prayer can be very helpful for patients dealing with cancer and its debilitating effects, even though it cannot cure the disease.

Scientific evidence for the mind-body connection: A growing body of research indicates that the mind exerts a powerful influence on the way a body responds to trauma and stress. Cancer creates a substantial amount of stress in the body, which in turn can be detrimental to the recovery process. Analysis of data from an online support group of breast cancer patients revealed that those who prayed or meditated had a more positive mental outlook and seemed to be more in control of their situation. Doctors have found that patients with advanced cancer who believe in and practice prayer and meditation cope well with the trauma from the disease and are often able to find meaning in their experience. Scientific evidence for the use of prayer alone in cancer therapy is not conclusive; however, many positive outcomes have been observed when it is used as an adjunct to conventional medical treatment. New studies on the positive correlation between prayer and recovery of patients with a strong faith in prayer suggest that it helps speed up the recovery process. Therefore, for patients with a strong faith, the integration of spiritual practices into their medical care is overall very beneficial to them.

Integrating prayer in medical care: For many years the medical community believed that there was no correlation whatsoever between spirituality and medicine. However, some physicians are beginning to acknowledge the existence of the mind-body connection in recovery, and a number of medical schools in the United States include a spirituality and prayer component in their medical curriculum as part of a complementary, adjunct strategy. Some hospitals include a spiritual representative as part of the patient's care team. Prayer and spirituality are an integral part of the lives of many cancer patients, and they also play an important role in dealing with issues of dying and death. Many medical institutions and physicians respect their patients' religious beliefs and help them incorporate them into their treatment regimen.

Mechanics of integrating prayer: Prayer can be practiced in many different ways, either alone or in a group, silently or with the accompaniment of music, with or without affiliation with any religion. Many cancer support groups use standard forms of prayer composed by religious leaders to pray for cancer patients. In addition, many hospitals have prayer rooms and contracts with clergy from various religious organizations to cater and minister to their patients' spiritual needs.

If faith plays a very important role in the life of a cancer patient and is not acknowledged by the care team while making decisions for treatment, conflicts can arise and channels of communication can be closed, resulting in a stressful situation that could be detrimental to the patient's health. When physicians inquire about and acknowledge a patient's spiritual beliefs in a nonjudgmental, sensitive manner, they set the stage for open communication and better decision making.

However, prayer should never be forced on patients, and spiritual practices should be incorporated into the treatment regimen only with their consent. On occasions when patients want to use prayer alone for their recovery and refuse or want to delay conventional medical treatment, it is the responsibility of the medical staff to explain the risks and serious health consequences involved in delaying or refusing treatment while simultaneously acknowledging the patient's religious beliefs respectfully.

Lalitha Krishnan, Ph.D.

▶ For Further Information

Dwyer, J. W., L. L. Clarke, and M. K. Miller. "The Effect of Religious Concentration and Affiliation on County Cancer Mortality Rates." *Journal of Health and Social Behavior* 31 (1990): 185-202.

Mytko, J. J., and S. J. Knight. "Body, Mind, and Spirit: Towards the Integration of Religiosity and Spirituality in Cancer Quality of Life Research." *Psycho-oncology* 8 (1999): 439-450.

Ott, Mary Jane. "Mind-Body Therapies for the Pediatric Oncology Patient: Matching the Right Therapy with the Right Patient." *Journal of Pediatric Oncology Nursing* 23, no. 5 (2006): 254-257.

▶ Other Resources

American Cancer Society
Spirituality and Prayer
http://www.cancer.org/docroot/ETO/content/ETO_5_3X_Spirituality_and_Prayer.asp

MedNet 2006
Effects of Prayer and Religious Expression Within Computer Support Groups on Women with Breast Cancer
http://www.mednetcongress.org/ocs/viewabstract.php?id=306

See also Cancer care team; Integrative oncology; Medical oncology; Pediatric oncology and hematology; Psycho-oncology; Psychosocial aspects of cancer; Stress management; Support groups.

▶ Preferred provider organizations (PPOs)

Category: Social and personal issues

Definition: Preferred provider organizations (PPOs) are health care delivery systems in which a third-party payer contracts with physicians, hospitals, and other providers to deliver health services to subscribers at a negotiated rate.

History: PPOs developed in the 1980's to address the escalating costs of health care services. Burdened with the increasing expense of health insurance for employees, businesses passed costs to the consumer in greater product or service prices. American businesses, finding it hard to compete in the growing international market, pushed insurance companies to decrease their premium rates.

Several models for health care delivery emerged to benefit the insurance companies, businesses, and health care providers. The PPO encouraged insurance companies and health care providers to negotiate lower product and service prices in return for a guaranteed group of subscribers. The result was reduced insurance premiums for the businesses, guaranteed customers for the health care providers, and a captive pool of subscribers for the insurance companies. Though somewhat changed beginning in the 1990's, the PPO model still functions on the same basic principles.

How PPOs work: PPOs are a blend of the traditional fee-for-service system and the health maintenance organization (HMO) model. PPOs have more relaxed rules and choices than the HMO model but can be more expensive to the subscriber. A list of physicians, hospitals, and other health care service and product providers is available to the subscriber as preferred providers or network providers. When the subscriber chooses a provider on the network list, most of the medical bill is covered. The subscriber may pay a minimum copayment (copay) and sometimes must reach a deductible out-of-pocket payment for certain services before costs are covered.

PPOs may require subscribers to choose primary care physicians to oversee their care. PPOs usually pay for preventive care, including screening tests such as mammograms. If the subscriber uses doctors or services not in the preferred network, PPOs usually cover some of the cost but at reduced rates, leaving the subscriber to cover the difference. This encourages the subscriber to use network providers.

How PPOs differ from HMOs: PPOs are attractive to cancer patients because they provide a wider range of services with more individual choices than HMOs. However, PPO subscribers pay for these advantages with higher premiums, copayments, and deductibles than those for HMO subscribers, who have low premiums, no or low copayments, and usually no deductibles. PPOs allow out-of-network care with higher subscriber copayments while HMOs do not cover out-of-network care unless preapproved or emergency related. PPO subscribers select their doctors with additional costs for out-of-network physicians; HMO subscribers choose their physicians from a restricted list of network providers and may find it difficult to receive a specialist referral. Individual choice of health care provider can increase the likelihood of continuity of care for the cancer patient.

Because cancer care can be expensive, cancer patients should research the difference in costs before going out of the PPO network for services. Cancer patients may need services that require preauthorization (preapproval) to be covered. If the patient (or doctor) does not obtain preapproval for the service or product, the PPO will not cover payment. Cancer patients might have to pay sizable costs for their health care services or products from their own financial means.

Cancer patients should consider what medications are covered by the PPO and at what price. HMOs may have a set drug formulary while PPOs use an open formulary, with access to more medications but with higher copayments for nonpreferred drugs. The PPO may offer more choices to cancer patients but at a higher price.

Marylane Wade Koch, M.S.N., R.N.

Questions Cancer Patients Should Ask About PPOs

Being informed can help cancer patients get the best care for a reasonable price. Cancer patients may have specific needs that require answers before joining a PPO. Seeking solutions to these questions can clarify any limitations before switching to a PPO:

- Can I choose from a list of doctors? Which ones are in the network plan and do they accept new patients?
- How do I get a referral to a specialist?
- What hospitals are on the covered network plan?
- What happens if I am out of town and need health care services?
- How do I receive emergency services through the PPO?
- Are preventive services covered? Which ones?
- Are there limits on services like cancer treatments, medical tests, mental health services, or prescription medications? Ask about any specific treatments, tests, or medications that apply to your cancer treatment such as chemotherapy, radiation therapy, stem cell transplants, and clinical trials.
- What will my monthly premium be?
- Is there a deductible? How much is it?
- Do I have to pay at the time of my doctor visits or will I receive a bill for care?
- What is the difference in costs if I go outside the network for services?
- Is there a maximum limit for my out-of-pocket expenses each year? Lifetime maximum limit for out-of-pocket expenses?
- Are my dependents covered?

▶ For Further Information

Calder, Kimberly J., and Karen Pollitz. *What Cancer Survivors Need to Know About Health Insurance*. Silver Springs, Md.: National Coalition for Cancer Survivorship, 2006.

Marcinko, David E. *Dictionary of Health Insurance and Managed Care*. New York: Springer, 2006.

Orin, Rhonda. *Making Them Pay: How to Get the Most from Health Insurance and Managed Care*. New York: St. Martin's Press, 2001.

Palmateer, Paige. "Interest Rises in Cancer Insurance." *Central New York Business Journal*, October 20, 2006.

▶ Other Resources

American Cancer Society
Medical Insurance and Financial Assistance for the Cancer Patient
http://www.cancer.org/docroot/MLT/content/MLT_1x_Medical_Insurance_and_Financial_Assistance_for_the_Cancer_Patient.asp?sitearea=&level=1

National Cancer Institute
Clinical Trials and Insurance Coverage: A Resource Guide
http://www.cancer.gov/clinicaltrials/learning/insurance-coverage

See also Chemotherapy; Clinical trials; End-of-life care; Financial issues; Health maintenance organizations (HMOs); Home health services; Insurance; Mammography; Managed care; Medicare and cancer; Prevention; Primary care physician; Screening for cancer; Second opinions; Survivorship issues.

▶ Pregnancy and cancer

Category: Social and personal issues

Definition: While pregnancy is not a risk factor for cancer, cancer can develop during pregnancy or the postpartum period in association with the hormonal changes in a woman's body. A woman with a diagnosis of cancer or who is a survivor of cancer, remitted or cured, should consult with her doctor regarding any potential impact of the disease or its treatment on the prospect of becoming pregnant, the expected course of a pregnancy, and the prospective outcome of a pregnancy.

Incidence, death, and survival statistics: Maternal malignancy occurs in approximately 1 in 1,000 to 1,500 pregnancies. Rarer is a malignancy present in the placenta or fetus originating from the maternal cancer. Among cancers occurring in pregnant and postpartum, lactating women, breast and cervical cancers are most common: Approximately half of cancer cases occurring during pregnancy are breast or cervical cancer, and leukemia and lymphoma account for approximately one-quarter of all malignancies during pregnancy. The incidence of breast cancer is 1 in 3,000 pregnancies, and the incidence of cervical cancer is 1 in 200 pregnancies. The incidence of these cancers during pregnancy may increase because of the trend of women bearing children when older. The average estimated incidence of ovarian tumors in pregnancy is 1 in 1,000 deliveries, with the majority being benign. The use of ultrasound in early fetal evaluation may contribute to the earlier detection and therefore increased incidence of ovarian cancer.

While rare, there may also be an increase in incidence of lung cancer during pregnancy due to smoking or delayed age of childbearing. Malignant melanomas, a serious type of invasive skin cancer, represent 8 percent of cancers diagnosed during pregnancy, and increased incidence is associated with a decrease in the age at which it is diagnosed (0.14 to 2.8 per 1,000 births). Hodgkin disease, a type of blood cancer, may occur in 1 per 1,000 to 1 per 6,000 of deliveries; the incidence of the disease is highest during a woman's childbearing years, ages twenty to forty. Non-Hodgkin lymphoma (NHL) is the fourth most common cancer in pregnant women. NHL has an age-dependent increase in incidence, however (with more cases occurring in midlife), and thus there are relatively few reports of its incidence during pregnancy.

Risk statistics: Various risk factors have been reported to increase the chance of a woman's developing cancer during pregnancy, including age, history of prior pregnancies, and factors associated with pregnancy.

Breast cancer risks. Women who have never been pregnant or who became pregnant after the age of thirty are at a slightly higher risk of developing breast cancer than women who became pregnant when younger than thirty. It is estimated that a woman who had her first child after the age of thirty-five has twice the risk of developing breast cancer as that of her counterpart under twenty years old. Some studies have shown that both pregnancy and breastfeeding may slightly reduce the risk for breast cancer because—particularly for those women who breast-feed between 1.5 and 2 years—these conditions reduce the number of menstrual cycles in a woman's life span. It has been reported that a pregnant woman has a 2.5-fold higher risk of being diagnosed with metastatic breast cancer and a decreased chance of being diagnosed with Stage 1 breast cancer (the early stage of invasive breast cancer), probably in part because of pregnancy-induced engorgement of the breast masking the detection of small lumps.

After giving birth, a woman is at increased risk of developing breast cancer for several years. A woman who took diethylstilbestrol (DES, a synthetic form of estrogen given during pregnancy between the early 1940's and 1971 to reduce the risk of repeated miscarriage or premature delivery) is at an increased risk of developing breast cancer. However, exposure to DES before birth in DES daughters does not appear to increase risk of breast cancer in these daughters.

It should be noted that there remain other risks for breast cancer that may place a woman at risk during her pregnancy, such as a family history of breast cancer in a first-degree relative, certain breast conditions, and the onset of menses before age twelve.

Cervical cancer risks. Pregnant woman infected with the human papillomavirus (HPV) may be at risk for cancer during pregnancy, although that is unlikely. HPV actually comprises a group of sexually transmitted viruses; the high-risk strains are thought to be the leading cause of cervical cancer and often may not present symptoms for some time following exposure to the virus. Some strains produce genital warts, which are very contagious. HPV-infected pregnant women with genital warts may experience growth in the warts during pregnancy because of the moist cervical environment in which the warts thrive, the hormonal changes attending pregnancy, and changes in the woman's immune system. Regular screenings for cervical cancer, physician-conducted breast examinations, and instruction in breast self-examinations are therefore important components of prenatal visits.

Although the presence of genital warts or abnormal cervical changes warrants medical follow-up, presence of HPV is unlikely to affect the pregnancy or the newborn's health. Also, while the genital warts may disappear on their own, or a pregnant woman may wait until after delivery for their removal, the warts can be removed safely during the pregnancy using conventional procedures such as cryotherapy or the loop electrical excisional procedure (LEEP).

Diagnosing and treating cancers during pregnancy: As a woman's breasts change and grow during pregnancy with the development of milk ducts, breasts feel lumpier and bumpier, rendering early detection of breast cancer during pregnancy difficult. However, 70 to 80 percent of painless lumps detected during or soon after pregnancy are noncancerous. Regular breast examinations should be conducted by the woman's doctor during prenatal visits, and pregnant women should conduct breast self-examinations regularly.

Nevertheless, a pregnant woman who detects a lump should visit the doctor promptly and request a diagnostic evaluation of any suspicious mass, rather than giving in to the temptation to delay until after childbirth. Mammography has not been found to harm the fetus for screening those who have signs or symptoms of a breast problem, and a mammogram can be taken as long as a lead shield is placed over the abdomen to block the effects of radiation. Because the accuracy of mammogram results during pregnancy is not as reliable as it is for nonpregnant women, ultrasound can be conducted before the mammogram to detect palpable lumps. A woman should also discuss with her doctor the use of magnetic resonance imaging (MRI). In the final analysis, however, a tissue biopsy—either needle or excisional—is the most accurate tool for diagnosing breast cancer, and it allows the physician to remove tissue from a suspicious mass at the same time. Although the resulting sample may be difficult to interpret during pregnancy, it offers the most conclusive results. Treatment of breast cancer during pregnancy should follow the standard for all women with modifications during pregnancy, such as avoiding chemotherapy during the first trimester.

Pregnant women with early-stage cervical cancer are often asymptomatic or may have symptoms similar to those of their nonpregnant counterparts, such as vaginal bleeding, pain, and discharge. Pregnant women with any suspicious lesions should see their doctor or prenatal provider for a Pap test with endocervical sampling and a biopsy of the lesion. Although pregnancy offers an opportunity for screening of cervical cancer during prenatal care, colposcopy (viewing the inside of the cervix with a microscope-like device) is technically more difficult; the complication rate following biopsy (if necessary) is higher, and vaginal bleeding due to cancer may be misdiagnosed as pregnancy related.

Although noninvasive cervical cancer is rare during pregnancy, if it is detected, treatment should be delayed until after childbirth. Studies have shown no adverse outcomes for the fetus or mother when treatment is delayed, and in fact it appears that a woman with a pregnancy-associated cervical cancer has an overall better prognosis than that of a nonpregnant woman (probably because of the likelihood of detecting any abnormalities in cervical cells during the course of regular prenatal visits). Despite the postponement of treatment, however, a pregnant woman with this diagnosis should see her doctor to be reevaluated because of the limitations in accurately diagnosing disease during pregnancy. Cervical cancer during pregnancy does not appear to adversely affect the newborn.

For a melanoma detected during pregnancy, standard treatment for early disease in pregnant women is surgery,

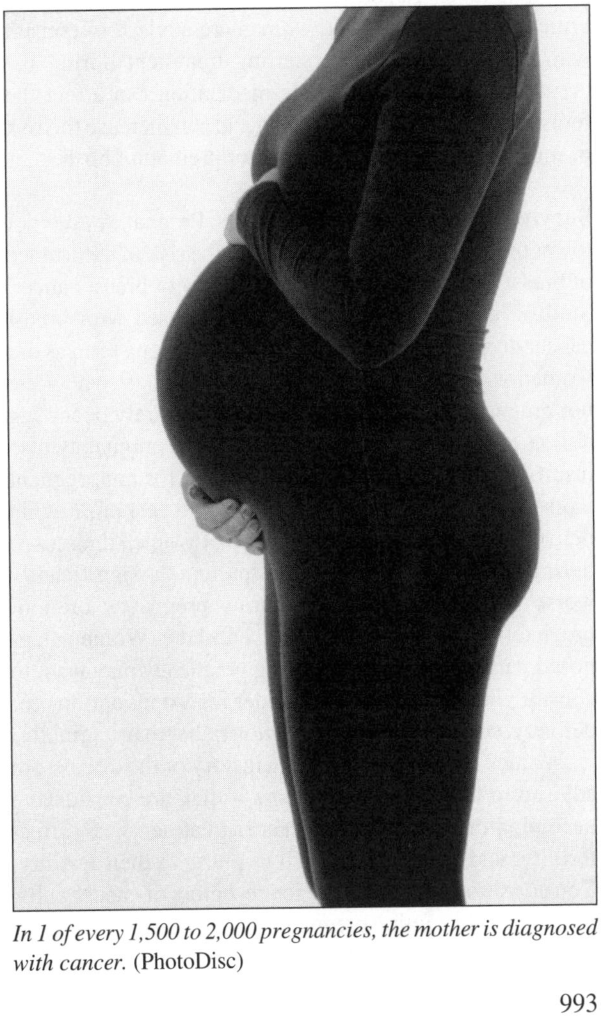

In 1 of every 1,500 to 2,000 pregnancies, the mother is diagnosed with cancer. (PhotoDisc)

as it would for nonpregnant women. Most studies of the effects of melanoma on the survival rate in pregnant women—when subjects were matched for age, anatomic site, and stage—show no difference in survival rates for pregnant as opposed to nonpregnant women.

Although Hodgkin disease is relatively rare in pregnant women, there are no standard guidelines for diagnosing and treating it during pregnancy. Typically, chemotherapy is delayed until after the first trimester and radiotherapy until after delivery. Breast-feeding is not recommended during active treatment for Hodgkin disease. There does not appear to be an effect of pregnancy on survival rates of women diagnosed with Hodgkin disease during pregnancy.

In general, factors to consider if a woman and her doctor are deciding whether to treat a cancer occurring during pregnancy include the gestational age of the fetus (the trimester of pregnancy), the location and type of cancer, how aggressively the cancer is growing, the stage of the cancer, and the overall health of the mother. Although some chemotherapies can be used after the first trimester, during critical fetal development, women are advised to consult with their doctors before starting treatment during the pregnancy. Chemotherapeutic medication can affect the fetus when it crosses the placenta and can increase the risk of miscarriage, low birth weight, or premature birth.

Survival perspective and prospects: Pregnancy does not lower the risk of survival or increase the risk of recurrence of breast cancer in women with a history of breast cancer. Studies have shown that women diagnosed with breast cancer during pregnancy did as well in the long term as did women with the same type and stage of cancer who were not pregnant when diagnosed. Although rarely occurring during pregnancy, cervical cancer during pregnancy also results in survival rates similar to those for nonpregnant women who were diagnosed at least five years following delivery. However, the survival rate of women diagnosed during the first six months postpartum is significantly worse than those diagnosed during pregnancy or nonpregnant counterparts diagnosed years later. Women diagnosed with cervical cancer during pregnancy may want to consult with their medical provider regarding options for delivery, such as by cesarean section rather than vaginally.

Women who have cancer or a history of the disease are advised to talk with their doctors if they are considering becoming pregnant. Certain cancer treatments can affect fertility, and women may wish to preserve their fertility. Considerations include estrogen receptors of cancer cells, difficulty in becoming pregnant, chemotherapy's effect on a woman's ovaries, and delaying childbearing until five years following treatment. Also, fertility treatment options for the woman with cancer or a history of cancer who wishes to become pregnant may be restricted due to the need to stimulate hormones during the course of most fertility treatments.

Susan H. Peterman, M.P.H.

▶ For Further Information

Adler, L., and P. Sykes. "How Little Is Known About Cervical Cancer in Pregnancy?" *Annals of Oncology (European Society for Medical Oncology)* 16, no. 3 (2005): 341-343.

Barnea, Eytan R., Eric Jauniaux, and Peter E. Schwartz, eds. *Cancer and Pregnancy*. London: Springer, 2001.

Koren, G., M. Lishner, and D. Farine, eds. *Cancer in Pregnancy: Maternal and Fetal Risks*. New York: Cambridge University Press, 1996.

Schover, Leslie R. *Sexuality and Fertility After Cancer*. New York: John Wiley & Sons, 1997.

▶ Other Resources

American Society of Clinical Oncology
http://www.asco.org

Leukaemia Research Foundation
http://www.lrf.org.uk

Mother Risk
http://www.motherrisk.org

Susan G. Komen for the Cure
http://www.cms.komen.org

See also Breast cancer in pregnant women; Cervical cancer; Childbirth and cancer; Diethylstilbestrol (DES); Fallopian tube cancer; Family history and risk assessment; Fertility drugs and cancer; Fertility issues; Fibroadenomas; Genetic testing; Gynecologic cancers; Gynecologic oncology; Hodgkin disease; Imaging tests; Magnetic resonance imaging (MRI); Mammography; Sexuality and cancer; Smoking cessation; Transvaginal ultrasound; Ultrasound tests.

▶ Premalignancies

Category: Diseases, symptoms, and conditions
Also known as: Premalignant lesions, dysplasia, neoplasia, neoplasms, dysplastic syndromes, neoplastic syndromes

Related conditions: Myelodysplastic syndromes in blood and bone marrow

Definition: Premalignancies are caused by the abnormal maturation of cells in a particular tissue. Premalignant cells are often immature and undifferentiated. An area with abnormal cells of this kind is called a premalignant lesion or a neoplasm. When the abnormal cells are limited to the tissue of origin, the condition is called dysplasia. Myelodysplastic syndromes arise when abnormal immature stem cells, called blasts, are present in the bone marrow or blood. In these syndromes, the abnormal blast cells crowd out the normal mature cells and platelets, resulting in anemia and a loss of immune function.

Risk factors: General risk factors for premalignancies include exposure to environmental pollutants and tobacco smoke, older age, and a family history of certain cancers (essentially, the same risk factors as for cancer development). Premalignancies for certain types of cancers have specific risk factors.

Epidermal premalignant lesions in the form of actinic keratosis are usually caused by sun damage, and basal cell lesions probably arise because of deoxyribonucleic acid (DNA) damage from ultraviolet radiation.

For colorectal cancer, people with a family history of premalignant lesions or polyps are at greater risk of having polyps and colorectal cancer. Individuals who have had inflammatory bowel disease (ulcerative colitis and Crohn disease) for more than eight years are also at greater risk of developing premalignant polyps and colorectal cancer.

Risk factors for gastrointestinal premalignant lesions include gastritis caused by infection with the bacterium *Helicobacter pylori* and gastroesophageal reflux disease (GERD), which can progress to a condition called Barrett esophagus, the only known premalignant condition for esophageal adenocarcinoma. Risk factors for Barrett esophagus are being a man, white, over fifty years old, a cigarette smoker, and obese, and having a history of reflux symptoms lasting more than five years.

Risk factors for myelodysplastic syndromes include being a man and over age sixty, having had prior treatment with chemotherapy or radiation therapy, and being exposed to tobacco smoke, pesticides, mercury, and lead.

Etiology and the disease process: Genetic abnormalities in the cell disrupt its normal maturation process, causing it to become premalignant. The traditional theory is that cancer progresses through a series of steps, from premalignant lesions to carcinoma in situ (localized cancer) and then to invasive carcinoma. Some researchers challenge this theory, arguing that most, if not all, of the molecular changes that occur in the cancer transformation process are present in premalignant lesions. For example, genetic analysis of premalignant lesions in mice has shown that gene abnormalities and changes in protein expression in the premalignant cells can be linked to the particular phenotype of the cancer cell (that is, the physical and biochemical characteristics of the cell). One study in mice showed that the molecular profiles (genes and proteins) of lesions in different stages of breast cancer had many similarities, suggesting that there may be a limited number of molecular changes associated with tumor progression.

Different cell types give rise to premalignant lesions in varied ways. In skin cancer, basal cell lesions are the most common type of premalignancy. These premalignant lesions occur in the basal epithelium of the skin, usually on the lower trunk and thighs. The premalignancies look like basal epithelium cells surrounded by a fibrous stroma and are thus called fibroepithelial premalignant tumors of Pinkus. Researchers have shown that the premalignant cells have abnormal cell cycle regulation, which most likely initiates their transformation from normal cells. In cancer progression, these abnormal basal cells grow aggressively until they predominate in the lesion, and the premalignant lesion becomes invasive basal cell epithelioma.

Other premalignant tumors occur in the epidermis. Epidermal premalignant lesions can take the form of Bowen disease, where abnormal cells are present throughout the epidermis and have the potential to develop into invasive squamous cell carcinoma. Bowen disease predominantly occurs in the lower limbs and resembles dermatitis or psoriasis, with scaly patches. Epidermal premalignant lesions can also be in the form of acitinic keratosis, where abnormal cells do not penetrate the entire epidermis and have a small probability (2 to 5 percent) of developing into cancer. Actinic keratosis is usually caused by sun damage.

Gastrointestinal premalignant lesions can arise from gastritis caused by infection with the bacterium *H. pylori*. Another condition that can result in a premalignancy is gastroesophageal reflux disease, which involves backflow of stomach acids up the esophagus, causing damage to the squamous epithelial cells lining the esophagus. This tissue damage can progress to a condition called Barrett esophagus, where normal esophageal squamous epithelial cells are replaced with specialized columnar epithelium containing goblet cells. This condition is often accompanied by dysplasia or metaplasia, and people with Barrett esophagus have a 0.5 percent risk of developing esophageal cancer (esophageal adenocarcinoma).

The etiology of colorectal cancer is still unclear, but it appears to involve a genetic component, with approximately 25 percent of colorectal cancer patients having a family member with the disease. Other factors such as diet, the composition of bile acids, and exposure to carcinogens are being studied. Individuals who have the rare familial adenomatous polyposis (FAP) syndrome, which is a hereditary genetic defect in which people develop hundreds to thousands of colorectal polyps at a young age, are at higher risk for developing colorectal cancer, and these individuals account for 1 percent of colorectal cancer cases annually.

Incidence: Incidence varies depending on the type of cell from which the premalignancy arises.

Symptoms: Symptoms vary depending on the organ in which the premalignant lesions occur. For example, Bowen disease predominantly occurs in the lower limbs and resembles dermatitis or psoriasis, with scaly patches. Actinic keratosis is characterized by epidermal premalignant lesions and can manifest as single or multiple scaly papules.

In the colon, premalignant lesions called polyps are often discovered during a routine colonoscopy. Other signs of polyps include blood in the stool. Removal of these premalignant polyps considerably decreases the probability of developing cancer.

Symptoms of myelodysplastic syndromes include shortness of breath (also known as dyspnea), fatigue, pale skin, bruising or bleeding readily, petechiae (pinpoint spots under the skin due to bleeding), fever, and frequent infections.

Screening and diagnosis: Routine skin examinations can detect premalignant skin lesions, which can then be excised before they can progress to skin cancer. The ABCD and seven-point checklists provide guidelines for classifying lesions according to their risk of developing into malignant melanoma. The ABCD checklist has four criteria: "A" for asymmetry (if the lesion is bisected, asymmetry of the two halves predisposes for malignancy), "B" for border irregularity (an uneven border is a risk factor), "C" for color variation (more than one color is a risk factor), and "D" for diameter (diameter greater than 6 millimeters, or mm, is a warning sign). The seven-point checklist for malignant melanoma includes three major signs (change in size, shape, or color) and four minor signs (inflammation, crusting or bleeding, sensory change, and a diameter of 7 mm or more). In addition to the criteria in these checklists, the shape of the lesion can be used as an indicator of malignancy. A more geometrically angular shape may be associated with a higher risk of malignant melanoma.

A range of screening and diagnostic tests help detect gastrointestinal lesions. Premalignancies associated with Barrett esophagus can be detected by means of endoscopic screening. Patients who are found to have Barrett esophagus and dysplasia can undergo treatment to prevent progression to esophageal cancer. For colorectal cancer screening, premalignant lesions (called polyps) are often discovered during a colonoscopy. They can also be found via sigmoidoscopy, in which a flexible tube with a camera is inserted into the rectum and lower colon. A small tissue sample can be taken at the same time. Another method of discovering polyps is the fecal occult blood test, which looks for blood in the stool. If blood is found, a colonoscopy is performed. Other methods include computed tomographic colonography (CTC; also known as "virtual" colonography), which involves scanning the colon by CT to produce a three-dimensional image that can be analyzed for polyps, and a double-contrast barium enema, in which barium is ingested by the patient and X rays are taken to look at the colon and rectum. Double-contrast barium enema testing is not as sensitive as a colonoscopy and is usually not used for screening.

Treatment and therapy: Skin lesions that are diagnosed as premalignant can be excised from the skin if they are basal cell derived, or they can be subjected to cryotherapy, excision, curettage, or topical 5-fluorouracil application if they are of the squamous cell carcinoma type.

Premalignant and malignant oral lesions can be treated with carbon dioxide laser surgery, a noninvasive method that is associated with less pain, bleeding, edema, and lower recurrence rates and risk of infection. Patients who are found to have Barrett esophagus and dysplasia can undergo ablative therapy, which includes acid-reducing drugs (including aspirin), proton pump inhibitors, antireflux surgery, or esophagectomy for more severe conditions.

For colorectal premalignancies, surgery is used to remove infected parts of the colon. For patients with familial adenomatous polyposis (FAP), sometimes the entire colon is removed (colectomy) to reduce the risk of cancer progression. Drugs such as the COX-2 inhibitors, including celecoxib (Celebrex) and sulindac (Clinoril), have the potential to reduce colorectal cancer risk and could be appropriate for some people.

Prognosis, prevention, and outcomes: Detecting premalignancies and treating them creates a much better prognosis than not detecting these tumors until they have become malignant or have metastasized. The timely treatment of premalignant lesions can allow patients to live disease-free for long period of time.

To help prevent premalignant skin lesions, people should avoid excessive ultraviolet light exposure by using sunscreen and protective clothing, staying out of the sun during peak ultraviolet-B radiation hours, and avoiding suntanning.

A diet high in fiber and low in fat may aid in the prevention of colorectal cancer. Individuals at risk for this type of cancer because of their family history or long-standing inflammatory bowel disease should regularly undergo colonoscopy to check for polyps, which helps prevent malignancies from developing. Other types of gastrointestinal premalignancies can be prevented by early treatment of infection with *H. pylori* and taking steps to prevent or alleviate gastroesophageal reflux.

Ing-Wei Khor, Ph.D.

▶ For Further Information

Cheah, P. Y. "Hypothesis for the Etiology of Colorectal Cancer: An Overview." *Nutrition and Cancer* 14 (1990): 5-13.

Chin, K., et al. "In Situ Analyses of Genome Instability in Breast Cancer." *Nature Genetics* 36 (2004): 984-988.

Dias Pereira, A., A. Suspiro, and P. Chaves. "Cancer Risk in Barrett's Oesophagus." *European Journal of Gastroenterology and Hepatology* 19 (2007): 915-918.

Ma, X. J., et al. "Gene Expression Profiles of Human Breast Cancer Progression." *Proceedings of the National Academy of Sciences of the United States of America* 100 (2003): 5974-5979.

Rustgi, A. K. "Hereditary Gastrointestinal Polyposis and Nonpolyposis Syndromes." *New England Journal of Medicine* 331 (1994): 1694.

Schuchert, M. G., and J. D. Luketich. "Management of Barrett's Esophagus." *Oncology (Williston Park)* 21 (2007): 1382-1389.

▶ Other Resources

GeneticHealth

Colon Cancer in People with FAP
http://www.genetichealth.com/CRC_FAP_FAP_and_Colon_Cancer.shtml

The Medical Group of Ohio

Do You Know Your ABCD's of Skin Cancer Detection?
http://www.themgo.com/DesktopDefault.aspx?tabid=153&itemid=1984&

Memorial Sloan-Kettering Cancer Center

Colorectal Cancer Screening Guidelines
http://www.mskcc.org/mskcc/html/65282.cfm#282976

Skin Cancer Foundation

http://www.skincancer.org

See also ABCD; Achlorhydria; Anemia; Barium enema; Barrett esophagus; Benign tumors; Biopsy; Bowen disease; Breast cancers; Cancer biology; Carcinomas; Cobalt 60 radiation; Colectomy; Colon polyps; Colonoscopy and virtual colonoscopy; Colorectal cancer; Crohn disease; Dysplastic nevus syndrome; Edema; Esophageal cancer; Esophagectomy; *Helicobacter pylori*; Hereditary mixed polyposis syndrome; Hereditary polyposis syndromes; Inflammatory bowel disease; Juvenile polyposis syndrome; Keratosis; Melanomas; Moles; Myelodysplastic syndromes; Oncology; Pancolitis; Polyps; Rectal cancer; Sigmoidoscopy; Skin cancers; Squamous cell carcinomas.

▶ Prevent Cancer Foundation

Category: Organizations

Also known as: Cancer Research and Prevention Foundation, Cancer Research Foundation of America (CRFA)

Definition: The Prevent Cancer Foundation is a nonprofit fund-raising organization that supports educational programs, cancer screenings, and research targeted at preventing cancers.

History: Carolyn Richardson Aldigé, a former endocrinology researcher, initiated the Cancer Research Foundation of America (CRFA) in 1985 after her father's death due to cancer. She felt that increased knowledge and use of prevention methods might effectively lessen the number of cancers and enhance survival. Aldigé, who became the foundation's president, designed CRFA to encourage and support cancer prevention research, educational resources, and screenings.

The CRFA's board of directors, medical advisory board, and scientific review panel oversee its work. In 2002, the CRFA became the Cancer Research and Prevention Foundation. Five years later, the organization's name changed again, becoming the Prevent Cancer Foundation. From 1985 to 2007, the organization secured approximately $95 million for its projects.

Education: The Prevent Cancer Foundation emphasizes public awareness of basic strategies—improving nutrition, changing habits regarding smoking and sun exposure, and engaging in exercise—to prevent cancer or control it after diagnosis. The foundation provides educational material on its Web site and pamphlets in English and Spanish. Its *Cancer Prevention Works*, an electronic newsletter, contains research updates, news, and advice.

The Prevent Cancer Foundation's educational exhibits include *Check Your Insides Out—From Top to Bottom*, which contains a twenty-foot-long, eight-foot-high Super Colon that people can enter to see examples of cancerous polyps. The foundation's *Save Your Skin* display emphasizes the dangers of ultraviolet (UV) rays. A computer program reveals the aging effects of UV rays on facial skin. Information provided by the foundation explains how to examine skin for malignancies and avoid UV damage.

During the 1990's, the Prevent Cancer Foundation introduced software for children called Dr. Health'nstein's Body Fun. Players virtually thrived or declined according to their decisions regarding what they ate, how much they exercised, and whether they used tobacco and other substances. The Prevent Cancer Foundation and Alabama public educators evaluated using Dr. Health'nstein's Body Fun technology for health education. Some California, Georgia, Massachusetts, and Arizona public schools have incorporated that software into their curricula.

The Prevent Cancer Foundation holds yearly national meetings for medical professionals. Its workshops demonstrate how new technologies might improve cancer prevention. It also cohosts the yearly Summit on Cancer Clinical Trials, which raises public awareness of trials and promotes participation.

Outreach: Foundation grants enhance screening availability by sponsoring displays at state fairs and such mobile health services as George Washington University Cancer Center's Mammovan, which screens uninsured women for breast cancer. Since 1994, the Prevent Cancer Foundation has funded ¡Celebremos la Vida! (let's celebrate life) to screen Hispanic women for cervical and breast cancers. The foundation provides money for the Cancer Preventorium, started by Elmer Huerta, a board member and physician, to screen both male and female Hispanics for cancer.

The Prevent Cancer Foundation sponsors Project Early Awareness, which provides breast education for minority teenage girls so that they can learn breast cancer screening methods and teach them to other young women. The foundation promotes Make the Connection, Make the Commitment, emphasizing the human papillomavirus (HPV) link to cervical cancer.

In March, 2000, the Prevent Cancer Foundation initiated National Colorectal Cancer Awareness Month. The foundation distributes buddy bracelets to encourage people to schedule colonoscopies.

The Prevent Cancer Foundation funds cancer education services for children and pediatric cancer research through Hope Street Kids and Tracy's Kids. The foundation supports the Congressional Families Action for Cancer Awareness Program, which stresses prevention.

Research: By 2007, the Prevent Cancer Foundation had funded an estimated 250 researchers affiliated with 150 academic institutions and medical and research centers. Twice yearly, the Prevent Cancer Foundation Scientific Review Panel, including representatives from the National Cancer Institute and major cancer centers, evaluates proposals. Any researcher who has received money from the tobacco industry cannot apply.

The Prevent Cancer Foundation provides funds for various grants financed with allied groups, including the American Society for Preventive Oncology. Starting in 2002, the American Association for Cancer Research (AARC)-Cancer Research and Prevention Foundation (CRPF) Award for Excellence in Cancer Prevention Research annually honored investigators.

Advocacy: The Prevent Cancer Foundation issues policy statements concerning cancer prevention issues. It has supported legislation regarding colorectal cancer and stem cell research and has urged medical professionals and pharmaceutical manufacturers to increase the availability of the human papillomavirus vaccine to uninsured and low-income young women.

Elizabeth D. Schafer, Ph.D.

▶ For Further Information

Geiger, Brian F., et al. "Using Technology to Teach Health: A Collaborative Pilot Project in Alabama." *Journal of School Health* 72, no. 10 (December, 2002): 401-407.

Lippman, Scott M., et al. "Cancer Prevention and the American Society of Clinical Oncology." *Journal of Clinical Oncology* 22, no. 19 (October 1, 2004): 3848-3851.

Sawyer, Kathy. "Breast Cancer Drug Testing Will Continue: Potential of Tamoxifen Is Said to Outweigh Risks." *Washington Post*, May 12, 1994, p. A3.

Trafford, Abigail. "On the Streets of Philadelphia, Prescriptions for Progress." *Washington Post*, August 8, 2000, p. Z5.

▶ Other Resources

Hope Street Kids
http://www.hopestreetkids.org

Prevent Cancer Foundation
http://www.preventcancer.org

Tracy's Kids
http://www.tracyskids.org

See also American Association for Cancer Research (AACR); American Cancer Society (ACS); American Institute for Cancer Research (AICR); Dana-Farber Cancer

Institute; Duke Comprehensive Cancer Center; Fox Chase Cancer Center; Fred Hutchinson Cancer Research Center; Jonsson Comprehensive Cancer Center (JCCC); M. D. Anderson Cancer Center; Mayo Clinic Cancer Center; Memorial Sloan-Kettering Cancer Center; National Cancer Institute (NCI); National Science Foundation (NSF); Robert H. Lurie Cancer Center.

▶ Prevention

Category: Lifestyle and prevention

Definition: Prevention of cancer can be defined as reducing cancer mortality by reducing the incidence of cancer.

Cancer in the United States: The National Cancer Institute issued a report in 2005 describing various statistical aspects of cancer in the United States. Overall death rates for the most common cancers, such as breast, lung, colorectal, and prostate, had declined. Survival rates for cancer patients were rising. The incidence of cancer had been stable since the 1990's. However, the prevalence of cancers such as melanoma of the skin and childhood cancers was increasing. Cancer remained the second leading cause of death in the United States. In 2003 more than half a million Americans had lost their lives to cancer.

Lowering the number of cases of cancer is a multifaceted process of avoiding exposures to known carcinogens, modifying lifestyle habits, and taking active steps to enhance the body's immune system. Although behaviors that help people avoid developing cancer, such as not smoking and lessening consumption of fat and alcohol, are on the rise in the United States, more needs to be done. Prevention generally falls into the categories of lifestyle, chemoprevention (use of vitamins and medicines), preventive surgery, screening, and environment. Prevention of cancer is an active process in which all Americans need to involve themselves to reduce their lifetime chance of cancer.

Research suggests that as much as two-thirds of all cancer can be prevented with lifestyle changes in daily living. Every day, each person makes choices that could increase or reduce that person's likelihood of developing cancer. No knowledge or program can prevent cancer on its own: People must make responsible choices and integrate them into their lifestyle.

Nutrition: Nutrition is a key part of cancer prevention. Much has been researched and written about the importance of nutrition. Although the relationship between diet and cancer is complex, numerous studies show that nutrition can make a difference in preventing cancer. The American Cancer Society promotes eating five to seven or more servings of fruits and vegetables each day as the single most important step people can take to prevent cancer. People can achieve this goal by eating vegetables and fruits at each meal and for snacks. Strawberries, raspberries, blueberries, and blackberries have cancer-fighting chemicals, as do citrus fruits such as oranges and grapefruit. Certain phytonutrients in vegetables, such as the indoles found in broccoli and cabbage, can help protect against cancer, especially hormone-related cancers. Generally the more color the vegetable has, the healthier and more protective it is. The likelihood of developing colon cancer and other gastrointestinal cancers may be decreased by eating dark green and yellow vegetables. Fruits and vegetables in their whole or natural form (fresh, frozen, dried, or canned) are more protective than supplements with dried extracts.

The nutritional aspect of prevention includes other foods besides fruits and vegetables. The use of whole-grain breads and cereals adds fiber to the diet. High-fiber diets increase motility of food through the colon and are thought to protect against colon cancer. Eating less meat may be accomplished by choosing beans as a protein source; meat consumption has been associated with colon and prostate cancer. Other foods, such as garlic, onions, soybeans, and ginger, are thought to protect against cancer by some experts. Herbal teas such as red clover or green tea have demonstrated promise in studies on cancer prevention.

How food is cooked can affect the nutrients or introduce carcinogens into the body. For example, meat protein cooked at high temperatures produces toxic substances. Studies have linked colorectal adenomas to red meat cooked at high temperatures. Processed meats and bacon contain carcinogens. Boiling vegetables can release nutrients into the water, so steaming is preferred to preserve the vitamins.

Studies have looked at the possibility of food preservatives and additives being carcinogenic, but the studies have not been conclusive. Foods are treated with chemicals to improve taste, increase shelf life, and allow them to be transported long distances in trucks. More than three thousand preservatives and additives are used in the U.S. food supply system. Some experts say that formaldehyde, a suspected carcinogen, is either contained in or released by some food preservatives and constitutes a hazard to humans; however, this has not been proven. Some people have chosen to minimize their exposure to additives and preservatives by eating more food in the raw state and purchasing organic foods and milk.

Exercise: Physical activity and exercise can help protect against developing certain cancers of the breast, colon, and prostate. The most recent guidelines by the Centers for Disease Control and Prevention (CDC) recommend that adults exercise moderately (for example, walking at a brisk pace) for a minimum of thirty minutes per day, five days per week, or exercise vigorously (for example, race-walking, jogging, or running) for a minimum of twenty minutes per day, three days per week. This recommendation complements the need to decrease the epidemic of obesity in the United States, as obesity is associated with increased risk of developing cancers of the colon and rectum, breast, prostate, kidney, and uterus (endometrium).

Alcohol: Alcohol use is associated with increased risk of mouth, esophagus (throat), larynx (voice box), and liver cancer. The amount of alcohol consumed affects the risk of cancer. Men are advised to have no more than two drinks per day and women no more than one drink per day. (One drink is 12 ounces of beer, 5 ounces of wine, or 1.5 ounces of 80-proof liquor.) Women who drink are at increased risk for breast cancer. When smoking is combined with excessive alcohol consumption, the risk is compounded. Excessive alcohol consumption can result in liver damage that affects the body's ability to excrete toxins and can effect cancer treatment. Wine is associated with an increased risk of upper digestive tract cancers in heavy users; however, some studies have shown that moderate consumption of red wine, which contains phytochemicals, may convey some cancer-fighting benefits.

Tobacco: Smoking and use of tobacco products is a choice made by many Americans. Smoking produces known carcinogens that can result in lung cancer as well as cancer of the upper respiratory tract (throat, mouth, and windpipe). Secondhand smoke (smoke in the environment that is inhaled by nonsmokers) can affect people's health, so many states and cities have banned smoking in restaurants or require them to have nonsmoking sections. Many states and cities also ban smoking in workplaces, bars, public buildings, and public gathering places. Though smoking overall is declining and death rates from lung cancer in men are declining, death rates from lung cancer in women have continued to rise.

Other methods of cancer prevention: Chemoprevention is a term that describes the use of natural or synthetic substances to avert cancer. Methods include the use of cancer-fighting nutrients (such as phytoestrogens) in food, herbs, and supplements that are believed to help prevent cancer. Medications such as tamoxifen or raloxifene to reduce the incidence of breast cancer, and vaccines such as the human papillomavirus (HPV) vaccine can prevent cervical cancer.

Preventive (prophylactic) surgery is useful in some cases for patients at high risk for cancer. Preventive procedures include removal of the breast (mastectomy), ovaries, and Fallopian tubes.

Cancer screening, a key part of cancer prevention, is covered by many insurance companies, including Medicare. Coverage may include mammograms for breast cancer, colorectal cancer diagnostic tests such as a colonoscopy, prostate-specific antigen (PSA) tests for prostate cancer, and Pap smears for cervical cancer. Early detection and treatment is one reason that cancer survival rates are rising.

Protective clothing and gear can help reduce the cancer risk from environmental hazards. Examples of cancer-causing substances that can be introduced into the workplace include silica from cement, wood dust, lacquers, wood finishes, paints, glues, solvents, asphalt, and pesticides. Wearing an appropriate mask and using proper ventilation can help decrease exposure to these toxins. Using the provided safeguards when taking (or giving) X rays in a hospital or at a dental office can decrease exposure to harmful radiation that can cause cancer. Those working outdoors and exposed to the sun's ultraviolet (UV) rays can minimize their risk of skin cancer by staying out of the sun in midday, using sunscreen, and wearing protective clothing and hats.

Cancer prevention requires vigilance on the part of each individual as well as businesses and the government. However, prevention is the best way to "treat" cancer and can save many lives.

Marylane Wade Koch, M.S.N., R.N.

▶ For Further Information

American Institute for Cancer Research. *Stopping Cancer Before It Starts: The American Institute for Cancer Research's Program for Cancer Prevention.* New York: St. Martin's Griffin, 2000.

Conley, Edward J. *The Breast Cancer Prevention Plan.* New York: McGraw-Hill, 2006.

National Cancer Institute. *Cancer Trends Progress Report 2005.* Bethesda, Md.: Author, 2005.

Verona, Verne. *Nature's Cancer Fighting Foods.* New York: Prentice Hall, 2001.

▶ Other Resources

American Institute for Cancer Research
http://www.aicr.org

Breast Cancer Prevention.com
http://www.breastcancerprevention.org

Cancer Index
Cancer Screening and Prevention
http://www.cancerindex.org/clinks4p.htm

Ohio State University: Extension Fact Sheet
Chemoprevention the Answer to Cancer?
http://ohioline.osu.edu/hyg-fact/5000/5051.html

Prevent Cancer Foundation
http://www.preventcancer.org

Smokefree.gov
http://www.smokefree.gov

World Health Organization
Cancer Prevention
http://www.who.int/cancer/prevention/en

See also Cancer care team; Carcinogens, known; Carcinogens, reasonably anticipated; Chemoprevention; Childhood cancers; Exercise and cancer; Fiber; Fruits; Garlic and allicin; Green tea; Infusion therapies; Nutrition and cancer prevention; Obesity-associated cancers; Pesticides and the food chain; Relationships; Smoking cessation; Sunscreens; Tobacco-related cancers; Wine and cancer.

▶ Primary care physician

Category: Medical specialties
Also known as: PCP, general practitioner, family practice specialist

Definition: A primary care physician is a doctor who diagnoses and treats common illnesses and medical conditions. A primary care physician is often the doctor who provides the initial, or first-contact, care when an individual feels ill. By considering the individual's health, well-being, and lifestyle, the primary care physician focuses on prevention rather than short-term acute care. There are four types of primary care in which a primary care physician may be certified: family practice medicine, pediatrics, obstetrics and gynecology, and internal medicine. A primary care physician is a generalist who does not specialize in diagnosing and treating a specific organ system, as does a cardiologist, neurologist, endocrinologist, and so on. Primary care physicians are also trained to counsel and educate patients about their disease, instruct in self-care, conduct preventive screenings, and administer immunizations.

Subspecialties: Internal medicine, family medicine, pediatrics, and obstetrics and gynecology

Cancers treated: All, especially skin, breast, and prostate cancers

Training and certification: A postgraduate primary care residency specialty program is three years in length and trains the internist in both ambulatory and hospital care. In addition to undergoing training in internal medicine practice, focusing on developing skills in diagnosing and treating a broad range of medical conditions, primary care physicians are trained in interviewing skills, recognizing and treating common psychiatric illnesses (primary or secondary to a primary medical condition), and counseling to promote behavior change. Primary care physicians are certified by their state licensing boards in their primary care specialties. The American Board of Medical Specialties (ABMS) oversees the ongoing evaluation and certification of specialists, thus setting standards for what is considered competency in practicing the medical specialty. The Accreditation Council for Continuing Medical Education (AACME) provides guidelines for continuing medical education required for primary care physicians to renew their licenses by ensuring that they maintain their competence and assimilate new knowledge to improve the care they provide patients.

Services and procedures performed: The primary care physician is trained in (but not limited to) the following: interviewing the patient and family for a medical history and current symptom history; conducting a comprehensive physical examination; mental health counseling relative to the medical condition; nutrition counseling; referring patients to labs for testing blood and other specimens, as well as interpreting the results from these tests; administering and reading X rays and results of other diagnostic tests; administering electrocardiograms and screening mammograms; instructing in self-exams; and consulting with specialists and other medical care providers.

Primary care physicians may be involved in early detection and treatment of all types of cancer, depending on the scope of the physician's practice, experience, and skills, as well as the needs of the patient and the patient's family. Primary care physicians act as gatekeepers who regulate access to medical specialists as needed. Since early detection and screening are critical to treatment and prognosis of cancers, the primary care physician is responsible for performing a thorough physical examination of the patient, taking a patient's medical history, and interviewing the patient to define the symptoms that have prompted the patient to seek care. Primary care physicians play a critical role in educating patients about risk factors (such as smoking, diet, occupational hazards, and other lifestyle factors) thought to contribute to developing cancers, and they teach patients to conduct self-examinations as appropriate.

Primary care physicians play a particularly important role in screening for those cancers for which preventive measures have proven effective, including but not limited to breast cancer (self-exam and mammography), cervical cancer (Pap testing), colorectal cancer (fecal occult blood test and sigmoidoscopy or colonoscopy for persons older than fifty), melanomas (skin cancer), and prostate cancer (prostate-specific antigen, or PSA, blood test and rectal exam). It has been reported that as many as 80 percent of individuals with common forms of cancer initially complain of symptoms to their primary care physicians. Studies have reported that women with breast cancer are more likely to be diagnosed earlier if they reside in areas with a rich supply of primary care physicians. Primary care physicians also can play a vital role in following cancer survivors, such as educating patients in behaviors that can reduce risk of recurring cancers and following up with maintenance visits.

The primary care physician will often refer a patient with a suspected cancer to a cancer specialist. Following referral, the primary care physician can continue to be involved in the care of the patient by communicating the diagnosis; forwarding all medical records containing family and symptom history, evaluations, procedures, and lab tests used for diagnosis; helping to set a treatment plan; coordinating specialty care; referring the patient and, as needed, the patient's family, for psychological support; treating illnesses secondary to the diagnosis and treatment of the cancer; scheduling follow-up visits for preventive care; and managing the side effects of the cancer and its treatment. Testimony to the importance of the primary care physician's role in diagnosing cancer are reports that a typical primary care physician will have three or four patients per year who have received a new diagnosis of cancer.

The benefits of having a primary care physician involved in ongoing cancer care are many. It has been reported that patients who are followed by a primary care physician as well as an oncologist or cancer specialist are more likely to receive preventive care and care for a noncancer chronic illness during the course of cancer treatment than are those who are followed only by an oncologist or cancer specialist. In addition, continuous primary care of patients who are being treated for a cancer primarily by a specialist can reduce visits to acute care or emergency room facilities and contribute to palliative care, which may enable the terminally ill cancer patient to die at home.

Although chemotherapy and radiation are usually directed by a subspecialist, the subspecialist may contact the primary care physician to manage potential adverse effects of treatment, such as vomiting and nausea, fever and neutropenia (a hematologic or blood disorder characterized by an unusually low number of neutrophils, a type of white blood cell that fights infection), fatigue, ongoing care following chemotherapy and radiation, sleep disturbances, exercise, depression, anxiety, pain, and ensuring that the patient maintains a healthy diet.

Related specialties and subspecialties: Primary care physicians may specialize in family medicine, geriatrics, pediatrics, obstetrics and gynecology, or preventive medicine. A variety of other medical care providers—such as nurse practitioners, registered nurses, physician assistants, and osteopaths—may provide primary care in their settings of practice or work in the setting.

Susan H. Peterman, M.P.H.

▶ For Further Information

Gore, Martin E., and Douglas Russell. *Primary Care and Cancer*. Edited by Paul F. Engstrom. New York: Informa Healthcare, 2003.

Hass, Jennifer, Celia Kaplan, et al. "Do Physicians Tailor Their Recommendations for Breast Cancer Risk Reduction Based on Patient's Risk?" *Journal of General Internal Medicine* 19, no. 4 (2004): 302-309.

Smith, George F., and Timothy R. Toonen. "Primary Care of the Patient with Cancer." *American Family Physician* 75, no. 8 (April 15, 2007): 1207-1214.

Summerton, Nicholas. *Diagnosing Cancer in Primary Care*. Abington, England: Radcliffe Medical, 1999.

▶ Organizations and Professional Societies

American Academy of Family Physicians
http://www.aafp.org
11400 Tomahawk Creek Parkway
Leawood, KS 66211-2672

American Association of Family Practice Physician Assistants
http://www.afppa.org
1905 Woodstock Road, Suite 2150
Roswell, GA 30075

American College of Physicians
http://www.acponline.org
190 N. Independence Mall West
Philadelphia, PA 19106-1572

Susan G. Komen for the Cure
http://cms.komen.org/komen/index.htm
5005 LBJ Freeway, Suite 250
Dallas, TX 75244

Other Resources

National Cancer Institute
http://www.cancer.gov

American Cancer Society
http://www.cancer.org

See also Gastrointestinal oncology; Gynecologic oncology; Health maintenance organizations (HMOs); Hematologic oncology; Managed care; Medical oncology; Neurologic oncology; Nutrition and cancer prevention; Nutrition and cancer treatment; Occupational exposures and cancer; Ophthalmic oncology; Pap test; Preferred provider organizations (PPOs).

Primary central nervous system lymphomas

Category: Diseases, symptoms, and conditions
Also known as: Primary cerebral lymphomas, non-Hodgkin lymphoma, reticulum cell sarcomas

Related conditions: Immunodeficient states including acquired immunodeficiency syndrome (AIDS), organ transplantation, prolonged immunosuppressive therapy, Wiskott-Aldrich syndrome, and Sjögren syndrome

Definition: Primary central nervous system lymphoma is a non-Hodgkin lymphoma, primarily B-cell type; it is a type of brain tumor that occurs in both normal and immunocompromised patients.

Risk factors: The main risk factor for primary central nervous system lymphoma is having AIDS.

Etiology and the disease process: Primary central nervous system lymphoma, if associated with AIDS, can manifest as poorly differentiated brain masses associated with hemorrhage and necrosis, composed of B cells (B lymphocytes), although T-cell lymphomas can also occur. It is thought that the dysfunction of suppressor T cells in AIDS patients leads to this B-cell lymphocytic cancer. In patients with normal immune systems, the brain tumor is usually more focal and well-circumscribed and is usually not associated with hemorrhage and necrosis.

Incidence: Primary central nervous system lymphoma makes up 1 to 2 percent of all intracranial neoplasms and 1 percent of all primary non-Hodgkin lymphomas. It occurs in 6 percent of patients with AIDS and is on the rise in both normal and immunocompromised patients, with a threefold increase since the late 1990's in patients with intact immune systems. The most common type to affect the brain is diffuse histiocytic lymphoma, also known as reticulum cell sarcoma. Because of the AIDS epidemic, primary central nervous system lymphoma is projected to become the most common primary malignancy of the brain.

Symptoms: Although primary central nervous system lymphoma can occur in all age groups, the average age at which it is diagnosed in normal adults is age sixty, but in immunocompromised patients it is found at the much younger average age of thirty-three. Its symptoms include headaches, seizures, focal neurologic impairment, and stupor.

Screening and diagnosis: Brain magnetic resonance imaging (MRI) findings often include periventricular and deep gray matter lesions with masses usually less than 2 centimeters (cm) in AIDS and greater than 2 cm in non-AIDS patients.

Treatment and therapy: Because this tumor is highly radiosensitive, radiotherapy is the treatment of choice, with regression of the tumor in most cases. Unfortunately, recurrence and progression typically occur after one year.

Prognosis, prevention, and outcomes: The prognosis is poor, with a median survival of thirteen and a half months after diagnosis.

Debra B. Kessler, M.D., Ph.D.

See also Brain and central nervous system cancers; Brain scan; Carcinomatous meningitis; Ependymomas; Gliomas; Hodgkin disease; Imaging tests; Lymphomas; Magnetic resonance imaging (MRI); Meningeal carcinomatosis; Non-Hodgkin lymphoma; Organ transplantation and cancer; Radiation therapies; Recurrence; Sjögren syndrome; Spinal cord compression.

Progesterone receptor assay

Category: Procedures
Also known as: PgR assay, hormone-response assay

Definition: A progesterone receptor assay is an immunoassay performed on sections from breast tumors removed during surgery or on small samples obtained with core needle biopsy.

Cancers diagnosed: Hormone-responsive breast cancer, ductal carcinoma in situ

Why performed: A progesterone receptor assay is used to determine whether a cancer is likely to respond to hormonal therapy.

Patient preparation: The assay is performed on sections of breast tumors removed during surgery or by needle biopsy. For needle biopsy, patients are usually asked not to use powder, deodorant, or perfume the day of the biopsy.

Steps of the procedure: Tumors that were removed during surgery are fixed and stained and then examined by a pathologist to determine whether the cells of the tumor express receptors for progesterone. For core needle biopsy, the patient is either upright or lying on her stomach. A local anesthetic is used to numb the breast, and a needle, which may be guided by X-ray imaging, is inserted into the breast mass. Samples of the mass are aspirated into the needle and then sent to a pathologist, who will stain the samples for the assay.

After the procedure: After surgery, the patient will be given specific instructions by the physician about activities. Patients can usually resume normal activity immediately after a needle biopsy.

Risks: For needle biopsy, the biopsied breast may occasionally show mild bruising.

Results: The progesterone receptor is a member of the steroid receptor superfamily of nuclear receptors. The steroid hormone progesterone binds to the receptor in the cell and regulates the expression of genes involved in growth and cell division. Expression of progesterone (PgR) or estrogen (ER) receptors in cancer cells indicates that they will respond to signals that inhibit their growth and division, including drugs that block signaling by estrogen and progesterone. The results are presented as positive or negative based on the number of hormone-responsive cells. A positive result, particularly in early-stage cancers that are both ER- and PgR-positive, suggests that a cancer will likely respond to hormonal (endocrine) therapies and generally signals a favorable prognosis. Such therapies may include removing the ovaries in premenopausal women, treating with an antiestrogen drug such as tamoxifen, or treating with an aromatase inhibitor to block the synthesis of estrogen by the body. A negative result on the progesterone receptor assay indicates that other types of treatments should be pursued.

Michele Arduengo, Ph.D., ELS

See also Adjuvant therapy; Breast cancers; Hormone receptor tests; Immunocytochemistry and immunohistochemistry; Leiomyomas; Meningiomas; Receptor analysis; Tumor markers.

▶ Prostate cancer

Category: Diseases, symptoms, and conditions
Also known as: Adenocarcinoma of the prostate

Related conditions: Benign prostatic hyperplasia (BPH), prostatitis

Definition: Prostate cancer is the growth of cancer cells in the prostate. A majority of prostate cancers start in the prostate gland. This type of cancer is referred to as an adenocarcinoma. There are other types of cancer cells that start in the prostate, but adenocarcinoma is the most common.

The prostate is a male reproductive gland, located in front of the rectum and below the bladder, that produces semen, the fluid that nourishes and transports sperm. The gland surrounds the urethra, the tube that carries urine outside the body. It is normally about the size and shape of a walnut.

Risk factors: The older a man gets, the higher his risk of getting prostate cancer. More than 70 percent of all diagnosed prostate cancer is found in men age sixty-five or older. Men with a family history of prostate cancer in an immediate relative, such as a father, brother, or son, are two to three times more likely to develop the disease. The disease is also more common among African American men, with more men in this racial group dying from the disease than in any other ethnic group. It is less common in men who are Hispanic, Asian, Native American, or from the Pacific Islands.

Etiology and the disease process: Prostate cancer is typically a slow-growing, silent disease that strikes older men. In fact, there are more men with prostate cancer who are never diagnosed and who never have symptoms than there

Incidence Rates of Prostate Cancer by Race, 2001-2005

Race	*Incidence per 100,000 Men*
All	163.0
Black	248.5
White	156.7
Hispanic	138.0
Asian	93.8
American Indian/Native Alaskan	73.3

Source: Data from National Cancer Institute, Surveillance Epidemiology and End Results, Cancer Stat Fact Sheets, 2008

are men diagnosed with the disease. However, some men develop an aggressive illness that can be life-threatening. There is not a clear understanding as to why some men develop an aggressive form of the disease while others may never know they have it.

Incidence: Prostate cancer is the second most common form of cancer among men in the United States—the most common is skin cancer—and the second leading cause of death, behind lung cancer. It is estimated that more than 235,000 men in the United States were diagnosed with this disease in 2006 and more than 27,000 men died from it.

Symptoms: Often, there are no symptoms until the disease has spread beyond the prostate, a condition called metastasis. Common symptoms may include frequent urination, a sudden urge to urinate, a weak urine stream, dribbling after urinating, straining to urinate, the inability to prevent urine leakage, or the sensation that the bladder is not empty even after urinating. Blood in the urine or semen, painful ejaculation, and pain in the lower back, hips, or thighs are also common complaints. The symptoms for prostate cancer are similar to those for the noncancerous conditions benign prostatic hyperplasia (BPH), prostatitis, or a urinary tract infection. If these symptoms occur, it is important to be checked by a doctor to determine the cause.

Screening and diagnosis: There are two tests commonly used to screen for prostate cancer: the prostate-specific antigen (PSA) blood test and the digital rectal exam (DRE). PSA is a protein produced by both normal and cancerous prostate cells that is released into the blood. This test measures the levels of PSA in the blood. High levels of PSA may be indicative of prostate cancer or noncancerous conditions.

For a digital rectal exam (DRE), the physician inserts a gloved, lubricated finger into the rectum to check the prostate for any unusual characteristics, such as an increase in size, nodules, or lumps. The benefit of the DRE as a screening tool for prostate cancer is that it can reach a part of the prostate gland where most cancers generally begin.

Men who are at high risk for the disease should begin testing with both a DRE and a PSA test at age forty-five. The recommended guidelines suggest testing for all other men beginning at age fifty.

If the PSA is high or there are suspicious findings during the DRE, additional testing is recommended. These tests may include a transrectal ultrasound or a biopsy. With a transrectal ultrasound, a small probe is inserted into the rectum to take ultrasound images of the prostate. If a suspicious area is found during the exam, a biopsy is taken.

The Prostate Gland

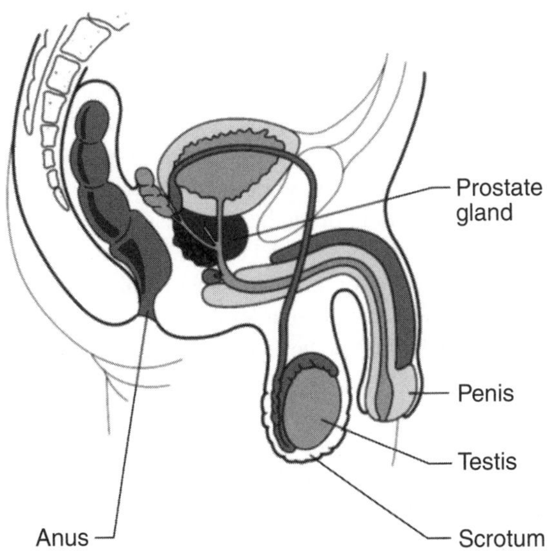

A biopsy is usually done with local anesthesia in a doctor's office. A small needle is inserted into the prostate to remove tissue samples. These samples are then examined under a microscope by a pathologist, a doctor who specializes in identifying diseases by examining tissues and cells, to determine if cancer cells are present and, if they are, how aggressive the disease may be.

When prostate cancer is diagnosed, it is given a Gleason score. The Gleason grade is a number between two and ten that reflects how closely the cancer cells resemble normal prostate tissue. In general, a low Gleason score suggests less aggressive tumors, and a higher Gleason score suggests more aggressive tumors.

The stage of the cancer refers to the extent of disease based on tumor location, size, number of tumors, and whether the cancer has spread outside the prostate gland to surrounding organs. Stages I and II refer to early-stage disease that is confined to the prostate. Stage III refers to locally advanced disease that has spread outside the prostate gland. Stage IV refers to cancer that has metastasized and possibly spread to the lymph nodes and other organs in the body.

Treatment and therapy: There are several treatment options, depending on age, overall health of the patient, and stage and grade of cancer. For men with local or locally advanced prostate cancer, treatment options generally include a radical prostatectomy, radiation therapy, hormone therapy, cryotherapy, and watchful waiting. Radical prostatectomy is surgical removal of the prostate gland and surrounding tissues. Radiation therapy is the administration of radiation energy to the prostate to destroy the cancer cells. Hormone therapy involves treatment to lower testosterone levels in the body, thereby reducing prostate cancer cell growth. Cryotherapy involves inserting a probe into the prostate to destroy cells by freezing the prostate gland. Watchful waiting, sometimes referred to as active surveillance, is monitoring the progression of the disease with regular examinations and testing. This option is usually recommended for men with other medical conditions or for those who would not tolerate surgery well.

For men with metastatic prostate cancer or men with returning cancer after surgery or radiation treatment, hormone therapy and chemotherapy are treatment options. Hormone therapy reduces prostate cancer cell growth, and chemotherapy destroys the cancer cells circulating throughout the body. Another option may be enrollment in ongoing clinical trials. Patients should discuss these options with their doctors and families to decide the best option to pursue.

Prognosis, prevention, and outcomes: Approximately 90 percent of prostate cancer is discovered in the early stages of the disease. When discovered at this stage, the five-year survival rate is almost 100 percent. When the cancer has spread to surrounding tissues or organs, the survival and cure rates vary, depending on the type and extent of disease.

As with other types of cancer, there is no definitive way to prevent prostate cancer. It is believed that good overall health; a diet low in fat and high in fruits, vegetables, and whole fibers; and plenty of exercise can strengthen the immune system and potentially slow the onset of cancer.

Vonne Sieve, M.A.

▶ For Further Information

Abdel-Wahab, May, and Orlando E. Silva, eds. *Prostate Cancer: A Practical Guide*. New York: Elsevier/Saunders, 2008.

American Cancer Society. *Quick Facts on Prostate Cancer: What You Need to Know—Now*. Atlanta: Author, 2007.

Bostwick, D. G., et al. "Human Prostate Cancer Risk Factors." *Cancer* 101, no. 10 (2004): 2371-2490.

Ellsworth, Pamela, John Heaney, and Cliff Gill. *One Hundred Questions and Answers About Prostate Cancer*. Sudbury, Mass.: Jones and Bartlett, 2003.

Metz, James M., and Margaret K. Hampshire. *Prostate Cancer*. New York: W. B. Saunders, 2008.

Tenke, P., J. Horti, P. Balint, and B. Kovacs. "Prostate Cancer Screening." *Recent Results in Cancer Research* 175 (2007): 65-81.

▶ Other Resources

American Prostate Cancer Initiative
http://www.americanprostate.org/involved.cfm

Cancer Research Institute
http://www.cancerresearch.org

National Cancer Institute
Prostate Cancer
http://www.nci.nih.gov/cancertopics/types/prostate

Prostate Cancer Foundation
http://www.prostatecancerfoundation.org

See also Benign prostatic hyperplasia (BPH); Carcinomas; Clinical trials; Digital rectal exam (DRE); Endorectal ultrasound; Gleason grading system; Metastasis; Prostate-specific antigen (PSA) test; Prostatectomy; Prostatitis; Proteomics and cancer research; Survival rates; Transrectal ultrasound; Watchful waiting.

▶ Prostate-specific antigen (PSA) test

Category: Procedures
Also known as: PSA blood test

Definition: The protein-specific antigen (PSA) test is a simple blood test used to screen for prostate cancer. PSA is a protein produced by both normal and cancerous prostate cells that is released into the blood. High levels of PSA may be indicative of prostate cancer, as well as other noncancerous conditions such as benign prostatic hyperplasia (BPH) or an infection or inflammation in the prostate. The first PSA test determines the baseline level. The PSA levels are compared each year and monitored for any changes.

Cancers diagnosed: Prostate cancer

Why performed: The benefit of this test is that it can detect signs of early-stage prostate cancer when there are no symptoms. When this cancer is treated in the early stages of the disease, there is a high probability of cure.

Prostate cancer is the second most common form of cancer among men in the United States—the most common is skin cancer—and the second leading cause of death behind lung cancer. It is estimated that nearly 235,000 men in the United States were diagnosed with this disease in 2006, and more than 27,000 men died from it.

Certain groups of men are at a greater risk of developing prostate cancer. Age is a risk factor; the older a man gets, the higher the risk of getting prostate cancer. More than 70 percent of all diagnosed prostate cancer is found in men sixty-five years of age or older. Men with a family history of prostate cancer in an immediate relative, such as a father, brother, or son, are two to three times more likely to develop the disease. It is also more common among African American men, with more men in this racial group dying from the disease than in any other ethnic group. It is less common in men who are Hispanic, Asian, Native American, or from the Pacific Islands.

Men who are at high risk for the disease should begin testing with both a digital rectal examination (DRE) and a PSA test at age forty-five. The recommended guidelines suggest testing for all other men beginning at age fifty. The test should be repeated yearly unless a medical provider suggests otherwise.

Patient preparation: No special preparation is needed for this blood test. There are indications that a recent urinary tract infection, a recent urinary catheter, prostate stones, a prostate massage, or a DRE right before the blood test may cause the PSA levels to rise. Therefore, it is recommended to avoid those situations before the blood test in order to avoid a false rise in PSA.

Steps of the procedure: Since this procedure is a blood test, it takes only a few minutes to perform. The blood is then sent to a laboratory for analysis. It may take a few days up to two weeks before the test results are available.

After the procedure: The patient can return to normal activity. It is important to follow up on the results of the blood test to ensure that the PSA levels are within normal limits.

Risks: No risks are associated with this procedure.

Results: There are several ways to interpret PSA results. A more traditional approach considers less than 4 nanograms per milliliter (ng/mL) to be normal, 4 to 10 ng/mL slightly elevated, 10 to 20 ng/mL moderately elevated, and over 20 ng/mL significantly elevated. Other physicians evaluate the PSA level based on age and suggest that the normal ranges vary by age group. For physicians who take that approach, less than 2.5 ng/mL is normal for men forty to forty-nine years old, less than 3.5 ng/ml is normal for men fifty to fifty-nine years old, less than 4.5 ng/mL is normal for men sixty to sixty-nine years of age, and less than 6.5 ng/mL is normal for men seventy or older.

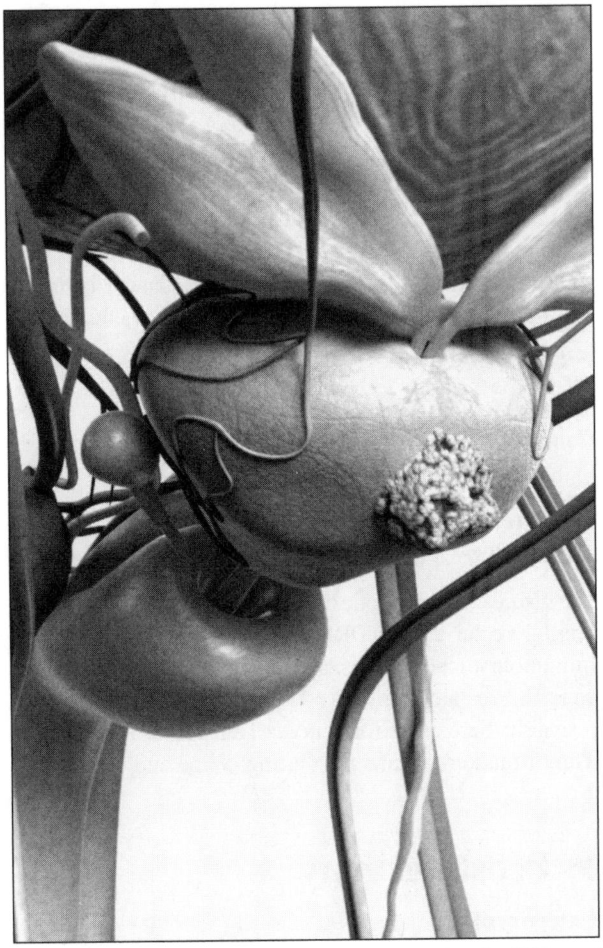

A prostate with a tumor on its posterior wall. (©MedicalRF.com/Corbis)

If the initial PSA level is found to be within normal limits, then one of the most important factors in determining whether prostate cancer is present is the change in PSA level from year to year. A dramatic rise in PSA levels from one screening to the next may be indicative of the presence of prostate cancer or other problems with the prostate. When the PSA level is elevated, it is important to have additional testing to determine the cause. Additional tests may include a transrectal ultrasound, in which a small probe is inserted into the rectum to take video images of the prostate, or a biopsy of the prostate, which involves inserting a needle into the prostate to take tissue samples. These samples are then checked for evidence of cancer.

Vonne Sieve, M.A.

▶ For Further Information

American Cancer Society. *Cancer Facts and Figures*. Atlanta: American Cancer Society, 2005.

Bostwick, D. G., et al. "Human Prostate Cancer Risk Factors." *Cancer* 101, suppl. 10 (2004): 2371-2490.

Ellsworth, Pamela, John Heaney, and Cliff Gill. *One Hundred Questions and Answers About Prostate Cancer*. Sudbury, Mass.: Jones & Bartlett, 2003.

U.S. Department of Health and Human Services. *United States Cancer Statistics: 1999-2002 Incidence and Mortality Web-Based Report*. Atlanta: Centers for Disease Control and Prevention and National Cancer Institute, 2005. Also available online at http://www.cdc.gov.

▶ Other Resources

Centers for Disease Control and Prevention

Cancer Prevention and Control

http://www.cdc.gov/cancer

Prostate Cancer Foundation

http://www.prostatecancerfoundation.org

See also Benign prostatic hyperplasia (BPH); Carcinomas; Digital rectal exam (DRE); Immunocytochemistry and immunohistochemistry; Pathology; Prevention; Prostate cancer; Prostatectomy; Prostitis; Proteomics and cancer research; Screening for cancer; Transrectal ultra sound; Tumor markers; Watchful waiting; Wine and cancer.

▶ Prostatectomy

Category: Procedures

Also known as: Radical prostatectomy, transurethral resection of the prostate (TURP)

Definition: Prostatectomy is the surgical removal of part or all of the prostate gland. A radical prostatectomy refers to removal of the prostate gland and surrounding tissue. A transurethral resection (TURP) refers to removal of part of the prostate.

Cancers treated: Prostate cancer

Why performed: A radical prostatectomy is performed to remove cancer that is confined to the prostate gland and surrounding area. This procedure is not usually done when cancer has spread beyond the prostate gland to distant tissues or organs.

A TURP is commonly done to relieve symptoms associated with benign prostatic hyperplasia (BPH). With BPH, the prostate gland is enlarged and squeezes the urethra, creating problems with urination. Removal of part of the prostate gland can usually alleviate those symptoms.

Patient preparation: Generally, no food or drink is consumed after midnight on the day before undergoing general anesthesia. The evening before a radical prostatectomy, a bowel preparation is usually taken to cleanse the colon.

Steps of the procedure: For a radical prostatectomy, the procedure varies depending on which method the surgeon uses: open, laparoscopic, or laparoscopically assisted prostatectomy. Typically, general anesthesia is used with all these procedures.

Open surgery involves an incision in the lower abdomen if the retropubic approach is done or in the groin between the anus and the penis for the perineal approach. The retropubic approach is most common and allows the surgeon to remove the prostate gland and the lymph nodes, if necessary, to be checked for cancer spread beyond the prostate. This approach allows the surgeon to attempt preservation of the nerves that help control bladder and sexual function. Lymph node removal can be done with the perineal approach, but a separate incision must be made, and preservation of sexual function is not possible. The open procedure can take from one and a half to four hours to complete.

With the laparoscopic and laparoscopically assisted approach, several small incisions are made in the lower abdomen. The laparoscope allows the surgeon to see inside the abdominal cavity and remove the prostate and surrounding tissue. With the robot-assisted procedure, the surgeon performs the procedure remotely with the use of a robot. Occasionally, a laparoscopic procedure may need to be converted to an open procedure if difficulty is encountered. This procedure may take four hours or more to perform.

No abdominal incision is needed for a TURP. A cutting instrument or a heated wire loop is inserted through the penis to the prostate gland to remove or destroy prostate tissue. The bladder is then flushed with sterile solution to remove the destroyed tissue from the body.

With all these procedures, a small flexible tube called a urinary catheter is inserted into the bladder and left in place to drain urine during the healing process.

After the procedure: An open prostatectomy is considered major abdominal surgery. Patients typically remain in the hospital from two to four days. Recovery time can be as long as twelve weeks. A laparoscopic procedure is less invasive. The hospital stay is usually two days, and recovery time averages two to four weeks. The urinary catheter is typically removed one to three weeks after the procedure.

With a TURP, the hospital stay is generally two to four days. The urinary catheter is generally left in place for one to three days after the procedure.

Risks: General complications from undergoing a major surgical procedure may include bleeding, blood clots, heart problems, infection, allergic reaction to anesthesia, and, in rare cases, death.

Short-term complications from a radical prostatectomy may include urinary incontinence, which is the inability to control the bladder. This condition generally improves, and full bladder control is regained over time. Long-term complications may include erectile dysfunction and urinary incontinence.

The risks from a TURP may include excessive bleeding, a urinary tract infection, or pain with urination. Some men temporarily develop problems as a result of the large amounts of irrigating fluid used to flush out the bladder. A more permanent condition that can develop is a stricture, a permanent narrowing of the urethra that can occur if the urethra is damaged during the procedure.

Results: When prostate cancer is confined to the prostate gland, the cure rate is very high. Five-year survival approaches 100 percent. Overall, prostatectomy success rates are about 76 to 98 percent for men with low-risk disease, 60 to 76 percent for men with moderate-risk disease, and 30 to 76 percent for men with high-risk disease. These rates vary depending on the surgeon's technique and experience with the procedure.

Erectile dysfunction is a common side effect. The nerves that control erections are located on both sides of the prostate gland and are easily damaged, or may be removed, during the procedure. Age and erectile function before surgery can affect the likelihood of problems after the procedure.

Urinary incontinence is another common problem with this procedure and includes occasional urine leakage to complete inability to control urine flow. In some cases, additional surgery may be necessary to correct the problem.

With a TURP, urination problems generally stop after the swelling has subsided.

After the surgical procedure, it is important for the patient to discuss monitoring his condition with additional testing to ensure that the problems have not returned.

Vonne Sieve, M.A.

▶ For Further Information

Ellsworth, Pamela, John Heaney, and Cliff Gill. *One Hundred Questions and Answers About Prostate Cancer.* Sudbury, Mass.: Jones & Bartlett, 2003.

Marks, Sheldon. *Prostate Cancer: A Family Guide to Diagnosis, Treatment, and Survival.* Cambridge, Mass.: Fisher Books, 2000.

Wainrib, Barbara, et al. *Men, Women, and Prostate Cancer: A Medical and Psychological Guide for Women and the Men They Love.* Oakland, Calif.: New Harbinger, 2000.

See also Benign prostatic hyperplasia (BPH); Carcinomas; Exenteration; Infection and sepsis; Obesity-associated cancers; Prostate cancer; Psychosocial aspects of cancer; Sexuality and cancer; Urinary system cancers; Urologic oncology.

▶ Prostatitis

Category: Diseases, symptoms, and conditions
Also known as: Prostatodynia, chronic pelvic pain syndrome

Related conditions: Urinary tract infection, benign prostatic hyperplasia, prostate cancer

Definition: Prostatitis is inflammation of the prostate gland. The prostate is a reproductive gland in men that produces semen, the fluid that nourishes and transports sperm. It is about the size and shape of a walnut and is located below the bladder. The gland surrounds the urethra, the tube that carries urine outside the body.

Risk factors: Prostatitis is more common in men under age forty or men who have recently experienced a bladder infection or obstruction (such as a tumor or stone), a urethral catheterization, an enlarged prostate, or a suppressed immune system. Some sexually transmitted diseases increase the risk of developing prostatitis.

Etiology and the disease process: Inflammation of the prostate can be caused by an acute or chronic bacterial infection or a nonbacterial infection. It may also be caused by abnormal nerve or muscle development in the pelvic region, a condition called prostatodynia. If an acute infection is left untreated, it may develop into a chronic condition.

Incidence: Prostatitis is a common problem in adult men, encompassing about 40 percent of visits to a urologist.

Symptoms: The symptoms for acute and chronic bacterial infections may include fever; frequent, painful, and difficult urination; pain in the pelvic region and lower back; and painful ejaculation. The symptoms for other forms of prostatitis can be nonspecific and mimic other conditions but are generally associated with pain in the pelvic region and lower back.

Screening and diagnosis: Acute bacterial prostatitis is diagnosed with the appearance of white blood cells and bacteria in the urine. Chronic bacterial prostatitis, a rare condition, is diagnosed after a prostate massage is performed;

fluid samples are taken and examined for the presence of prostatic bacteria. Nonbacterial prostatitis is not well understood and may be caused by infectious agents such as viruses, physical abnormalities, physical activity, or muscle spasms. It can be difficult to diagnose because the symptoms are often similar to those associated with other conditions.

Treatment and therapy: Treatment for bacterial prostatitis includes administration of an antibiotic, which generally resolves the problem. Lifestyle changes, pain relievers, muscle relaxants, and physical therapy are sometimes used to treat other forms of prostatitis.

Prognosis, prevention, and outcomes: Proper hygiene and avoiding sexual activity with a partner with a bacterial infection may help prevent bacterial prostatitis. The most effective way to prevent a chronic condition is to seek treatment when the symptoms first appear.

Vonne Sieve, M.A.

See also Bacteria as causes of cancer; Benign prostatic hyperplasia (BPH); Fever; Infection and sepsis; Prostate cancer; Prostate-specific antigen (PSA) test; Risks for cancer; Transrectal ultrasound; Urethral cancer; Urologic oncology.

▶ Proteasome inhibitors

Category: Chemotherapy and other drugs
ATC code: 101XX

Definition: Proteasome inhibitors are small-molecule drugs that target the proteasome, a large protein complex responsible for the degradation of unwanted proteins in the cell. Certain proteins are marked for proteasomal degradation by ubiquitination, the process of adding multiple ubiquitin molecules to the protein. Ubiquitinated proteins are recognized by the proteasome, allowing for the degradation of specifically targeted proteins. Cells rely on the proteasome to maintain a proper balance of particular proteins, as well as to remove damaged protein. Because the proteasome is an essential component for many cellular processes, including cell division and survival, it is an attractive target for actively growing cancer cells.

Cancers treated: Multiple myeloma, mantle cell lymphoma

Subclasses of this group: Synthetic inhibitors, natural inhibitors

Delivery routes: Intravenous (IV) injection

How these drugs work: Proteasome inhibitors are targeted therapies with specificity for the proteasome protein complex. These agents act by binding to the proteasome, impairing its ability to degrade proteins in the cell. Because degradation of excess and damaged proteins is a necessary function for normal cellular processes such as cell proliferation, these inhibitors can induce death in actively dividing malignant cells.

The only proteasome inhibitor currently approved to treat patients with cancer is bortezomib (Velcade). Bortezomib is administered by IV injection, at a recommended dosage of twice weekly for two weeks, followed by a rest period. Several cycles of this therapy may be given.

Other compounds have been discovered to have proteasome inhibitory activity, but these agents are not currently indicated for the treatment of cancers. Ritonavir is an antiretroviral drug used in human immunodeficiency virus (HIV) therapy. Preclinical studies have shown that ritonavir may have activity against brain tumor cells. Lactacystin is a natural proteasome inhibitor primarily used in laboratory settings.

Side effects: Bortezomib, the only proteasome inhibitor currently improved as an antineoplastic agent, is generally safe and well tolerated. The predominant side effects noted with bortezomib therapy are weakness, diarrhea and constipation, nausea and vomiting, and peripheral neuropathy, a tingling in the hands and feet. Additionally, myelosuppression such thrombocytopenia and neutropenia has been noted.

Lisa M. Cockrell, B.S.

See also Antineoplastics in chemotherapy; Chemotherapy; Diarrhea; Gastrointestinal complications of cancer treatment; HIV/AIDS-related cancers; Lymphomas; Mantle cell lymphoma (MCL); Moles; Multiple myeloma; Myeloma; Nausea and vomiting; Neutropenia; Thrombocytopenia.

▶ Protein electrophoresis

Category: Procedures
Also known as: Serum protein electrophoresis (SPEP)

Definition: Protein electrophoresis is a laboratory test used to measure the amounts of major proteins in a patient's blood serum, urine, or cerebrospinal fluid.

Cancers diagnosed: Most metastatic cancers, especially multiple myeloma

Why performed: Serum protein electrophoresis is used to screen for cancer or evaluate the extent of an existing cancer, particularly multiple myeloma. It can also be used to identify other diseases, including kidney, liver, intestinal, and immune disorders, as well as malnutrition. These disorders are associated with abnormal levels of different blood proteins, which can be detected by electrophoresis.

Patient preparation: There is no special preparation for this procedure. Patients undergo a normal blood test and should tell their physicians which prescription medications they are taking.

Steps of the procedure: A physician or nurse will draw blood from a vein in the patient's arm in an outpatient setting. The blood sample is transferred to the laboratory, where it is centrifuged to separate serum, the plasma without clotting factors, from the blood cells. Blood proteins are retained in the serum. A small amount of serum is then transferred to an electrophoretic paper or gel such as cellular acetate or agarose, respectively. Since proteins are charged molecules and vary in size, they will migrate differentially when a current is applied to the electrophoretic field. A fluorescent agent that binds to proteins is added to the serum for illumination. The result is a gradient of separated bands, or fractions, of proteins. A laboratory specialist studies an image of the gel to determine the relative concentrations of different proteins in the blood serum.

After the procedure: A bandage is applied to the patient's arm at the puncture site, and the patient can go home.

Risks: No risks are associated with protein electrophoresis. A blood draw, however, may cause minor bleeding or bruising at the puncture site. The patient may also feel light-headed, and there is a possibility of fainting after the blood draw.

Results: The major blood proteins consist of albumin and globulins. There are four types of globulin proteins: alpha-1 globulins, alpha-2 globulins, beta globulins, and gamma globulins. Normally, albumin makes up more than half of the proteins in the blood serum and is important for normal tissue growth. High levels of albumin proteins are a result of dehydration, while low levels suggest inflammatory disease, liver disease, malnutrition, or a kidney disorder. High levels of alpha-1 globulins (alpha-1 antitrypsin, thyroid-binding globulin, and transcortin) may indicate acute inflammatory disease and malignancies, while a low level can indicate liver disease. The levels of certain alpha-2 globulins (ceruloplasmin, alpha-2 macroglobulin, and haptoglobulin) can aid in cancer diagnosis. For example, a low level of haptoglobin may indicate tumor metastasis or liver disease. Variations in other alpha-2 globulin levels may indicate inflammation, nephrotic syndrome, or hemolysis, which is the loss of hemoglobin from red blood cells. High levels of beta globulin (transferrin and beta lipoprotein) can indicate biliary cirrhosis, hyperthyroidism, diabetes mellitus, and carcinoma in some cases, while decreased levels indicate malnutrition. High levels of gamma globulins (various antibodies) are the most indicative of cancers such as multiple myeloma, lymphocytic leukemia, or malignant lymphoma. In addition, high levels can indicate Hodgkin disease, connective tissue disorders, and chronic or acute infections. A patient whose serum protein electrophoresis yields abnormal results will be referred to a hematologist-oncologist.

Bharat Burman, B.A.

▶ For Further Information

Aziz, Khalid, and George Y. Wu. *Cancer Screening: A Practical Guide for Physicians*. Totowa, N.J.: Humana Press, 2002.

Hoffman, Ronald, et al. *Hematology: Basic Principles and Practice*. 4th ed. Philadelphia: Churchill Livingstone, 2005.

Keren, David F. *High-Resolution Electrophoresis and Immunofixation: Techniques and Interpretation*. 2d ed. Boston: Butterworth-Heinemann, 1994.

O'Connell, T. X., et al. "Understanding and Interpreting Serum Protein Electrophoresis." *American Family Physician* 71, no. 1 (January 1, 2005): 105-112.

Wallach, Jacques. *Interpretation of Diagnostic Tests*. 8th ed. Philadelphia: Wolters Kluwer Health/Lippincott Williams & Wilkins, 2007.

▶ Other Resources

American Cancer Society
How Is Multiple Myeloma Diagnosed?
http://www.cancer.org/docroot/CRI/content/CRI_2_4_3X_How_is_multiple_myeloma_diagnosed_30.asp?sitearea=

National Cancer Institute
Screening and Testing to Detect Cancer
http://www.cancer.gov/cancertopics/screening

See also Immunoelectrophoresis (IEP); Lactate dehydrogenase (LDH) test; Multiple myeloma; Myeloma.

▶ Proteomics and cancer research

Category: Cancer biology

Definition: The term "proteome" was coined in 1994 to describe the study of all the protein forms expressed within an organism, tissue, or group of cells as a function of time, age, state, and external factors. Many technological advances have led to the emergence of the discipline termed proteomics, which is now widely employed in the cancer field.

Background: Many scientists are using the rapidly emerging technologies of proteomics in an effort to identify new cancer biomarkers, specific protein species in the body that are helpful for disease prediction or treatment, and to understand the underlying mechanisms associated with cancer onset and progression. These technologies are also being applied to drug development and the identification of patients who might benefit from targeted therapies. Proteomics integrates some key fundamental technologies such as high-throughput protein separation and profiling, mass spectrometry, large databases, and bioinformatics tools to analyze and extract information from these databases.

Scientific rationale: After the human genome was sequenced, it consisted of fewer genes than scientists had expected—approximately 30,000, about twice as many genes as a worm or fly. This raised the question of how human complexity can be explained by a genome with such a relatively small number of genes. Scientists realized that such complexity is achieved in part by the economical use of genes. The effective number of distinct protein species present in a cell is greatly increased through a wide variety of ways in which proteins can be modified after being synthesized, collectively called posttranslational modifications. These modifications range from the addition of biochemical functional groups such as phosphate groups (resulting in phosphorylation) and carbohydrate groups (resulting in glycosylation), the addition of other proteins or peptides, chemical changes to the amino acids of the protein, and structural changes to the protein such as formation of disulfide bridges or proteolytic cleavage of the protein.

Besides their ability to undergo modifications, another characteristic of proteins is their dynamic state. They have the ability to constantly move around and bind to other proteins or cellular components. Proteins are able to respond quickly to a changing cellular environment, and they play an important role in the elaborate communication pathways within and between cells. A cell's complement of proteins in their specific posttranslationally modified forms is increasingly being recognized as playing an important role in many cellular processes and states, including cancer.

Scientists believe that cancer develops through a multistep process involving the accumulation of genetic alterations that lead to altered gene expression patterns, protein structures, and functions. Because the transformation of a normal cell to a cancerous one involves changes in the proteins present in the cell, the aim of proteomics in cancer research is to monitor these changes and use the information to provide valuable information that may aid diagnosis, prognosis, and monitoring response to therapy.

One goal of proteomics in cancer research is to define the expression patterns of proteins that are expressed at different levels in cells in different physiological states, such as cancer cells compared with noncancerous cells, or late-stage cancer cells compared with early-stage cancer cells. Another goal is the identification of tumor markers, proteins that are associated with particular types of cancer. Ideally, such markers would be sensitive, selective, and measurable by a noninvasive procedure (such as by analysis of blood or urine). In addition, the emergence of proteomics offers the promise of helping to elucidate the complex molecular events involved in cancer, as well as those that control clinically important tumor behaviors such as metastases, invasion, and resistance to therapy. Biomarkers may also be used to help devise optimal therapeutic treatment plans for different patient subsets and to monitor the effect of treatment.

Technologies: Proteomics consists of sample preparation, protein separation, and protein identification. Since the late 1990's, mass spectrometry has increasingly become the method of choice for analyses of complex protein samples. Mass spectrometry is a technique that generates electrically charged fragments from the proteins present in the mixture and measures particular properties of those fragments. The end product is a spectrum or chart with a series of peaks. The size of the peaks and the distance between them provide a "fingerprint" of the sample. Mass spectrometry offers the ability to measure, rapidly and inexpensively, thousands of proteins in a few drops of blood. The entire process, from collection of a few drops of blood to analyzing the "fingerprint," can take less than one minute. Hundreds of samples can be analyzed sequentially and very small amounts of protein can be detected.

The spectrum obtained from mass spectrometry experiments is difficult to analyze manually, but computers are being used to analyze such patterns and distinguish small differences in patterns between patients. Bioinformatics tools are the computer-based algorithms that are used to convert raw proteomics data into a useful form that can be analyzed, compared, interpreted, and stored in large databases.

Of particular interest in the field of proteomics research are high-throughput technologies that are capable of simultaneous and rapid analysis of multiple samples. One example is microarray technology, an automated technique for the simultaneous analysis of thousands of different samples affixed to a thumbnail-sized "chip" of glass or silicon.

Examples of tumor markers: The tumor marker prostate-specific antigen (PSA) is indispensable in the management of prostate cancer. Patients at high risk for primary liver cancer are screened by the tumor marker alpha-fetoprotein, in combination with ultrasonography, a regimen that has been shown to result in earlier detection and therefore more effective treatment and longer survival for patients with this type of cancer. Available screening tests for ovarian cancer include the biomarker cancer antigen 125 (CA 125), which has also proved to be a useful marker for monitoring response to chemotherapy. A rapid fall in the CA 125 level during chemotherapy predicts a favorable prognosis. In another example for ovarian cancer, a blood test for the levels of four proteins (leptin, prolactic, osteopontin, and insulin-like growth factor II) has been shown to discriminate with high accuracy between patients with early ovarian cancer and those who were disease free.

Challenges: The identification of large numbers of proteins from complex biological samples is a continuing challenge in this field. Techniques to address this challenge are evolving quickly. The biological variability among patient samples and the large concentration range over which proteins can be present also present challenges to deducing diagnostic patterns that are unique to specific types of cancer. The fast pace of technological innovation in this area should result in the identification of new biomarkers for different cancers and their use to improve diagnosis and treatment.

Standardization of proteomics techniques is needed to allow for the reproducibility required for medical applications. A large knowledge base is needed to allow for the accurate interpretation of proteomics data. Large databases, such as the publicly available Protein Atlas, are being assembled. Frozen tissue banks will be useful to preserve tissue samples for future analysis and comparison of samples taken at different times.

The main bottlenecks for proteomics research are the rapid accumulation of data and the lack of suitable computational tools for analysis. Data are being collected at a faster pace than researchers can validate, interpret, and integrate with other known data. Software tools are needed in all areas of data analysis, including data collection, searching, evaluation, archiving, and retrieval.

Prospects: With the ongoing rapid technological developments in this field, the prospects for identification of new highly sensitive and specific biomarkers for different cancers and their use for making significant contributions to the understanding, diagnosis, and treatment of cancer patients seems very hopeful.

Jill Ferguson, Ph.D.

▶ For Further Information

Brusic, V., O. Marina, C. J. Wu, and E. L. Reinherz. "Proteome Informatics for Cancer Research: From Molecules to Clinic." *Proteomics* 7 (2007): 976-991.

Cho, W. C. S. "Contribution of Oncoproteomics to Cancer Biomarker Discovery." *Molecular Cancer* 6 (2007): 25-37.

Liang, S.-L., and D. W. Chan. "Enzymes and Related Proteins as Cancer Biomarkers: A Proteomic Approach." *Clinica Chimica Acta* 381 (2007): 93-97.

Pastwa, E., S. B. Somiari, M. Czyz, and R. I. Somiari. "Proteomics in Human Cancer Research." *Proteomics—Clinical Application* 1 (2007): 4-17.

Reid, J. D., C. E. Parker, and C. H. Borchers. "Protein Arrays for Biomarker Discovery." *Current Opinion in Molecular Therapeutics* 9 (2006): 216-221.

Wu, W., W. Hu, and J. J. Kavanagh. "Proteomics in Cancer Research." *International Journal of Gynecological Cancer* 12 (2002): 409-423.

▶ Other Resources

The Human Genome/Wellcome Trust
Proteomics and Cancer
http://genome.wellcome.ac.uk/doc_WTD020926.html

National Cancer Institute
Clinical Proteomic Technologies for Cancer
http://proteomics.cancer.gov

See also Alpha-fetoprotein (AFP) levels; American Association for Cancer Research (AACR); CA 125 test; Cancer biology; Chemotherapy; Pathology; Prostate-specific antigen (PSA) test; Screening for cancer; Tumor markers.

▶ Proton beam therapy

Category: Procedures

Definition: Proton beam therapy is a procedure for delivering targeted radiation therapy using protons instead of the electrons used by traditional radiation therapies.

Cancers treated: Primarily cancers of the prostate, lung, head, neck, and brain

Why performed: Proton beam therapy, like traditional radiation therapy, is performed to kill cancer cells. It may be performed as a primary treatment for a tumor, to kill any cancer cells that remain after surgical cancer treatment, or in addition to other cancer treatment options. Proton beam therapy is only offered at a few locations in the United States, and for many cancers it is still considered an experimental treatment.

Proton beam therapy is a site-specific therapy, so it is designed to treat cancers that have not spread to large areas or throughout the body. It is mainly used to treat cancers occurring in the prostate, lung, head, neck, and brain, although it is being tested in clinical trials for use on cancers occurring in many other areas as well.

Patient preparation: The patient should discuss with the cancer care team any necessary preparation for the specific procedure that he or she is undergoing. Necessary preparation may vary depending on the type of cancer being treated and the patient's previous response to any radiation therapy.

Steps of the procedure: Proton beam therapy uses high-speed protons to kill cancer cells, instead of the electrons used by most radiation therapy techniques. Atoms are made up of a nucleus of protons and neutrons surrounded by orbiting electrons. Protons have a positive charge, neutrons have no charge, and electrons have a negative charge. When free protons come very close to an atom, the electrons orbiting the nucleus are attracted to the positive charge of the protons. The electrons are then pulled out of their orbits. This is called ionization of the atom. Atoms that have been ionized are not as stable as normal atoms.

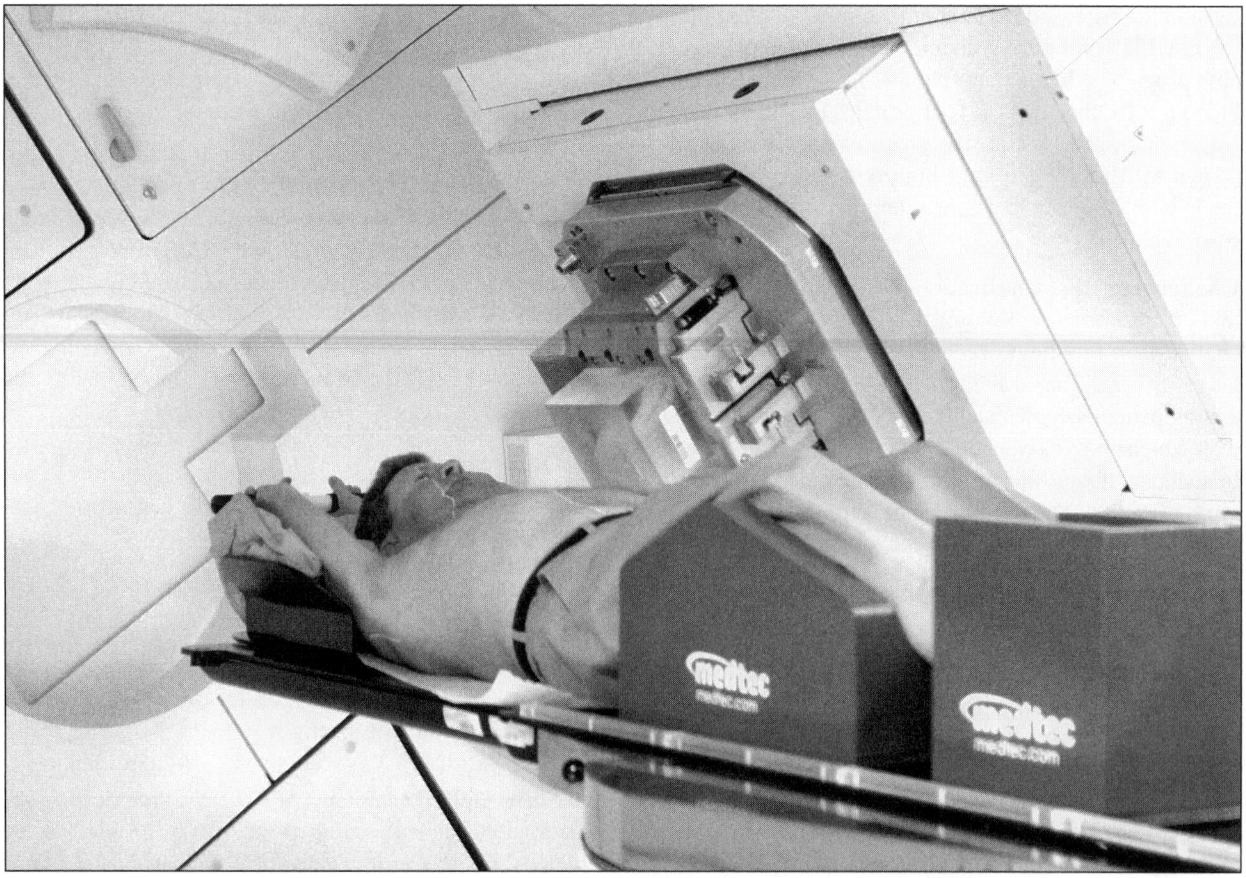

A lung cancer patient receives proton beam therapy. (AP/Wide World Photos)

This change to the atom means that changes also occur to the molecule of which the atom is part, and eventually to the cell of which the molecule is part. If the cell cannot repair the damage caused, then it eventually dies.

Proton beam therapy begins with protons traveling around a synchrotron, a machine that makes the protons go very fast and energizes them. The protons are then sent through vacuum tubes to the machine that actually aims them at the area of the patient that will receive the radiation. The patient is positioned and held still so that the proton beam can be aimed as accurately as possible. Complex computer technology helps the doctors and technicians aim the proton beam very accurately so that it hits as little healthy tissue as possible.

The protons are released in a directed stream toward the cancer cells. The protons are traveling very quickly at first, but they slow down as they get closer to the cancer. When they are traveling fast, they do not have a very strong effect on the atoms they are passing. When they are slower, however, they have an extremely strong effect. This is one reason that proton beam therapy causes less damage to healthy cells than does traditional radiation therapy. Traditional radiation therapy uses X rays, which strongly affect all the cells with which they come into contact, which makes it hard to deliver enough radiation to the cancer cells without also killing healthy cells. With proton beam therapy, doctors aided by computers can determine the right way to release the protons so that they have the maximum impact just as they come into contact with the cancer cells. Proton beam therapy may need to be repeated one or more times depending on the size and type of the cancer and other factors.

After the procedure: After proton beam therapy, many individuals experience no negative side effects. Some individuals, however, may experience pain, fatigue, nausea, or diarrhea.

Risks: The risks associated with proton beam therapy are believed to be somewhat lower than those associated with traditional radiation therapy for most people. This is the case because proton beam therapy causes less damage to surrounding healthy cells, so healthy tissue is less likely to be significantly damaged. Some of the risks of proton beam therapy include nausea, diarrhea, and fatigue. Damage to healthy tissue is still a possible risk of proton beam therapy.

Results: The goal of proton beam therapy is generally to destroy a tumor, to reduce the size of a tumor, to reduce related symptoms, or to kill any residual cancer cells left after a tumor has been surgically removed. Success rates for proton beam therapy can vary drastically depending on the type of cancer, its size, and how far it has spread. It is generally found to be successful at reducing the side effects usually associated with traditional radiation therapy. If the procedure is done to completely destroy a tumor or residual cancer, then the procedure is generally considered to have been successful if the cancer does not return for five years or more. If the procedure was done to reduce tumor size, then it is considered successful if quality of life is improved.

Helen Davidson, B.A.

▶ For Further Information

Barton-Burkey, Margaret, and Gail M. Wilkes. *Cancer Therapies*. Sudbury, Mass.: Jones and Bartlett, 2006.

Chan, Helen S. L. *Understanding Cancer Therapies*. Jackson: University of Mississippi Press, 2007.

DeLaney, Thomas F., and Hanne M. Kooy, eds. *Proton and Charged Particle Radiotherapy*. Philadelphia: Lippincott Williams & Wilkins, 2008.

Haas, Marilyn L., et al. *Radiation Therapy: A Guide to Patient Care*. St. Louis: Mosby/Elsevier, 2007.

▶ Other Resources

The National Association for Proton Therapy
http://www.proton-therapy.org

See also Afterloading radiation therapy; Brain scan; Cancer care team; External beam radiation therapy (EBRT); Gastrointestinal complications of cancer treatment; Meningiomas; Nausea and vomiting; Neurologic oncology; Radiation oncology; Radiation therapies; Virus-related cancers.

▶ Proto-oncogenes and carcinogenesis

Category: Cancer biology
Also known as: Precursors of oncogenes

Definition: Proto-oncogenes are cellular genes that may be transformed into oncogenes (cancer-causing genes). Proto-oncogenes provide signals that promote the division and specialization of normal cells or regulate programmed cell death (apoptosis). Changes in their genetic sequence or their expression level due to chromosomal translocation, point mutation, or amplification can trigger a sequence of events leading to the neoplastic transformation (abnormal growth) of a cell and subsequently to tumor formation.

Particularly at risk are persons carrying chromosomal translocations or molecular rearrangements in their genome and persons infected with distinct viruses: Epstein-Barr virus (EBV) in Burkitt lymphoma, sinonasal lymphoma, and lymphomas in immunocompromized patients; human T-cell lymphotropic virus type 1 (HTLV-1) in adult T-cell lymphoma/leukemia; and human herpesvirus 8 (HHV-8) in body-cavity-based lymphomas in patients infected with the human immunodeficiency virus (HIV).

Etiology and symptoms of associated cancers: B-cell lymphomas are caused by malignant B-cell lymphocytes. Through a chromosomal translocation, the *BCL2* proto-oncogene may become rearranged, resulting in overexpression of its protein product. The protein product blocks apoptosis, thereby enabling continued growth of the malignant B cells.

T-cell lymphomas show a high frequency of a characteristic chromosomal translocation, resulting in the combination of the *NPM1/ALK* genes and a fused oncogenic protein product.

Nephroblastoma (Wilms' tumor) is the most common malignant tumor of the kidney in children. Mutations of the *WT1* proto-oncogene are found in approximately 20 percent of Wilms' tumors, half of which additionally carry mutations in *CTNNB1*, a proto-oncogene encoding beta-catenin.

Plasmacytomas frequently show chromosomal translocations resulting in dysregulation of oncogenes followed by proliferation of a plasma cell clone. Genomic instability leads to further mutations and translocations.

The oncogene *CCND1* product cyclin D1 is overexpressed in 45 to 50 percent of primary ductal mammary carcinomas, in part because of amplification of the region of the genome where the proto-oncogene is located. Other oncogenes that play roles in mammary carcinomas are *HER2/neu* (*ERBB2*), *MYC* (*c-myc*), and *WNT1*.

History: Oncogenes were first discovered in certain retroviruses and were later identified as cancer-causing agents in many animals. In 1976 it was demonstrated by J. Michael Bishop and Harold Varmus that cancer-causing genes (oncogenes) carried by certain viruses are derived from normal genes (proto-oncogenes) present in the cells of their host. Further research showed that such genes can cause cancer even without viral involvement. By 2008 scientists had identified more than one hundred oncogenes in animals.

Nicola E. Wittekindt, Dr.Sc. (ETH Zürich)

See also Burkitt lymphoma; Cancer biology; Carcinogens, known; Carcinogens, reasonably anticipated; Carcinomas; Endocrine cancers; Epstein-Barr virus; Free radicals; Gene therapy; Genetics of cancer; Giant cell tumors (GCTs); HIV/AIDS-related cancers; *HRAS* gene testing; Leukemias; Lymphomas; Mesothelioma; Mitochondrial DNA mutations; Molecular oncology; *MYC* oncogene; Nephroblastomas; Oncogenes; Oncogenic viruses; Viral oncology; Virus-related cancers; Wilms' tumor.

▶ Psycho-oncology

Category: Medical specialties

Definition: Originally, psycho-oncology was a subspecialty of oncology that investigated, assessed, and treated the social and psychological aspects of having cancer. Psycho-oncology evolved to include the study and amelioration of pain stemming from cancer and its treatments, subjective emotional responses to receiving and carrying the diagnosis (anxiety, depression, degree of hope/hopelessness, delirium), application of patients' effective coping, functional status and quality of patients' lives, role of spiritual and philosophical beliefs, management of stress on caregivers and professional staffs, and the interactions between psychological and emotional factors on immune systems.

Subspecialties: Behavioral medicine, health psychology, medical-liaison psychiatry/psychology, pain management, psycho-immunology, psychoneuroimmunology, psychosomatic medicine, psychosocial medicine, psychospirituality

Cancers treated: All

Training and certification: Because psycho-oncology is a clinical and research application of professional training, there is not a universally accepted academic credential although training programs exist at most major cancer treatment centers. Professional organizations promoting the work of psycho-oncology include the American Psychosocial Oncology Society, the British Psychosocial Oncology Society, and the International Psycho-oncology Society. Their membership consists of oncologists, psychiatrists, and allied health professionals.

Those practicing or researching psycho-oncology come from several professional disciplines that apply their training to the psychological and psychosocial treatment of cancer patients and their families: residency-trained physician oncologists, residency-trained physician psychiatrists, clinical health psychologists, nurse practitioners, medical social workers, and pastoral counselors. (Pastoral counselors are not routinely required to possess a state license.) Professionals follow the individual requirements of their disciplines regarding obtaining licenses to practice their specialty independently, privileges to treat patients from the institutions where they practice, and specialty board certification (where applicable) and maintaining (renewing) board certification.

Specific training in psycho-oncology usually occurs as an elective track or certificate program at the major cancer treatment centers for professionals in training there. Psycho-oncology is not typically a requirement of curricula in oncology, psychiatry, health psychology, or social work. Therefore, people who engage in its practice are generally those who have actively sought out training, reflecting a high degree of interest and commitment.

The National Comprehensive Cancer Network (NCCN) is an organization representing nearly all the major comprehensive cancer care centers in North America. It has produced standards for psychosocial cancer care and clinical practice guidelines for those involved in providing psycho-oncology services, including nonlicensed professionals such as pastoral counselors. Institutional regulatory and oversight bodies such as the Joint Commission of Accreditation of Heathcare Organizations (JCAHO), the American Osteopathic Association (AOA), and governmental departments of health have not yet fully incorporated these guidelines or psycho-oncological care itself as standard criteria for providing treatment to cancer patients.

Reimbursement for and revenue generation by psycho-oncology interventions is meager relative to other cancer treatment modalities such as surgery, radiation oncology, and chemotherapy. When institutions reassess fiscal priorities, psycho-oncology services and programs are often among the first to be discontinued.

Services and procedures performed: Historically, receiving a cancer diagnosis was equivalent to receiving a terminal diagnosis. In a humanely motivated effort to protect patients from completely losing hope and entering a state of despair, a cancer diagnosis routinely was not revealed to patients, though families were generally told. In the mid-1970's people began to believe that it was generally more harmful to patients to keep their diagnosis a secret, an idea that was supported by studies on patients' psychological reactions to having and being treated for cancer conducted at Memorial Sloan-Kettering Cancer Center in New York and the Massachusetts General Hospital in Boston. Early services in psycho-oncology promoted telling the truth to patients, encouraging patients with similar diagnoses to meet for emotional support, disseminating treatment information, and educating professionals about quality-of-life considerations and the values in comfort care over curative intervention among grave prognostic cases. These growing changes in the environment of cancer treatment were concurrent with improvements in actual cancer treatments and growing survival rates. In the twenty-first century, psycho-oncology professionals provide multiple services under the umbrella of engaging the psychological and psychosocial aspects of having cancer.

Psycho-oncology researchers have developed many instruments that assess a wide range of patients' reactions to cancer, including pain, anxiety, depression, and delirium. These instruments assist with evaluating the efficacy of interventions and provide quantitative parameters through which ongoing research in psycho-oncological methods can be tracked and understood. Preexisting psychological "tests" or instruments were not normed on populations that were this medically ill and routinely overreported patients' experiences. Researchers have developed scales derived from patient responses to sets of questions that are cancer specific.

Psycho-oncology's contribution to outcomes research (whether a new treatment, drug, or procedure is effective, worth the costs and risks, and so on) has moved it beyond whether the intervention increases survival to include consideration of whether the survival is worth having—it asks the question whether sustaining this life allows the patient to enjoy a high enough quality of life. In the twenty-first century, oncological treatments must not only reduce tumor growth but also promote sufficient functional status for them to be considered efficacious and beneficial. "Quality-adjusted life years" is a widely cited statistic combining survivability (how much time the treatment adds to patients' lives) with measures of patients' quality of life. Mortality rate statistics are inadequate by themselves.

Psycho-oncology practitioners who perform consultation-liaison services commonly treat adjustment disorders that arise in cancer patients. In effect, they treat not the disease but the disturbed emotions that understandably arise in the face of coping with cancer. They treat not cancer, but patients' reactions to having cancer.

Health psychologists' study of how patients cope with illness and comply with treatment plans has become a standard component of what psycho-oncologists work to facilitate in their patients: adaptive patterns of feeling, thinking, and behaving in facing cancer and its treatments and informed compliance with treatment plan options. Psycho-oncology practitioners unite understanding patients' subjective experiences without judgment or reprimand, respect for patients' rights to react in the way they do, and compassionate positive regard for their emotional suffering with the focused treatment of the cancer itself.

Practitioners of psycho-oncology also focus on preventive and behavioral health measures, helping patients effect lifestyle changes to reduce the risk of developing or exacerbating cancer. Reducing sun exposure and high-fat, high-calorie food intake; eliminating tobacco use; and achieving and maintaining healthy levels of exercise can reduce cancer risk.

Psycho-oncology's contribution to cancer treatment includes the provision of comfort and palliative care so that patients who are terminally ill do not suffer needlessly as a result of aggressive or invasive treatments that prolong life at the cost of reducing functional ability. Helping patients and their loved ones deal with life-threatening disease means that psycho-oncologically oriented treatments encourage inclusion of patients' spiritual beliefs, religious practices, and search to find meaning when death is inevitable.

Finally the high emotional demands of dealing with life and death, the uncertainty of treatments, and cancer-caused physical and emotional pain profoundly affect not only patients but also health care professionals and caregivers. Psycho-oncology interventions include protocols and strategies to avoid provider burnout and depression.

Paul Moglia, Ph.D.

▶ For Further Information

Barraclough, Jennifer. *Cancer and Emotion: A Practical Guide to Psycho-Oncology*. New York: Wiley, 1999.

Bearison, David J., and Raymond K. Mulhern, eds. *Pediatric Psychooncology: Psychological Perspectives on Children with Cancer*. New York: Oxford University Press, 1999.

Holland, Jimmie C., et al., eds. *Psycho-Oncology*. New York: Oxford University Press, 1998.

Lewis, Clare E., Jennifer Barraclough, and Rosalind O'Brien. *The Psychoimmunology of Cancer*. New York: Oxford University Press, 2002.

▶ Organizations and Professional Societies

American Psychosocial Oncology Society
http://www.apos-society.org
2365 Hunters Way
Charlottesville, VA 22911

American Society of Clinical Oncology
http://www.asco.org
1900 Duke Street, Suite 200
Alexandria, VA 22314

National Comprehensive Cancer Network
http://www.nccn.org
500 Old York Road, Suite 250
Jenkintown, PA 19046

▶ Other Resources

British Psychosocial Oncology Society
http://www.bpos.org

International Psycho-oncology Society
http://www.ipos-society.org

National Breast Cancer Coalition
http://www.natlbcc.org

See also Anxiety; Cancer care team; Depression; Exercise and cancer; Immune response to cancer; Medical oncology; Oncology social worker; Pain management medications; Prayer and cancer support; Psychosocial aspects of cancer; Stress management; Support groups.

▶ Psychosocial aspects of cancer

Category: Social and personal issues

Definition: Psychosocial aspects of cancer involve the full array of behavioral, cognitive, emotional, and social factors associated with the disease. Included are the coping mechanisms patients employ in dealing with the physical and emotional stressors caused by the illness and its treatment.

Reactions to cancer diagnosis: Despite significant advances in treatment and steadily increasing rates of survival, cancer is perceived by most to be a frightening and painful disease. Receiving the diagnosis of cancer evokes the possibilities of disabling illness, suffering, changes in appearance and physical abilities, altered social and professional goals, loss of personal control and independence, and even death. Shock, emotional "numbing," and denial are common responses to the diagnosis. Treatment of the disease may be associated with unpleasant and often severe side effects such as pain, disfigurement, fatigue, and nausea. Not surprisingly, cancer diagnosis typically engenders distress, and patients commonly experience at least periodic feelings of hopelessness, fear, and dysphoria during the course of their illness. Although a minority of cancer patients develop psychiatric illnesses, many experience unpleasant psychological or social problems that hinder coping skills and quality of life. The manner in which patients adapt to cancer is determined by individual and family characteristics, illness-related factors, and cultural and societal influences.

Individual and family characteristics: The developmental stage of the patient at the time that cancer is diagnosed and treated influences how the illness is perceived and which developmental tasks may be disrupted. For example, cancer treatment in childhood or adolescence involving changes in appearance, pain, or weakness can hinder self-confidence and make social development more difficult. In early adulthood, illness-related disruptions can affect job performance and modify career goals and perceptions of self-worth. In later adulthood, cancer can markedly alter financial status and long-awaited expectations for retirement years.

Other factors influencing the extent that cancer affects psychosocial functioning include personality, emotional maturity, coping style, and prior experience with illness. General coping tasks of all cancer patients involve regulating stress and anxiety caused by the diagnosis and treatment requirements; adapting to changes in social, familial, and occupational roles; coping with new role demands associated with being a patient, including participating in treatment efforts, maintaining a sense of self-worth, continuing relations with family and friends (such as spouses and employers); and developing acceptance and satisfaction with post-illness circumstances. Personality variables such as optimism, flexibility and openness to change, emotional expressiveness, and acceptance of emotional support appear to help with coping. For some, prior exposure to a serious illness—whether their own illness or that of someone close to them—makes adaptation to cancer more difficult. A history of psychiatric illness before cancer diagnosis also appears to be a risk factor for poor coping. Some cancer patients, including those without prior psychiatric histories, develop psychiatric illness in response to stressors associated with cancer. The most common of these are depression and anxiety. Left untreated, these conditions can markedly reduce patients' quality of life, adherence to treatment regimens, and overall adaptation to cancer. Fortunately, effective medicines and psychological therapies exist to treat psychiatric illness in cancer patients.

In most cases, cancer affects all members of a patient's family, and the response of the family in turn affects the patient's adaptation to the illness. Family members' reactions to a diagnosis of cancer can be extreme and sometimes mirror the struggles and adaptive demands experienced by the patient. Parents of children with cancer are faced with unusually difficult challenges; however, most are able to effectively deal with the worry, family disruption, and myriad behavioral and emotional demands that accompany the diagnosis. A family's makeup, relationships, cohesiveness, communication patterns, and especially level of support have been identified as factors contributing to cancer patients' psychosocial response to their illness. The impact of serious illness frequently alters family members' roles and responsibilities, necessitating adaptation to these changes.

Families are the primary providers of support to most patients, and a family environment characterized by high levels of communication and emotional expressiveness, along with low levels of conflict, predicts better adjustment in cancer patients. Having a family that is critical, emotionally distant, or unresponsive to patient distress appears related to poorer patient adaptation to the challenges of cancer. Patients who lack support from family or friends may benefit from participating in support groups in terms of improved mood, coping skills, pain tolerance, and general mental health.

Illness-related factors: Disease-related factors contributing to psychosocial adaptation to cancer include the type, stage, and location of the disease; its symptoms; treatment demands and side effects; and the prognosis for rehabilitation, cure, or survival.

Certain types of cancer appear to be particularly potent in producing emotional distress in patients. For example, the diagnosis of breast cancer and awareness of associated treatments and potential side effects (such as surgical intervention and disfigurement, chemotherapy and hair loss, radiation and infertility) can be profoundly disturbing to many women, especially those of childbearing age. Other types of cancer associated with behavioral or lifestyle factors (such as smoking and lung cancer) may produce debilitating guilt and self-reproach in the patient. For most, initial emotional turmoil gives way to a return to more normal coping strategies and gradual adaptation to the demands of their health status.

Pain, diminished strength and physical abilities, and attendant loss of independence are some of the symptoms associated with cancer that require psychosocial adaptation in patients. For those patients who have a realistic hope of cure, unpleasant or painful treatment side effects, such as nausea, weakness, vomiting, or hair loss, are endured with the hope of long-term benefits. Counseling, meditation, support groups, and medication may be employed to assist the patient in controlling psychological symptoms stemming from treatment. Because patients are increasingly surviving cancer, there is greater awareness of how individuals adapt to life after their illness. Many survivors find positive aspects to their experience with illness, including examining life goals and searching for more meaningful pursuits and spiritual growth. Many survivors struggle with anxiety associated with fears of recurrence of the disease or how they will cope as they resume roles and activities disrupted by their illness. Although successful coping is seen in most individuals, some experience esteem issues, grief, difficulties with intimacy, and a heightened sense of vulnerability even after several years of survival.

In terminal cases, the transition from active treatment to palliative or comfort care, and the attendant confrontation with the inevitability of death, can be very difficult for patients and their friends and family. Reactions to this change often involve shock and denial of physical realities. Similar to what is seen at initial diagnosis, after a period of distress, most patients draw on their usual means of coping and adapt to new therapeutic goals such as pain control, comfort care, and maximizing quality of life. Increasingly, terminal care is provided at the homes of patients, with benefits to the patient and family resulting from greater comfort and closeness during the patient's final days. Progress in the control of symptoms of advanced illness (such as pain) has significantly improved the quality of life for many patients and thereby facilitated psychosocial adjustment to end-of-life issues.

Cultural and societal influences: Cultural and societal factors that influence adaptation to cancer change as knowledge, perceptions, and beliefs about the illness evolve. Historically, when effective treatment options were limited and a culture of paternalism held sway in medicine, the diagnosis of cancer was kept from individuals, because the disease typically led to death and patient awareness was viewed as merely adding to the suffering. Treatment advances, coinciding with overall efforts in medicine to increase patient participation in medical care, have curtailed this practice. Improved patient-physician communication and a greater sense of autonomy and control in the patient are some of the benefits of this change. Increased public access to medical information (such as via the Internet) has led to heightened awareness of cancer and has reduced the prevalence of some associated myths (for example, that cancer is a contagion), which previously contributed to stigmatizing those with the disease. Greater exposure to accurate information regarding treatment alternatives for many forms of cancer has led to a generally less grim view of the disease by the general public. Consequently, reflexive catastrophic emotional responses to the diagnosis may be reduced. However, overall increases in optimism regarding cancer may be tempered in some cases by access to starkly realistic prognostic and treatment information associated with the more virulent types of the disease. Also, access to inaccurate sources of information, such as those erroneously attributing the cause of cancer to inadequate personality traits or "toxic" relationships, may unnecessarily add to the psychological burden of the patient. Greater awareness and cultural acceptance of mental health problems and the availability of effective treatment has increased the likelihood of cancer patients receiving care for depression and anxiety. Treatment of these conditions has been found to improve the quality of life of cancer patients.

Paul F. Bell, Ph.D.

▶ For Further Information

Gatchel, Robert, and Mark Ooordt. *Clinical Health Psychology and Primary Care*. Washington, D.C.: American Psychological Association, 2003.

Goldman, Larry, Thomas Wise, and David Brody. *Psychiatry for Primary Care Physicians*. Chicago: American Medical Association, 1998.

Kufe, Donald W., et al., eds. *Holland Frei Cancer Medicine 7*. 7th ed. Hamilton, Ont.: BC Decker, 2006.

▶ Other Resources

American Cancer Society
Counseling, Psychological, and Social Services
http://www.cancer.org/docroot/PED/content/PED_13_3x_Counseling_Psychol_and_Social_Services.asp?sitearea=PED

Cancer Coping Center
http://www.cancercopingcenter.com

National Cancer Institute
Coping with Cancer
http://www.cancer.gov/cancertopics/coping

National Institutes of Health
Cancer: Coping with Cancer
http://health.nih.gov/result.asp/105

See also Aging and cancer; Anxiety; Cancer care team; Cancer education; Case management; Childhood cancers; Cognitive effects of cancer and chemotherapy; Complementary and alternative therapies; Counseling for cancer patients and survivors; Depression; Elderly and cancer; End-of-life care; Fatigue; Fertility issues; Financial issues; Grief and bereavement; Palliative treatment; Personality and cancer; Prayer and cancer support; Primary care physician; Psycho-oncology; Rehabilitation; Relationships; Self-image and body image; Sexuality and cancer; Singlehood and cancer; Smoking cessation; Stress management; Support groups; Transitional care.

▶ Radiation oncology

Category: Medical specialties
Also known as: Radiotherapy oncology

Definition: Radiation oncology is the treatment of cancers using radiation, including therapeutic high-dose, high-energy forms of ionizing radiation, to shrink tumors and kill cancer cells. As one of the four major approaches to the treatment of cancer (along with surgery, chemotherapy, and biological therapy), radiation oncology is at the forefront of cancer treatment and research.

Subspecialties: Clinical radiation therapy, radiation and cancer biology, radiation physics

Cancers treated: Many cancers, but particularly cancers of the brain, head and neck, lung, breast, prostate, skin, rectum, cervix, and uterus, as well as lymphomas and sarcomas

Training and certification: The structure of accredited radiation oncology programs and residencies varies. In North America, most radiation oncologists have completed a radiation oncology residency in a program approved by the American Council of Graduate Medical Education (ACGME), the American Board of Radiology (ABR), or the Royal College of Physicians and Surgeons of Canada.

Radiation oncologists must possess a broad and deep command of both cancer biology and imaging technology. They study the etiology of cancer; its evaluation, diagnosis, and treatment in a clinical setting; the ways radiation interacts with various cancers at all levels, from molecular to multicellular; the physics of radiotherapeutic technologies and associated machines such as linear accelerators and hyperthermia devices; techniques such as interstitial brachytherapy, intraoperative radiotherapy, and stereotactic radiosurgery; and a host of other disciplines associated with radiation therapy, such as nuclear medicine, oncology, diagnostic radiology, and surgical pathology.

During postdoctoral training, students may elect to focus on research, as in radiation biology; on the integration of advanced technologies and radiation physics with clinical research; or on clinical practice. Most residencies in clinical radiation oncology require at least three, more often four, years to complete, usually following a first postgraduate year (PGY-1) of surgical, medical, or flexible internship.

After receiving their primary certification, radiation oncologists usually must renew certification every several years, depending on their subspecialties. The American Board of Radiology, for example, requires its diplomates to satisfy its "maintenance of certification" (MOC) program to maintain their primary certification.

Services and procedures performed: All radiation oncologists participate in the evaluation, staging, treatment, and therapy of their patients. They are the overseers of the cancer patient's radiation oncology team, ensuring the precision and accuracy of radiation treatment, and they work with physicians treating the patient's cancer in other ways. Throughout the course of radiation therapy, radiation oncologists are responsible for monitoring the patient's progress, side effects, and treatment to meet two goals: that the cancer is effectively halted or reduced in size, and that the patient's comfort is at the same time adequately addressed. The balance of these objectives is essential to achieving the best outcome.

Radiation oncologists head a team of medical professionals who together design and deliver the patient's radiation treatments. In concert with the patient's primary oncologist, the radiation oncologist learns about the specifics of the patient's cancer to determine the role radiation therapy will play in its treatment, then meets with the patient to evaluate his or her probable response to radiation therapy. Along with a radiation physicist and a dosimetrist, the radiation oncologist will then design the treatment plan, which involves simulations, immobilization devices, calculating radiation dosages, and conducting periodic checks to confirm accurate delivery of treatment.

The types of procedures radiation oncologists design and perform with the radiology team fall into two major categories. In the various forms of external beam radiation, the most common type of radiotherapy, the radiation oncologist uses a machine similar to an X-ray machine to direct high-energy X and gamma rays to the specific area of the body where the tumor resides. Treatments are given on a daily basis, usually for one to eight weeks and sometimes more than once a day, depending on the tumor and its aggressiveness.

Brachytherapy—also known as internal, implant, interstitial, or intracavitary radiation therapy—is the other main form of radiotherapy. The radiation oncologist implants, in the form of capsules called needles or seeds, a small amount of a radioactive substance in the body near the tumor while the patient is under general anesthesia. Among the radioactive materials used are cesium, iridium, iodine, phosphorus, and palladium.

Other procedures include electron therapy, including total skin treatment; radioimmunotherapy, in which monoclonal antibodies are enlisted to deliver the radiation by binding to the tumor cells; proton beam therapy, which uses protons to deliver higher doses of radiation to tumors

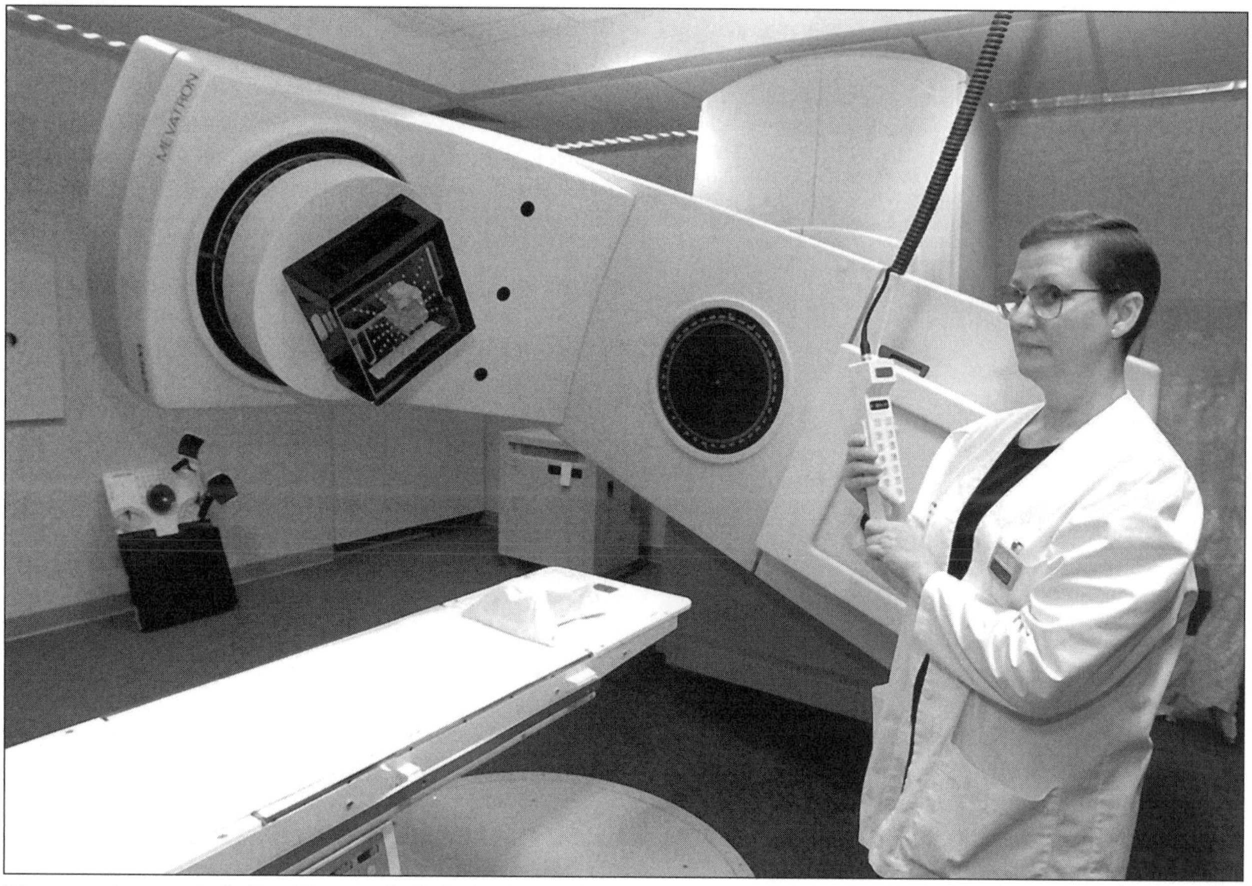

Linear accelerators, including this one at St. Catherine Hospital in Garden City, Kansas, are used in radiation therapy. (AP/Wide World Photos)

than can be accomplished using conventional X and gamma radiation; neutron therapy, which can work in oxygen-free environments, such as the depths of a large tumor, to deliver radiation to cancers that cannot be treated by other forms of radiation; and stereotactic radiosurgery, such as the Gamma Knife, used to treat head and neck cancers by delivering a very high dose of radiation targeted directly at a tumor and sparing surrounding, healthy tissue.

Finally, radiation oncologists offer palliative treatment for those whose outcome is not expected to be survival but whose pain can be ameliorated by halting the growth of a tumor or shrinking its size.

Related specialties and subspecialties: Many radiotherapy subspecialists work with the radiation oncologist. While radiation oncologists oversee care and integrate it with that of surgeons, chemotherapy oncologists, and other physicians, the day-to-day application of radiotherapy to the patient's tumor is often carried out by others on the radiology team.

First, radiation physicists, certified by the American Board of Radiology or the American Board of Medical Physics, work directly with the radiation oncologist, oversee dosimetrists, develop quality-control programs for procedures, and perform safety tests on equipment. Their education usually consists of four years of college, two to four years of graduate school, and one or two years of clinical physics training.

Radiation therapists, under the supervision of radiation oncologists, administer the daily treatments, keep records, and check the performance of machines. They typically have two to four years of college education and have been certified by the American Registry of Radiologic Technologists. Many states also require licensing for radiation therapists.

Dosimetrists calculate dosages and durations of radiation with the goal of doing the greatest damage to the tumor while limiting damage to normal tissue. Because of the complexity of determining treatment dosages, dosimetrists often start as radiation therapists and, with additional training, advance to dosimetry. There are also intensive dosimetry programs lasting one to two years. Dosimetrists are certified by the Medical Dosimetrist Certification Board.

Radiation oncology nurses are charged with caring for radiation patients from before the beginning of treatment through its completion. They are also the patient's first line of communication regarding what to expect during the procedure and how to identify and evaluate side effects. All radiation oncology nurses are registered nurses, and most are also accredited in the specialty of oncology nursing, which requires the completion of a master's degree program.

Christina J. Moose, M.A.

▶ For Further Information

Cukier, Daniel. *Coping with Chemotherapy and Radiation Therapy*. 4th ed. New York: McGraw-Hill, 2004.

Delfino, Michelangelo, and Mary E. Day. *We Live and Die by Radiation*. Mountain View, Calif.: MoBeta, 2006.

Leibel, Steven A. *Textbook of Radiation Oncology*. 2d ed. Philadelphia: Saunders, 2004.

Parker, Robert G. *Radiation Oncology for Cure and Palliation*. New York: Springer, 2003.

Schlegel, W., et al., eds. *New Technologies in Radiation Oncology*. New York: Springer, 2006.

▶ Organizations and Professional Societies

American Board of Radiology
http://www.theabr.org/index.htm
5441 East Williams Boulevard, Suite 200
Tucson, AZ 85711

American College of Radiology
http://www.acr.org
1891 Preston White Drive
Reston, VA 20191

American Society for Therapeutic Radiology and Oncology
http://www.astro.org
P.O. Box 631567
Baltimore, MD 21263

International Radiosurgery Support Association
http://www.irsa.org
30905 Hoffman Street
Harrisburg, PA 17110

National Association for Proton Therapy
http://www.proton-therapy.org
7910 Woodmont Avenue, Suite 1303
Bethesda, MD 20814

▶ Other Resources

Radiation Oncology Online Journal
http://www.rooj.com/default.htm

RT Answers
http://www.rtanswers.org

See also Afterloading radiation therapy; Boron neutron capture therapy (BNCT); Brachytherapy; Cobalt 60 radiation; External beam radiation therapy (EBRT); Ionizing radiation; Iridium seeds; Linear accelerator; Nuclear medicine scan; Proton beam therapy; Radiation therapies; Radiopharmaceuticals; Stereotactic needle biopsy; Stereotactic radiosurgery (SRS); X-ray tests.

▶ Radiation therapies

Category: Procedures
Also known as: Radiotherapy, external beam radiation therapy (EBRT), internal beam radiation therapy (IBRT), systemic radiation therapy, stereotactic radiosurgery, afterloading radiation, implants, brachytherapy, tomotherapy, proton therapy, intensity-modulated radiation therapy (IMRT), image-guided radiation therapy (IGRT), Mammosite therapy, radioimmunotherapy

Definition: Radiation therapy uses high doses of radiation to kill cancer cells and prevent metastasis (the spread of disease). Most cancers may be treated with one or more of the three types of radiation therapy. About 50 to 60 percent of all cancers may be treated by radiation therapy during the initial treatment phases, and an additional 12.5 percent of patients may need a second course of treatment later in their disease to manage symptoms caused by the growth of their tumor. The radiation oncologist, with other physicians involved in the care of the patient, will determine if the patient's cancer is appropriately treated with radiation.

Cancers treated: Most, such as breast, prostate, thyroid, and gynecological cancers

Why performed: Radiation therapies are performed to kill, stop, or slow the growth of cancer cells in the body. Cancer is usually treated with surgery, chemotherapy, and radiation, which is called multimodal therapy. Radiation, as a component of this combined approach to care, may be used before, during, or after surgery; in combination with chemotherapy; or alone. Some patients who are not able to tolerate aggressive surgeries or chemotherapies may benefit, to some degree, from radiation therapy. Many patients develop side effects from their cancers that may be treated with radiation. Spinal cord compression or bony metastases may be treated to reduce paralysis or pain.

There are three ways to administer radiation to a patient. When a machine outside the body delivers radiation to a tumor inside the body, the process is called external beam radiation therapy (EBRT). Internal beam radiation therapy (IBRT) uses sources, applicators, or a high-dose remote afterloader to place radioactive material in the body near the cancer site. Systemic radiation therapy uses a radioactive substance that is injected or swallowed and then travels to cancer cells in tissues of the body.

EBRT uses X-ray beams that may be given by a linear accelerator, a machine that generates high-energy radiation beams; by a machine with a radioactive source, cobalt 60; by a tomotherapy unit, which is a linear accelerator coupled with a computed tomography (CT) scanner that delivers radiation in spirals around the body; or by a robotically controlled accelerator that delivers radiation while tracking and controlling for patient movement or organ movement during the treatment. Proton beam therapy, one of the newer of the external beam radiation therapies, uses a machine that generates protons to damage the deoxyribonucleic acid (DNA) of cancer cells. With proton therapy, the radiation beam of protons enters the body with a low dose of radiation, deposits its highest dose at the site being treated, and then stops without traveling through the body.

Advances in external beam therapy, based on the ability to better plan therapies, continue to develop rapidly. Conformal radiation therapy (3D-CRT) develops a three-dimensional model of the tumor and then uses shaped beams to treat the cancer from several directions. Intensity-modulated radiation therapy (IMRT) uses sophisticated treatment planning to vary the strength of the radiation beam in an attempt to lessen damage to the normal tissues surrounding the tumor. Tomotherapy is considered a type of IMRT and image-guided radiation therapy (IGRT), as the beams spiral around the body, allowing for precise and focused radiation beams based on data from a CT scan. IGRT is used to visualize the tumor location prior

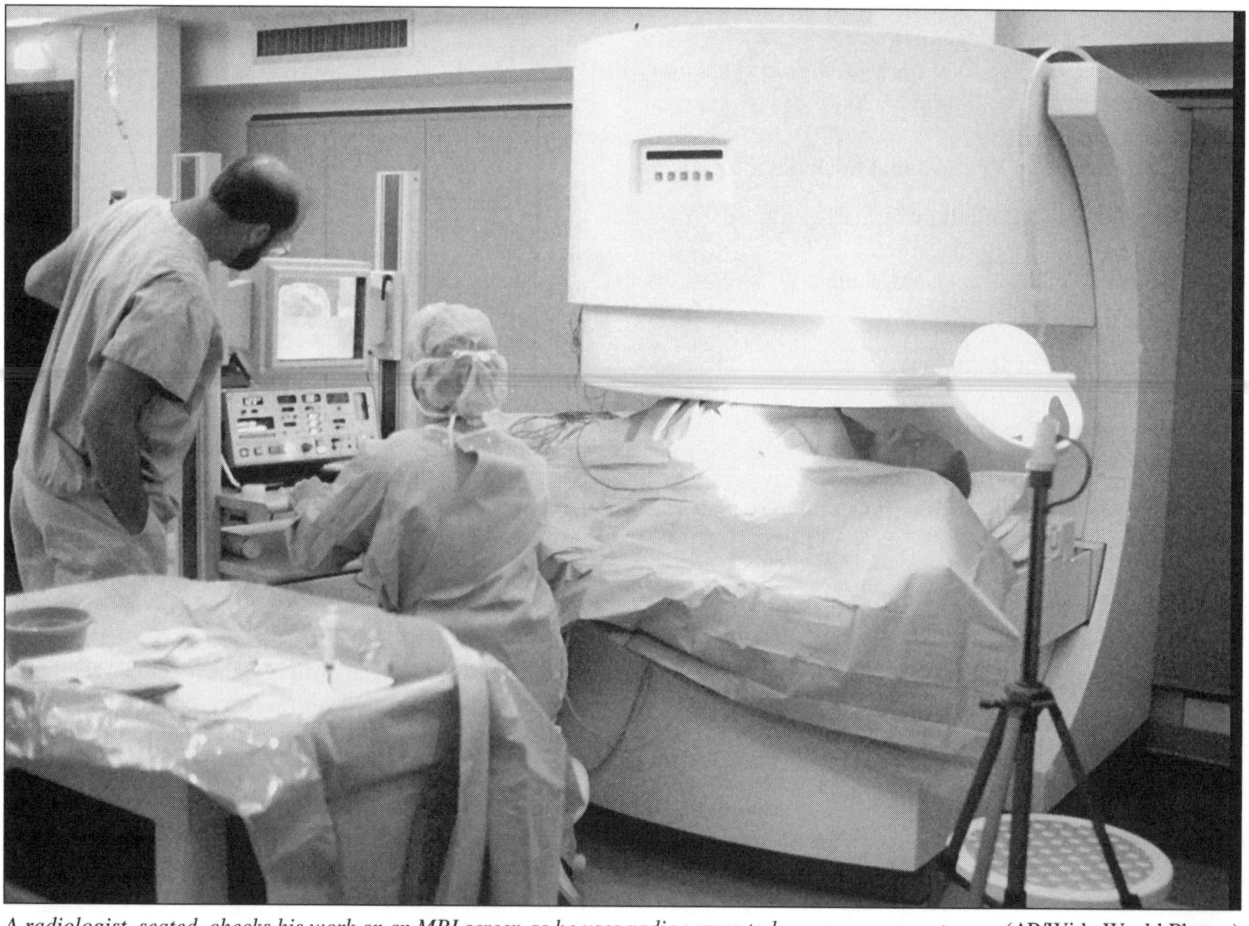

A radiologist, seated, checks his work on an MRI screen as he uses radio waves to burn a cancerous tumor. (AP/Wide World Photos)

to treatment, as tumor movement occurs daily, and to control for tumor movement with respiration (respiratory gating). In addition to a CT scan, ultrasound may be used.

Stereotactic radiosurgery is a type of radiation therapy that delivers a large, precise dose to a defined tumor site. It is most commonly used for brain tumors, but applications in the abdomen and other sites are being explored. A cobalt 60 source machine is used with a head frame for brain tumors, and a robotically control linear accelerator may be used for both brain tumors and tumors outside the head (extracranial tumors). It is called radiosurgery because of its accuracy. The radiation beam is considered as accurate as a knife (or scalpel) and may treat tumors that surgeons cannot reach using traditional surgical techniques.

Intraoperative radiation therapy is used at the time of surgery to deliver external beam radiation directly to the tumor during the surgical procedure. The surgeon locates the cancer and moves normal tissues and organs out of the way, and then an accelerator delivers radiation directly to the tumor. The patient is asleep (under anesthesia) during the procedure, which is done in a special lead-lined operating room.

IBRT is delivered by several methods and is often referred to as brachytherapy. IBRT using a remote-controlled machine called a high-dose remote afterloader (HDR) unit sends high-dose radioactive material through catheters or needles placed in the patient for a period of minutes, and then the sources are withdrawn, so that the patient is not radioactive. When patients are exposed to radiation sources for a period of hours or days, the process is called low-dose-rate brachytherapy. Applicators or cases that house radioactive sources are placed in the patient and left for a prescribed period of time. The area around the patient is considered radioactive until the source is removed. Therefore, staff must limit their exposure to the patient, and visitors are not allowed. Permanent brachytherapy is a type of low-dose therapy in which radioactive seeds are placed in the patient and remain while giving off low doses of radiation for weeks or months. The patient gives off some radioactivity in very small doses. The primary safety consideration is to keep children away from the area of the implant. For example, a man undergoing permanent brachytherapy for prostate cancer must not allow children to sit on his lap.

Systemic radiation therapy is given as a capsule or liquid swallowed by the patient, or it may be given in a vein (injected intravenously). The radioactive liquid then moves throughout the body. The patient may stay in a special room in the hospital, and body fluids are handled carefully, as the radiation materials are eliminated from the body through urine, saliva, and sweat. When the radioactivity has dipped to safe levels, the patient may be discharged from the hospital. In some cases, the patient may be able to go home after treatment with special instructions about handling wastes.

Breast cancer is one of the most commonly treated cancers using external beam radiation therapy. Use of an HDR unit decreases the treatment time of several weeks to just five days. This procedure is often referred to as Mammosite therapy, named for the company that initially developed the procedure for commercial use. Prostate cancer may also use external beam radiation, an HDR unit, or implantable seeds (low-dose brachytherapy) to kill cancer cells. Thyroid cancer is often treated with radioactive iodine, a systemic radiation therapy in a liquid form that is swallowed by the patient. Gynecological cancers may be treated with an HDR unit or low-dose brachytherapy with an applicator that is left in for a period of time.

Patient preparation: The radiation oncologist, a physician with specialized training in radiation therapy care, will see the patient in a consult visit to determine if radiation therapy is appropriate for his or her cancer. Patients are generally referred to the radiation oncologist by the patient's surgeon or medical oncologist. The physicians treating the patient will discuss whether external, internal, or systemic radiation is most appropriate. Prior to receiving treatment, patients have a simulation using a CT scanner or fluoroscopic simulator to allow the physician to visualize the area to be treated. A simulation may take up to two hours. To assist in positioning the patient for treatment, small marks may be placed on the skin. Later in the treatment room, the marks will be used with wall-mounted positioning lasers to place the patient in the correct position to receive the treatment. The simulation data are used to plan the radiation dose amounts to be given by the linear accelerator, the HDR unit, or any other source of radiation, such as implantable seeds. The simulation information is given to the physicist and dosimetrist, who load the data into a sophisticated treatment-planning computer. The physician then verifies the treatment site, the treatment plan, and the radiation dose to be given.

Steps of the procedure: The steps of the radiation treatment will depend on the type of radiation therapy that the patient receives. Regardless of whether external, internal, or systemic therapy is used, treatment planning is still the key to accurate radiation placement and dosing. For external beam therapy, the treatment plan will outline the patient position on the treatment table, determine the shape of the beam, define the number of treatments to be given, and prescribe the daily and cumulative doses the patient is to receive. The patient has four to six weeks of treatment depending on the treatment plan, five days a week, with two days a week off for normal cells to rest and recover. If an HDR unit is to be used, then catheters may be implanted at the time of surgery, or hollow needles may be placed just before the treatment. HDR treatments usually take place once or twice a day for approximately five days.

For patients receiving internal radiation, a simulation and treatment plan are still necessary. For low-dose brachytherapy, such as prostate seed implants, additional imaging studies may be needed. Seeds are implanted during a surgical procedure with the patient under general anesthesia. Low-dose brachytherapy, such as used in gynecological cancers, may use applicators that are placed in a treatment room and then loaded with the radioactive source. Patients receiving systemic radiation also need treatment planning to determine the amount of radioactive liquid needed to treat the cancer.

After the procedure: Most external beam treatments are done on an outpatient basis, and the patient may leave immediately after the daily treatment. Patients are not radioactive during treatments. A few external beam treatments, such as intraoperative radiation therapy and select stereotactic radiosurgery, may require hospitalization. Internal beam radiation treatments may be done on either an inpatient or an outpatient basis, depending on the method used to deliver the radiation therapy. If an HDR unit is used to deliver high-dose radiation, then the patient may be able to go home between treatments. If the internal beam radiation therapy requires that the radioactive source stay in the patient for a period of hours or days, then the patient is usually hospitalized, as the bodily fluids are emitting radioactive waste. Systemic radiotherapy may be either inpatient or outpatient in nature.

Risks: The risks from radiation depend on the site being treated and the type of radiation therapy being used. EBRT is a local treatment, so risks involve the area around the site being treated. For example, if abdominal radiation is used, then bowel and bladder problems may develop. Skin reactions, similar to sunburn, may occur. Hair loss, called alopecia, may occur if radiation is given to the head or other body areas with hair follicles. Xerostomia, or dry mouth, may occur with radiation of the head and neck areas, and dental problems may also occur with this radiation site. Fatigue is often associated with any radiation procedure. Side effects usually go away within two to three months after therapy is completed. Late side effects, those developing six or more months after therapy is completed, may include infertility, lymphedema, joint pain, or other problems, as well as a risk of a second cancer due to the radiation. There is always a risk that not all cancer cells will be killed by the radiation.

Results: Cancer cell kill is expected after any method of radiation treatment.

Patricia Stanfill Edens, R.N., Ph.D., FACHE

▶ For Further Information

Penson, D. F., M. S. Litwin, J. L. Gore, et al. "Quality of Life After Surgery, External Beam Irradiation, or Brachytherapy for Early Stage Prostate Cancer." *Urologic Oncology* 25, no. 5 (September/October, 2007): 442-443.

Tao, Y., D. Lefkopoulos, D. Ibrahima, et al. "Comparison of Dose Contribution to Normal Pelvic Tissues Among Conventional, Conformal, and Intensity-Modulated Radiotherapy Techniques in Prostate Cancer." *Acta Oncologica*, September 28, 2007, 1-9.

▶ Other Resources

American Cancer Society
http://www.acs.org

American Society for Therapeutic Radiology Oncology
http://www.astro.org

Medline Plus
Radiation Therapy
http://www.nlm.nih.gov/medlineplus/radiationtherapy.html

National Cancer Institute
Radiation Therapy and You
http://www.cancer.gov

See also Accelerated partial breast irradiation (APBI); Afterloading radiation therapy; Angiography; Barium enema; Barium swallow; Bone scan; Boron neutron capture therapy (BNCT); Brachytherapy; Brain scan; Bronchography; Cobalt 60 radiation; Computed tomography (CT)-guided biopsy; Computed tomography (CT) scan; Cystography; Ductogram; Endoscopic retrograde cholangiopancreatography (ERCP); External beam radiation therapy (EBRT); Gallium scan; Gamma Knife; Hysterography; Imaging tests; Intensity-modulated radiation therapy (IMRT); Iridium seeds; Linear accelerator; Lymphangiography; Magnetic resonance imaging (MRI); Mammography; Microwave hyperthermia therapy; Nuclear medicine scan; Positron emission tomography (PET); Proton beam therapy; Radiation therapies; Radiofrequency ablation; Radionuclide scan; Radiopharmaceuticals; Stereotactic needle biopsy; Stereotactic radiosurgery (SRS); Thermal imaging; Thyroid nuclear medicine scan; Wire localization; X-ray tests.

Radical neck dissection

Category: Procedures
Also known as: Classical radical neck dissection

Definition: A radical neck dissection is a surgical procedure that involves the excision of a primary malignant cancer and several adjacent head and neck structures (salivary glands, sternocleidomastoid muscle, cervical lymph nodes, fatty tissue, jugular vein, and spinal accessory nerve).

Cancers treated: Squamous and basal cell carcinomas of the head and neck, lymphoma, thyroid carcinoma, metastatic cancer

Why performed: On gross examination of the neck, masses that preserve the outer tissue can suggest a benign tumor but cannot eliminate the possibility of cancer. Microscopically, benign tumor cells have an increased, orderly growth while malignant cells have an increased, disorderly growth and large nuclei relative to the surrounding cytoplasm. Cervical lymph node samples possessing cancerous cells strongly suggest microscopic spread outside the neck.

Extensive infiltration of the neck by a tumor can affect breathing, speech, and movement as well as blood circulation to the head. Surgery may be necessary to restore the function of the affected structures. The procedure is performed when malignant cancer has spread to adjacent facial and neck structures. Introduced in 1906 by George W. Crile, it remains the standard surgical treatment for metastasis.

Patient preparation: Surgical risk assessment, tissue biopsy, and computed tomography (CT) and/or magnetic resonance imaging (MRI) are done.

Steps of the procedure: A hockey-stick-shaped incision is made over the anterolateral neck. The superficial neck muscle (platysma) is cut and retracted. The submandibular gland and duct, lymph nodes, a segment of the facial artery, and the tail of the parotid gland are removed or ligated. The sternocleidomastoid muscle is cut above the clavicle and retracted. The posterior omohyoid, anterior trapezius, spinal accessory nerve, jugular vein, surrounding lymph nodes, and the upper border of the sternocleidomastoid are ligated, cut, and removed.

After the procedure: The patient is monitored until stable. A breathing tube may be put in place to protect the airway until the wound heals. Food intake may be withheld for at least twenty-four hours after the operation. The patient may be discharged if stable after a few days.

Risks: Bleeding is the most common complication because of the dense capillary network around the head and neck. Breathing problems, infections, formation of an abnormal connection between the esophagus and the trachea, shoulder muscle paralysis, and significant disfigurement can also occur.

Results: Although neck dissection has veered toward preserving function, radical neck dissection remains a sound surgical option for advanced stages of cancer.

Aldo C. Dumlao, M.D.

For Further Information

Brockstein, Bruce, and Gregory Masters, eds. *Head and Neck Cancer*. Boston: Kluwer Academic, 2003.

Kelloff, Gary, Ernest T. Hawk, and Caroline C. Sigman. *Cancer Chemoprevention*. Totowa, N.J.: Humana Press, 2004.

Thaller, Seth R., and W. Scott McDonald. *Facial Trauma*. Miami: Informa Health Care, 2004.

See also Basal cell carcinomas; Benign tumors; Carcinomas; Computed tomography (CT) scan; Imaging tests; Infection and sepsis; Lymphomas; Magnetic resonance imaging (MRI); Metastasis; Metastatic squamous neck cancer with occult primary; Oral and maxillofacial surgery; Salivary gland cancer; Thyroid cancer.

Radiofrequency ablation

Category: Procedures
Also known as: RFA, thermal ablation

Definition: Radiofrequency ablation is the application of high-energy radio waves (radiofrequency thermal energy) through a catheter probe to heat and destroy abnormal tissues. As a cancer treatment, radiofrequency ablation is used to ablate (destroy) cancerous tumors by directing the radiofrequency heat directly to the tumor, causing the cancerous cells to die.

According to the Society of Interventional Radiology, radiofrequency energy is safer than many cancer therapies because it is absorbed by living tissues as simple heat, and the heat generated by radiofrequency does not alter the basic chemical structure of cells.

Radiofrequency ablation technology was originally developed for the treatment of cardiac arrhythmias in the early 1990's and has since been used as a cancer treatment after clinical studies proved its efficacy. The technology is approved by the Food and Drug Administration (FDA).

Radiofrequency applications vary, depending on the

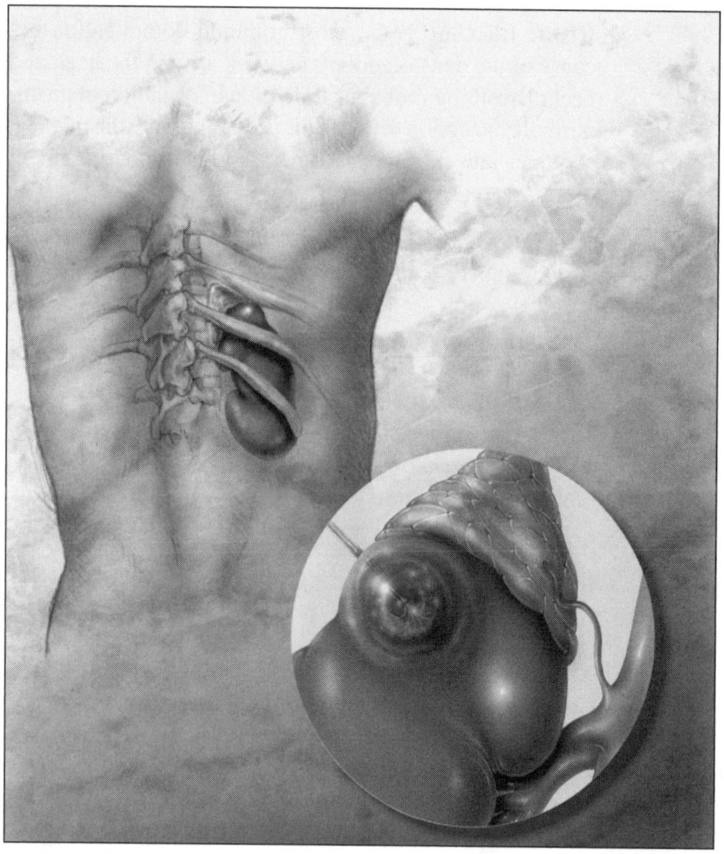

Radio frequency catheter ablation of a kidney tumor (inset); the kidney in the body (background). (© Kevin A. Somerville/Phototake—All rights reserved)

type of catheter used and the dose of energy applied. Newer RFA applications involve ablation with multiple electrodes to treat large or multiple tumors and ablation with liposomal therapy, a method of delivering heat-activated chemotherapy drugs via synthetic capsules called liposomes. The coating on the liposome capsules allows the medication to remain in the circulation for a longer period of time, so the drugs selectively target cancer cells and decrease the side effects for healthy tissue.

Cancers treated: Primary and metastatic liver cancer, early-stage breast cancer, lung cancer, bone cancer, prostate cancer, and kidney and adrenal gland cancers; RFA is also being investigated as a treatment option for many other cancers

Why performed: Radiofrequency ablation is a minimally invasive, percutaneous procedure that offers an alternative treatment option for some patients with tumors that cannot be surgically removed, for patients who are not surgical candidates because of comorbid conditions or other risk factors, or for those who desire a less invasive treatment. In some cases, radiofrequency ablation can be used to ease certain side effects of cancer treatment, such as chronic pain caused by some cancers. Radiofrequency ablation may be used in combination with chemotherapy or other cancer treatments to improve a patient's quality of life and survival.

The recommendation for radiofrequency ablation is dependent on the type of cancer, the patient's overall medical condition, the number of tumors, and the tumor size and location.

Patient preparation: Tests performed before the procedure include positron emission tomography (PET) testing and computed tomography (CT) scanning. Radiofrequency ablation does not interfere with most standard cancer therapies and can be performed for some patients who are actively receiving chemotherapy.

A few days before the procedure, patients must stop taking aspirin and products containing aspirin, ibuprofen, and anticoagulants, as directed by the physician. Other anticoagulant medications may be prescribed if necessary before the procedure. Antiarrhythmic medications may also need to be discontinued. Patients with diabetes may need to adjust their diabetes medications, insulin dosages, or meal plan, as directed by the physician. Patients must not eat or drink for eight hours beforehand.

Patients should remove all makeup and nail polish. The patient will change into a hospital gown before the procedure.

Steps of the procedure: An intravenous (IV) line is inserted into a vein in the patient's arm to deliver medications. A sedative is usually given before the procedure so that the patient will be in a form of light sleep during the procedure. General anesthesia is used in some cases. An interventional radiologist usually performs the procedure, although a surgeon can also do so.

If general anesthesia is not used, then a local anesthetic is injected into the procedure site to numb the area. A thin, needlelike probe is placed through a puncture or small incision in the skin and is guided by ultrasound or CT into the core of the tumor. Once it is in place, thin, hook-shaped wires (tines) on the end of the probe extend upon deployment to an area beyond the diameter of the tumor. Localized radiofrequency energy is transmitted through the probe, which is attached to a radiofrequency generator. Energy is applied for ten to fifteen minutes to each targeted area, thereby heating and destroying the tissue. The temperature of the applied energy is carefully controlled; beyond 60 degrees Celsius, cells begin to die, resulting in an area of tissue death surrounding the probe. The probe may be deployed more than once for tumors larger than 3 centimeters.

Multiple tumors may be treated during the ablation procedure. A small region of normal cells around the tumor (margin) is also heated and destroyed with the goal of eradicating cancer in surrounding tissues. The procedure lasts from two to four hours.

After the procedure: The RFA probe is removed and pressure is applied to the insertion site to prevent bleeding. No stitches are needed unless a small incision was made. A small sterile dressing (bandage) will cover the insertion site. The patient may need to stay in bed from one to six hours after the procedure to prevent bleeding.

Most patients stay in the hospital overnight for observation after the procedure, but some patients go home the same day of the procedure. The patient may experience discomfort for two to three days afterward. Pain medication may be prescribed, or the patient may take acetaminophen (Tylenol) to relieve discomfort as needed.

The patient should not drive or operate machinery for eight hours after the procedure. Within twenty-four hours, the patient is usually able to return to light activity but should avoid vigorous physical activity and heavy lifting after the procedure, as directed by the physician. The average recovery time is from three to seven days, after which the patient may resume regular activities. The recovery time for radiofrequency ablation is much faster than that for surgical treatment, which can take from two to three months for full recovery.

Patients usually have a follow-up CT or magnetic resonance imaging (MRI) scan one week after the procedure to evaluate the effectiveness of the treatment. Thereafter, follow-up CT scans and blood tests are performed every three months or more frequently, based on the patient's condition.

Risks: The risks of radiofrequency ablation vary in relation to the type of cancer being treated and the area that is being ablated. For example, the risks of RFA applications for lung cancer include pleural effusion and pneumothorax. The risks of RFA applications for liver cancer include portal vein thrombosis, liver abscess, or acute renal insufficiency. The physician performing the procedure will discuss the potential risks of the procedure with the patient, depending on the type of cancer that is being treated.

The rate of overall complications is 1 to 4 percent, according to the Society of Interventional Radiology, depending on the disease treated and the patient's overall health. Most complications are minor and are often relieved on their own without further treatment or intervention. The risk of infection is rare, since there is no open wound associated with the procedure.

Results: Radiofrequency ablation is a safe and effective treatment option. Tumors from 1 to 10 centimeters in size can be successfully treated with radiofrequency ablation. A tumor or lesion that is successfully ablated should be reduced in size, or disappear altogether, and show no blood flow on follow-up CT scans. In addition to other cancer treatments, radiofrequency ablation can reduce the size of an inoperable tumor. RFA also can ease tumor-related symptoms, such as flushing, diarrhea, or hypertension, that are associated with some hormone-secreting tumors.

Long-term outcomes following radiofrequency ablation are promising. Based on literature reviews, complete tumor ablation with low recurrence rates can be achieved, particularly for smaller cancers. Research is ongoing to evaluate the long-term outcomes of the procedure. For example, RFA in combination with standard radiation therapy has shown two-year and five-year survival rates of 50 and 39 percent, respectively, for the treatment of Stage I and Stage II non-small-cell lung cancer. Research shows the local recurrence rate after RFA of colorectal cancer liver metastases averages less than 10 percent. Recurrence rates are related to the lesion size.

Repeat radiofrequency ablations can be performed for patients who develop new or recurrent tumors. Radiofrequency ablation does not preclude patients from undergoing other cancer treatments if necessary.

Angela M. Costello, B.S.

▶ For Further Information

Ellis, Lee M., et al. *Radiofrequency Ablation for Cancer: Current Indication, Techniques, and Outcomes.* New York: Springer, 2003.

Patti, Jay W., et al. "Radiofrequency Ablation for Cancer-Associated Pain." *The Journal of Pain* 3, no. 6 (2002): 471-473.

Phillips, Carmen. *Radiofrequency Ablation Making Inroads as Cancer Treatment.* Bethesda, Md.: National Cancer Institute, 2005. Also available online at http://www.cancer.gov.

Wood, B. J., et al. "Percutaneous Tumor Ablation with Radiofrequency." *Cancer* 94, no. 2 (2002): 443-451.

▶ Other Resources

American Cancer Ablation Centers
http:///www.cancerablation.com

American Society of Clinical Oncology
http://www.asco.org

Society of Interventional Radiology
http://www.sirweb.org

See also Adenoid cystic carcinoma (ACC); Adrenal gland cancers; Bone cancers; Bone scan; Breast cancers; Carcinoid tumors and carcinoid syndrome; Computed tomography (CT) scan; Hyperthermia therapy; Liver cancers; Lung cancers; Prostate cancer; Virus-related cancers.

▶ Radionuclide scan

Category: Procedures
Also known as: Nuclear medicine scan

Definition: A radionuclide scan is the detection of electromagnetic radiation, usually gamma rays, emitted from an injected radioactive tracer that has been taken up by an organ in the body to be studied, with the goal of producing an image. The most common radioisotope used is technetium 99m, whose gamma rays are absorbed by a sodium iodide crystal detector. The radiation absorbed by this detector is used to generate an image that is interpreted by a radiologist or nuclear medicine physician. The exceptions are positron emission tomography (PET) scanning, which uses positron emission; gallium scanning, which uses gallium as the radionuclide; and some thyroid imaging, which uses iodine.

Cancers diagnosed: Virtually all types of cancer, especially metastases

Why performed: A radionuclide scan is used to diagnose primary and secondary cancer (bone scan, iodine scan, PET scan) and to diagnose various ailments, including but not limited to the following: hypothyroidism or hyperthyroidism (thyroid scan), bone fractures and bone infection (bone scan), kidney obstruction (renal scan), inflammatory disorders such as sarcoid and fever of unknown origin (gallium scan), cardiomyopathy multiple uptake gated acquisition (MUGA scan), coronary artery disease (cardiac single photon emission computed tomography, or SPECT) pulmonary embolus (lung scan), and Alzheimer's disease (brain SPECT).

Patient preparation: The preparation for a radionuclide scan is minimal to none; the scan is usually performed as an outpatient procedure. For some procedures, the patient may be asked to fast several hours prior to the scan.

Steps of the procedure: The radioisotope is prepared by the technologist and injected into a peripheral vein by the radiologist or nuclear medicine physician. The patient is then placed supine on a table under a gamma camera that houses the detectors. The scan time is usually about one hour.

After the procedure: The scan is generated by the computer attached to the camera and read by the radiologist the same day. The patient will need to contact his or her doctor for the radiologist's report and any follow-up therapy.

Risks: The risks of this type of scan include minor pain or bruising at the injection site. If the patient is pregnant, then the scan should be avoided if possible, since the radiation dose, although small in most cases, is not negligible. Radioactive iodine should not be administered to a pregnant patient because of risk to the fetus.

Results: The scan results are dependent on the type of scan performed and the reason for the study.

Debra B. Kessler, M.D., Ph.D.

See also Appendix cancer; Bone scan; Electromagnetic radiation; Gallium scan; Imaging tests; Ionizing radiation; Nuclear medicine scan; Positron emission tomography (PET); Thyroid cancer.

▶ Radiopharmaceuticals

Category: Chemotherapy and other drugs
ATC code: V10

Definition: Radiopharmaceuticals are a class of therapeutic drugs that carry a radioactive isotope in trace quantities. These drugs deliver radiation to kill a targeted region of malignant cells.

Cancers treated: Various cancers metastasizing to bone tissues, especially prostate cancer and thyroid cancer, B-cell non-Hodgkin lymphoma, and polycythemia vera

Subclasses of this group: Radioisotopes of iodine, phosphorous, rhenium, samarium, strontium, and yttrium

Delivery routes: These drugs are administered intravenously, orally in capsule or liquid form, or through a direct injection to the site of cancer, on an inpatient or outpatient basis, depending on the specific drug, the type of cancer,

Common Radiopharmaceuticals Used in Cancer Therapy

Drug	*Brands*	*Delivery Mode*	*Cancers Treated*
Iodine 131 (^{131}I), sodium iodide		Oral	Thyroid cancer
Phosphorus 32 (^{32}P), sodium phosphate, chromic phosphate		Oral, IV	Polycythemia vera; bone metastases; cancers causing malignant ascites, pleural effusion, pericardial effusions, and brain cysts
Rhenium 186 (^{186}Re) HEDP		IV	Bone metastases; breast cancer
Samarium 153 (^{153}Sm) EDTMP	Quadramet	Injection	Bone metastases
Strontium 89 (^{89}Sr), strontium chloride	Metastron	Injection	Bone metastases
Yttrium 90 (^{90}Y) ibritumomab tiuxetan	Zevalin	IV	B-cell non-Hodgkin lymphoma

and its location. When possible, these drugs are best delivered directly to the tumor site to limit damage to normal cells.

How these drugs work: Initially, radiopharmaceuticals were developed to diagnose various medical problems, including tumors. Using radiographic imaging, nuclear medicine specialists detect the radiation emitted by these drugs and track their activity within an organ. Since the 1980's, the role of radiopharmaceuticals has been expanded to palliation and therapy of metastatic cancers. In this case, a slightly larger amount of the radioactive isotope is used to destroy a group of cancerous cells by interfering with cell division. Instead of photons (used for imaging), the drugs emit beta particles and gamma rays that damage the machinery needed for mitosis. The radioactive isotope is attached to a carrier molecule that is capable of targeting a specific organ or group of cells. For example, radiopharmaceuticals for bone cancer therapy have a mineral-like carrier molecule taken up by bone tissues.

Radiopharmaceuticals for specific organs may have a monoclonal antibody that recognizes the cell surface receptors of certain tissue cells. Once the drug reaches its target area, the isotope emits radiation slowly over short distances. The half-life, or time required for half of the radiation to be emitted, for these drugs is two to fifty days, depending on the isotope.

In almost all cases, radiopharmaceuticals are used when chemotherapy has failed, or in conjunction with second-line chemotherapy. Radiopharmaceuticals are especially helpful in cancers that have metastasized to neighboring bones, such as prostate and thyroid cancers. Studies have shown that these drugs are valuable in palliative care for patients experiencing pain from cancerous bone tissue, resulting in better disease management and improved quality of life.

Side effects: The side effects of radiopharmaceuticals vary depending on the specific radioactive isotope, its dosage, and the individual patient's physical condition. An excessive dose of these drugs may result in toxicity that affects normal cells as well as malignant cells, which could lead to an intensification of the cancer. The most common side effect of radiopharmaceuticals, however, is a decrease in the patient's white blood cell and platelet counts. Other common side effects include black or bloody stools, coughs, fevers or chills, back or side pain, difficulty in urination, unusual bleeding or bruising, and nausea and vomiting. Less common side effects include bone pain and irregular heartbeat. Patients who take iodine 131 for thyroid cancer may also experience loss of taste and tenderness in the salivary glands and neck. Since children and older adults are particularly sensitive to radiation, they may experience more side effects during and after treatment with radiopharmaceuticals.

Bharat Burman, B.A.

▶ For Further Information

Ballantyne, Jane C., ed. *The Massachusetts General Hospital Handbook of Pain Management*. 3d ed. Philadelphia: Lippincott Williams & Wilkins, 2006.

Leibel, Steven A., and Theodore L. Phillips, eds. *Textbook of Radiation Oncology*. 2d ed. Philadelphia: Saunders, 2004.

Parker, R. G., N. A. Janjan, and M. T. Selch. *Radiation Oncology for Cure and Palliation*. New York: Springer, 2003.

▶ Other Resources

Radiation Oncology Online Journal
http://www.rooj.com/default.htm

Society of Radiopharmaceutical Sciences
http://www.srsweb.org

See also Bone cancers; Chemotherapy; Imaging tests; Non-Hodgkin lymphoma; Nuclear medicine scan; Prostate cancer; Radiation oncology; Thyroid cancer; X-ray tests.

▶ Radon

Category: Carcinogens and suspected carcinogens
RoC status: Known human carcinogen since 1994
Also known as: Radon-222, thoron (radon-220), actinon (radon-219)

Related cancers: Lung cancer

Definition: Radon is an invisible, odorless, radioactive gas produced naturally from uranium in rocks and soil. Except for areas rich in uranium-ore deposits, radon is usually present at low levels in water, soil, and outdoor air. It decays spontaneously to form solid radioactive products called radon daughters that emit ionizing radiation, mostly as alpha particles and gamma radiation. Radon gas may seep into buildings from underlying soil and accumulate at dangerous levels in indoor spaces. Its levels can be measured by using radon test kits.

Exposure routes: Inhalation, ingestion

Where found: Uranium mines and mills, hard-rock mines, phosphate mines, granite formations, groundwater, soil, air, building materials

At risk: Workers in uranium mining and milling, workers in iron-ore and fluorite mining, general population exposed to indoor radon levels of 4 picoCurie per liter (pCi/L) or higher

Etiology and symptoms of associated cancers: Radon is the second leading cause of lung cancer after cigarette smoking and accounts for 15 percent of lung cancers worldwide. Most of the risk to humans is from inhaled radon daughters that can lodge in the lungs and emit energetic particles. Damage to epithelial cells in lung tissue can eventually lead to cancer. For smokers, the risk of lung cancer is even greater because of the synergistic effects of radon and smoking.

The deadliest of all cancers, lung cancer has an overall five-year survival rate of less than 15 percent. Radon-related lung cancers include squamous cell carcinoma, adenocarcinoma, and large-cell carcinoma. In its early stages, lung cancer may be asymptomatic or have nonspecific symptoms (weight loss, fatigue, and fever). By the time symptoms develop that are suggestive of the disease (chronic coughing, shortness of breath, hoarseness, bloody sputum, difficulty swallowing, wheezing, and chest pain), the cancer has usually spread to other organs.

History: Once produced commercially for use in radiotherapy, radon is used mostly in research. Scientists established radon's carcinogenicity primarily from occupational studies conducted between the 1950's and 1980's that revealed high mortality rates from lung cancer among underground uranium miners. In 1984 exposure to radon in buildings came to be recognized as a potential health hazard. In the Indoor Radon Abatement Act of 1988, the U.S. Environmental Protection Agency (EPA) recommended that indoor radon levels not exceed average levels outdoors (about 0.4 pCi/L). This standard is one tenth of the recommended safety level for homes.

Anna Binda, Ph.D.

See also Air pollution; Benzene; Bronchoalveolar lung cancer; Carcinogens, known; Carcinogens, reasonably anticipated; Ionizing radiation; Lung cancers; Occupational exposures and cancer; Risks for cancer.

▶ *RB1* gene

Category: Cancer biology
Also known as: Retinoblastoma 1 (including osteosarcoma), OSRC

Definition: The *RB1* gene (a tumor-suppressor gene), which is 180 kilobase pairs with 27 exons, can become inactivated and cause retinoblastoma, a rare childhood cancer of the retina, occurring from in utero to about five years of age.

Gene location and function: The retinoblastoma gene, *RB1*, is on chromosome 13q14.2. This ubiquitously expressed gene codes for a 110 KDa tumor suppressor (pRB), which regulates cell division. The retinoblastoma protein regulates the progression of cells through the cell cycle and the exiting of differentiating cells from the cell cycle. This protein controls cell cycle by sequestering transcription factors and by deacetylating histones, involved in gene silencing. To lose the tumor-suppressor ability, both copies of the *RB1* gene must be mutated. Individuals with an inherited form of retinoblastoma have a germ-line mutation of one *RB1* gene. During development, the second copy of the *RB1* gene is mutated; control of the cell cycle is lost, and tumors develop. These tumors may be in both eyes. Other individuals have sporadic retinoblastoma in which mutations occur in the same somatic cell to inactivate both copies of the *RB1* gene. Sporadic retinoblastoma is often in only one eye.

***RB1* gene inactivation:** Causes of *RB1* gene inactivation include chromosome rearrangements of the 13q14 region; nucleotide changes, loss of heterozygosity (loss of the normal copy); and CpG hypermethylation in the *RB1* promoter region (which silences the gene).

Molecular screening: Methods to screen for *RB1* gene mutations include multiplex polymerase chain reaction (PCR) sequencing of the gene, a protein truncation test, and methylation analysis. The usual clinical screening for retinoblasoma requires examination of the eyes under anesthesia. Molecular screening could eliminate anesthesia-related risks and reduce the financial and psychological costs of clinical screening. Individuals without germline *RB1* mutations will not need the clinical screening. Fetuses that have highly penetrant germ-line mutations could be delivered early and treated sooner to save their vision. People with inherited forms of retinoblastoma (have one defective *RB1* gene) have an increased risk of developing other cancers, such as those of the bladder, pineal gland, bone, and skin.

Incidence: Retinoblastoma accounts for 3 percent of cancers in children under the age of fifteen. The frequency of retinoblastoma is about 1 in 20,000. About 60 percent of those with retinoblastoma have *RB1* mutations only in the tumor and not in other cells. Some 40 percent of retinoblastoma cases are hereditary. Of hereditary cases, 90 percent are due to new mutations occurring near the time of conception; 10 percent are due to a mutation inherited from a parent.

Susan J. Karcher, Ph.D.

See also Cancer biology; Childhood cancers; Fibrosarcomas, soft-tissue; Oncogenes; Pineoblastomas; Retinoblastomas; Simian virus 40; Tumor-suppressor genes.

▶ Receptor analysis

Category: Procedures
Also known as: Receptor status test

Definition: Receptor analysis refers to diagnostic testing procedures carried out on cells or tissues to determine the abundance or functional integrity of specific receptors.

Cancers diagnosed: Breast cancer, colorectal cancer, prostate cancer, lung cancer, leukemia

Why performed: Many factors that stimulate cell growth start the mitogenic cascade by binding to specific cellular receptors, and one of the hallmarks of cancer is cell growth in the absence of these factors. This observation points to the critical role that receptors play in tumor cell growth and provides the basis for selecting among drug regimens that target receptor-signaling pathways. Breast cancer is the most prominent tumor type in which receptor analysis plays a role, but abnormal growth factor receptors may also be a feature of other solid tumors (colorectal, prostate, lung) and some hematologic (blood) malignancies.

Patient preparation: Tissue samples are required and are obtained as part of tumor resection surgery or biopsy. Procedures done under general anesthetic require an overnight fast. Receptor analysis is performed on tumor tissue that is removed, and the patient requires no special or additional postoperative care. Sample collection in leukemia and lymphoma patients is by a simple blood draw, which requires no fasting or special postvenipuncture care.

Steps of the procedure: After the appropriate tumor tissue samples are collected by the surgeon or phlebotomist, receptor analysis proceeds by fixing and processing the tissue for immunohistochemistry (IHC) or deoxyribonucleic acid (DNA) sequence analysis. IHC involves placing a very thin slice of tumor on a microscope slide and incubation with antibody preparations that react with the receptors of interest. After a washing step, other reagents are added that bind to the antireceptor antibodies and lead to chemical reactions that produce a visible color in cells that have the receptors. Pathologists then examine the tissue to determine the percentage of tumor cells that express the receptor. In breast cancer, receptors for estrogen and progesterone are routinely determined by IHC, as is the orphan receptor HER2/neu (Erb B2). IHC is also used to determine androgen receptor expression in prostate cancer. In lung and colorectal cancer, DNA sequence analysis is done to characterize mutations in the epidermal growth factor receptor (EGFR). In suspected lymphoproliferative disorders, analysis of the T-cell receptor gene by polymerase chain reaction can be used to determine monoclonal expansion (a sign of malignancy).

After the procedure: The operative or biopsy site is kept clean and dry to avoid infection. No special instructions regarding receptor analysis are required.

Risks: The risks and side effects of the sample acquisition procedure may be significant; however, receptor analysis itself carries no additional risk to the patient. Some assays for the estrogen receptor have large interlaboratory variability and high false negative rates for tumors with low receptor expression.

Results: In general, retention of normal receptor status by malignant cells is a favorable prognostic sign and forms the basis for a range of endocrine-based therapeutic options. In breast cancer patients, 25 to 35 percent of patients are expected to have amplified HER2/neu receptors, and a humanized monoclonal antibody to HER2 overexpressing breast cancer cells inhibits growth of the cells. The antibody trastuzumab (marketed as Herceptin) increases the clinical benefit of first-line chemotherapy in metastatic breast cancer that overexpresses HER2. Breast cancers that express estrogen and progesterone receptors may grow in response to these hormones, and patients may therefore benefit from antiestrogen drugs such as tamoxifen.

In prostate cancer cells, androgen receptors (ARs) are often overexpressed, and loss of the receptors is an unfavorable sign. AR-positive prostate cancer patients can be treated with leuprolide, which acts at the pituitary to decrease the secretion of gonadotropins. Lower gonadotropin levels result in lower androgen levels, which slows the growth of AR-positive tumor cells.

Tumors that are found to overexpress the EGFR may be treated with cetuximab, a monoclonal antibody that competitively inhibits the receptor, or with small molecules that inhibit the kinase activity of the receptor.

Tumors can express a wide variety of other growth factor receptors, notably those for insulin-like growth factor I (IGF-I) and for vascular endothelial growth factor (VEGF). Inhibiting these receptors with specific compounds is a promising area of cancer research.

John B. Welsh, M.D., Ph.D.

▶ For Further Information

Carpenter, G., ed. *The EGF Receptor Family: Biologic Mechanisms and Role in Cancer*. Amsterdam: Elsevier Academic Press, 2004

Chang, J., et al. "Prediction of Clinical Outcome from Primary Tamoxifen by Expression of Biologic Markers in Breast Cancer Patients." *Clinical Cancer Research* 6 (2000): 616-621.

Chen, W. Y., and G. A. Colditz. "Risk Factors and Hormone-Receptor Status: Epidemiology, Risk-Prediction Models and Treatment Implications for Breast Cancer." *Nature Clinical Practice Oncology* 4 (2007): 415-423.

Schally, A. V., and A. M. Comaru-Schally. "Hypothalamic and Other Peptide Hormones." In *Holland-Frei Cancer Medicine 7*, edited by D. W. Kufe et al. Hamilton, Ont.: BC Decker, 2006.

Sequist, L. V., et al. "Molecular Predictors of Response to Epidermal Growth Factor Receptor Antagonists in Non-Small-Cell Lung Cancer." *Journal of Clinical Oncology* 25 (2007): 587.

Slamon, D., et al. "Use of Chemotherapy Plus a Monoclonal Antibody Against HER2 for Metastatic Breast Cancer That Overexpresses HER2." *New England Journal of Medicine* 344 (2001): 783-792.

Taube, S. E., et al. "Cancer Diagnostics: Decision Criteria for Marker Utilization in the Clinic." *American Journal of Pharmacogenomics* 5 (2005): 357-364.

Wang, Y., et al. "Inhibition of the IGF-I Receptor for Treatment of Cancer: Kinase Inhibitors and Monoclonal Antibodies as Alternative Approaches." *Recent Results in Cancer Research* 172 (2007): 59-76.

See also Androgen drugs; Antiestrogens; Biopsy; Breast cancer in children and adolescents; Breast cancer in men; Breast cancer in pregnant women; Breast cancers; Bronchial adenomas; Colorectal cancer; Colorectal cancer screening; Epidemiology of cancer; HER2/neu protein; Hormone receptor tests; Leukemias; Lung cancers; Lymphomas; Medical oncology; Monoclonal antibodies; Oncology; Progesterone receptor assay; Prostate cancer; Rectal cancer; Risks for cancer.

▶ Reconstructive surgery

Category: Procedures
Also known as: Plastic surgery, cosmetic surgery

Definition: Reconstructive surgery is surgery to rebuild areas lost as a result of cancer or cancer treatment, as well as injury.

Cancers treated: Many different types of cancers, especially breast and skin cancers

Why performed: Reconstructive surgery may be performed to correct problems caused by cancer or cancer treatment. It is often performed to restore better functioning to the affected area. It can also be performed for cosmetic reasons. When it is done for cosmetic reasons, it is usually performed to restore a more symmetrical appearance, to reduce the signs left by cancer and cancer treatment, and to improve self-esteem.

Patient preparation: Patient preparation depends in large part on the procedure that is being done. Preparation before surgery generally includes not eating or drinking any fluids for a certain number of hours before the surgery, stopping certain medications such as blood thinners, or beginning to take medications such as antibiotics to help prevent infection. The surgeon and the surgeon's health care team will provide the patient with the necessary information about what to do, and what not to do, in the hours, days, and weeks before the surgery. In some cases, mental health support may be suggested for before the surgery, as well as afterward, if the surgery is going to make a great change in the individual's appearance.

Steps of the procedure: The steps of reconstructive surgery will vary depending on the type of surgery. For many types of surgery, there will be more than one option, and the surgeon will decide which one to use based on the desires of the patient, the patient's health level, body type, and other factors.

Most reconstructive surgery involves using skin, fat, muscle, or tissue from one area of the body and moving it to another location to reconstruct the desired area. Sometimes prosthetics are used in addition to the material from another area of the patient's body. For example, one possible method of breast reconstruction involves using some tissue from the patient in addition to an implant made of saline.

Five main types of procedures are used during cancer treatment and afterward. The first type is a simple closure of the wound area, in which the wound created by the removal of cancerous tissue is closed using sutures. This generally allows for healing with minimal scarring and a coloration that matches the surrounding skin.

If the area removed is too large to be closed using sutures, then a skin graft might be used. In this procedure, skin is removed from another site on the patient's body and is placed over the area that needs to be closed. A donor site will usually be selected for the best possible match of coloration to the recipient area, and minimal visibility.

When more than just skin is desired, a local flap may be used. The surgeon will take skin and tissue from an area next to the site of the wound and move it over the wound. The flap remains connected to its original surroundings by veins and arteries.

If a local flap is not available or appropriate for some reason, then the surgeon may decide to use a pedicle flap, a section of tissue that is removed from one area but left attached to the blood supply in that area. The flap is anchored to the recipient site with its original source of blood still intact.

The other alternative is to use a free flap. A free flap is completely removed from the donor site, including the severing of all arteries and veins. The flap is then moved to the recipient site and connected. This is generally a longer and more complex surgery than a local or pedicle flap, because the surgery team must use microsurgery to connect the flap to the adjacent area so that blood can flow in and out of the tissue, keeping it alive.

After the procedure: The aftercare for reconstructive surgery will vary depending on the type of procedure and the area of the surgery. Usually there will be a hospital stay of short to moderate duration after the procedure, although some more minor procedures may be performed on an outpatient basis. Healing will take varying lengths of time depending on the type of procedure used and the location on the body of the surgery. For most reconstructive surgeries, as with most surgeries, it will take a few weeks or longer for the patient to return to their normal level of activity.

Some reconstructive surgeries can be followed up at a later time, generally after the wound has mostly or completely healed, with additional cosmetic procedures. For example, after breast reconstruction, the nipple can be reconstructed at a later time, after the breast itself has healed. Additionally, tattooing of the nipple and areole can be done at a later time to try to match the existing breast as nearly as possible.

Risks: There are risks associated with any kind of surgical procedure. The risks of reconstructive surgery are generally low when the procedure is performed by a certified reconstructive surgeon who is experienced in the procedure. A patient who has questions about the surgeon's training, qualifications, or experience with the type of procedure being considered should never hesitate to ask.

The risks associated with reconstructive surgery are generally the same as those associated with any other type of surgery, including excessive bleeding, infection, pooling of blood beneath the skin, bruising, and problems with wound healing. Procedures that are done under general anesthesia have the risks associated with general anesthesia, including changes in blood pressure or heart rhythm. Complications from general anesthesia are generally rare, although certain diseases and conditions can increase these risks.

Reconstructive surgery is generally considered to be relatively low risk for individuals who are otherwise in reasonably good health. Certain diseases and conditions can interfere with the healing process or can cause an increased risk of complications. Individuals who have high blood pressure, diabetes, or immune system problems or who have conditions that affect the blood's ability to clot may be at increased risk of complications. Individuals who smoke may be required to quit smoking for a few months before the surgery to decrease the likelihood of side effects or complications and to increase the body's ability to heal effectively. This kind of requirement generally depends on the specific surgeon who is doing the procedure. In general, individuals who smoke have a more difficult time healing completely after surgery and may have increased visibility of scars.

In addition to the risks associated with any type of surgery, each reconstructive procedure may have its own associated risks. For example, there is a small risk of breast implant rupture associated with breast reconstruction. Individuals should talk carefully with their surgeons and any other health care providers to discuss all the possible risks associated with the specific procedure that they are considering before making a final decision.

Results: Reconstructive surgery is often very successful. It is important, however, for the individual to talk to his or her surgeon about what realistic expectations for the procedure should be, as the results of reconstructive surgery can vary. Nearly all procedures will result in some scarring, which will usually fade with time but never disappears completely. Reconstructive surgeries often cannot change some things with which the individual was unhappy before the cancer. In many cases, the procedure is a large improvement, but the reconstruction is not a 100 percent perfect match because of a number of factors. In cases of skin grafts, the area from which the skin is taken is usually not a perfect match in terms of pigmentation and tone for the area to which it is moved. For breast reconstruction, the reconstructed breast is often a close match, but not a perfect match, of the other breast. The more realistic the expectations of the reconstructive procedure, the more likely the individual is to be satisfied with the results.

Helen Davidson, B.A.

▶ For Further Information

Berry, Daniel J., and Scott P. Steinmann. *Adult Reconstruction*. Philadelphia: Lippincott Williams & Wilkins, 2007.

Kryger, Zol B., and Mark Sisco, eds. *Practical Plastic Surgery*. Austin: Landes Bioscience, 2007.

Park, Stephen S. *Facial Plastic Surgery: The Essential Guide*. New York: Thieme, 2005.

Sarwer, David B., and Thomas Pruzinsky, eds. *Psychological Aspects of Reconstructive and Cosmetic Plastic Surgery: Clinical, Empirical, and Ethical Perspectives*. Philadelphia: Lippincott Williams & Wilkins, 2006.

▶ Other Resources

American Society of Plastic Surgeons
http://www.plasticsurgery.org

See also Aids and devices for cancer patients; Basal cell carcinomas; Breast reconstruction; Exenteration; Eyelid cancer; Fibrosarcomas, soft-tissue; Gynecologic oncology; Head and neck cancers; Infection and sepsis; Lip cancers; Orthopedic surgery; Otolaryngology; Psychosocial aspects of cancer; Risks for cancer; Sexuality and cancer; Skin cancers.

▶ Rectal cancer

Category: Diseases, symptoms, and conditions
Also known as: Colorectal cancer

Related conditions: Colon cancer

Definition: The rectum is the last 8 inches of the colon (large intestine). Almost all (98 percent) of rectal cancers are adenocarcinomas. Adenocarcinomas are cancers that begin in cells that line internal organs of the body, in this case, the lining of the rectum. Since the colon and rectum are continuous, cancer may develop in both places simultaneously. Often colon and rectal cancer are talked about together as colorectal cancer because their causes and treatments are similar.

Risk factors: Rectal cancer usually develops slowly, so more than 90 percent of newly diagnosed cases occur in people over age fifty. In addition to age, diet is a major risk factor. The link between diet and rectal cancer is well established. Rectal cancer is more likely to develop in people who eat large amounts of animal fats (such as red meat) and saturated vegetable oils (such as corn oil but not olive or fish oils). It has been shown, for example, that Africans who eat mainly a plant-based diet have low levels of colorectal cancer, but when these people move to Western countries and adopt a meat-based diet, their incidence of colorectal cancer rises to the same level as that of other people living in these countries.

Other lifestyle factors that increase the risk of rectal cancer include heavy alcohol use, smoking, obesity, and lack of physical exercise. A family history of colorectal cancer or a history of many polyps developing in the colon and rectum, especially at an early age, also increase the risk of rectal cancer. Although risk factors are important screening tools, about three-quarters of people who develop rectal cancer have no specific risk factors.

Etiology and the disease process: The exact cause of rectal cancer is unknown, but both genetics and the environment play a role in its development. The cells lining the colon and rectum are replaced about every six days. These cells develop in interior tissue layers and work their way to lining the rectum, after which they stop dividing. Cancer develops when these cells continue to divide after reaching the rectal lining. The cells then form tumors that grow into the rectal wall. Researchers have found that cells lining the wall of the rectum must develop at least four genetic defects to become cancerous.

Incidence: The American Cancer Society estimates that about 41,400 new cases of rectal cancer occurred in 2007 and that rectal cancer causes about 16,000 deaths annually. The lifetime risk of developing cancer of either the colon or rectum is nearly 6 percent.

Rectal cancer is more common in industrialized countries than in developing countries. It affects slightly more men than women and is highest among Jews of Eastern European descent (Ashkenazi Jews). Most people diagnosed with colorectal cancer are over age sixty, although people who are genetically predisposed to the disease may develop it in childhood or early adulthood.

Age-Adjusted Death Rates for Colorectal Cancer by Race, 2001-2005

	Deaths per 100,000 People	
Race	*Men*	*Women*
All races	22.7	15.9
Black	31.8	22.4
White	22.1	15.3
American Indian/Alaska Native	20.5	14.2
Hispanic	16.5	10.8
Asian/Pacific Islander	14.4	10.2

Source: Data from National Cancer Institute, Surveillance Epidemiology and End Results, Cancer Stat Fact Sheets, 2008

Note: The overall age-adjusted death rate from colorectal cancer was 18.8 per 100,000 people.

Symptoms: Rectal cancer often has few symptoms until the disease becomes advanced. The most common symptoms include changes in bowel activity (constipation or diarrhea), blood in the stool, abdominal pain, a continuous feeling that the rectum is full, and general fatigue.

Screening and diagnosis: Abnormal cells gradually become cancerous over ten to fifteen years, so screening is an essential part of prevention and early treatment. Individuals with no specific risk factors should be screened beginning at age fifty, while those with specific risk factors (such as a family history of polyps) should discuss earlier screening with their doctor. A colonoscopy is used to detect polyps (growths) or abnormalities in the rectal lining. If abnormalities are detected, a biopsy (tissue sample) is taken and the tissue examined under the microscope for cancer. An ultrasound of the rectum may also be done to determine how far the cancer has spread.

Rectal cancer is evaluated using the four-stage TNM (tumor/lymph node/metastasis) system. Tumors are graded based on their invasiveness, with T1 indicating penetration into the layer below the surface lining and T4 indicating invasion of the tumor into other organs. Lymph nodes (N) are graded for involvement, with higher numbers indicating greater spread of the disease. Metastasis is evaluated as either absent (M0) or present (M1). Combining this information results in cancer stages designated as I (least advanced) to IV (most advanced).

Treatment and therapy: Treatment depends on the stage of the cancer. People who have only surgery have a 30 to 50 percent chance of developing additional colorectal cancer. Radiation and chemotherapy used in conjunction with surgery decrease the likelihood of recurrence. Radiation may be used both before and after surgery. Chemotherapy involves administration of multiple antineoplastic drugs.

Prognosis, prevention, and outcomes: Survival rates depend on the stage at which the cancer is detected. Five-year survival rates are as follows: Stage I, 72 percent; Stage II, 54 percent; Stage III, 39 percent, and Stage IV, 7 percent. With widespread screening leading to early treatment, survival rates continue to improve.

Martiscia Davidson, A.M.

▶ For Further Information

Delaini, Gian D., ed. *Rectal Cancer: New Frontiers in Diagnosis, Treatment, and Rehabilitation*. New York: Springer, 2005.

Levin, Bernard, ed. *American Cancer Society's Complete Guide to Colorectal Cancer*. Atlanta: American Cancer Society, 2006.

Pochapin, Mark B. *What Your Doctor May Not Tell You About Colorectal Cancer: New Tests, New Treatments, New Hope*. New York: Warner Books, 2004.

▶ Other Resources

American Cancer Society

All About Colon and Rectal Cancer
http://www.cancer.org/docroot/CRI/CRI_2x.asp?sitearea=LRN&dt=10

Colon Cancer Alliance

http://www.ccalliance.org

National Cancer Institute
Colon and Rectal Cancer
http://www.cancer.gov/cancertopics/types/colon-and-rectal

See also Abdominoperineal resection (APR); Adenocarcinomas; Adenomatous polyps; Anal cancer; Anoscopy; *APC* gene testing; Bethesda criteria; Colectomy; Coloanal anastomosis; Colon polyps; Colonoscopy and virtual colonoscopy; Colorectal cancer; Colorectal cancer screening; Colostomy; Computed tomography (CT) scan; Crohn disease; Cyclooxygenase 2 (COX-2) inhibitors; Desmoid tumors; Diarrhea; Digital rectal exam (DRE); Diverticulosis and diverticulitis; *DPC4* gene testing; Duodenal carcinomas; Endorectal ultrasound; Enteritis; Enterostomal therapy; Epidermoid cancers of mucous membranes; Family history and risk assessment; Fecal occult blood test (FOBT); Gardner syndrome; Gastric polyps; Gastrointestinal cancers; Gastrointestinal complications of cancer treatment; Gastrointestinal oncology; Hemorrhoids; Hereditary cancer syndromes; Hereditary mixed polyposis syndrome; Hereditary polyposis syndromes; Inflammatory bowel disease; Juvenile polyposis syndrome; *MLH1* gene; *MSH* genes; Nuclear medicine scan; Peutz-Jeghers syndrome (PJS); *PMS* genes; Polyps; Rectal cancer; Small intestine cancer.

▶ Recurrence

Category: Diseases, symptoms, and conditions
Also known as: Return of cancer, metastases

Related conditions: Metastasis

Definition: When cancer returns after a period of remission, it is called a recurrence. Cancer can come back months or years after the original diagnosis.

Risk factors: An oncologist will assess the patient's risk of recurrence based on several factors. Tumor cells are graded based on how closely they resemble normal cells when viewed under a microscope. The less like normal cells, the higher the grade and the greater the likelihood the cancer will recur. If cancer is found in the lymph nodes, the risk of recurrence is greater, even if the cancerous lymph nodes are removed.

Etiology and the disease process: A recurrence happens because cancer cells were left behind when the patient was first treated. These cells may have remained at the original site or may have traveled to another location in the body.

Incidence: The incidence of recurrence varies greatly for different cancers and with the presence or absence of risk factors.

Symptoms: Some general symptoms may indicate that cancer has recurred: for example, a new lump or swelling somewhere in the body, back pain, shortness of breath, weight loss, pain or weakness in the arms or legs, or a new onset of headaches. The specific symptoms of a recurrence will depend on the type of cancer.

Screening and diagnosis: Based on the oncologist's assessment of the risk of recurrence, a patient will be given a schedule for follow-up care. Such care will include regular doctor visits and tests specific to the type of cancer previously diagnosed.

Treatment and therapy: Treatment will vary according to the type of cancer and how widespread the recurrence is. Surgery is an option for some types of cancer, and most patients will receive some form of chemotherapy, radiation therapy, or hormonal therapy. The drugs used to treat a recurrence are frequently different from the drugs used to treat the original cancer. Patients with advanced cancer may want to consider entering a clinical trial to evaluate an experimental therapy.

Prognosis, prevention, and outcomes: Prognosis after a recurrence of cancer will depend on a number of factors, including whether the cancer returned in the same location in the body (local recurrence) or at another site (distant recurrence). Generally speaking, the prognosis is poorer for cases of distant recurrence. A recurrence cannot always be prevented; however, abiding by recommended follow-up care guidelines are the best way to ensure that any recurrence will be caught early.

Melanie Hawkins, B.S.N., R.N., O.C.N.

See also Chemotherapy; Clinical trials; Cobalt 60 radiation; Hormonal therapies; Lumps; Nutrition and cancer prevention; Oncology; Risks for cancer; Staging of cancer; Weight loss.

▶ Rehabilitation

Category: Procedures

Definition: Rehabilitation aims to treat the physical, emotional, and psychological limitations often experienced by cancer patients. The goal of rehabilitation is to help the individual with cancer participate as fully and independently as possible in daily life. During rehabilitation, the cancer

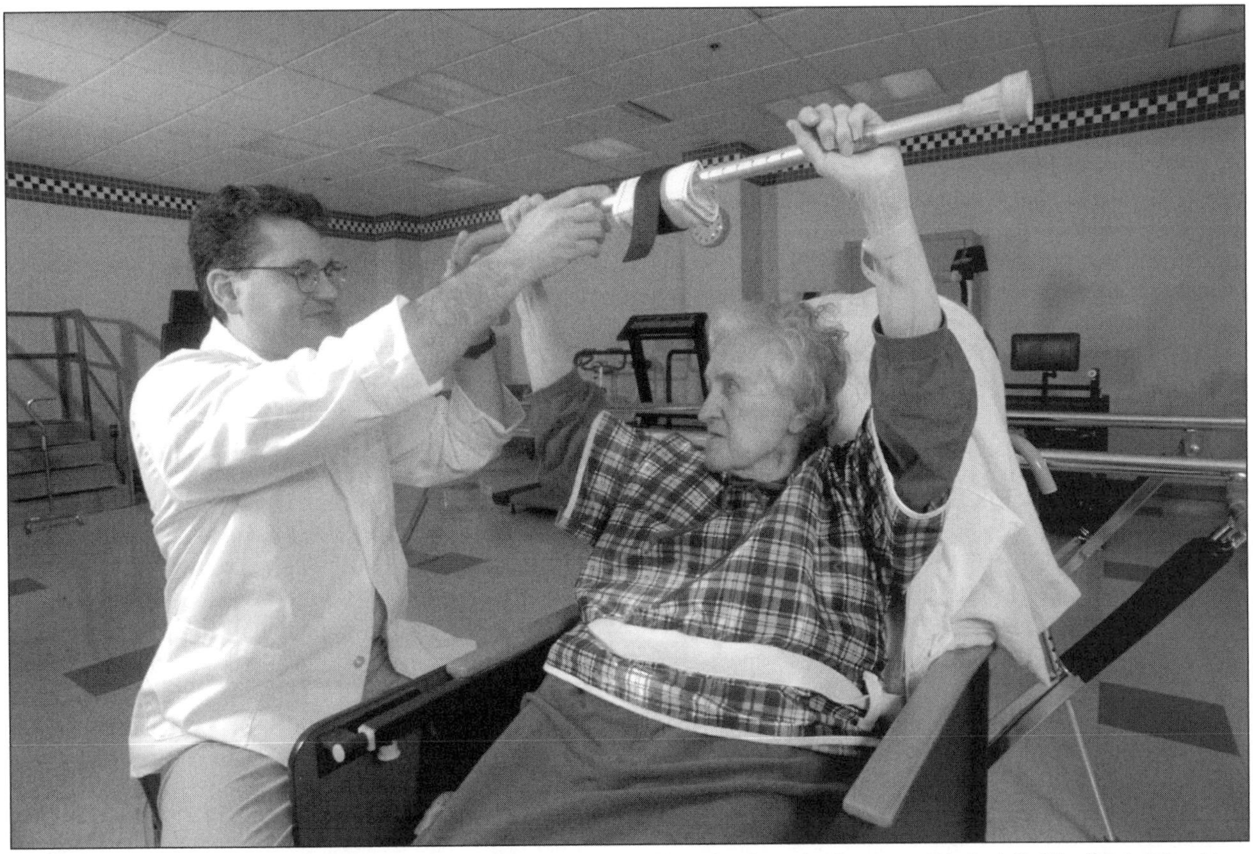

Rehabilitation enables the patient with cancer to participate as fully and independently as possible in daily life. (Digital Stock)

patient works to regain skills and abilities that were lost through the effects of cancer or cancer treatment.

Cancers treated: All types of cancers beginning before, during, or after cancer treatment

Why performed: The specific goals of rehabilitation are different for each individual. In general, the goal of rehabilitation is to allow the individual to function as fully and independently as possible. The rehabilitation team will include different allied health professionals depending on the goals and needs of the individual. Often the rehabilitation team will include many health professionals, such as a physical therapist, an occupational therapist, a rehabilitation nurse, a psychologist or psychiatrist, a nutritionist or registered dietician, the individual's physician or oncologist, pain management specialists, a case manager, and home health workers.

The rehabilitation team will work together with the patient and the patient's family and loved ones to help the patient regain as high a degree of functioning as possible. The specific activities included in the rehabilitation plan usually comprise dressing, bathing, cooking, eating, and other activities of daily living. Some individuals may receive help recovering the ability to drive, take public transportation, or other aspects of mobility.

For individuals whose job skills were affected by cancer or cancer treatment, regaining the skills necessary to return to a job is usually considered a high priority. An occupational therapist or other member of the rehabilitation team may help the individual determine what skills are required, work to improve those skills, and seek ways to modify the employment environment so that the individual may return to work sooner.

The individual may have goals in addition to those necessary for return to employment or for daily living. Many recreation and leisure activities that were formerly pleasurable may become difficult or impossible because of cancer or cancer treatment. Rehabilitation therapists listen to the patient to address additional goals, such as the ability to go camping or sailing, play sports, or play music.

Patient preparation: Before beginning to meet with a rehabilitation specialist, it may help the patient to consider specific goals for rehabilitation. Making a list of activities or skills on which the patient would like to work can help the rehabilitation therapist look beyond the activities of daily living to other activities important in that individual's life. Goals can be very specific, such as being able to knit or type again, or more general, such as being able to play with children or grandchildren.

The patient preparation required before the individual rehabilitation sessions will vary depending on the type of therapy. The rehabilitation specialist will give the patient specific information about what steps to take before a session, which may include things such as doing gentle stretches to warm up or even mentally preparing to meet the challenges that rehabilitation therapy provides.

Steps of the procedure: The steps of rehabilitation are very individualized. They depend on the type of therapy that is being done and on the specific needs and goals of the patient. Rehabilitation therapy often breaks down the goal activity or skill into smaller parts or steps and then works on one step at a time. For example, an occupational therapist who is helping a cancer patient regain the ability to feed himself may work on the action of bringing the food to the mouth as one activity, the act of using a spoon or fork to scoop food as a separate activity, and the act of cutting food as yet a separate skill. As these different aspects of the skill of feeding oneself are mastered, they can be combined into more complex sequences of actions.

Another way of approaching rehabilitation can be from the standpoint of increasing the day-to-day abilities of the patient in the affected areas. In this case, the rehabilitation therapist might focus on getting food from the plate or bowl and into the mouth using the hands and then slowly add skills, such as beginning to help the patient use a spoon, then a fork, and then working on cutting food.

Rehabilitation also often helps to identify assistive devices that individuals can use to help them accomplish various tasks. In some cases, these devices are only necessary for a short time; in other cases, they will be used by the individual for the rest of his or her life. For instance, a rehabilitation specialist may help an individual regain the ability to walk using a walker, or may help an individual who had a leg amputated master the use of a prosthetic leg.

After the procedure: The steps after rehabilitation will vary depending on the type of therapy performed. After therapy that involves physical activity or exercise, a series of stretches and cooldown activities is usually performed. Often the rehabilitation therapist will assign the individual exercises or activities to practice each day, sometimes several times a day, before the next session. This approach can help to ensure that the progress made during the session is maintained until the next session. The patient's family members or caregivers may be shown how to help the individual complete these exercises.

Rehabilitation therapy may be continued for weeks, months, or even longer. When the therapy has ended, the therapist may give the patient a list or set of exercises or activities to continue to do to help keep up the skills that were gained during therapy, or to help the patient continue to make improvements.

Risks: The risks associated with rehabilitation are generally mild but are different for different forms of rehabilitation therapy. There are some risks that during physical therapy individuals may strain or pull muscles, or otherwise overextend or injure themselves, especially if the proper stretching and warmup routine is not followed before the therapy. Risks of occupational therapy and other forms of rehabilitation therapy that involve the patient working to perform certain actions or movements, such as the movements of dressing or bathing, may also result in strain or injury if the individual pushes too hard to accomplish the task before his or her body is ready. An individual working on regaining the ability to walk may fall if not carefully monitored. Generally, these and other physical risks from rehabilitation are very low if the therapy is overseen by a qualified health professional.

There may also be some emotional risks relating to rehabilitation. The issues discussed with a psychologist or psychiatrist can often be painful or upsetting as they help the individual with cancer work through the fear, uncertainty, and feelings of hopelessness that often accompany cancer diagnosis and treatment. Although discussions with a psychologist or therapist can often be very upsetting, they can usually help the patient deal effectively with these new emotions.

Results: The results of rehabilitation are usually very positive. With consistent effort by the patient and the rehabilitation team, many skills and abilities that have been lost can be regained. Many people can return to jobs and activities in which they would not have been able to participate without rehabilitation. Psychological and emotional rehabilitation is usually effective at helping the individual regain a positive outlook and overcome the fear and unhappiness often associated with cancer and cancer treatment. A comprehensive rehabilitation plan that involves many different allied health professionals, as well as family, friends, or other caregivers, is often especially effective.

It is important for the rehabilitation team to help the patient develop a realistic view of the amount of work required by rehabilitation, the length of time that it will take to reach rehabilitation goals, and what rehabilitation goals are likely to be realistic overall. Having realistic expectations can help reduce frustrations and negative feelings that may occur during the rehabilitation process as hurdles are met and overcome.

Helen Davidson, B.A.

▶ For Further Information

Davis, Carol M., ed. *Complementary Therapies in Rehabilitation.* 2d ed. Thorofare, N.J.: Slack, 2004.

Galvin, Jan C., and Scherer Marcia J., eds. *Evaluating, Selecting, and Using Appropriate Assistive Technology.* Austin, Tex.: Pro-Ed, 2004.

Macky, Hazel, and Susan Nancarrow. *Enabling Independence: A Guide for Rehabilitation Workers.* Malden, Mass.: Blackwell, 2006.

Stidwill, Howard. *Exercise Therapy and the Cancer Patient: A Guide for Health Care Professionals and Their Patients.* Belgium, Wisc.: Champion Press, 2005.

▶ Other Resources

National Rehabilitation Information Center
http://www.nairc.com

See also Aids and devices for cancer patients; Amputation; Cancer care team; Case management; Cognitive effects of cancer and chemotherapy; Cordectomy; Exercise and cancer; Head and neck cancers; Home health services; Limb salvage; Nutrition and cancer treatment; Occupational therapy; Pain management medications; Self-image and body image; Transitional care.

▶ Relationships

Category: Social and personal issues

Definition: Cancer can affect a person's relationships with others in many significant ways. The diagnosis can bring fear, anxiety, concern for the future, sadness, confusion, and many other emotions. Any time of high emotion and stress can cause tension in even the strongest relationships. During treatment there may be changing roles and responsibilities at home and at work that can lead to stress and tension. Even after successful treatment, when life may be returning to normal, changes in roles and expectations can lead to frustration and conflict. Although cancer can put an enormous strain on relationships, it can also make them stronger, as families work together, priorities and values are reassessed, and friends and families show their love and support for one another.

Spouses: A cancer diagnosis can put a lot of strain on a relationship. There may be fear, anxiety, and sadness on the spouse's part as the person is forced to contemplate the possibility of losing the individual who has been diagnosed. Roles within the relationship may change, as the person who was once the primary caregiver may now be the one who receives the caregiving. Also, the spouse may face a huge increase in responsibilities as that person assumes the tasks of taking the partner to treatment or to various doctors' offices, being supportive, and doing any household tasks the individual with cancer can no longer do. If the patient can no longer work, the spouse may have to work longer hours or take an additional job.

Talking about fears, frustrations, and other feelings can be an extremely important part of maintaining a good relationship during cancer treatment. Although a cancer diagnosis can bring strain to a relationship, it can also cause people to reevaluate their priorities and spend more time together, or to remember how important they are to each other. Working together through cancer can be difficult, but it can also bring incredible strength to a relationship. Gay and lesbian couples may have an even more difficult time because medical personnel may not allow them access to their hospitalized partner and may not permit them to make any decisions regarding care, especially if some family members are not aware of the relationship. Finding a cancer care team that is respectful of the relationship and being honest about feelings can help to reduce the impact of some of these possible issues.

Children: When a parent has cancer, it can be very difficult for the parent to decide how much to tell children about the cancer itself, treatments the parent may be undergoing, the prognosis, how life for the family may be changing, and all of the other issues that the family will be facing. Deciding what to tell a child depends on a number of factors, including the child's age and maturity and the parent's comfort level in talking with the child.

Many parents are hesitant to tell children that a parent has been diagnosed with cancer. Often parents do not want the children to worry or be afraid. It is normal for a child to feel upset, confused, or worried when told that a parent has been diagnosed with cancer. However, often if a child is not told, the resulting anxiety and worry will be even worse. Children are aware when something is wrong in the family from a very young age. They can be aware of a parent's stress or anxiety and may believe that things are much worse than they actually are. Telling a child the truth about the situation in a way that is age appropriate can help quell some fears that are unfounded and also help the child cope with fears and feelings that are realistic.

The sense of trust that develops between a parent and child is extremely important. If a child finds out about a parent's cancer diagnosis from another source, it can be difficult or nearly impossible for the parent to regain that sense of trust. It is hard to keep a secret from children if many other people know. Other family members or adults in the child's life who know about the diagnosis may bring it up. The child may even overhear a parent talking about cancer. Children who find out indirectly may not even let their parents know that they are aware of the cancer but instead may feel alone and try to cope with their fears and sadness on their own.

If it is a brother or sister who has been diagnosed with cancer, it may be even more important to let siblings know what is going on in a way that they can understand. This way, parents and other caregivers can help them express their fears and concerns and provide support for their ill sibling.

No matter who in the family has been diagnosed with cancer, it can make relationships between children and their parents strained. Children may act out their fears and frustrations in many different ways, including clinging to a parent, withdrawing from the family, being irritable, or acting younger than their age. When parents are under extreme stress and have fears of their own, it can be difficult to maintain a close positive relationship with their children. Allowing children to provide assistance so that they feel they are helping the family and providing truthful information that they can understand can help alleviate some of these pressures.

Coworkers: Relationships between coworkers can vary dramatically from person to person and workplace to workplace. Some coworkers are close friends who discuss intimate details of their lives during breaks and after work, and some coworkers discuss only business and never personal subjects of any kind. Because these differences exist before a cancer diagnosis, relationship changes in the workplace may be hard to predict.

Some coworkers may have misunderstandings about cancer, such as a belief that it is contagious, which may cause them to react in unexpected ways. Other people may be fearful of talking to the person with cancer for fear of saying the wrong thing. Tension can also occur in the workplace if the person with cancer has to miss a lot of time for treatment or can no longer perform all of the assigned duties. Even if a coworker does not blame the person with cancer, having an increased workload can be frustrating.

Like other relationships, those at work often can benefit from openness and truthfulness. Cancer patients should tell only those people with whom they are comfortable sharing this fact, but often at least their immediate supervisor will need to know so that patients can schedule their work around treatments and follow-up appointments. If cancer patients are comfortable talking to coworkers and letting them know that they appreciate their concern and that it is okay to talk about it, it can help everyone at the workplace improve their relationships and may clear up some misunderstandings.

Extended family and friends: When a person has been diagnosed with cancer, relationships with extended family and friends may change dramatically. Some people who were not especially close friends may become invaluable sources of help during the stressful time. Unfortunately, others may draw away from the person with cancer, and might show that they are not as good friends as was once thought. Many people are not sure what to say or how to help. If the person with cancer feels comfortable, letting friends and relatives know ways that they can help, such as picking up a child from school, helping with the housework, or just coming for a visit, can make people feel needed and more comfortable.

Helen Davidson, B.A.

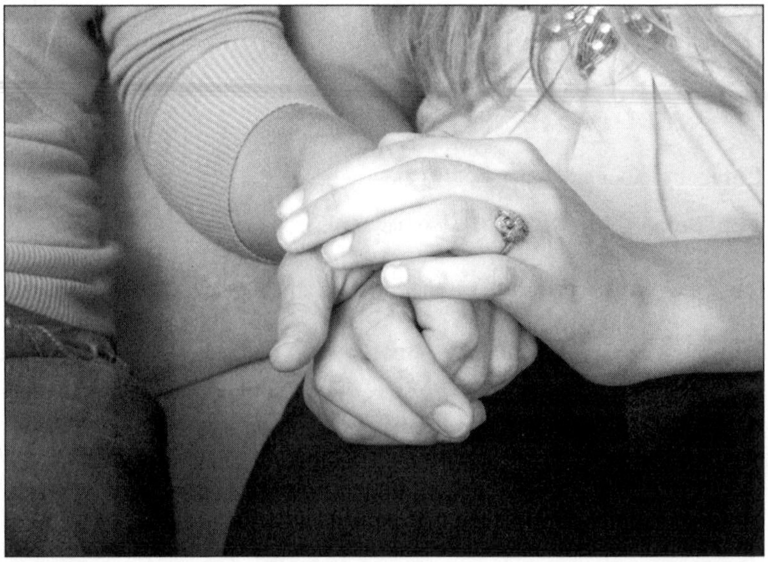

The relationships, or bonds with other people, that a cancer patient has may undergo some changes and strains during and after treatment; often they are strengthened. (©Nicholas Sutcliffe/Dreamstime.com)

▶ For Further Information

Fincannon, Joy L., and Katherine V. Bruss. *Couples Confronting Cancer: Keeping Your Relationship Strong.* Atlanta: American Cancer Society, 2003.

Harpham, Wendy Schlessel. *When a Parent Has Cancer: A Guide to Caring for Your Children.* New York: Perennial Currents, 2004.

Jennings, Lesajean McDonald. *A Guide for Men as They Walk Through the Experience of Breast Cancer with the Women in Their Lives: Specifics to Support Emotional and Relationship Health.* Auburn Hills, Mich.: Jessies Legacy, 2004.

Knox, Sally M. *The Breast Cancer Care Book: A Survival Guide for Patients and Loved Ones.* Grand Rapids, Mich.: Zondervan, 2004.

National Cancer Institute. *Taking Time: Support for People with Cancer and the People Who Care About Them.* Bethesda, Md.: Author, 2003.

▶ Other Resources

American Cancer Society
http://www.cancer.org

National Cancer Institute
http://www.cancer.gov

The Wellness Community
http://www.thewellnesscommunity.org

See also Aging and cancer; Anxiety; Breast cancer in men; Breast cancer in pregnant women; Cancer care team; Caregivers and caregiving; Long-distance caregiving; Psychosocial aspects of cancer; Sexuality and cancer; Singlehood and cancer; Stress management; Vasectomy and cancer; Young adult cancers.

▶ Renal pelvis tumors

Category: Diseases, symptoms, and conditions
Also known as: Gurnistical tumors

Related conditions: Renal cell carcinomas, kidney cancer

Definition: Renal pelvis tumors are masses that develop in the center of the kidney and can become malignant (cancerous).

Risk factors: Risk factors for renal tumors include smoking, misusing certain pain medicines over an extended period of time, and having certain genetic conditions, such as von Hippel-Lindau disease or hereditary papillary renal cell carcinoma.

Etiology and the disease process: Renal pelvis tumors develop in the kidney tubule (or renal tubule), which is the portion of the kidney constituting the basic filtration unit of the kidney.

Incidence: Renal pelvis tumors affect less than 1 percent of the population, with approximately 40,000 people diagnosed with cancer. It predominantly affects men over the age of fifty-five.

Symptoms: Symptoms of renal pelvis tumors include blood in the urine, a noticeable lump in the abdomen, pain in the side or back, weight loss, and anemia.

Screening and diagnosis: Diagnosis of renal pelvis tumors is confirmed with a physical exam, urinalysis, and urine cytology tests. The urinalysis determines if abnormalities, such as blood, protein, sugar, and solids, exist in the urine. Urine cytology is a microscopic examination of urine to detect any abnormal cells that have sloughed off the walls of the bladder or kidney and been released in the urine. If necessary, cytoscopy is performed with a very narrow tube with a light and camera inserted through the urethra to examine the inside of the bladder and ureter. Further imaging studies can help determine if the cancer has spread to other layers of the organs or beyond the urinary tract. Tumors found in the collecting duct are transitional or medullary carcinomas.

If bladder or kidney cancer is suspected, a physician may order a computed tomography (CT) scan, pyelography, or biopsy. The CT scan provides a three-dimensional view of the urinary tract to determine if any masses or tumors exist. Pyelography involves injecting a special dye into the vein or urethra and examining a series of X rays to determine if abnormalities exist. The biopsy is typically performed during cytoscopy, and abnormal cells can be detected with a microscope.

The staging of the disease according to the National Cancer Institute is as follows:

- Stage I: The tumor is 7 centimeters (cm) or smaller and is found only in the kidney.
- Stage II: The tumor is larger than 7 cm and is found only in the kidney.
- Stage III: Cancer is found in the kidney and in one nearby lymph node; or in an adrenal gland or in the layer of fatty tissue around the kidney and may be found in one nearby lymph node; or in the main blood vessels of the kidney and may be found in one nearby lymph node.
- Stage IV: Cancer has spread beyond the layer of fatty tissue around the kidney and may be found in one nearby lymph node; or to two or more nearby lymph nodes; or

to other organs, such as the bowel, pancreas, or lungs, and may be found in nearby lymph nodes.

Treatment and therapy: Renal pelvis tumors that are noncancerous can be closely monitored for an increase in size or for malignant development. If necessary, they can be removed with surgery. Malignant renal tumors do not respond to chemotherapy or radiation therapy, and therefore surgery is required to remove the cancerous tumor.

Renal pelvis tumors are sometimes also treated with immunotherapy, which stimulates the patient's immune system to recognize tumor cells as targets and to attack the malignant tumor cells. This is accomplished by administering therapeutic antibodies to enable the immune system to destroy tumor cells.

Prognosis, prevention, and outcomes: If renal pelvis tumors are treated early, the prognosis is very good. However, because symptoms often go unnoticed, diagnosis is not usually made until the cancer is in later stages, resulting in a mortality rate of nearly 30 percent of people diagnosed with malignant renal tumors.

Robert J. Amato, D.O.

▶ For Further Information

Figlin, Robert A., ed. *Kidney Cancer*. Boston: Kluwer Academic, 2003.

Kurth, K. H., G. H. J. Mickisch, and Fritz H. Schroder, eds. *Renal, Bladder, Prostate, and Testicular Cancer: An Update*. New York: Parthenon, 2001.

Patel, Uday, ed. *Carcinoma of the Kidney*. New York: Cambridge University Press, 2008.

▶ Other Resources

American Cancer Society

Detailed Guide: Kidney Cancer

http://www.cancer.org/docroot/cri/content/cri_2_4_1x_what_is_kidney_cancer_22.asp

Kidney Cancer Association

http://www.kidneycancer.org/

National Cancer Institute

Kidney Cancer

http://www.nci.nih.gov/cancertopics/types/kidney

See also Adrenal gland cancers; Angiogenesis inhibitors; Corticosteroids; Endocrine cancers; Hereditary leiomyomatosis and renal cell cancer (HLRCC); Hereditary papillary renal cell carcinomas; Kidney cancer; Nuclear medicine scan; Smoking cessation; Urinary system cancers; Von Hippel-Lindau (VHL) disease.

Incidence Rates of Kidney and Renal Pelvis Cancer by Race, 2001-2005

	Incidence per 100,000 People	
Race	*Men*	*Women*
All races	18.3	9.2
Black	21.3	10.1
American Indian/Alaska Native	19.5	12.7
White	18.8	9.5
Hispanic	17.4	9.6
Asian/Pacific Islander	9.1	4.6

Source: Data from National Cancer Institute, Surveillance Epidemiology and End Results, Cancer Stat Fact Sheets, 2008

Note: The age-adjusted incidence rate from cancer of the kidney and renal pelvis was 23.2 per 100,000 people per year.

▶ *Report on Carcinogens* (RoC)

Category: Carcinogens and suspected carcinogens
Also known as: RoC

Definition: The *Report on Carcinogens* (RoC) is a U.S. government document, issued by the National Toxicology Program (NTP) of the U.S. Department of Health and Human Services (DHHS), which identifies and profiles substances that are known to cause cancer or that are reasonably anticipated to cause cancer in a significant number of persons residing in the United States. It is published every two years by the Department of Health and Human Services to comply with the Public Health Service Act, Section 301(b)(4). The first edition was published in 1980.

Content: The RoC lists substances for which there is published scientific evidence establishing a relationship between exposure to the substance and the development of cancer. The substances are categorized as "known to be human carcinogens" or "reasonably anticipated to be human carcinogens" based on human and laboratory animal studies and epidemiological studies.

The report presents information on each substance. It identifies regulations and guidelines pertaining to the substance and discusses how they decrease the risk of exposure. All substances nominated for review are included in the report with explanations of why they were included in or excluded from the list.

Review process: The process begins with a substance being nominated for review. Requests for RoC nominations are published in the Federal Registry. Sources include the public, other agencies, and reviews of scientific literature.

A nomination is reviewed by several scientific committees within the Department of Health and Human Services. These committees consider background information, additional literature searches, and public comments when making their recommendations. The secretary of the department makes the final review and approval before submitting the report to Congress.

Affiliated agencies: Agencies that are involved with the nomination and review process are the Agency for Toxic Substances and Disease Registry (ATSDR), the Consumer Product Safety Commission (CPSC), the Environmental Protection Agency (EPA), the Food and Drug Administration (FDA), the National Center for Environmental Health (NCEH), the National Institute for Occupational Safety and Health (NIOSH), the Occupational Safety and Health Administration (OSHA), the National Institutes of Health (NIH), the National Cancer Institute (NCI), and the National Institute of Environmental Health Sciences/NTP (NIEHS/NTP).

Limitations: The RoC will not include a substance if exposure is limited to a small number of people. The report does not discuss the benefits of a substance versus its risk of causing cancer. It does not provide the specific conditions under which a substance will cause cancer to develop.

The focus of the report is to present technical and scientific information—the supported facts—and not to discuss the many variables involved for cancer to develop.

Carol Ann Suda, B.S., M.T. (ASCP), S.M.

See also Air pollution; Asbestos; Carcinogens, known; Carcinogens, reasonably anticipated; Cigarettes and cigars; Dioxins; National Cancer Institute (NCI); Occupational exposures and cancer; Pesticides and the food chain.

▶ Resveratrol

Category: Lifestyle and prevention
Also known as: Trans-3,4’,5-trihydroxystilbene, polyphenolic phytoalexin

Definition: Resveratrol is a compound manufactured by plants as part of their defense mechanism against disease. These compounds, which belong to the stilbene chemical classification, are also known as polyphenolic phytoalexins.

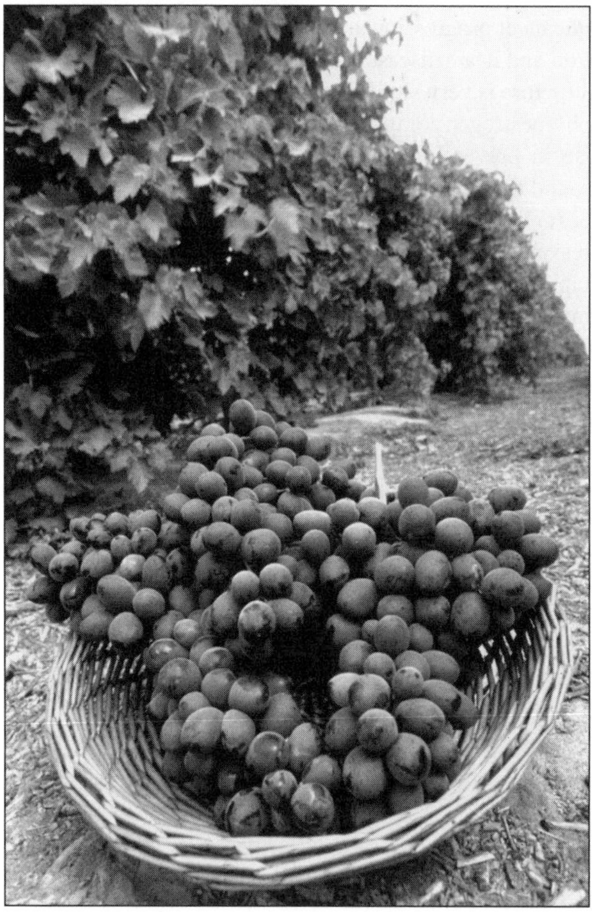

Red grapes are a good source of resveratrol, thought to have cancer-preventing properties. (U.S. Department of Agriculture)

Resveratrol has become synonymous with cancer prevention and is thought to have protective antioxidant, anti-inflammatory, and life-extending properties.

Cancers treated or prevented: Leukemia, prostate cancer, breast cancer, stomach cancer, colon cancer, pancreatic cancer, thyroid cancer, skin cancer

Delivery routes: Oral via food and dietary supplements; significant food sources include red grapes, red wines, red and purple grape juice, berries (including raspberries, blueberries, cranberries, and bilberries), peanuts, and peanut butter

How this substance works: Resveratrol is a stilbene compound manufactured by plants as a defense mechanism against diseases. It is primarily found in red grape skins, and laboratory experiments find that it functions as an antioxidant against cell-damaging free radicals. It has also been found to prevent some cancers, slow or halt the stages of cancer progression and metastasis, decrease inflammation and heart disease, and extend life span. Its chemical structure is very similar to estrogen, and it is considered a phytoestrogen compound. While it has shown some promise in preventing estrogen-sensitive cancers, one study found that it actually stimulated the growth of breast cancer cells. While only a small number of studies have tested resveratrol in humans, initial results show that the body rapidly metabolizes it. Thus, blood levels of resveratrol may not reach the protective levels that have been observed in the lab setting and it may only provide limited health benefits to humans. Recommended doses for resveratrol have yet to be determined.

Side effects: Caution is advised for individuals with food allergies or sensitivities to resveratrol-containing foods. There have been no reported side effects or drug interactions, but women with a history of estrogen-sensitive cancers are advised to avoid resveratrol dietary supplements because of its estrogen-like chemical structure. Individuals taking anticoagulant, antiplatelet, or nonsteroidal anti-inflammatory drugs (NSAIDs) should also avoid dietary supplements, as high doses of resveratrol may increase the risk of bleeding. Unsafe intake of alcohol should be avoided, as it may increase cancer risk as well as other health risks.

Alice C. Richer, R.D., M.B.A., L.D.

See also Antioxidants; Beta-carotene; Bioflavonoids; Calcium; Carotenoids; Chemoprevention; Coenzyme Q10; Complementary and alternative therapies; Cruciferous vegetables; Curcumin; Dietary supplements; Essiac; Free radicals; Fruits; Garlic and allicin; Glutamine; Green tea; Herbs as antioxidants; Isoflavones; Lutein; Lycopene; Nonsteroidal anti-inflammatory drugs (NSAIDs); Nutrition and cancer prevention; Phenolics; Phytoestrogens; Wine and cancer.

▶ Retinoblastomas

Category: Diseases, symptoms, and conditions
Also known as: Cancer of the retina

Related conditions: Second extraocular tumors or cancer, trilateral retinoblastomas (pineoblastomas)

Definition: Retinoblastomas are rare cancers (malignant tumors) of the retina of the eye in young children. The retina is the innermost light-sensitive layer of the eye wall and is responsible for vision. There are two types of retinoblastoma, bilateral (affects both eyes) and unilateral (affects one eye). The bilateral type is hereditary and affects 25 percent of children with retinoblastoma. The unilateral type is not hereditary and occurs during prenatal development. The unilateral type affects 75 percent of children with retinoblastoma.

Risk factors: There are no risk factors for retinoblastoma; however, this disease creates a risk of a secondary cancer as it can spread outside the eye to other parts of the body. More children with the bilateral type have died from a second tumor than from the original retinoblastoma. Retinoblastoma also places patients at risk of developing other types of cancer.

Etiology and the disease process: During prenatal development of a child, the youngest cells (retinoblasts) divide and redivide to form the differentiated cells of the retina. Sometimes gene mutations occur, causing an abnormality in chromosome 13. This causes some retinoblasts to multiply uncontrolled, creating a tumor of undifferentiated cells: a retinoblastoma. From this point onward, the retinoblastoma is classified into bilateral and unilateral types. The uncontrolled tumor can fill the entire orbit and glaucoma can develop, which can cause pain and vision loss. If the condition remains untreated, the cancer can spread through the brain and spinal cord and then to other parts of the body (second tumor).

Incidence: Generally 200 to 300 children per year are diagnosed with retinoblastoma in the United States; the disease occurs equally in boys and girls. The rate of incidence is higher in infants (newborn to one year) and younger children, and lower in older children (between two and twelve years). About 95 percent of children diagnosed with the disease are younger than five.

Symptoms: The most common symptom (60 percent) is leukocoria, a white pupil or white reflex. The second is strabismus (crossed eyes), which accounts for 20 percent of cases, and third, inflammation (red irritation and swelling) around the eyes, 10 percent.

Screening and diagnosis: The main screening by an ophthalmologist is to check for a normal red reflex in the eye (normally blood vessels in the back of the eye reflect red). If white reflex (cat's-eye reflex) is observed, it is due to leukocoria. The doctor will also examine the corneal light reflex to check for strabismus and look for inflammation around the eyes or vision problems, including a decrease in vision. A blood test may be performed to check for deoxyribonucleic acid (DNA) mutations.

Diagnosis of retinoblastoma is confirmed by ophthalmoscopic examination, ultrasound, computed tomogra-

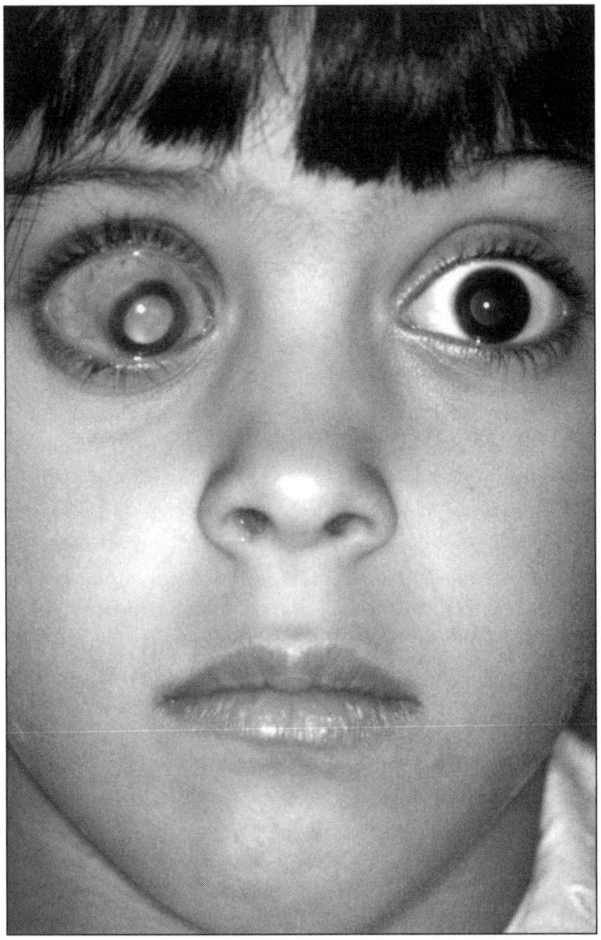

Retinoblastoma. (Custom Medical Stock Photo)

phy (CT) and magnetic resonance imaging (MRI) scans, and if absolutely necessary, spinal tap and bone marrow biopsy.

The following are the three stages of retinoblastoma:

- Stage I: Intraocular; the tumor remains inside the eye.
- Stage II: Extraocular; the tumor spreads outside the eye or to another part of the body (second tumor).
- Stage III: Recurrent; cancer returns in the eye or another part of the body after being treated. The hereditary form of retinoblastoma can recur years after treatment.

Treatment and therapy: Treatment depends on the size of the tumor. For tumors less than 3 millimeters (mm) in diameter and 2 mm in thickness, photocoagulation, a laser treatment, is used to kill blood vessels that nourish the tumor. If the tumor is less than 5 mm in diameter and 3 mm in thickness, cryotherapy is used to freeze the cancer cells. Chemotherapy (oral or intravenous) can also be used to kill cancer cells. When the tumor is less than 16 mm in diameter and 8 mm in thickness, radiation therapy is used. Radiation therapy can consist of an external beam of X rays or internal radiation (plaque radiotherapy). In plaque radiotherapy, radioactive material is placed near the tumor to kill cancer cells.

When all other treatments fail to control the tumor, pain, and blindness, enucleation, or surgical removal of the eye, is performed to save the child's life.

Prognosis, prevention, and outcomes: The disease was nearly always fatal one hundred years ago. The prognosis improved from an 80 percent survival rate in the 1960's to more than 95 percent in the 1990's. Retinoblastoma is highly curable if diagnosed and treated early. The prognosis for vision and a second tumor depends on the stage of the disease and treatment efficacy.

Retinoblastoma cannot be prevented, because of its genetic component; however, the defective gene can be detected through tests of amniotic fluid, which allows for the option of terminating the pregnancy. Another option is in vitro fertilization, in which an embryo without the defective gene can be implanted in the womb.

Arun S. Dabholkar, Ph.D.

▶ For Further Information

Albert, Daniel M., and Arthur Polans, eds. *Ocular Oncology*. New York: Marcel Dekker, 2003.

Melamud, Alex, Rakhee Palekar, and Arun Singh. "Retinoblastoma." *American Family Physician* 73, no. 6 (2006): 1039-1044.

Parker, James N., and Philip M. Parker, eds. *The Official Parent's Sourcebook on Retinoblastoma: Directory for the Internet Age*. San Diego, Calif.: Icon Health, 2005.

▶ Other Resources

Genetics Home Reference
Retinoblastoma
http://ghr.nlm.nih.gov/condition=retinoblastoma

Ocular Oncology at Bascom Palmer Eye Institute
http://www.eyecancermd.org/retinoblastoma/index.html

Retinoblastoma.com
http://retinoblastoma.com/retinoblastoma/

See also Cancer biology; Childhood cancers; Computed tomography (CT) scan; Eye cancers; Genetics of cancer; Oncogenes; Ophthalmic oncology; Pineoblastomas; *RB1* gene; Sarcomas, soft-tissue; Tumor-suppressor genes; Virus-related cancers.

▶ Rhabdomyosarcomas

Category: Diseases, symptoms, and conditions
Also known as: Embryonal rhabdomyosarcomas, alveolar rhabdomyosarcomas, botryoid rhabdomyosarcomas, soft-tissue sarcomas

Related conditions: Li-Fraumeni syndrome, Beckwith-Wiedemann syndrome, Costello syndrome

Definition: Rhabdomyosarcomas are soft-tissue, malignant tumors that develop from cells called rhabdomyoblasts, which normally develop into skeletal, cardiac, and smooth muscles. This cancer develops from embryonal cells and is more common in children than in adults.

Risk factors: There are no known environmental factors that increase the risk of rhabdomyosarcoma. There is some evidence that suggests that an increased risk of rhabdomyosarcoma occurs with certain related, inherited conditions. These syndromes are rare, but children may inherit an increased risk of the tumor when these diseases are present. There is no evidence that lifestyle-related risk factors, including use of drugs or X rays during pregnancy, have an impact on rhabdomyosarcoma.

Etiology and the disease process: There is no known cause for most cases of rhabdomyosarcoma, but it is assumed that there is a genetic component. With embryonal rhabdomyosarcomas, research has demonstrated that a small piece of deoxyribonucleic acid (DNA) on chromosome 11 may be missing.

Incidence: The annual incidence of rhabdomyosarcoma is 4.5 cases per 1 million children under the age of fourteen. These cases represents 3.5 percent of all malignancies in children under the age of fourteen. The ratio of boys to girls is 1.5:1.

Age-Specific Annual Incidence Rates for Rhabdomyosarcoma, 1975-1995

Age (years)	*Incidence per 1 Million Children*
5 and under	6.4
5-9	4.4
10-14	3.1
15-19	3.6

Source: L. A. G. Ries et al., eds., *Cancer Incidence and Survival Among Children and Adolescents: United States SEER Program, 1975-1995*, NIH Pub. No. 99-4649 (Bethesda, Md.: National Cancer Institute, SEER Program, 1999)

Symptoms: The symptoms of rhabdomyosarcoma depend on the initial site of the tumor. Tumors on the trunk, groin, arms, or legs may be first noticed as swelling that causes little or no pain. Tumors that grow inside the abdomen or pelvis may cause nausea, vomiting, difficulties with bowel and bladder function such as constipation or frequent urination, and pain. These symptoms are caused by pressure on internal organs. Masses that grow in the bladder or vagina may cause bleeding. Tumors in the ear or in the sinuses have symptoms similar to ear infections or sinus infections and cause pain in the area affected. A rhabdomyosarcoma of the eye, or orbital area, may cause the eye to bulge, or the child may appear cross-eyed.

If the tumor goes undetected for a period of time, the child may develop symptoms of fatigue, cough, weight loss, enlarged lymph nodes, and generalized muscle weakness. This may indicate that the rhabdomyosarcoma has already metastasized (spread) to other parts of the body.

Screening, diagnosis, and staging: There is no screening test for rhabdomyosarcoma. If a family has a history of cancer, particularly childhood cancer, it is important to tell the pediatrician at the first visit. Parents should take note of any unusual lumps, swellings, or blood in the stool or urine, as many tumors are picked up by parents bathing the child or changing a diaper. Children should be taken to the doctor if they complain of persistent pain in any area or if a bump or swelling does not go away.

Diagnosis begins with imaging (X-ray) studies, as tumors may be hidden or hard to see. Tests may include ordinary X rays, computed tomography (CT) scans, a magnetic resonance imaging (MRI) scan, a bone scan, and a positron emission tomography (PET) scan. These scans can detect the location of the tumor, reveal any spread to other areas, and in the case of the PET scan, determine whether the tumor may be cancer. A biopsy, the removal of a small piece of the tumor for review under the microscope by a pathologist, usually follows imaging studies. A bone marrow biopsy is done once the diagnosis of rhabdomyosarcoma is made to determine if the tumor has spread.

Staging rhabdomyosarcoma is important to determine the treatment needed to best effect cure. Generally staging begins with the pathology review and initial biopsy or surgery. Staging is done in two ways: clinical groups I-IV and TNM (tumor/lymph node/metastasis) stages I-IV. Clinical group staging is based on how much of the tumor is removed during the initial surgery and knowledge of the extent of the disease. The TNM stage is determined by size

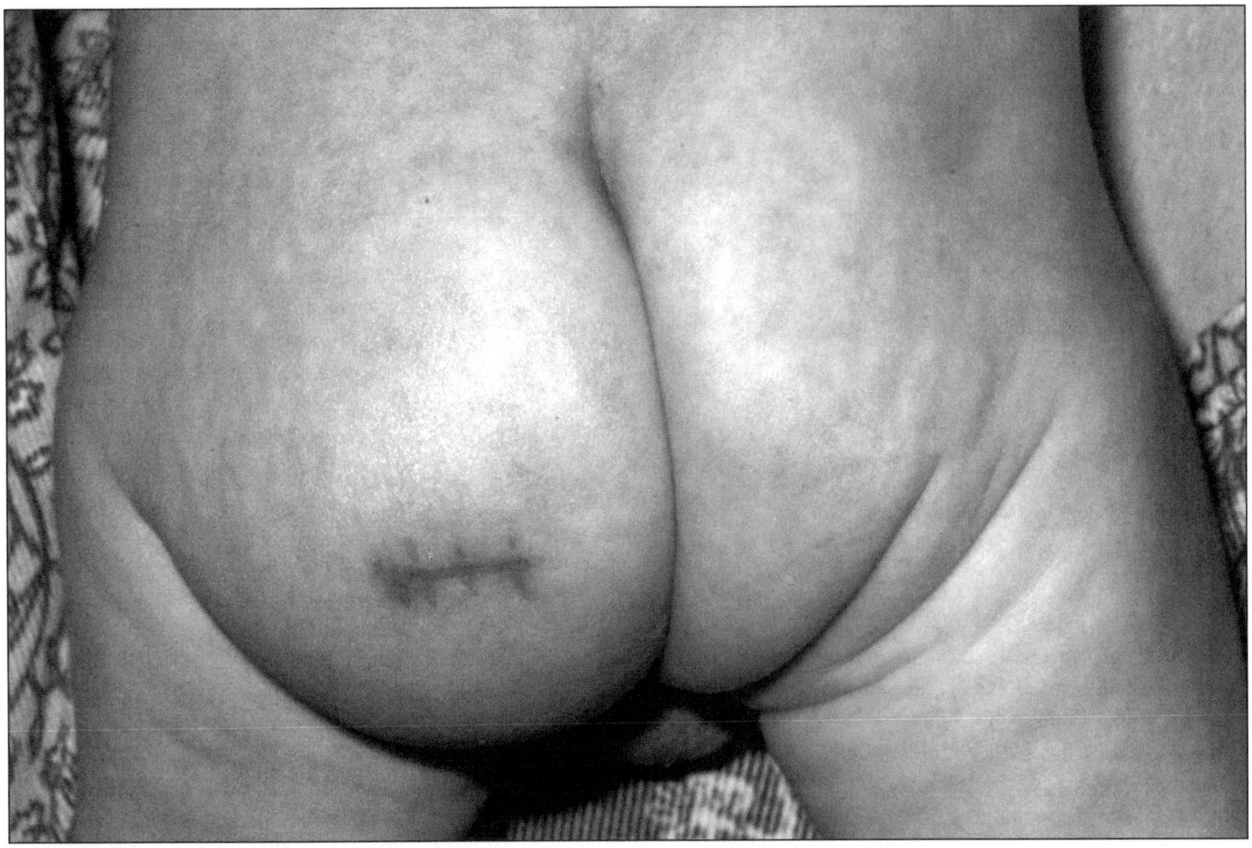

Rhabdomyosarcoma was biopsied from the buttock of this two-month-old baby boy. (Dr. P. Marazzi/Photo Researchers, Inc.)

and type of the tumor (T), spread to lymph nodes (N) and distant organs, and metastases (M). Once the clinical group and TNM stage are determined, patients are categorized as low, intermediate, or high risk.

Treatment and therapy: Surgery is the initial treatment of choice to remove as much of the rhabdomyosarcoma as possible. If surgery may be disfiguring or damaging, only partial tumor removal is possible. Chemotherapy is used to kill any cells remaining after surgery or to attack cells that may have spread elsewhere in the body. Radiation therapy may be used, especially if part of the tumor has been left behind after surgery or the tumor has metastasized. A team will make the best treatment decisions for the child based on staging, location of the tumor, and other factors.

Prognosis, prevention, and outcomes: The prognosis for rhabdomyosarcoma depends on the stage at diagnosis, the site and the size of the tumor, the success of surgical removal, and whether the tumor has spread. Approximately 70 percent of children diagnosed will be disease-free at five years, and rhabdomyosarcoma is considered a curable disease. Depending on the site of surgery, there may be residual damage to the patient such as loss of an eye or other body part or organ. There is no way to prevent rhabdomyosarcoma.

Patricia Stanfill Edens, R.N., Ph.D., FACHE

▶ For Further Information

Magne, N., and C. Haie-Meder. "Brachytherapy for Genital-Tract Rhabdomyosarcoma in Girls: Technical Aspects, Reports, and Perspectives." *Lancet Oncology* 8, no. 8 (August, 2007): 729-739

Rodeberg, D. A., C. Erskine, and E. Celis. "In Vitro Induction of Immune Responses to Shared Tumor-Associated Antigens in Rhabdomyosarcoma." *Journal of Pediatric Surgery* 42, no. 8 (August, 2007): 1396-1402

▶ Other Resources

American Cancer Society

Detailed Guide: Rhabdomyosarcoma
http://www.cancer.org/docroot/CRI/content/CRI_2_4_1X_What_is_rhabdomyosarcoma_53.asp

National Cancer Institute
Childhood Rhabdomyosarcoma
http://www.cancer.gov/cancertopics/types/childrhabdomyosarcoma

See also Alveolar soft-part sarcomas; Amputation; Beckwith-Wiedemann syndrome (BWS); Breast cancer in children and adolescents; Childhood cancers; Fibrosarcomas, soft-tissue; *HRAS* gene testing; Limb salvage; Orbit tumors; Pleuropulmonary blastomas; Sarcomas, soft-tissue; Testicular cancer; Tumor markers; Vaginal cancer.

▶ *RhoGD12* gene

Category: Cancer biology
Also known as: Guanine nucleotide binding protein, tumor-suppressor gene

Definition: *RhoGD12* is an oncogene, the product of which suppresses the metastatic potential of several types of tumors, including those of the bladder, lung, prostate, ovarian, breast, and colon. The *RhoGD12* gene is expressed within a variety of neoplastic cells. The method of regulation of expression of the gene is unknown. Tumors that have undergone metastasis appear to downregulate the gene, while increased expression is correlated with reduced levels of metastasis.

Significance: Mortality associated with cancer can be the result of two separate but interrelated processes: growth of the primary tumor and metastasis of the growth to distal sites, potentially any organ in the body, which may result in damage to that organ. Removal of the primary tumor by surgery may eliminate one growth, but if metastasis has taken place, the tumor may recur at other sites, potentially proving fatal. Elimination of metastatic growth sites has been addressed using chemotherapy, a method of treatment that may have significant side effects.

The discovery of the *RhoGD12* suppressor gene potentially opens another method to limit metastasis. The gene product has been found to suppress metastasis, apparently by interfering with the function of endothelin, a member of a protein family involved in cell signaling and cell dissemination from primary tumors.

Endothelin-1 was found to be overexpressed in several forms of cancers, but particularly in ovarian cancers, and appears to play an important role in the development of these forms of cancers. Measurement of endothelin-1 in abdominal fluids may potentially represent a screening mechanism for early-stage cancer. Because it appears to be an important factor in the metastasis of these neoplasms, use of the RhoGD12 gene product has the potential of suppressing metastasis, providing a means to treat these diseases.

History: In 2002 cancer researchers attempted to correlate the likelihood of metastasis of various types of neoplasms with the expression of specific genes. Using a technique known as microarray analysis, a method to measure expression of large numbers of genes in a cell, it was discovered that the level of expression of one specific gene, now called *RhoGD12*, correlated with lack of metastasis. That is, the greater the level of expression, the less likely metastasis would take place.

Richard Adler, Ph.D.

See also Bladder cancer; Breast cancers; Cancer biology; Chemotherapy; Colorectal cancer; Lung cancers; Metastasis; Oncogenes; Oncogenic viruses; Ovarian cancers; Prostate cancer; Proto-oncogenes and carcinogenesis; Tumor-suppressor genes.

▶ Richter syndrome

Category: Diseases, symptoms, and conditions
Also known as: Diffuse large-cell lymphoma, diffuse large B-cell lymphoma, Richter transformation, Richter's syndrome

Related conditions: Chronic lymphocytic leukemia (CLL), high-grade non-Hodgkin lymphoma (NHL)

Definition: Richter syndrome, named after Maurice Nathaniel Richter, an American pathologist, is a very rare type of cancer that primarily affects adults and can be found most often in women. Only 10 percent of patients diagnosed with Richter syndrome are under the age of fifty. Leukemia is a cancer of the white blood cells, and Richter syndrome is an advanced type of lymphocytic leukemia that starts in the bone marrow as chronic lymphocytic leukemia but develops or transforms into diffuse large-cell lymphoma. This transformation of the cancer type is very aggressive and has the ability to travel through the blood and access the entire body. When chronic lymphocytic leukemia transforms into diffuse large-cell lymphoma, it does so quickly and causes sudden deterioration of the patient's health, which leads to an extreme exacerbation of symptoms and often to death of the patient.

Risk factors: To develop Richter syndrome, a person first must have chronic lymphocytic leukemia, a rare cancer of the blood. Of those patients with chronic lymphocytic leukemia, those who smoke or have had exposure to pesticides and radiation, as well as those who have family members with chronic lymphocytic leukemia, are more likely to develop Richter syndrome. Some genetic influence may also play a role in the transformation of chronic lymphocytic leukemia to diffuse large-cell lymphoma. It is important to remember, however, that these risk factors are not determinant but have been shown to be possibly related to Richter syndrome.

Etiology and the disease process: There is no known cause for Richter syndrome. Onset of Richter syndrome or of the transformation of chronic lymphocytic leukemia to diffuse large-cell lymphoma is thought to be typically brought about by a variation in the patient's lymphocytes accompanied by rapid tumor growth, swelling of lymph nodes, fever, and weight loss caused by a reduction in appetite.

Incidence: Cases of Richter syndrome are extremely rare, occurring in only 2 to 3 percent of patients with the aggressive form of non-Hodgkin lymphoma, chronic lymphocytic leukemia. This translates to approximately 1 in 20 patients whose chronic lymphocytic leukemia will transform into diffuse large B-cell lymphoma.

Symptoms: Symptoms of lymphoma include swelling of the lymphatic system, particularly swelling of the lymph nodes in the neck, armpit, or groin. Symptoms of Richter syndrome often include fatigue, decreased appetite, fever, night sweating, weight loss, and breathlessness.

Screening and diagnosis: Screening for Richter syndrome is performed on patients with chronic lymphocytic leukemia who are judged to be at risk to develop the syndrome. Diagnosis of Richter syndrome is done through microscopic examination of cells and biopsy of the bone marrow of a select "flat" bone, including bones of the rib, hip, and shoulder. Further tests include blood tests, bone scans, and X rays to assess the cancer and its spread within the body.

Treatment and therapy: Treatment for Richter syndrome is typically chemotherapy; however, because this cancer is very aggressive, chemotherapy often is not successful. Bone marrow transplantation is also a potential treatment, but this option is rare and usually occurs within clinical trials.

The two medications typically used to treat diffuse large-cell lymphoma are doxorubicin and cyclophosphamide. These drugs are often used in combination with radiation. Another popular treatment option is called the R-Chop regimen, which consists of a monoclonal antibody and four types of chemotherapy. Monoclonal antibodies are used to improve the body's immune response. Additionally, supportive therapies, such as steroids, are used to help alleviate the side effects of the aggressive medicinal regimen.

Prognosis, prevention, and outcomes: Prognosis for Richter syndrome is survival for less than one year following diagnosis, as patients with Richter syndrome typically do not respond well to treatment because of the advanced state of their cancer, as well as their depressed immune response. As genetic factors play a role in this cancer, prevention steps are limited but include maintaining a healthy lifestyle without the use of tobacco products and without exposure to pesticides, herbicides, and radiation.

Anna Perez, M.Sc.

▶ For Further Information

Catovsky, D., J. Fooks, and S. Richards. "Prognostic Factors in Chronic Lymphocytic Leukaemia: The Importance of Age, Sex, and Response to Treatment in Survival—A Report from the MRC Chronic Lymphocytic Leukemia 1 Trial." *British Journal of Haematology* 72 (1989): 141-149.

Robertson, L. E., et al. "Richter's Syndrome: A Report on Thirty-nine Patients." *Journal of Clinical Oncology* 11 (1993): 1985-1989.

Rodriguez, J., et al. "Allogenic Haematopoietic Transplantation for Richter's Syndrome." *British Journal of Haematology* 110 (2000): 897-899.

Souhami, Robert L., et al., eds. *Oxford Textbook of Oncology*. 2d ed. New York: Oxford University Press, 2002.

Tsimberidou A. M., and M. J. Keating. "Richter Syndrome: Biology, Incidence, and Therapeutic Strategies." *Cancer* 103 (2005): 216-228.

▶ Other Resources

American Cancer Society
Chronic Lymphocytic Leukemia
http://www.cancer.org/docroot/CRI/content/CRI_2_4_4X_Chronic_Lymphocytic_Leukemia_62.asp

Leukemia and Lymphoma Society
http://www.leukemia-lymphoma.org

Lymphoma Information Network
http://www.lymphomainfo.net

National Cancer Institute
http://www.cancer.gov

See also Chronic lymphocytic leukemia (CLL); Clinical trials; Leukemias; Lymphomas; Medical oncology; Non-Hodgkin lymphoma; Oncology.

▶ Risks for cancer

Category: Lifestyle and prevention

Definition: Risk is defined as the probability that exposure to a hazard will result in a negative outcome, such as the occurrence of cancer. Although cancer is one of the most feared diseases in the modern world, the majority of cancer risks can be reduced through simple lifestyle choices.

Concepts of risk: There are several concepts of risk. Absolute risk is defined as the probability that an event will occur over a defined period. Age-specific lifetime risk estimates are a type of absolute risk. For example, a woman may have a cumulative 30 percent lifetime risk of breast cancer but only have a 5 percent chance of developing the disease in the next five years. Risk is frequently described in epidemiological studies (studies of population-wide patterns of disease) using a ratio known as a relative risk (RR), which compares the incidence of disease in people who have a certain risk factor, such as family history, to those who do not have the risk factor (control group). Many studies of cancer risk factors have found higher or lower relative risks that are so slight that they could be the result of random chance. These are referred to as statistically insignificant. When assessing risk, it is also important to know the effect size, rather than just a percentage increase in risk. For example, an increase in risk from 1 to 2 percent is a much less significant finding than an increase in risk from 20 to 40 percent, yet both increases in risk could be reported in the media as a 50 percent increase in risk.

Risk perception: Risk means different things to different people. Experts often see risk differently from the average person, because experts tend to evaluate risk based on statistics and technical information. The average person, however, may judge risks based on technical information and many other factors, such as how familiar the risk is, whether the risk can be controlled, the catastrophic potential of the outcome, and the voluntariness of the exposure. Men and women also tend to perceive risk very differently, which may be related to how much power individuals feel they have over their exposure to hazards. Many people are willing to tolerate a higher level of risk from activities seen as beneficial or enjoyable, such as smoking and drinking. The perceived risk goes down as the perceived benefit goes up.

Because cancer is so common, represents such a burden on society, and is a highly dreaded disease, public health researchers are very interested in understanding risk factors for cancer. One of the most important messages coming out of this research since the early 1980's is that the majority of risks for cancer can be mitigated through lifestyle changes.

Tobacco use: Tobacco use is responsible for about one-third of all cancer deaths. The use of tobacco not only greatly increases the risk for lung cancer but also appears to influence the risk for cancer of the larynx, oral cavity, esophagus, bladder, kidney, pancreas, stomach, and cervix. Women who smoke are at a higher risk of developing lung cancer than male smokers, as are heavy smokers—for example, a person who smokes forty cigarettes a day for twenty years is at higher risk than one who smokes twenty a day for forty years. No matter how long or how much a person has used tobacco, it is never too late to quit: The risk of cancer begins to decrease as soon as tobacco use stops.

Cigars and pipes are often seen as less harmful than cigarettes. However, even if cigar and pipe smokers do not inhale, they are at increased risk for cancer of the oral cavity and lungs. Pipe smokers also are at increased risk for lip cancers in areas where the pipe stem rests. Using chewing tobacco and dry snuff increases the risk of cancer in the cheek, gums, and lips.

Diet and obesity and overweight: Poor diet, overweight, and obesity are responsible for about 30 percent of cancer deaths. Diets low in vegetables, fruits, whole grains, and beans and high in animal protein and fat have been convincingly linked to higher risk for many cancers, including those of the colon, rectum, stomach, and esophagus. However, the link between diet and breast cancer risk is unclear. Some researchers have found associations with fat intake and increased risk, while others have not. Similarly, while fiber intake was once thought to protect against colon cancer, the evidence now is inconclusive.

High fat intake is a major risk factor for cancers. In the large, well-known Nurses' Health Study, which followed more than 87,000 women for up to twenty-four years, researchers compared the occurrence of breast cancers in women who ate the most animal fat to women who ate the lowest amount and found a statistically significant relative risk of 1.33 (33 percent increased risk). Plant fats, such as those from avocados and walnuts, do not appear to increase the risk of cancer.

Processed meats, such as bacon, hot dogs, and sausage, may be particularly risky to eat. In a study that followed nearly 200,000 men and women for seven years, people who consumed the most processed meats increased their risk of pancreatic cancer by 68 percent over those who consumed few or no meat products. Other studies have shown increased risk of stomach and colorectal cancers associated with eating processed meats, pork, and red meat. Preparing meat at high temperatures (for example, grilling or using a wok) can create higher levels of cancer-causing substances in the meat. These studies suggest that eating red meat, processed meats, and pork should be limited to two to three times a week at most, particularly in childhood, when eating habits are being established.

A poor diet increases the risk of overweight and obesity, which are responsible for about 10 percent of cancer deaths in men and 15 percent in women. Researchers have identified three major ways that excess weight—especially in the midsection—may increase cancer risk. One is that body fat secretes substances that seem to promote inflammation throughout the body, increasing the chance of deoxyribonucleic acid (DNA) damage that allows cancer to start. The second is that being overweight can lead to higher blood levels of insulin and insulin-related growth factors, which promote the development of some cancers. Third, excess body fat also changes the levels of several reproductive hormones, such as estrogen and testosterone.

Preventing weight gain is best, but losing excess body fat also seems to lower cancer risk. In the Nurses' Health Study, postmenopausal women who lost 22 pounds or more and kept it off had a 30 percent lower breast cancer risk than postmenopausal women who did not lose weight. Another major study, the Iowa Women's Health Study, followed more than 33,000 women for up to fifteen years. Women who lost weight after menopause had a 23 percent lower risk of breast cancer compared with women who gained weight throughout adulthood. Women who began to lose weight before menopause reduced their risk even more. Losing weight benefits men as well: Among almost 70,000 men in the Cancer Prevention Study II, those who lost at least 11 pounds over a ten-year period had a 16 to 17 percent overall lower risk of prostate cancer and 42 percent lower risk of aggressive forms of prostate cancer.

Lack of exercise: Sedentary lifestyles are responsible for an estimated 5 percent of cancer deaths. Since regular physical activity helps prevent obesity, an indirect association between physical activity and cancer risk has been hypothesized for some time. The understanding that activity level itself is directly linked to cancer risk is new in the last several years. Physical activity changes the body's levels of hormones, insulin, and other growth factors, improves the immune system, and has an anti-inflammatory effect, all of which may help prevent cancer.

Studies consistently show that after controlling for weight, colon cancer risk drops 40 to 50 percent with exercise. Similarly, regular moderate exercise may reduce risk of breast cancer 30 to 40 percent, with greater benefits after menopause. Exercise may also independently lower the risk of prostate, lung, endometrial, ovarian, and kidney cancers, although confirming studies are needed.

Environmental hazards: Environmental hazards that increase the risk of cancer include radon, asbestos, certain chemicals (such as pesticides), and aflatoxins. Environmental hazards, combined, are blamed for about 7 percent of cancer deaths. Many of these hazards are related to occupational exposure. For example, people who work with herbicides are at increased risk of lymphoma, and construction workers are at higher risk of lung cancer from asbestos. Asbestos exposure is also related to an increased laryngeal cancer incidence, and exposure to cement dust raises the risk for pharyngeal cancer. Radon, a naturally occurring radioactive material, is known to increase the risk of lung cancer among underground miners exposed to high levels. Household levels of radon exposure have not been shown to increase lung cancer risk.

Aflatoxins are naturally occurring toxins produced by certain species of fungus, which are found on foods such as corn, peanuts, various other nuts, and cottonseed. High-level aflatoxin exposure is a risk factor for liver cancer, and infection with hepatitis B increases this risk. Food-borne aflatoxin exposure is most common in Africa, China, and Southeast Asia.

The average American is very concerned about carcinogens, and believes that the current risk from potentially carcinogenic chemicals, such as pesticides or cleaning agents, is unacceptably high. Up to 70 percent of Americans say they try to avoid contact with chemicals and chemical products in everyday life. Although it is not possible to know for sure, the best guess is that about 2 to 3 percent of cancer deaths are caused by carcinogenic chemicals.

Genetics: About 5 to 10 percent of cancer deaths are related to genetic factors and factors present at birth. A family history of any cancer raises a person's risk, but the increase varies by type of cancer. Breast-ovarian cancer syndrome results from mutations in the *BRCA1* or *BRCA2* gene. People with this mutation have an 80 to 90 percent lifetime risk of breast cancer and a 20 to 60 percent chance of developing ovarian cancer. Men with this syndrome have an elevated risk of prostate cancer, and both sexes are at increased risk of melanoma and pancreatic cancer. Hereditary forms of colon cancer, melanoma, pancreatic cancer, and brain cancers are also known.

Both low and high birth weight have both been identified as risk factors for testicular cancer. Among men, but not women, being relatively short at birth is associated with increased risk of colorectal cancer in adulthood. Because studies that follow people from birth for sixty to eighty years are expensive and logistically difficult, very little research has been done on other possible risk factors that are present at birth.

Viral and bacterial infections: About 5 percent of cancer deaths are related to viral infections. Several different types of infections raise a person's cancer risk. For example, people infected with one of the viruses that cause hepatitis are more susceptible to liver cancer and lymphoma. Chronic infection with *Helicobacter pylori*, a bacterium that lives on the lining of the stomach, increases risk for stomach cancer and lymphoma. Human immunodeficiency virus (HIV) and Epstein-Barr virus are linked to lymphoma as well. People with inflammatory bowel disease have above-average rates of colon cancer. Cervical and anal cancers are associated with the human papillomavirus (HPV). The risk is greater for people who have chronic, untreated infections, so screening for viruses to catch them early is important in preventing cancer.

Alcohol: Alcohol use is associated with increased risk for mouth, esophageal, laryngeal, pharyngeal, breast, and liver cancers. About 3 percent of cancer deaths are related to alcohol consumption. Alcohol may increase cancer risk in several ways: It may reduce the body's ability to absorb vitamins, raise the level of hormones in the body, or suppress the immune system. There may be some association with diet as well, since heavy drinkers tend to have poorer diets than abstainers. All types of alcohol—beer, wine, and liquor—increase risk equally.

People who drink more than three drinks a day are at the highest risk. One study says that for the average woman, having just one drink a day increases the lifetime risk of breast cancer from 1 in 8 (12.5 percent) to about 1 in 7 (about 14.25 percent). Moderate alcohol intake (two drinks a day for men and one a day for women) may have cardiovascular benefits for men over age fifty and women over age sixty that outweigh the increased risk of cancer, although people who do not drink should not start in the hope of gaining cardiovascular benefits.

Screening: Although screening does not, by itself, prevent cancer, it does reduce the risk of advanced or late-stage cancer. The earlier a case of cancer is detected, the better the chances of survival. There are simple screening tests for many common cancers, including breast, prostate, ovarian, colorectal, and oral.

Lisa M. Lines, M.P.H.

▶ For Further Information

Colditz, Graham A., and Cynthia J. Stein. *Handbook of Cancer Risk Assessment and Prevention*. Boston: Jones and Bartlett, 2004.

Pensiero, Laura, Michael Osborne, and Susan Oliviera. *The Strang Cancer Prevention Center Cookbook: A Complete Nutrition and Lifestyle Plan to Dramatically Lower Your Cancer Risk*. New York: McGraw-Hill, 2004.

Ropeik, D., and G. M. Gray. *Risk: A Practical Guide for Deciding What's Really Safe and What's Dangerous in the World Around You*. Boston: Houghton Mifflin, 2002.

Slovic, P. *The Perception of Risk*. London: Earthscan, 2000.

▶ Other Resources

American Cancer Society
Who Is at Risk?
http://www.cancer.org/docroot/WHO/WHO_0.asp

American Institute for Cancer Research
Recommendations for Cancer Prevention
http://www.aicr.org/site/PageServer?pagename=dc_home_guides

Siteman Cancer Center, Washington University School of Medicine
Your Disease Risk
http://www.yourdiseaserisk.wustl.edu/

See also Air pollution; Asbestos; Cancer education; Carcinogens, known; Carcinogens, reasonably anticipated; Cell phones; Chewing tobacco; Cigarettes and cigars; Developing nations and cancer; Dioxins; Family history and risk assessment; Genetics of cancer; Geography and cancer; Native North Americans and cancer; Obesity-associated cancers; Occupational exposures and cancer; Pesticides and the food chain; Plasticizers; Prevent Cancer Foundation; Radon; *Report on Carcinogens* (RoC); Tobacco-related cancers.

▶ Robert H. Lurie Cancer Center

Category: Organizations

Definition: The Robert H. Lurie Cancer Center of Northwestern University is a university-based comprehensive cancer center located in Chicago. The Feinberg School of

Medicine on Northwestern University's Chicago campus, basic science research labs at both the Chicago and Evanston campuses, and five affiliated teaching hospitals are integrated to provide state-of-the-art cancer care.

Founding and history: The Cancer Center was established at Northwestern University in 1974. In 1991 the Cancer Center was dedicated as the Robert H. Lurie Cancer Center of Northwestern University, and in 1998 the name was changed to the Robert H. Lurie Comprehensive Cancer Center of Northwestern University, reflecting the designation from the National Cancer Institute as a comprehensive cancer center. In 1987 Robert H. Lurie, for whom the center is named, began treatment for advanced colon cancer at the center. Lurie was forty-six years old at the time of his diagnosis, and he was at the peak of a successful career in real estate. Lurie exemplified an individual who believed in living life to the fullest and in not giving in to his illness. Before he died in 1990, Robert Lurie and his wife, Ann, determined they would endow the center to further cancer research. The decision to use Robert Lurie's name for the center reflects that individual's tenacious battle with cancer and is meant to symbolize the center's dedication to the research and treatment of individuals dealing with cancer. Ann Lurie has continued her involvement in the cause of cancer research and treatment; in addition to the endowment of the Robert H. Lurie Comprehensive Cancer Center, she has made a gift to Children's Memorial Hospital to establish a new medical center, scheduled to open in 2012 on Northwestern University's Chicago campus, for the care of children and for pediatric research initiatives.

Current facilities: An outpatient clinical cancer center in downtown Chicago, the collaboration of the Robert H. Lurie Comprehensive Cancer Center of Northwestern University and the Northwestern Medical Faculty Foundation, was opened in 2003. All physicians at the cancer center are faculty of the Feinberg School of Medicine. The cancer center provides oncology diagnostic and treatment services as well as patient access to clinical trials. The Division of Hematology/Oncology (for cancers and disorders of the blood), the Division of Surgical Oncology (for cancers of skin, breast, and the gastrointestinal system), and the Division of Gynecology Oncology (for cancers of the female reproductive system) are housed in the cancer center.

Clinical inpatient treatment and clinical research is conducted at the teaching hospitals affiliated with the Feinberg School of Medicine. The hospitals included are Northwestern Memorial Hospital, Rehabilitation Institute of Chicago, Jesse Brown VA Medical Center, and Children's Memorial Hospital.

Research: Basic science research laboratories for the cancer center are on the Evanston, Illinois, campus of Northwestern University. The three divisions of the research center are the Basic Sciences Division, the Clinical Sciences Division, and the Cancer Prevention and Control Division. The Basic Sciences Division has research programs in viral oncogenesis; tumor invasion, metastasis and angiogenesis (TIMA); hormone action and signal transduction in cancer; cancer genes and molecular targeting; and cancer cell biology. The Clinical Sciences Division has breast cancer, prostate cancer, and hematologic malignancies research programs. The Cancer Prevention and Control Division researches the preventive themes of epidemiology, chemoprevention, biomarkers and early detection, and behavioral science and the cancer control themes of the costs and patterns of oncology treatments, measurement, analysis and interpretation of quality of life, and palliative and rehabilitation oncology.

A collaboration of the Robert H. Lurie Cancer Center and Northwestern University's International Institute for Nanotechnology, Northwestern University Center of Cancer Nanotechnology Excellence (NU-CCNE) was established in 2005. This center is funded by the National Cancer Institute. The NU-CCNE includes scientists, cancer biologists, engineers, and clinicians working together toward the research goal of designing and testing nanomaterials and nanodevices for their application in the setting of clinical care for cancer screening, diagnosis, and treatment. Clinical research is conducted in the inpatient and outpatient facilities of the cancer center with access to clinical trials.

Specialization: Two Specialized Programs of Research Excellence (SPORE) at the Robert H. Lurie Comprehensive Cancer Center—the Breast Cancer SPORE and the Prostate Cancer SPORE—are supported by the National Cancer Institute. The cancer center has a program for stem cell transplantation and is known for its research in hematologic malignancies. The Genetic Testing and Counseling Services provide a full range of genetic counseling, testing, screening, and research. The pediatric oncology program includes specialists in the treatment of children with leukemia, brain and spinal cord tumors, and other solid tumors. A special program of palliative care is offered at the cancer center; the program includes consultation services, an acute inpatient palliative care unit, and a home hospice program.

Vicki Miskovsky, B.S., R.D.

▶ For Further Information

Dollinger, M. *Everyone's Guide to Cancer Therapy: How Cancer Is Diagnosed, Treated, and Managed Day to Day,* 4th ed. Kansas City, Mo.: Andre McMell, 2002.

Leonard, John P., and Morton Coleman. *Hodgkin's and Non-Hodgkin's Lymphoma.* New York: Springer, 2006.

Waller, Alexander, and Nancy L. Caroline. *Handbook of Palliative Care in Cancer.* 2d ed. Boston: Butterworth-Heinemann, 2000.

▶ Other Resources

National Cancer Institute
Cancer Centers Program
http://cancercenters.cancer.gov/cancer_centers/rhiccc.html

National Comprehensive Cancer Network
Robert H. Lurie Comprehensive Cancer Center
http://www.nccn.org/members/profiles/northwestern.asp

Robert H. Lurie Comprehensive Cancer Center
http://www.cancer.northwestern.edu/home/index.cfm

See also American Association for Cancer Research (AACR); American Cancer Society (ACS); American Institute for Cancer Research (AICR); Clinical trials; Genetic counseling; National Cancer Institute (NCI); Prevent Cancer Foundation.

▶ Rothmund-Thomson syndrome

Category: Diseases, symptoms, and conditions
Also known as: RTS, Rothmund dystrophy, Thomson's disorder, poikiloderma congenitale

Related conditions: RAPADILINO syndrome, Baller-Gerold syndrome

Definition: In 1868, August von Rothmund, a German ophthalmologist, published an account of a syndrome that included cataracts, a depressed nasal bridge, and skin degeneration, with familial links. Then, in both 1923 and 1936, Matthew S. Thomson, a British dermatologist, reported a disorder with the same defining characteristics. After some controversy over whether the reports described the same disorder, the disease became known as Rothmund-Thomson syndrome. As suggested by the time elapsed between Rothmund's and Thomson's accounts, Rothmund-Thomson syndrome is extremely rare. It is an inherited disorder that affects many body systems and is usually diagnosed during early infancy, typically between the ages of three and six months.

Risk factors: Family history is the only known risk factor for Rothmund-Thomson syndrome. The disorder is inherited as an autosomal recessive trait, which means that both parents of an affected child have one copy of the defective gene that is responsible for the disorder but do not have the disorder themselves. If both parents have one copy of the defective gene, each of their children has a 25 percent chance of having both defective genes and the disorder, a 25 percent chance of not having the gene, and a 50 percent chance of having one defective gene, like the parents.

Etiology and the disease process: The defective gene responsible for Rothmund-Thomson syndrome is called adenosine triphosphate (ATP)-dependent deoxyribonucleic acid (DNA) helicase Q4, or *RECQ14*. To date, it is the only gene that has been associated with Rothmund-Thomson syndrome, although it is commonly believed that there are others. Mutations in *RECQ14* have been detected in about 66 percent of affected individuals.

At birth, an affected child's skin appears normal. Usually, by the age of six months, a characteristic rash has developed on the child's face and later spreads to the buttocks and extremities. The rash eventually changes into a chronic pattern of several skin abnormalities, collectively known as poikiloderma. At birth, and as the child ages, many other abnormalities may be diagnosed, including skeletal defects, growth delays, vision disturbances, and possibly bone and skin cancers. The clinical features, disease progression, and severity can vary from case to case.

Incidence: Only about 300 cases of Rothmund-Thomson syndrome have been reported in scientific literature. It does not seem to affect one group more than another, as it has been found in all races and many nationalities. More than 90 percent of patients develop the characteristic skin symptoms by their first birthday.

Symptoms: The initial rash that is characteristic of most cases of Rothmund-Thomson syndrome begins as abnormally red, swollen patches, usually on the face, that are accompanied by blistering and abnormal accumulations of fluid between the layers of tissue under the skin. Additional areas of the body become involved as the disorder progresses, including the arms, legs, hands, feet, and buttocks. Eventually, a collective group of findings, known as poikiloderma, begins. The swollen skin begins to shrink, groups of small blood vessels widen abnormally, and patchy areas of abnormally decreased or increased coloration appear. Skin that is exposed to the sun usually shows greater abnormalities, and the individual can develop thickened skin or cancerous skin changes later in life.

Skeletal abnormalities may be present from birth or develop as the child grows. They include unusually small, short hands and feet and underdeveloped or absent thumbs and forearm bones. The development of osteosarcoma, a bone cancer, can occur later in life. Affected individuals may also have characteristic abnormalities of the head and face, including a prominent forehead, sunken nasal bridge, and a protruding lower jaw. Growth delays can lead to shortened height. Some other common characteristics of Rothmund-Thomson syndrome that may begin in childhood include gray, sparse hair; absent eyebrows and eyelashes; cataracts; excessive cavities and unusually small or missing teeth; and abnormally developed nails. Irregular menstruation in women and delayed sexual development and reduced fertility in both sexes can also occur because of deficient activity of the ovaries in women or testes in men.

Screening and diagnosis: The only way to screen for Rothmund-Thomson syndrome is genetic testing for family members of affected individuals. The diagnosis of Rothmund-Thomson syndrome is usually based on physical examination and family history. Some skin cell and lymphocyte tests may show changes that have been seen with Rothmund-Thomson syndrome, but they are not considered diagnostic. Testing to determine the extent of the disorder and monitoring for complications includes X rays for skeletal abnormalities, routine eye examinations for the early diagnosis of cataracts, endocrine tests, and a complete blood count.

Treatment and therapy: Treatment of Rothmund-Thomson syndrome primarily involves annual physical examinations to monitor for skin and bone changes as well as complications that develop as the person ages, such as endocrine deficiencies. Cataracts should be removed if they decrease vision. For cosmetic purposes, skin conditions can be treated with a variety of medications or laser therapy. People who develop cancer should receive treatment based on the type of cancer.

Prognosis, prevention, and outcomes: Rothmund-Thomson syndrome usually is not a life-threatening disease unless the individual develops bone cancer or allows skin cancer to go untreated. Use of sunscreen and avoiding repeated or excessive sun exposure are recommended. There is no prevention or cure for the disorder.

Dorothy P. Terry, R.N.

▶ For Further Information

Broom, M. A., et al. "Successful Umbilical Cord Blood Stem Cell Transplantation in a Patient with Rothmund-Thomson Syndrome and Combined Immunodeficiency." *Clinical Genetics* 69, no. 4 (April, 2006): 337-343.

Kumar, P., et al. "Late-Onset Rothmund-Thomson Syndrome." *International Journal of Dermatology* 46, no. 5 (May, 2007): 492-493.

Wang, L. L., et al. "Association Between Osteosarcoma and Deleterious Mutations in the *RECQ14* Gene in Rothmund-Thomson Syndrome." *Journal of the National Cancer Institute* 95, no. 9 (May 7, 2003): 669-674.

▶ Other Resources

Genetics Home Reference

Rothmund-Thomson Syndrome
http://ghr.nlm.nih.gov/condition=rothmund thomsonsyndrome

National Organization for Rare Disorders

Rothmund Thomson Syndrome
http://www.rarediseases.org/search/rdbdetail_abstract.html?disname=Rothmund%20Thomson%20Syndrome

See also Bone cancers; Bone scan; Childhood cancers; Complete blood count (CBC); Computed tomography (CT) scan; Dermatology oncology; Ewing sarcoma; Eye cancers; Eyelid cancer; Family history and risk assessment; Genetic testing; Genetics of cancer; Ophthalmic oncology; Skin cancers; Stem cell transplantation; Sunscreens.

▶ Salivary gland cancer

Category: Diseases, symptoms, and conditions
Also known as: Parotid gland cancer

Related conditions: Throat, neck, and mouth cancers

Definition: Salivary gland cancer is cancer that develops in the glands found in the mouth, nose, sinuses, and larynx (voice box) that secrete saliva.

Risk factors: The main risk factor for developing salivary gland cancer is exposure to radiation in the head and neck. This exposure often occurs for other medical conditions. Workplace exposure to certain metal dusts and silica dust also increase the likelihood of developing salivary gland cancer. Tobacco use increases the risk of developing squamous cell salivary gland cancer as well as squamous cell cancers of the throat and mouth. A few studies suggest that a diet high in animal fat and low in vegetables or a family history of salivary gland cancer are risk factors, but these studies have not been conclusive, and these risk factors appear minor compared with radiation exposure.

Etiology and the disease process: The salivary glands produce saliva that contains enzymes to help digest food. There are three pairs of major salivary glands. The largest are the parotid glands located in front of and below each ear. The paired sublingual salivary glands are found under the tongue, and the pair of submandibular salivary glands are located below the jawbone. There are also between six hundred and one thousand microscopic glands, called minor salivary glands, located in the lining of the mouth, the nose, sinuses, and larynx.

About 80 percent of all salivary tumors develop in the parotid glands and another 10 to 15 percent develop in the submandibular glands. Most of the tumors that develop in these salivary glands are benign (not cancerous). Tumors that begin in the minor salivary glands are usually malignant (cancerous). Malignant tumors are classified as low grade if they grow slowly and high grade if they grow aggressively and rapidly.

Salivary glands contain a mix of several different types of cells. Each type of cell gives rise to a different type of tumor. About a dozen specific types of cancer can develop in these glands. There are four major types of salivary gland cancer.

Mucoepidermoid carcinomas usually develop in the parotid glands. They may form low-grade or high-grade tumors.

Acinic cell carcinomas also start in the parotid gland. They usually grow slowly but also tend to invade surrounding tissues.

Adenoid cystic carcinomas are low-grade but persistent tumors that often cause the cancer to recur after surgery.

Polymorphous low-grade adenocarcinomas usually begin in the minor salivary glands and grow slowly.

There are another half a dozen or so rare or very rare malignant carcinomas that can develop in the salivary glands. Of these, sebaceous adenocarcinoma, oncocytic carcinoma, and salivary duct carcinoma tend to have the worst outcomes. Basal cell adenocarcinomas, clear cell carcinomas, cystadenocarcinomas, and mucinous adenocarcinomas tend to be curable or have good outcomes. Other rare salivary gland cancers include squamous cell carcinoma, undifferentiated carcinomas, and mixed malignant carcinomas, all of which tend to be high-grade, aggressive cancers.

Incidence: Salivary cancer is rare, as most tumors that form in the salivary glands are benign. The American Cancer Society estimates that between 2 and 3 people per 100,000 population develop salivary gland cancer each year. Of these cancers, 85 percent are in the parotid gland. Most people are first diagnosed with salivary gland cancer

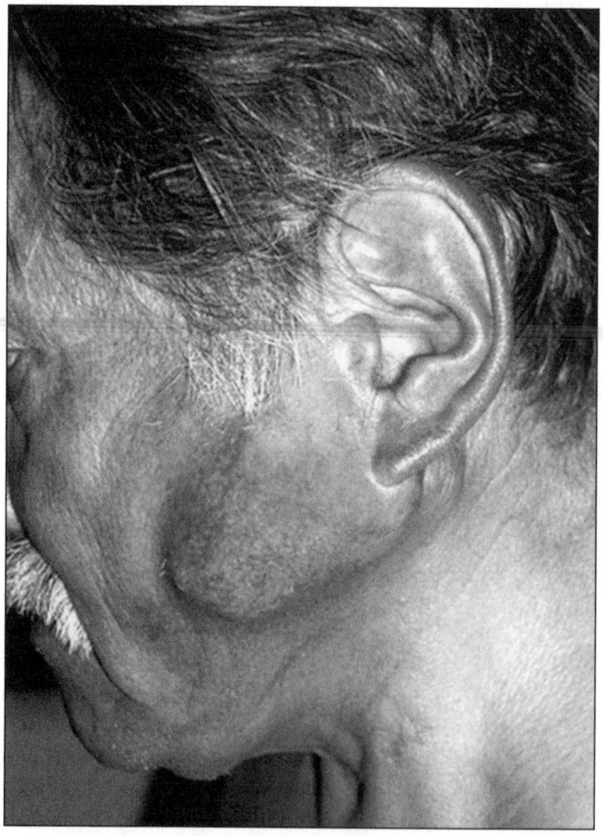

A man with a parotid gland tumor. (Scott Camazine/Photo Researchers, Inc.)

Distribution and Five-Year Survival Rates for Salivary Gland Cancer by Histology, 1988-2001

Histology	*Total Cases (%)*	*Survival Rate (%)*
Squamous cell carcinoma	17.1	45.6
Adenocarcinoma	15.2	59.9
Adenoid cystic carcinoma	13.5	84.1
Mucoepidermoid carcinoma, poorly differentiated	13.2	90.4
Acinic cell carcinoma	12.4	95.8
Mucoepidermoid carcinoma, other	6.7	66.1
Malignant mixed tumor	5.2	82.2
Mucoepidermoid carcinoma, well differentiated	3.3	98.6
Other	13.3	N/A

Source: Data from L. A. G. Ries et al., eds., *Cancer Survival Among Adults: U.S. SEER Program, 1988-2001—Patient and Tumor Characteristics*, NIH Pub. No. 07-6215 (Bethesda, Md.: National Cancer Institute, 2007)

between the ages of fifty and seventy, although this cancer occasionally can develop in children and young adults.

Symptoms: Salivary gland cancer often shows no symptoms in its early stages. The most common symptom is a lump on the face or neck or in the mouth. Other symptoms include pain in these areas and numbness or weakness on one side of the face. These symptoms also can be caused by a variety of other conditions unrelated to salivary gland cancer.

Screening and diagnosis: Although there is no specific screening for salivary gland cancer, many cases are first detected during routine dental examinations. Diagnosis begins with a complete physical examination and patient history. This is followed by a series of imaging scans. These may include magnetic resonance imaging (MRI) and a computed tomography (CT) or computed axial tomography (CAT) scan. These scans help provide a three-dimensional view of soft tissue within the body. An ultrasound helps to pinpoint tissue of different densities and helps locate the tumor. A positron emission tomography (PET) scan uses a small amount of radioactive glucose (sugar) to locate tumors. Malignant cells divide faster than healthy cells and use more glucose, making them show up as bright spots on the scan. Diagnosis is confirmed by a fine needle aspiration biopsy, in which a sample of tissue is removed and examined for malignant cells under a microscope.

Salivary gland cancer is staged using the TNM system where T stands for the size of the tumor, N stands for the degree to which the cancer has spread to the nearby lymph nodes, and M stands for whether the cancer has spread (metastasized) to distant sites. The stages for salivary gland cancer are as follows:

- Stage 1: The tumor is less than 2 centimeters (cm) in diameter and has not spread to nearby tissue, lymph nodes, or distant sites.
- Stage II: The tumor is larger than 2 cm but less than 4 cm and has not spread to nearby tissue, lymph nodes, or distant sites.
- Stage III: The tumor is larger than 4 cm or has grown into nearby tissue, but has not spread to the lymph nodes. Alternately a tumor of any size that has spread to lymph nodes on the same side of the neck as the tumor is considered as Stage III.
- Stage IV: The tumor is of any size but has invaded nearby structures (bones, skin, and so on) and lymph nodes, or has spread to distant sites.

Treatment and therapy: Treatment depends on the stage of the cancer and the health of the patient. Surgery is generally recommended for Stage I, II, and III salivary gland cancer. For Stage I, the cancer and the salivary gland are usually removed. For Stage II, the surgeon removes more facial tissue and may remove some lymph nodes in the neck on the same side as the tumor. For Stage III cancer, the tumor, some tissue, and lymph nodes on both sides of the neck are removed. Surgery may damage nerves in the face and neck. This may cause difficulty eating and speaking and can be quite disfiguring.

Radiation therapy is usually done after surgery, especially if the cancer cannot be completely removed. Chemotherapy is sometimes done after Stage III surgery, although this is not yet standard procedure. Stage IV cancer can rarely be cured. Radiation therapy and drugs are used to relieve pain and improve quality of life. Some experimental chemotherapy may be used.

Prognosis, prevention, and outcomes: It is important to remember that most tumors arising in the salivary glands are not cancerous. Malignant tumors of the salivary gland make up less than 1 percent of all tumors found in the body. Whether a salivary gland cancer can be cured depends on the specific cell type of the cancer, whether the tumor is high grade or low grade, and the degree to which the cancer has invaded nearby tissues or spread to other parts of the body. Squamous cell cancer, for example, has a poor outcome, with a five-year survival rate of only about 25 percent. The best outcomes are associated with slow-growing, low-grade tumors that are diagnosed early. The worst outcomes are associated with late-stage aggressive high-grade tumors. According to the American Cancer Society, overall five-year survival rates for all salivary gland cancers by stage are Stage I, 86 percent; Stage II, 66 percent; Stage III, 53 percent; and Stage IV, 32 percent.

Avoiding unnecessary radiation exposure to the head and neck and workplace exposure to nickel alloy dust, silica dust, and similar fine metal or mineral dusts is the best way to prevent most salivary gland cancers. Avoiding all tobacco products also helps reduce the risk of squamous cell salivary gland cancer.

Martiscia Davidson, A.M.

▶ For Further Information

Brockstein, Bruce, and Gregory Masters, eds. *Head and Neck Cancer*. Boston: Kluwer Academic, 2003.

Carper, Elise, Kenneth Hu, and Elena Kuzin. *One Hundred Questions and Answers About Head and Neck Cancer*. Sudbury, Mass.: Jones and Bartlett, 2008.

Icon Health. *The Official Patient's Sourcebook on Salivary Gland Cancer: A Revised and Updated Directory for the Internet Age*. San Diego, Calif.: Author, 2004.

Myers, Eugene N., et al., eds. *Cancer of the Head and Neck*. 4th ed. Philadelphia: Saunders, 2003.

▶ Other Resources

American Cancer Society

Detailed Guide: Salivary Gland Cancer
http://www.cancer.org/docroot/CRI/CRI_2_3x.asp?dt=54

National Cancer Institute

Salivary Gland Cancer Treatment
http://www.cancer.gov/cancertopics/pdq/treatment/salivarygland

See also Adenoid cystic carcinoma (ACC); Cell phones; Chewing tobacco; Computed tomography (CT) scan; Dry mouth; Head and neck cancers; Mucosa-associated lymphoid tissue (MALT) lymphomas; Nasal cavity and paranasal sinus cancers; Occupational exposures and cancer; Oral and maxillofacial surgery; Oral and oropharyngeal cancers; Radical neck dissection; Radiopharmaceuticals; Sjögren syndrome; Taste alteration; Throat cancer; Tobacco-related cancers; Young adult cancers.

▶ Salpingectomy and salpingo-oophorectomy

Category: Procedures
Also known as: Unilateral or bilateral salpingo-oophorectomy

Definition: Salpingectomy is the surgical excision of one or both Fallopian tubes to diagnose suspicious tubo-ovarian masses that are, or may become, cancerous; salpingo-oophorectomy includes surgical excision of one or both ovaries for the same reason.

Cancers diagnosed or treated: Invasive cervical, uterine, and ovarian cancers; hydatidiform mole; rarely, Fallopian tube cancer

Why performed: Salpingectomy is performed in order to remove and examine tubal or tubo-ovarian masses suspicious for cancer and to determine the extent of malignant disease spread. These masses may be fluid-filled (cystic), solid, or mixed and can also be hormone-secreting or hormone receptive. A salpingo-oophorectomy is often performed alongside a hysterectomy in women who are postmenopausal and are suspected of having an endometrial, tubal, and/or ovarian mass at risk for encroaching on other pelvic organs. It is also performed in women of childbearing age who have a suspected malignancy and have completed their families. Women with localized, unilateral disease who still wish to bear children may have only the diseased Fallopian tube and ovary removed, although this is not recommended in the light of the more common occurrence of disease in both tubes and ovaries. Salpingo-oophorectomy may also be done to remove masses of an infectious origin (for example, tubo-ovarian abscess caused by pelvic inflammatory disease) or endometriosis that has irreversibly damaged these organs. A bilateral salpingo-oophorectomy is performed prophylactically when patients are at high risk for developing gynecologic cancers associated with *BRCA1* and *BRCA2* gene mutations, particularly ovarian and breast cancers.

Patient preparation: The patient undergoes preoperative evaluation for any contraindications to the procedure (such as a pregnancy test) and evaluation of coexisting diseases to determine her fitness to undergo surgery and general anesthesia. Patients are instructed to take nothing per mouth the night before the procedure.

Steps of the procedure: After the patient is anesthetized, placed in the lithotomy position, and the vagina, external genitalia, pubic area, and inner thighs have been surgically prepped and draped, a transverse or vertical incision is made above the pubic bone. An incision extended up to the level of the umbilicus is preferred, as it provides a wider surgical field and provides a wider incision through which a large mass can be removed. The incision is taken down to the pelvic cavity. The uterine and ovarian vessels are identified, dissected, and separated from the ureters. The supporting broad, round, and suspensory ovarian ligaments of the Fallopian tubes and ovaries with their vessels are then dissected, isolated, cut, and ligated. In a simultaneous hysterectomy, the uterus and uterine vessels are also dissected away from other pelvic structures, cut, and ligated. When disease extending outside the reproductive tract is suspected, biopsies of suspicious lesions, sampling of lymph nodes around the pelvis and abdominal aorta, and abdominal cavity washings are done.

Laparoscopic removal of the Fallopian tubes and ovaries is done in conjunction with a hysterectomy. It is done through two small abdominal incisions through which sleeved trochars accommodating a scope and any of several instruments for probing, grasping, cutting, and cauterizing are inserted. The uterus, Fallopian tubes and ovaries, vessels, and ligaments are dissected, cut, and ligated. The organs are removed vaginally, and the remaining vaginal cuff is closed off.

After the procedure: The patient is monitored in the postanesthesia care unit until she is fully awake and her vital signs are stable. Once the patient is stable in unit, she may be discharged to the gynecologic ward for postoperative monitoring. Once the patient is stable, ambulatory, urinating, and eating, she may be discharged home after a few days.

Risks: The most significant risk of a salpingectomy is an ectopic pregnancy. Other risks include deep vein thrombosis, pulmonary embolism, perforation of the bladder or bowel, and intractable bleeding.

Results: Cross-sectional examination of both grossly normal and diseased Fallopian tubes should be done, documenting size, depth of penetration, and location along the length of the specimen, although primary tubal cancers account for only 0.1 to 1.8 percent of all female reproductive tract cancers. When a mass encompassing both Fallopian tube and ovary is encountered intraoperatively, it is presumed to be of ovarian origin until proven otherwise during pathological examination, where tubal tissue is recognized within the mass. A gross and microscopic examination of tubal or ovarian masses may reveal whether they are cancerous by evaluating individual cells and the tissue architecture for signs of cancerous changes. On gross examination, masses that preserve the outer tissue surrounding the ovaries can suggest no malignancy but cannot eliminate the possibility of early invasive cancer. Central necrosis and hemorrhage may be present in large tumors as they outgrow their blood supply but do not necessarily imply malignancy, as they can occur in both benign and malignant masses. Microscopic changes pointing to a nonmalignant origin of the tumor include increased but orderly growth of ovarian cells but no elements of disordered growth of abnormal cells and distortion of the tissue architecture. Microscopic examinations that reveal disordered

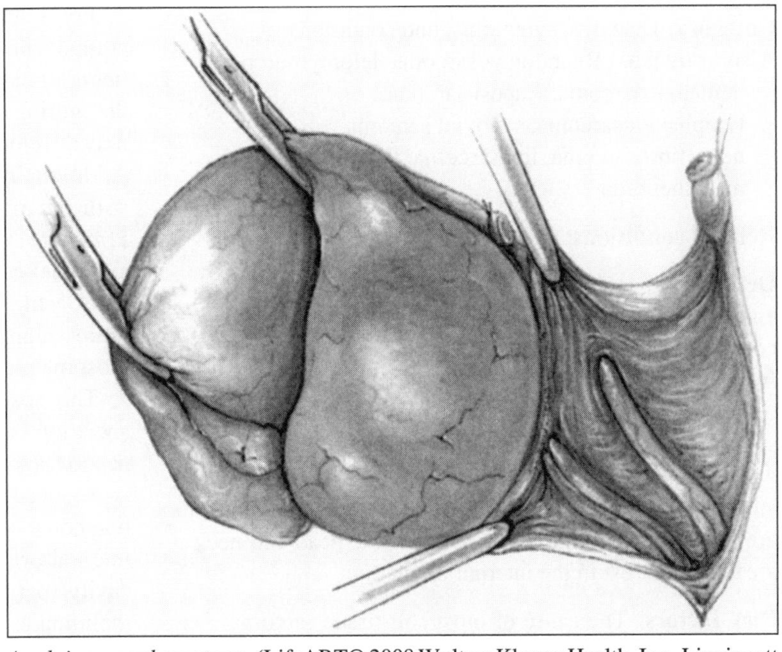

A salpingo-oophorectomy. (LifeART© 2008 Wolters Kluwer Health, Inc.-Lippincott Williams &Wilkins. All rights reserved.)

growth and abnormal cells of tubal or ovarian origin are suggestive of Fallopian tube cancer or ovarian cancer. An invasive hydatidiform mole that has spread from the uterus can exhibit characteristic cells and tissues of placental and fetal origin. Lymph node samples and washings from the abdominal cavity possessing cancerous cells strongly suggest microscopic spread outside the reproductive tract.

Aldo C. Dumlao, M.D.

▶ For Further Information

Haas, Adelaide, and Susan L. Puretz. *The Woman's Guide to Hysterectomy: Expectations and Options*. Berkeley, Calif.: Celestial Arts, 2002.

Memorial Sloan-Kettering Cancer Center. "Cancer-Reducing Benefits of Preventive Surgery May Be Specific to Gene Mutation." *Science Daily*, June 5, 2006. Also available at http://www.science daily.com.

Rosenthal, Sara M. *The Gynecological Sourcebook*. 4th ed. New York: McGraw-Hill, 2003.

See also *BRCA1* and *BRCA2* genes; Cervical cancer; Fallopian tube cancer; Gynecologic cancers; Hydatidiform mole; Hysterectomy; Hystero-oophorectomy; Laparoscopy and laparoscopic surgery; Oophorectomy; Ovarian cancers; Pregnancy and cancer; Risks for cancer; Uterine cancer.

▶ Sarcomas, soft-tissue

Category: Diseases, symptoms, and conditions

Also known as: Rhabdomyosarcoma, leiomyosarcoma, hemangiosarcoma, Kaposi sarcoma, lymphangiosarcoma, synovial sarcoma, neurofibrosarcoma, liposarcoma, fibrosarcoma, mesothelioma

Related conditions: Osteosarcoma, bone cancer

Definition: Sarcomas are divided into two categories: sarcomas of bone and sarcomas of soft tissue. Soft-tissue sarcomas describe a class of malignant tumors that develop from connective tissue, which usually derives from an embryonic layer called mesoderm, is involved in structural support, and is found in linings or coverings of muscle, organs, nerves, and joints. These sarcomas can develop in any part of the body. However, more than half arise in the arms or legs, just under 20 percent in the head and neck area, and the rest in the internal organs.

Risk factors: The cause of most soft-tissue sarcomas is unknown; however, for some, there may be an association with heredity, radiation therapy, immune disorders, or en-

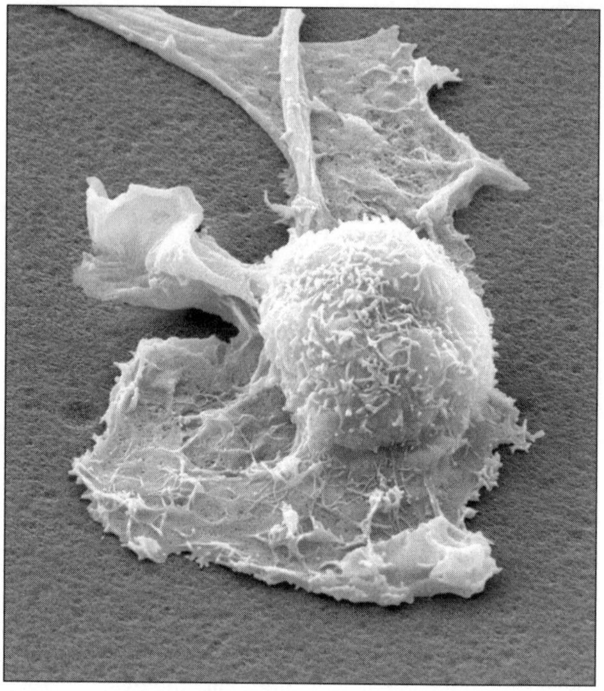

A scanning electron micrograph of a sarcoma cell. (Steve Gschmeissner/Photo Researchers, Inc.)

vironmental factors. For example, sarcomas may follow radiation therapy used in treating thyroid disease, breast cancer, lymphoma, or tuberculosis of the skin. Historically, sarcoma develops about ten years after such treatment.

For some soft-tissue sarcomas, there is an inherited component. Heredity plays a part in about 5 percent of patients stricken with neurofibromatosis, a benign but often disfiguring condition of the nerves in which the sarcoma may develop in the surrounding connective tissue sheaths. Additionally, there is an increased sarcoma risk associated with inherited diseases such as Gardner syndrome, Li-Fraumeni syndrome, intestinal polyposis, tuberous sclerosis, basal cell nevus syndrome, and retinoblastoma. Genetic testing has linked soft-tissue sarcoma with a mutated tumor-suppressor gene in some cases and heritable chromosome rearrangement in others.

The most prominent environmental risk factor is the association between asbestos and mesothelioma. The connection is so strong, in fact, that it is unlikely that the disease is produced in any other way. The mesothelium is a protective connective tissue lining covering most of the body's internal organs, including lungs (pleura), the abdominal cavity (periosteum), and the heart (pericardium). Mesothelioma usually occurs in job-related settings where asbestos dust is prevalent. Some investigators have named vinyl chloride, dioxin, and herbicides containing the chemical phenoxyacetic acid as causative agents for other soft-tissue sarcomas, but the association is weak.

Viruses are the cause of Kaposi sarcoma in people with defective immune systems. Kaposi sarcoma usually involves the skin but may affect other areas as well.

Etiology and the disease process: Whatever its origin or cause, a sarcoma begins as a solid mass that grows from a central point outward with the least mature elements on the periphery. Surrounding the mass is a pseudocapsule, which is composed of compressed tumor cells bordered by inflammatory cells and fibrous components. The degree of pseudocapsule containment may have important implications on the progress of the tumor and the prognosis of the disease. Sarcomas generally are contained within anatomical borders such as muscle sheaths, but as the disease progresses, these borders are challenged and the tumor grows into new compartments until these are also breached. Compartmental breakdown poses special challenges for the surgeon and radiologist.

Incidence: Soft-tissue sarcoma is a relatively uncommon malignancy representing about 1 percent of all cancers. It has an annual incidence in the United States of just under 9,300 cases, with women affected slightly less than men. Approximately 3,500 people die of soft-tissue sarcoma annually. The average occurrences of the most prevalent forms are fibrosarcoma, 23 percent; liposarcoma, 19 percent; rhabdomyosarcoma, 13 percent; synovial sarcoma, 8 percent; and neurofibrosarcoma, 5 percent of total soft-tissue sarcomas.

Symptoms: Symptoms will vary with the location, size, and type of the soft-tissue sarcoma. For example, a sarcoma may appear as a seemingly harmless lump under the skin or as an abdominal growth that exhibits symptoms only after it becomes quite large. As the sarcoma grows and presses on nearby organs, nerves, muscles, or blood vessels, symptoms will correspond to the degree of interference with those tissues. For example, pressure on the nerves may result in pain or paralysis, while interference with the blood supply may cause an accumulation of fluid in the surrounding tissue spaces (edema). Similarly, restriction in mobility follows joint involvement, and internal growths may cause obstructions of the bowel, urinary tract, or chest cavity. As the tumor progresses, signs such as weight loss, fever, and fatigue may become apparent. Additionally, specific endocrine gland involvement may cause goiter, hypoglycemia, or pituitary dysfunction.

Screening and diagnosis: Early detection brings the most favorable result. However, the tumor is usually painless and often will grow unobserved. Once a tumor is suspected, imaging tests such as computed tomography (CT) or magnetic resonance imaging (MRI), radioisotope studies, and tissue biopsy will help define its aggressiveness and characteristics. Additionally, arteriograms are useful in defining the extent of tumor growth and in outlining the irregularity of the vascular network. Chest films using CT scans are essential in evaluating metastatic spread to the lungs.

The pathologist examining the biopsy tissue pays close attention to how fast the cells are dividing and compares the tissue's structure to the surrounding normal tissue. The information from the biopsy report allows for formal grading and staging of the sarcoma. All the information from the biopsy, imaging, staging, and past experience sets the best course of treatment and gives an estimate of the patient's prognosis.

The pathologist grades the sarcoma according to the degree of new blood vessels supplying the tumor, how far it has reached into surrounding tissues, how fast the cells are dividing (mitosis), and their degree of structural abnormality. The grading systems vary somewhat according to the parameters set by the Musculoskeletal Tumor Society (MTS) or the American Joint Committee (AJC), but both are a measure of the tumor's aggressiveness.

Common Sarcomas

Sarcoma	*Tissue*	*Typical Location*
Fibrosarcoma	fibrous tissue	arms, legs, trunk
Hemangiosarcoma	blood vessels	arms, legs, head, trunk
Kaposi sarcoma	blood vessel walls	general locations
Leiomyosarcoma	smooth muscle	uterus, gastrointestinal tract, blood vessel linings
Liposarcoma	fatty tissue	arms, legs, trunk
Lympangiosarcoma	lymph vessels	arms, or area exposed to radiation
Mesothelioma	mesothelium	lungs, heart, intestine
Neurofibrosarcoma	peripheral nerves	arms, legs, trunk
Rhabdomyosarcoma	skeletal muscle	arms, legs
Synovial sarcoma	synovial tissue	joints

Staging further defines the tumor by characterizing its aggressiveness and anatomic profile. The designation T1 indicates a tumor less than 5 centimeters (cm), T2 more than 5 cm, and T3 signifies the invasion of major blood vessels, nerves, or bones. The letter N describes the presence or absence of metastasis to the local lymph nodes and respectively receives an N1 or N0 description. Similarly, M1 or M0 represents the presence or absence, respectively, of metastasis to distant areas. The sarcoma is staged from IA through IVB depending on severity. For example, at the lower end of the system the tumor might receive the most favorable grade (G) of 1A and its GTNM parameters might look like this: G1, T1, N0, M0. At the opposite extreme, the GTNM description would have this designation: G3, T3, N1, M1.

Treatment and therapy: The staging system combined with tumor location sets the course of treatment. The treatment decisions incorporate surgery, radiation therapy, and possibly chemotherapy in a multidisciplinary approach. Typically, surgery alone is reserved for grade 1 tumors, where the surgeon is able to incise the tissue using wide margins. Generally, however, surgery alone invites recurrence. Combining surgery with radiation allows for less radical surgery and may eliminate the need for such debilitating outcomes as amputation.

Soft-tissue sarcomas are not always what they seem. They may appear well encapsulated, but there is no true capsule, and the surgeon must resect the tumor beyond its apparent margins. This requires using wide or even radical incisions when extracting the tumor and may include limb amputation. In the past, less aggressive surgical removal resulted in recurrence in almost a third of the cases, effectively doubling the likelihood of metastasis. Conversely, aggressive surgery combined with radiation therapy and possibly chemotherapy results in recurrence rates as low as 5 percent.

Like surgery, radiation therapy usually targets a larger area than seems affected. Past experience with sarcomas dictates the total destruction of the primary tumor, as any recurrence is associated with metastasis and a poor prognosis. Because of this, maintaining function or anatomical form is an important but secondary consideration. Soft-tissue sarcomas tend to grow along fascial planes, which are the connective tissue surrounding muscles, bones, organs, nerves, blood vessels, and other structures, and accordingly, this is factored in during treatment. Radiation therapy may be used before or after surgery, and there are advantages and disadvantages to each, but the effectiveness is the same.

Beyond traditional radiation therapy, techniques using intraoperative irradiation and interstitial implantation are coming into use. Intraoperative radiation therapy (IORT) sends a concentrated beam of radiation directly into the exposed sarcoma during surgery. This technique allows doctors to administer high doses of radiation to tumors without exposing nearby healthy organs to radiation. Interstitial implantation is a radiotherapeutic technique in which the physician implants radioactive isotopes directly into tissue.

Chemotherapy, although gaining status with newer drug combinations, still has limited use and has resulted in mixed outcomes when applied to soft-tissue sarcomas. The four-drug program CYVADIC—cyclophosphamide, vincristine, doxorubicin (Adriamycin), dacarbazine (DTIC-Dome)—has yielded some encouraging results, as has the combination of methotrexate and cisplatin, especially in more advanced sarcomas. Although chemotherapy results in mixed outcomes, it has found a place when used for limb salvage together with surgery and irradiation.

Newer forms of therapy being investigated include angiogenesis inhibitors that block the formation of blood vessels feeding the tumors and biological therapies that enlist the body's own immune system in the fight against the disease.

Prognosis, prevention, and outcomes: Prognosis depends on the health of the patient; the size, location, type, grade, and stage of the tumor; and whether the tumor has recurred. For example, sarcomas of the arms or legs respond better than those of other locations, and older patients generally have a poorer result. When the tumor is still small and localized, the five-year survival rate is about 90 percent. As the tumor becomes more aggressive, survival becomes increasingly difficult. Recurrence rates rise considerably when the tumor exceeds 10 cm in diameter, and beyond 20 cm, there is little hope of containment. Location of the tumor is critical. When tumors arise in the extremities, they are usually noticed earlier, are easier to remove surgically, and are more amenable to radiation therapy. Conversely, tumors in the pelvis, chest, paraspinal region, neck, and abdomen pose greater barriers to complete resection and effective radiation therapy. In general, lymph node metastasis is uncommon, with an overall incidence of 5 to 15 percent.

According to the National Cancer Institute (NCI), the five-year survival rate for sarcomas as a group is 68 percent. Included in the overall picture is a five-year survival rate of 84.1 percent for localized sarcomas; 61.5 percent for regional stage sarcomas; 16.3 percent for sarcomas with distant spread; and 54.3 percent for unstaged sarcomas. Over 90 percent of those living beyond five years reach the ten-year mark. Considering this, the NCI states that survival beyond five years is tantamount to being cured. Specifically, the metastasis-free survival rates are 75 percent for all grade 1 tumors, 71 percent for grade 2 tumors, and 41 percent for grade 3 tumors.

Richard S. Spira, D.V.M.

▶ For Further Information

Albritton, K. H. "Sarcomas in Adolescents and Young Adults." *Hematology/Oncology Clinics of North America* 19 (2005): 527-546.

Geisinger, K. R., et al. "Soft-Tissue Sarcoma." *New England Journal of Medicine* 353 (2005): 2303-2304.

Ghert, M. A., et al. "The Surgical and Functional Outcome of Limb-Salvage Surgery with Vascular Reconstruction for Soft-Tissue Sarcoma of the Extremity." *Annals of Surgical Oncology* 12 (2005): 1102-1110.

Liu, J., et al. "Wild-Type *p53* Inhibits Nuclear Factor-κB-Induced Matrix Metalloproteinase-9 Promoter Activation: Implications for Soft-Tissue Sarcoma Growth and Metastasis." *Molecular Cancer Research* 4 (2006): 803-810.

Meyer, W. H., and S. L. Spunt. "Soft-Tissue Sarcomas of Childhood." *Cancer Treatment Reviews* 30 (2004): 269-280.

Zhang, L., et al. "Vascular Endothelial Growth Factor Overexpression by Soft-Tissue Sarcoma Cells: Implications for Tumor Growth, Metastasis, and Chemoresistance." *Cancer Research* 66 (2006): 8770-8778.

▶ Other Resources

MayoClinic.com
Soft-Tissue Sarcoma
http://www.mayoclinic.com/health/soft-tissue-sarcoma/DS00601

National Cancer Institute
Soft-Tissue Sarcoma
http://www.cancer.gov/cancertopics/types/soft-tissue-sarcoma

See also Alveolar soft-part sarcomas; Bone cancers; Childhood cancers; Computed tomography (CT) scan; Endotheliomas; Ewing sarcoma; Fibrosarcomas, soft-tissue; Gallium scan; Gastrointestinal stromal tumors (GISTs); Hemangiopericytomas; Hemangiosarcomas; Hyperthermic perfusion; Li-Fraumeni syndrome (LFS); Limb salvage; Liposarcomas; Malignant fibrous histiocytoma (MFH); Mesenchymomas, malignant; Rhabdomyosarcomas; Spinal axis tumors; Synovial sarcomas; Tumor lysis syndrome; Young adult cancers.

▶ Saw palmetto

Category: Lifestyle and prevention; complementary and alternative therapies

Also known as: *Serenoa repens*, *Sabal serrulatum*, Permixon

Definition: Saw palmetto, or *Serenoa repens*, is a small fan palm native to the Atlantic and Gulf coastal plains that can be found as far inland as southern Arkansas. The olive-sized fruit of this plant is enriched with fatty acids and phytosterols, and its extracts have been the subject of research for the treatment of certain cancers, especially prostate cancer.

Cancer treated or prevented: Prostate cancer

Delivery route: Oral by capsule

How this substance works: Used as an herbal supplement, saw palmetto is considered to be safe, effective, and relatively inexpensive. It enjoys widespread use in the United States but is also popular in Germany and France for the treatment of prostate disorders.

Saw palmetto inhibits 5-alpha-reductase, an enzyme that converts testosterone into its most potent form, dihydrotestosterone (DHT). Its effects have been compared to Proscar (finasteride), which is a prescription drug that results in the shrinkage of an enlarged prostate, a condition called benign prostatic hyperplasia (BPH). While studies of the efficacy of saw palmetto are somewhat inconsistent, it largely lacks the adverse side effects of Proscar, such as decreased libido and gastrointestinal irritation. The most studied form is Permixon, which is made by using hexane as a solvent in the extraction process of the sterols and fatty acids found in the dried fruits of the saw palmetto berry. Other mixtures include ethanol, methanol, or less commonly nettle root or pumpkin seed oils. Although the extract is much studied, it is not fully understood which are its active components, but phytosterols and fatty acids seem to be the most proficient at treating symptoms.

Similarly, the mechanism by which saw palmetto actually works is yet unclear. Some suggest that it acts as an anti-inflammatory, blocks the chemical conversion of testosterone to DHT, or promotes prostate epithelial involution. Whichever is correct, studies have shown that saw palmetto relieves symptoms caused by prostate disorders, including decreased urine stream and flow, post-voidance dribbling, overflow incontinence, and excessive retention of urine in the bladder. Relief of prostate swelling aids a return to sexual function, which also contributes to the popular use of saw palmetto among older men.

Not all studies agree on the therapeutic efficacy of saw palmetto; a double-blind, randomized study by Dr. Stephen Bent of the University of California, San Francisco, and his coworkers that was funded by the National Institutes of Health (NIH) and the National Center for Complementary and Alternative Medicine (NCCAM) found that saw palmetto was no more effective in reducing symptoms associated with BPH than a placebo. This raises the question of whether it is a medically useful substance.

Overall, the Moores Cancer Center of the Medical Center of the University of California, San Diego, states that "this treatment modality is thought to manage symptoms of cancer, side effects from conventional therapies and/or control pain." Researchers warn, however, that saw palmetto should be used as a supplement to cancer treatment, not in place of standard therapy.

Side effects: Almost all patients reported that adverse side effects were mild and infrequent, differing little from those reported after placebo use. Some reports indicate that saw palmetto can cause gastrointestinal distress, but this can largely be alleviated by taking saw palmetto with food.

Dwight G. Smith, Ph.D.

See also Complementary and alternative therapies; Fruits; Herbs as antioxidants; Nonsteroidal anti-inflammatory drugs (NSAIDs); PC-SPES; Prostate cancer.

▶ Schwannoma tumors

Category: Diseases, symptoms, and conditions
Also known as: Schwann cell tumors

Related conditions: Malignant peripheral nerve sheath tumors (MPNSTs), neurofibromatosis, schwannomatosis

Definition: Schwannoma is a benign (noncancerous) encapsulated solitary tumor formed by Schwann cells of the peripheral nerves: cranial nerves, spinal nerves, and autonomic nerves. Schwannomas generally occur in the head, neck, and upper and lower limbs. A common cranial nerve schwannoma is the vestibular schwannoma (unilateral and nonhereditary), which affects the eighth cranial nerve, which governs hearing and balance. Other schwannommas include trigeminal, facial, and hypoglossal. Less than 1 percent of schwannomas become cancerous. When schwannomas are found in children, they are usually associated with neurofibromatosis. Schwannomatosis is newly identified neurofibromatosis of multiple schwannomas.

Risk factors: There are no known risk factors for schwannomas.

Etiology and the disease process: The etiology of schwannomas is unknown. The nerve fiber, or axon, of peripheral nerves is sheathed in glial cells called Schwann cells. Sometimes Schwann cells abnormally proliferate to form a tumor, or schwannoma. The cells of schwannomas are spindle-shaped neoplastic Schwann cells.

Incidence: Schwannoma is generally a disease of adults and can commonly occur between the ages of forty and sixty. The incidence rate for vestibular schwannoma is 1 per 100,000 people per year.

Symptoms: Schwannomas are generally slow-growing, small, painless tumors, although sometimes they can be painful and be as large as 10 centimeters. Subcutaneous tumors (under the skin) can be palpated during physical examination. In vestibular schwannoma, additional symptoms are hearing loss, dizziness, and ringing in the ears. Other cranial nerve schwannomas can have symptoms related to the function of that nerve.

Screening and diagnosis: A medical history and physical examination of the patient plus X rays, ultrasound, computed tomography (CT) scans, magnetic resonance imaging (MRI) scans, and biopsy are used to diagnose schwannoma. Vestibular schwannoma also requires a hearing test (audiogram). According to the World Health Organization (WHO), schwannoma is a grade I tumor, and malignant peripheral nerve sheath tumors are grades III and IV.

Treatment and therapy: Chemotherapy is usually not effective. Radiotherapy and surgery are the main treatments. Rarely occurring malignant tumors may also require chemotherapy.

Prognosis, prevention, and outcomes: Schwannomas cannot be prevented. Prognosis is good with early diagnosis and surgery but worsens if the tumor is detected at a later state. For example, an untreated vestibular schwannoma can cause pressure on the neighboring facial nerve, causing paralysis of the face on the affected side, and can further press on the brain stem, even resulting in death. The recurrence rate of malignant peripheral nerve sheath tumors after surgery is high.

Arun S. Dabholkar, Ph.D.

See also Acoustic neuromas; Brain and central nervous system cancers; Computed tomography (CT) scan; Fibrosarcomas, soft-tissue; Gliomas; Magnetic resonance imaging (MRI); Mediastinal tumors; Neurofibromatosis type 1 (NF1); Orbit tumors; Spinal axis tumors.

▶ *SCLC1* gene

Category: Cancer biology
Also known as: Small-cell carcinoma of lung, small-cell lung cancer (SCLC)

Definition: The *SCLC1* gene is located on a region on the short arm of chromosome 3 that is frequently deleted in neoplastic lung cells associated with small-cell carcinomas, cells of epithelial origin.

Significance: Approximately 110,000 cases of small-cell carcinomas of the lung are diagnosed annually, accounting for some 60 percent of all forms of lung cancer diagnosed yearly. Small-cell carcinomas of the lung are most commonly associated with people exposed to airborne carcinogens, particularly those associated with cigarette smoke. This form of lung cancer is particularly aggressive and has undergone metastasis at the time of diagnosis. SCLC cells frequently express a number of unusual neuroendocrine markers, including dopa-decarboxylase (DDC), and evidence suggests that these cells originate from a form of neuroendocrine cells that differentiate into epithelial cells in the lung.

Cancer cells in general arise from mutations that disrupt normal regulation of cell divisions, frequently at the level of internal cell signaling. Expression of neuroendocrine markers in SCLC neoplasms appears to affect the *RHOA* (*ras* homolog) family of genes in particular, the products of which are part of the signaling mechanism to stimulate cell division. Other oncogenes also appear to be altered in cell lines originating from SCLC neoplasms.

Regulation of oncogenes in a cell in part involves the production of tumor suppressors, proteins that either regulate oncogene expression or serve as stop signals to prevent the cell from undergoing replication. The region of the short arm on chromosome 3 that is deleted, 3p14-23, and specifically the *SCLC1* gene, appears to encode one or more tumor suppressors.

Deletions of this region of chromosome 3, the region which encodes the *SCLC1* gene, appears to take place during the early stages of formation of the neoplasm. Whether the deletion is required for development of this form of cancer is unknown, but this specific mutation seems to occur in nearly all cases of SCLC that have been analyzed. The mechanism of the deletion is also unknown.

History: The presence of this particular deletion in small-cell carcinomas of the lung was first noted in 1982. Scientists had established a number of lung-cancer cell lines in the laboratory, the purpose of which was to study characteristics unique to each group; twelve lines originated as SCLC cases. All were observed to have the same deletion on chromosome 3, while cells from other lines did not.

Richard Adler, Ph.D.

See also Bronchial adenomas; Bronchoalveolar lung cancer; Cancer biology; Cigarettes and cigars; Lambert-Eaton syndrome (LEMS); Lung cancers.

▶ Screening for cancer

Category: Procedures; lifestyle and prevention
Also known as: Testing, cancer detection

Definition: Screening tests are tests or procedures that can detect the presence of a specific cancer in persons who are not experiencing any symptoms.

Cancers diagnosed: The most common cancer screenings detect breast, cervical, colorectal, and prostate cancer. Some require a blood test, while others require more extensive screening procedures.

Why performed: The purpose of screening tests is to allow early identification of cancer and prevent the progression of any existing cancer. Screening and early detection can save human lives, minimize the trauma of cancer illness, and conserve limited health care resources spent on costly cancer therapies.

People participate in screenings for various reasons. Sometimes they see screening as a preventive measure, and sometimes they undergo screening because they are at high risk for a cancer. Often health-conscious people participate in routine cancer screenings, and their health insurance pays the bill. Medicare (health insurance for older adults and the disabled) Part B covers certain key preventive cancer screening tests such as colorectal screening, mammograms, Pap smears and pelvic examinations, and prostate cancer screenings within certain parameters.

Screening for cancer offers many advantages for the public. Screening can save the life of someone who may have died without early intervention. When cancer is discovered, treatment can be started immediately and decrease the possibility of radical surgery or therapy. Early intervention also results in lower health care costs. A primary advantage is that the person who receives negative (benign) results has peace of mind that, at that point in time, cancer is not present. This is reassuring for anyone but especially for someone with a family history of cancer or who has other high risks for cancer.

However, the disadvantage of screening is that some false negatives may occur so the person does not believe there is a problem even when symptoms surface. Con-

Two Grading Systems for Sarcomas

American Joint Committee (AJC)
G1 Low-grade
G2 Moderately differentiated
G3 Poorly differentiated

Musculoskeletal Tumor Society (MTS)
G1 Well-differentiated
G2 High-grade

versely, "false positives" can cause undue anxiety until further tests confirm there is no cancer. Sometimes the screening finds a cancer that is not treatable or is so advanced that the screening does not alter the negative outcome for the person. Another disadvantage is that borderline reports from cancer screenings can result in excessive testing and associated costs.

Breast self-exam (BSE): Breast cancer can be detected through several screening tests. One is palpation of the breast tissue through a monthly breast self-examination (BSE). Palpation is a noninvasive way to examine and screen for abnormalities in the breast such as cysts, lumps, or thickening. The patient can be taught to do an examination of her breasts each month and note visual or palpable changes in the breasts.

Patient preparation. The patient should stand unclothed from the waist up and view her breasts in a mirror. The best time to complete an examination is a few days after the completion of the menses, when swelling and tenderness are lessened.

Steps of the procedure. A breast self-examination is a five-step process:

- The woman observes her breasts in the mirror, with her hands on her hips, for any visual changes in color, shape, and size. She looks for dimpling, swelling, or puckering of the skin as well as changes in the nipples or redness or rash on the breast.
- She raises her arms over her head and observes the same as above.
- She gently squeezes the nipples and observes for any liquid or discharge. (None should be present unless the woman is breast-feeding.)
- She lies down and examines each breast with the opposite hand in a circular pattern, starting at the nipple and working outward. She palpates all breast tissue from the collarbone to the abdomen and from the armpit to the cleavage area.
- She palpates the breast again in a sitting or standing position in the same pattern. Some women find that the examination is best completed when the skin is wet and slippery, such as in the shower.

After the procedure. The woman should record any observation and the date of each examination in a journal to be sure that it is completed monthly, preferably after the menses. This simple screening can detect early changes in the woman's breasts.

Risks. None.

Results. The woman makes an appointment with her health care provider if abnormalities are noted. She should schedule her annual examination with the health care provider, which includes a clinical breast exam (CBE).

Mammograms: A screening mammogram uses X rays to detect breast cancer. Mammography offers a noninvasive way to screen the breasts for cancer. A screening mammogram is useful when a woman has no history of problems with her breasts. Two X-ray views are taken of each breast. Scheduling the mammogram a week after the menses can decrease the patient's discomfort, as hormonal soreness or tenderness is less at that time. An annual screening mammogram is recommended primarily for women over the age of forty. A screening mammogram can detect suspicious areas that may be breast cancer long before a mass can be palpated.

Patient preparation. The patient should avoid use of powders, deodorant, or lotion before the mammogram, since particles from these products can be viewed as abnormalities on the X ray. The patient completes paperwork such as her history, last menses, risk factors, childbearing, surgeries, implants, birth control, hormone therapy, or any problems. The patient undresses from the waist up and wears an examination gown into the X-ray room. The patient can expect the X rays to take about a half hour.

Steps of the procedure. The patient stands in front of the X-ray machine. A radiology technician exposes one breast at a time and places it on a film holder; the breast is compressed for a few seconds between the holder and a plastic paddle to take the X ray. Good compression is necessary for accurate X rays. Next the patient moves her side toward the machine, and the breast is compressed from the side. The X ray is repeated.

After the procedure. A radiologist reads the X ray either immediately or at a later time, depending on the facility's availability to the radiologist.

Risks. The risk of radiation exposure through a screening mammogram is considered minimal. Most authorities agree that the benefit of screening for breast cancer outweighs the risk of low-dose radiation.

Results. Screening mammograms do not detect breast cancer 100 percent accurately. A normal result means that the mammogram detects no abnormalities, though a cancer can be hidden in dense breast tissue. Screening mammograms may be read as borderline, which may suggest that further testing (such as a diagnostic mammogram, ultrasound, or biopsy) is indicated to confirm the diagnosis of breast cancer.

Pap smear: The Pap smear is a screening test to detect changes in the cervix that may lead to cervical cancer in women. Early detection can increase the chance of successful treatment. All women need this screening examination, including sexually active women over the age of eighteen and those at risk for cervical cancer, such as women who had a previous abnormal pap smear. This test is usually performed during the woman's annual gynecological exam.

Patient preparation. The woman should avoid douching or using any vaginal medications within forty-eight hours of the test. For accurate results, she should avoid intercourse within twenty-four hours of the screening. Optimal time for a Pap smear is at midcycle of the menses; a Pap smear cannot be performed during the menses. The woman should empty her bladder before the test to decrease discomfort.

Steps of the procedure. The Pap smear does not take long to perform. The patient lies on her back with her knees bent and her feet slightly apart. The health care provider will lubricate a speculum (an instrument that holds the walls of the vagina apart) and place it into the vagina. The patient will feel pressure as the provider swabs the cervix for a sample to examine. The sample is swabbed on a glass slide and sprayed with preservative. The slide is sent to the lab for microscopic examination for abnormal cells.

After the procedure. There are usually no side effects of this test. The lab results will be sent to the patient.

Risks. One risk is a false positive, which would lead to further testing, or a false negative, which might cause the person to ignore other warning signs of cervical cancer.

Results. Results are categorized as negative if no abnormal cells are seen. The patient usually receives a written notification of the results. Patients need to seek further testing from their health care provider for abnormalities.

Fecal occult blood, sigmoidoscopy, colonscopy: Colon cancer is the third leading cause of cancer death in the United States today. The first screening test for colon cancer is the fecal occult blood sample. This test detects blood in the stool. The next screening is a sigmoidoscopy or colonoscopy. Regular rectal and colon screening is advised in persons over fifty years of age and in those at high risk. This includes a fecal test annually, a sigmoidoscopy every five years, and a colonoscopy every ten years after age fifty-five.

Patient preparation. Certain medications (aspirin and aspirin products, ibuprofen products, iron tablets, and vitamin supplements) should be avoided for a week before screening. Prescribed medications can usually be taken, but the physician should be consulted. A sigmoidoscopy or colonoscopy requires preparation of the bowel. The exact preparation used may vary by provider preference, but these preparations usually include a diet of clear liquids for twenty-four hours prior to the test as well as a liquid laxative about two to four hours before the examination.

Steps of the procedure. Both a sigmoidoscopy and colonoscopy require the insertion of a rigid or flexible tube that contains a lens and a light into the colon. The provider can visualize the rectum, lower colon (or sigmoid colon), or upper colon.

After the procedure. Patients may need someone to drive them home after this test, especially if they have sedation. The patient can experience some soreness and mild cramping due to the air that was injected into the colon for the test, but this condition improves as the air is passed. No other aftercare is required.

Risks. A slight risk of bleeding is possible, especially when the patient has decreased clotting capacity. A perforated (torn) colon is a serious but rare complication following a sigmoidoscopy or colonoscopy.

Results. A normal result is one where the colon walls are smooth and without polyps, inflammation, or tumors. An abnormal result would be present when the colon shows precancerous polyps or tumors. A biopsy and surgical removal of the polyps or tumors would be scheduled.

Digital rectal exam (DRE) and prostate-specific antigen (PSA) blood test: Prostate cancer is the second leading cause of death in men sixty-five years of age or older. By the age of fifty, men should have screening tests for prostate cancer; in high-risk men, screening should start at the age of forty-five. The main screening tests for prostate cancer are digital rectal exam (DRE) and the prostate-specific antigen (PSA) blood test. The prostate is the male reproductive organ located under the bladder and in front of the rectum.

Patient preparation. No special preparation is required.

Steps of the procedure. For the digital rectal exam, the patient is dressed in an examination gown and placed in a relaxed position (such as lying on his side or resting over an exam table) with the rectum accessible. The doctor inserts a well-lubricated, gloved finger into the rectum and feels the size of the prostate.

After the procedure. No residual patient discomfort occurs.

Risks. None.

Results. If abnormal results are reported from either the digital rectal exam or prostate-specific antigen test, the patient will need further testing to confirm a cancer diagnosis.

Marylane Wade Koch, M.S.N., R.N.

▶ For Further Information

Finkel, Madelon L. *Understanding the Mammography Controversy: Science, Politics, and Breast Cancer Screening*. Westport, Conn.: Praeger, 2005.

Miller, Anthony B., ed. *Advances in Cancer Screening*. Boston: Kluwer Academic, 1996.

Querna, Elizabeth. "Breast Cancer Screening: What Is the Best Way to Find Out If You Have the Disease?" *U.S. News & World Report*, September 9, 2004.

▶ Other Resources

Centers for Disease Control

National Breast and Cervical Cancer Early Detection Program

http://www.cdc.gov/cancer/nbccedp/about.htm

MayoClinic.com

Prostate Cancer Screening: Should You Get a PSA test?

http://www.mayoclinic.com/health/prostate-cancer/HQ01273

National Cancer Institute

Screening and Testing to Detect Cancer

http://www.cancer.gov/cancertopics/screening

See also Biopsy; Bone scan; Brain scan; Breast self-examination (BSE); Breast ultrasound; Clinical breast exam (CBE); Colorectal cancer screening; Complete blood count (CBC); Core needle biopsy; Genetic testing; Imaging tests; Magnetic resonance imaging (MRI); Mammography; Nuclear medicine scan; Pap test; Positron emission tomography (PET); Radionuclide scan; Testicular self-examination (TSE); Ultrasound tests; Urinalysis; X-ray tests.

▶ Second opinions

Category: Social and personal issues

Definition: A second opinion is a medical diagnosis from a health care professional who was not the patient's initial source of information. There are two types of second opinions. In one, the patient gives the second doctor all previous medical test results, sharing information and concerns from the first doctor. In the other, the patient sees the second doctor and starts over with all new testing, so that the new opinion is not influenced by that of the first doctor. This is difficult to do if the two doctors are in the same health maintenance organization (HMO), as the medical records within an organization are shared information.

Other sources of advice: Before, or in addition to, asking another doctor for an opinion, patients can review their test results and ask their health provider questions about them. Patients may want to determine how likely false positives and false negatives are for the tests that they took. Cancer patients can use readily available resources to help evaluate their medical condition: Internet (WebMD, Mayo Clinic, American Cancer Society, National Cancer Institute), books (local bookstore, public library, medical or hospital library), and pamphlets from cancer organizations, cancer hospitals, or government sources (American Cancer Society, Centers for Disease Control and Prevention).

Friends and relatives who have had cancer may be able to provide advice, although specificity may be lacking. Alternative medicines and treatments may offer another perspective on cancer, although many may lack scientific evidence as to their efficacy. Media can serve as a source of information about current medical advances and new treatments for cancer. Information on clinical trials is available through the registry of federally and privately supported clinical trial conducted in the United States and worldwide provided by the U.S. National Institutes of Health.

Financial and insurance issues: Second opinions are usually not covered by insurance. Patients should call their insurance company to determine if second opinions are covered and what the cost would be for retesting and reevaluation. Some insurance plans require preauthorization for some tests, which may take several weeks. Preauthorization may also be needed if patients wish to see a specialist in their particular cancer. Patients are advised to keep a list of names, phone numbers, and conversations to avoid insurance confusion.

Time factor: The severity or extent of the cancer can make it necessary that the patient start treatment as soon as possible, leaving little time for a second opinion. Patients are advised to take the earliest appointments possible, so that a second opinion does not delay treatment too much.

The final decision: Cancer patients must feel at ease with their final decisions and be willing to live with the consequences, whether the outcome is positive or negative. Second opinions, particularly where cancer is concerned, can facilitate confidence in these decisions, allowing patients to trust their chosen medical team, as they will be working together for an extended period of time.

Suzette Buhr, R.T.R., C.D.A.

See also Cancer care team; Clinical trials; Elderly and cancer; Financial issues; Health maintenance organizations (HMOs); Insurance; National Cancer Institute (NCI); Preferred provider organizations (PPOs).

▶ Self-image and body image

Category: Social and personal issues

Definition: Self-image refers to a person's perception of his or her personality and physical, mental, spiritual, and social characteristics. Body image contributes to self-image and refers to how people view their physical appearance and functioning.

Cultural influences: In contemporary culture, physical appearance influences how individuals perceive themselves and how others judge them. Messages from popular media celebrate physical beauty and encourage people to aspire to idealized standards of appearance. Body image has a strong influence on most people's overall self-image, and physical changes can powerfully affect how they view themselves. People with cancer commonly experience changes in their bodies resulting from the disease and its treatments. Changes may involve physical appearance, how a person feels, or how well they function. The extent to which these changes influence cancer patients' images of themselves and their bodies is influenced by factors such as the severity and permanence of these changes, the stage of life in which they occur, and the personality traits of the individual.

Changes in appearance: Visible changes in appearance, stemming from the cancer itself or from its treatment, can profoundly affect body image. Overt changes may cause cancer patients to be highly focused on appearance and hypersensitive to attention from others (such as questions about health). Insecurity over appearance often leads to distress and diminished body image. Hidden or less visible changes in appearance (such as breast or testicle removal and surgical scarring) can still cause significant anxiety, alter self-perceptions, and lead to a person's avoiding interactions and intimacy with friends and family at a time when social and family support is a vital component to successfully coping with cancer.

Changes in how the body feels: Illness-related factors (such as pain) and treatment side effects (such as fatigue) can significantly affect how cancer patients feel about themselves and their bodies. Activities previously accomplished with ease may be markedly more difficult or even impossible to perform because of pain or reduced strength. These experiences can sap cancer patients' confidence and lessen views of themselves as competent, effective, and independent individuals. Cancer patients may feel "betrayed" by their bodies and perceive themselves as deficient, even after surviving their illness.

Changes in functioning: Changes in body functioning caused by cancer can also affect people's self-perceptions. Some types of cancer may result in the loss of limbs or other body parts and markedly alter independence and functionality. Cancer treatment may change how patients eliminate body waste and necessitate the use of colostomy bags (for bowel movements) or urostomy bags (for passing urine). Other treatments can cause sterility or alter sexual functioning. These circumstances can shake the foundation of patients' self-perceptions and require considerable ongoing coping and adaptation.

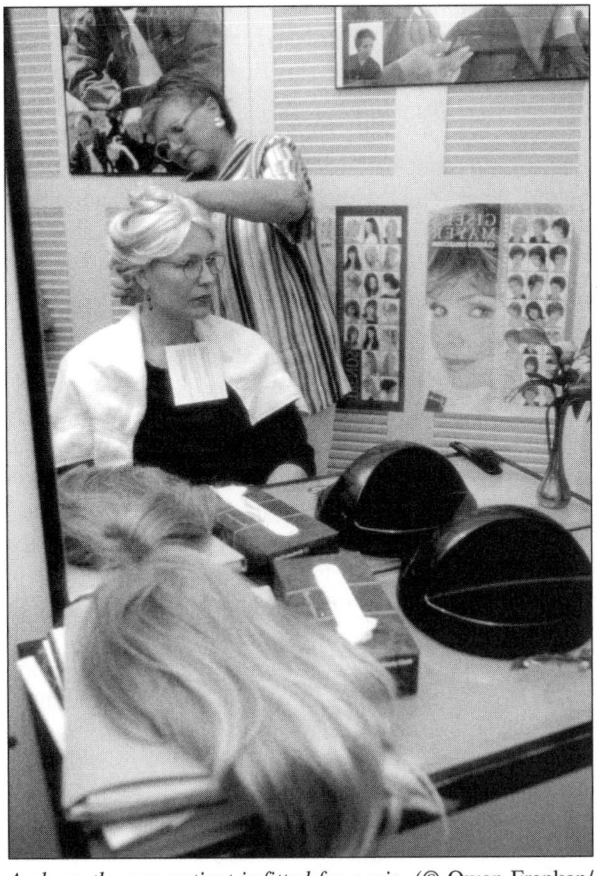

A chemotherapy patient is fitted for a wig. (© Owen Franken/ Corbis)

Permanence of changes: Whether physical changes caused by cancer are temporary or permanent affects the extent to which these changes alter body image. For most patients with cancer, altered self-perceptions resulting from temporary physical changes, such as hair loss or weight loss, are limited to the duration of treatment. Most regain former perceptions of their body and self when these changes disappear. Some individuals continue to struggle with altered body image and view themselves as "damaged" even after treatment has ended. Permanent physical changes resulting from cancer typically have a bigger impact on body image. A period of bereavement, involving initial shock, "numbing," anger, and denial, may be seen in some patients. Most patients employ coping mechanisms developed before their illness to adapt to their altered physical state. Other patients have significant long-term struggles in dealing with their changed appearance or functioning and may develop psychiatric illnesses such as anxiety and depression.

Developmental considerations: The age and developmental level at which cancer occurs influence patients' self-perceptions. Cancer-related factors causing children and adolescents to feel nauseated or weak or to look sick or what the young person perceives as different from others can make it hard for them to develop healthy self-images and body images. Young adults with cancer may feel unattractive and "damaged" and fear that they will never find a mate. Older adults with cancer may fear abandonment from loved ones or loss of social or occupational standing resulting from looking unhealthy. Cancer and associated functional loss in geriatric patients may bolster established fears of losing control and independence.

Personality factors: Personality, coping style, and self-perceptions before the illness influence how cancer affects people's self-image. People who are optimistic, flexible, emotionally expressive, and willing to accept emotional support appear to adapt best to stressors caused by cancer, including those related to body image. Also, those with a robust self-esteem before their illness appear to cope well. People whose feelings of self-worth were closely tied to their appearance before they developed cancer, who have difficulty accepting emotional support, and who have histories of psychiatric illness appear to have the most difficulty adapting to physical changes associated with their illness.

Management approaches: A number of approaches have been identified to assist individuals with cancer to maintain or enhance their self-image and body image. Participation in support groups in which cancer patients and survivors discuss their experience with illness and share methods of coping has been found to promote healthy adaptation. Using wigs, hats, scarves, or makeup may boost confidence in appearance and increase social interaction and acceptance of support. Participating in treatment and rehabilitation efforts and developing alternate interests and skills to take the place of those that are no longer possible as a result of cancer can increase physical confidence. Keeping a healthy diet, engaging in exercise, and maintaining good sleep habits help those with cancer reestablish a sense of control over their bodies. Finally, cancer patients and survivors struggling with self-image and body image concerns or psychiatric illness are advised to seek or be referred for mental health care, as a number of effective psychological and medical treatments exist.

Paul F. Bell, Ph.D.

▶ For Further Information

Gatchel, Robert, and Mark Ooordt. *Clinical Health Psychology and Primary Care*. Washington, D.C.: American Psychological Association, 2003.

Goldman, Larry, Thomas Wise, and David Brody. *Psychiatry for Primary Care Physicians*. Chicago: American Medical Association, 1998.

Sadock, Benjamin James, and Virginia Alcott Sadock. *Kaplan and Sadock's Synopsis of Psychiatry: Behavioral Sciences—Clinical Psychiatry*. 10th ed. Philadelphia: Wolter Kluwer/Lippincott Williams & Wilkins, 2007.

▶ Other Resources

American Cancer Society

Look Good . . . Feel Better

http://www.cancer.org/docroot/ESN/content/ESN_3_1X_Look_Good_Feel_Better.asp?sitearea=EMP

Cancer.Net

Self-Image and Cancer

http://www.ascocancerfoundation.org/patient/Coping/Emotional+and+Physical+Matters/Self-Image+and+Cancer

See also Aging and cancer; Aids and devices for cancer patients; Amputation; Breast reconstruction; Counseling for cancer patients and survivors; Exercise and cancer; Fatigue; Hereditary polyposis syndromes; Ileostomy; Limb salvage; Nausea and vomiting; Personality and cancer; Psychosocial aspects of cancer; Rehabilitation; Sexuality and cancer; Sterility; Stress management; Support groups; Young adult cancers.